11th EDITION

CLINICIAN'S POCKET REFERENCE

The Scut Monkey Book

Published continuously since 1979, with the mission of providing medical students, residents, practicing physicians, and health care providers with the essential and up-to-date information to learn the basics of excellence in patient care

EDITED BY

LEONARD G. GOMELLA, MD, FACS

The Bernard W. Godwin, Jr., Professor and Chairman
Department of Urology
Jefferson Medical College
Thomas Jefferson University
Philadelphia, Pennsylvania

STEVEN A. HAIST, MD, MS, FACP

Professor of Medicine and Residency Program Director
Department of Internal Medicine
University of Kentucky Medical Center
Lexington, Kentucky

Based on a program originally developed
at the University of Kentucky College
of Medicine Lexington, Kentucky
WWW.THESCUTMONKEY.COM

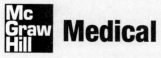

Mc Graw Hill Medical

New York   Chicago   San Francisco   Lisbon   London
Madrid   Mexico City   Milan   New Delhi   San Juan
Seoul   Singapore   Sydney   Toronto

The McGraw·Hill Companies

Clinician's Pocket Reference, 11th Edition

1 2 3 4 5 6 7 8 9 0 DOC/DOC 0 9 8 7 6

ISBN-13: 978-0-07-145428-5; ISBN-10: 0-07-145428-4
ISSN: 1041-1348

Notice

Medicine is an ever-changing science. As new research and clinical experience broaden our knowledge, changes in treatment and drug therapy are required. The authors and the publisher of this work have checked with sources believed to be reliable in their efforts to provide information that is complete and generally in accord with the standards accepted at the time of publication. However, in view of the possibility of human error or changes in medical sciences, neither the editors nor the publisher nor any other party who has been involved in the preparation or publication of this work warrants that the information contained herein is in every respect accurate or complete, and they disclaim all responsibility for any errors or omissions or for the results obtained from use of the information contained in this work. Readers are encouraged to confirm the information contained herein with other sources. For example and in particular, readers are advised to check the product information sheet included in the package of each drug they plan to administer to be certain that the information contained in this work is accurate and that changes have not been made in the recommended dose or in the contraindications for administration. This recommendation is of particular importance in connection with new or infrequently used drugs.

This book was set in Times Roman by Silverchair Science + Communications, Inc.
The editors were Jim Shanahan and Harriet Lebowitz.
The production supervisor was Phil Galea.
The text designer was Marsha Cohen/Parallelogram Graphics.
The indexer was Pamela Edwards.
RR Donnelley was printer and binder.

This book is printed on acid-free paper.

To Tricia, Leonard, Patrick, Andrew, Michael, Aunt Lucy, and PJ

To Meg, Sarah, and Will

"We don't drive the trucks, we only load them."

Nick Pavona, MD
UKMC Class of 1980

DEA: MB2596786

NPI: 1528335130

LIC: PA6048609

CONTENTS

Editorial Board vii–ix
Preface xi–xii
Abbreviations xiii–xxi
"So You Want to Be a Scut Monkey":
An Introduction to Clinical Medicine xxiii–xxx

1. History and Physical Examination 1
2. Chartwork 25
3. Differential Diagnosis: Symptoms, Signs, and Conditions 33
4. Laboratory Diagnosis: Chemistry, Immunology, Serology 47
5. Laboratory Diagnosis: Clinical Hematology 91
6. Laboratory Diagnosis: Urine Studies 105
7. Clinical Microbiology 117
8. Blood Gases and Acid–Base Disorders 163
9. Fluids and Electrolytes 179
10. Blood Component Therapy 195
11. Nutritional Assessment, Therapeutic Diets, and Infant Feeding 207
12. Enteral and Parenteral Nutrition 225
13. Bedside Procedures 241
14. Pain Management 323
15. Imaging Studies 341
16. Introduction to the Operating Room 355
17. Suturing Techniques and Wound Care 361
18. Respiratory Care 377
19. Basic ECG Reading 383
20. Critical Care 403
21. Common Medical Emergencies 455
22. Commonly Used Medications 475

Appendix 649
Index 669
Commonly Used Emergency Care Medications
(inside front and back covers)

EDITORIAL BOARD

PREFACE

Since 1979, students, residents, practicing physicians, nurses, and other allied health professionals have turned to the "Scut Monkey Book" for learning the essential information on basic patient care. The *Clinician's Pocket Reference* is based on a University of Kentucky manual entitled *So You Want to Be a Scut Monkey: Medical Student's and House Officer's Clinical Handbook.* The "Scut Monkey" program at the University of Kentucky College of Medicine was first held in the summer of 1979 and was developed by the Class of 1980 to help ease the sometimes frustrating transition from the preclinical to the clinical years of medical school. Based on detailed surveys from the University of Kentucky and 44 other medical schools, the essential information and skills that students should be familiar with at the start of their clinical years was developed.

The "Scut Monkey" program was developed around this core and consisted of a simple reference manual and a series of workshops conducted at the start of the third year. Held originally as a pilot program for the University of Kentucky College of Medicine Class of 1981, the program has become an annual event. Each new fourth-year class traditionally takes the responsibility of orienting the new third-year students in basic skills. The program is successful because it was developed and taught *by students for other students.* Over the years, students have been the main source of feedback for the book, critical to its longevity. Information on the rising third-year "Scut Monkey" orientation program is available from Dr. Todd Cheever, Assistant Dean for Academic Affairs at the University of Kentucky College of Medicine in Lexington.

Over the last ten editions, the book has been continually updated to reflect the dynamic changes in medical care. Because of the demand, it is now on a two-year revision cycle to keep the information as up to date as possible. An attempt is made to cover the most frequently asked basic management questions that are normally found in many different sources such as procedure manuals, laboratory manuals, drug references, and critical care manuals, to name a few. This book is not meant as a substitute for specialty-specific reference manuals; the core information presented is the essential foundation for the new medical student or health care provider beginning to learn hands-on patient care.

The book is designed to represent common medical practices around the country. Over the years, contributors from dozens of medical centers have enhanced the content of the book. The *Clinician's Pocket Reference* has been translated into many foreign languages, including Japanese, Chinese, Korean, Portuguese, and Spanish. The "Scut Monkey" was honored to have been asked by Warner Brothers, the producers of the TV show "ER," to be one of the prop books used on their series. The companion manual, the mini-pocket *Clinician's Pocket Drug Reference 2007,* has been well received and is in its sixth edition this year.

We would like to express special thanks to our wives and children for their patience and long-term support of the "Scut Monkey" project. Our thanks to the team at McGraw-Hill, in particular Editors Jim Shanahan and Harriet Lebowitz, for keeping this book as one of their high priority publications. A special thanks to our administrative assistant Denise Tropea for her support.

A word of eternal gratitude to the past administration of the University of Kentucky College of Medicine: Drs. Kay Clawson, Terry Leigh, and Roy Jarecky, and the then very young faculty member Dr. Richard Braen, who took a chance and supported a group of third-year medical students who wanted to try something a "little bit different" way back in 1978. Thanks also to the hundreds of past contributors, Dr. Michael Olding, and readers who have helped to establish the "Scut Monkey Book" as one of the enduring references for students and residents worldwide. Every medical student at the University of Kentucky College of Medicine since 1979 has received a courtesy copy of this book as a small token of our appreciation for the University's dedication to producing outstanding and caring physicians who serve patients in the Commonwealth and beyond.

We look forward to your comments and suggestions because they allow us to keep the book up to date and useful, an effort that would be impossible if it were not for our readers. We hope this book will not only help you learn some of the basics of the art and science of medicine but also allow you to care for your patients in the best way possible.

Leonard G. Gomella, MD
Philadelphia, Pennsylvania
leonard.gomella@jefferson.edu

Steven A. Haist, MD
Lexington, Kentucky
sahaist@email.uky.edu

Visit our web site www.thescutmonkey.com for complimentary enhanced content for this edition of the *Clinician's Pocket Reference*.

ABBREVIATIONS

The following are common abbreviations used in medical records and in this edition:

÷: divided dose
↓: decrease(d), reduce, downward
×: times for multiplication sign
↑: increase(d), upward (as in titrate upward)
/: per
+/–: with or without
+: with
<: less than, younger than
>: more than, older than
~: approximately
≈: approximately equal to
AAA: abdominal aortic aneurysm
A–a gradient: alveolar-to-arterial gradient
A/A index: ankle/arm index
AADC VAN DISSL: mnemonic for Admit/Attending, Diagnosis, Condition, Vitals, Activity, Nursing procedures, Diet, Ins and outs, Specific medications, Symptomatic medications, Labs
AAS: acute abdominal series
A&B: apnea and bradycardia
A/B index: ankle/brachial index
AB: antibody, abortion, antibiotic
ABD: abdomen
ABG: arterial blood gas
ABMT: autologous bone marrow transplantation
ac: before eating (ante cibum)
AC: assist controlled, air conduction
ACCP: American College of Chest Physicians
ACE: angiotensin-converting enzyme
Ach-ase: acetylcholinesterase
ACLS: Advanced Cardiac Life Support
ACS: acute coronary syndrome, American Cancer Society, American College of Surgeons
ACT: activated coagulation time
ACTH: adrenocorticotropic hormone, corticotropin
ADH: antidiuretic hormone
ADHD: attention-deficit hyperactivity disorder

ad lib: as much as needed (ad libitum)
ad lib: as often as desired
ADR: adverse drug reaction
AED: automated external defibrillator
AEIOU TIPS: mnemonic for Alcohol, Encephalopathy, Insulin, Opiates, Uremia, Trauma, Infection, Psychiatric, Syncope (diagnosis of coma)
AF: afebrile, aortofemoral, atrial fibrillation
AFB: acid-fast bacilli
AFP: alpha-fetoprotein
A/G: albumin/globulin ratio
AHA: American Heart Association
AHF: antihemophilic factor
AI: aortic insufficiency
AIDS: acquired immunodeficiency syndrome
AJCC: American Joint Committee on Cancer
AKA: above-the-knee amputation, also known as
ALL: acute lymphocytic leukemia
ALS: amyotrophic lateral sclerosis
ALT: alanine aminotransferase
AM: morning
AMA: American Medical Association
amb: ambulate
AMI: acute myocardial infarction
AML: acute myelocytic leukemia, acute myelogenous leukemia
AMMoL: acute monocytic leukemia
amp: ampule
AMP: adenosine monophosphate
ANA: antinuclear antibody
ANC: absolute neutrophil count
ANCA: antineutrophil cytoplasmic antibody
ANLL: acute nonlymphoblastic leukemia
ANS: autonomic nervous system
AOB: alcohol on breath
AODM: adult-onset diabetes mellitus
AP: anteroposterior, abdominal-perineal
APAP: acetaminophen
APL: acute promyelocytic leukemia
aPPT: activated partial thromboplastin time

APSAC: anisoylated plasminogen streptokinase activator complex

APUD: amine precursor update (and) decarboxylation

Ara-C: cytarabine

ARB: angiotensin II receptor blocker

ARD: antibiotic removal device

ARDS: adult respiratory distress syndrome

ARF: acute renal failure

AS: aortic stenosis

ASA: American Society of Anesthesiologists

ASAP: as soon as possible

ASAT: aspartate aminotransferase

ASCVD: atherosclerotic cardiovascular disease

ASD: atrial septal defect

ASHD: atherosclerotic heart disease

ASO: antistreptolysin O

AST: aspartate aminotransferase

ATG: antithymocyte globulin

ATN: acute tubular necrosis

ATP: adenosine triphosphate

AUC: area under the curve

A–V: arteriovenous

AV: atrioventricular

A–Vo$_2$: arteriovenous oxygen

AZT: azidothymidine (zidovudine)

B: band neutrophils

B I&II: Billroth I and II

B. burgdorferi: Borrelia burgdorferi

BACOD: bleomycin, doxorubicin (Adriamycin), cyclophosphamide, vincristine (Oncovin), dexamethasone

BACOP: bleomycin, doxorubicin (Adriamycin), cyclophosphamide, vincristine (Oncovin), prednisone

BAL: bronchoalveolar lavage

BAS: body surface area

BBB: bundle branch block

BC: bone conduction

BCAA: branched-chain amino acid

BCG: bacille Calmette-Guérin

BE: barium enema

BEE: basal energy expenditure

bid: twice/day

bili: bilirubin

BKA: below-the-knee amputation

BLS: basic life support

BM: bone marrow, bowel movement

BMD: bone mineral density

BMR: basal metabolic rate

BMT: bone marrow transplantation

BOM: bilateral otitis media

BOO: bladder outlet obstruction

BP: blood pressure

BPH: benign prostatic hypertrophy

BPM: beats per minute

BR: bed rest

BRBPR: bright red blood per rectum

BRP: bathroom privileges

BS&O: bilateral salpingo-oophorectomy

bs, BS: bowel sounds, breath sounds

BSA: body surface area

BUN: blood urea nitrogen

BW: body weight

Bx: biopsy

c: with (*cum*)

C. difficile: Clostridium difficile

Ca: calcium

CA: cancer

CAA: crystalline amino acid

CABG: coronary artery bypass graft

CAD: coronary artery disease

CAF: cyclophosphamide, doxorubicin (Adriamycin), 5-fluorouracil

CALGB: Cancer and Leukemia Group B

cAMP: cyclic adenosine monophosphate

Cao$_2$: arterial oxygen content

CAP: carcinoma of prostate

caps: capsule(s)

CAT: computed axial tomography

CBC: complete blood count

CBG: capillary blood gas

CC: chief complaint, clinical clerk

CCB: calcium channel blocker

CCI: corrected count increment (platelets)

CCO: continuous cardiac output

Co$_2$: capillary oxygen content

CCU: clean-catch urine, cardiac care unit

CCV: critical closing volume

CD: continuous dose

CDC: Centers for Disease Control and Prevention

CEA: carcinoembryonic antigen

CEP: counterimmunoelectrophoresis

CF: cystic fibrosis

CFU: colony-forming unit(s)

CGL: chronic granulocytic leukemia

CH$_{50}$: (total serum) hemolytic complement

CHD: coronary heart disease

CHF: congestive heart failure

CHO: carbohydrate

CHOP: cyclophosphamide, doxorubicin, vincristine (Oncovin), prednisone

CI: cardiac index

CIEP: counterimmunoelectrophoresis

circ.: circulating

CIS: carcinoma in situ

CK: creatine kinase

CK-MB: isoenzyme of creatine kinase with muscle and brain subunits

CKI: cyclin-dependent kinase inhibitor

Cl: chlorine

CLL: chronic lymphocytic leukemia

CML: chronic myelogenous leukemia

CMV: cytomegalovirus

CN: cranial nerve

CNS: central nervous system

CO: cardiac output
C/O: complaining of
COAD: chronic obstructive airway disease
COLD: chronic obstructive lung disease
COMT: catechol-*o*-methyltransferase
conc: concentrate
cont inf: continuous infusion
COPD: chronic obstructive pulmonary disease
COX-2: cyclooxygenase-2
CP: chest pain, cerebral palsy
CPAP: continuous positive airway pressure
CPK: creatinine phosphokinase
CPP: central precocious puberty
CPR: cardiopulmonary resuscitation
CPT: Current Procedural Terminology
CR: controlled release
CrCl: creatinine clearance
CREST: calcinosis cutis, Raynaud disease, esophageal dysmotility, syndactyly, telangiectasia
CRF: chronic renal failure
CRH: corticotropin-releasing hormone
CRP: C-reactive protein
C&S: culture and sensitivity
CSA: cyclosporine
CSF: cerebrospinal fluid, colony-stimulating factor
C-spine: cervical spine
CT: computed tomography
CV: cardiovascular
CVA: cerebrovascular accident, costovertebral angle
CVAT: costovertebral angle tenderness
CVH: common variable hypogammaglobulinemia
Cvo_2: oxygen content of mixed venous blood
CVP: central venous pressure
CXR: chest x-ray
d: day
D: diarrhea
D_{50}: 50% dextrose solution
DAG: diacylglycerol
DAP: diastolic pulmonary artery pressure
DAT: diet as tolerated
DAW: dispense as written
D/C: discontinue
D&C: dilation and curettage
DC: discontinue, discharge, direct current
ddI: dideoxyinosine
DDx: differential diagnosis
DEA: US Drug Enforcement Administration
DES: diethylstilbestrol
DEXA: dual-energy x-ray absorptiometry
DFA: direct fluorescent antibody
DHEA: dehydroepiandrosterone
DHEAS: dehydroepiandrosterone sulfate
DI: diabetes insipidus

DIC: disseminated intravascular coagulation
DIP: distal interphalangeal joint
DIT: diiodotyrosine
DJD: degenerative joint disease
DKA: diabetic ketoacidosis
D_5LR: 5% dextrose in lactated Ringer solution
DM: diabetes mellitus
DMARD: disease-modifying antirheumatic drug
DMSA: dimercaptosuccinic acid
DN: diabetic nephropathy
DNA: deoxyribonucleic acid
DNP: deoxyribonucleic protein
DNR: do not resuscitate
Do_2: oxygen delivery
DOA: dead on arrival
DOCA: deoxycorticosterone acetate
DOE: dyspnea on exertion
DOPA: dihydroxyphenylalanine
DP: dorsalis pedis
2,3-DPG: 2,3-diphosphoglycerate
DPL: diagnostic peritoneal lavage
DPT: diphtheria, pertussis, tetanus
DR: delayed release
DRG: diagnosis-related group
DS: double strength
DSA: digital subtraction angiography
DTPA: diethylenetriamine-pentaacetic acid
DTR: deep tendon reflex
DVT: deep venous thrombosis
D_5W: 5% dextrose in water
Dx: diagnosis
Dz: disease
E: eosinophils
E. coli: Escherichia coli
EAA: essential amino acid
EBL: estimated blood loss
EBV: Epstein–Barr virus
EC: enteric-coated
ECC: emergency cardiac care
ECG: electrocardiogram
ECOG: Eastern Cooperative Oncology Group
ECT: electroconvulsive therapy
EDC: estimated date of confinement
EDTA: ethylenediamine tetraacetic acid
EDVI: end-diastolic volume index
EFAD: essential fatty acid deficiency
EIA: enzyme immunoassay
ELISA: enzyme-linked immunosorbent assay
EMD: electromechanical dissociation
EMG: electromyelogram
EMIT: enzyme multiplied immunoassay technique
EMS: emergency medical system, eosinophilia-myalgia syndrome

EMV: eyes, motor, verbal response (Glasgow Coma Scale)
ENA: extractable nuclear antigen
ENT: ear, nose, and throat
eod: every other day
EOM: extraocular muscle
EPO: erythropoietin
EPS: extrapyramidal symptoms
EPSP: excitatory postsynaptic potential
ER: endoplasmic reticulum, emergency department, extended release
ERCP: endoscopic retrograde cholangiopancreatography
ERV: expiratory reserve volume
ESR: erythrocyte sedimentation rate
ESRD: end-stage renal disease
ET: endotracheal
EtOH: ethanol
ETT: endotracheal tube
EUA: examination under anesthesia
ExU: excretory urogram
Fab: antigen-binding fragment
FANA: fluorescent antinuclear antibody
FBS: fasting blood sugar
Fe: iron
FEV_1: forced expiratory volume in 1 s
FFP: fresh frozen plasma
FHR: fetal heart rate
FIGO: Fédération Internationale de Gynécologie et d'Obstétrique
FIO_2: fraction of inspired oxygen
FRC: functional residual capacity
FSH: follicle-stimulating hormone
FSP: fibrin split product
FTA-ABS: fluorescent treponemal antibody-absorbed
FTT: failure to thrive
FU: follow-up
5-FU: fluorouracil
FUO: fever of unknown origin
FVC: forced vital capacity
Fx: fracture
Fxn: function
G: gravida
G6PD: glucose-6-phosphate dehydrogenase
GABA: gamma-aminobutyric acid
GAD: glutamic acid decarboxylase
GC: gonorrhea (gonococcus)
G-CSF: granulocyte colony-stimulating factor
GDP: guanosine diphosphate
gen: generation
GERD: gastroesophageal reflux disease
GETT: general by endotracheal tube (anesthesia)
GF: growth factor
GFR: glomerular filtration rate
GGT: gamma-glutamyltransferase
GH: growth hormone
GHB: gamma hydroxybutyrate

GHIH: growth hormone-inhibiting hormone
GI: gastrointestinal
GM-CSF: granulocyte-macrophage colony-stimulating factor
GNID: gram-negative intracellular diplococci
GnRH: gonadotropin-releasing hormone
GOG: Gynecologic Oncology Group
gr: grain
GSP: glycated serum protein
GSW: gunshot wound
gt, gtt: drop, drops (*gutta*)
GTP: guanosine triphosphate
GTT: glucose tolerance test
GU: genitourinary
GVHD: graft-versus-host disease
GXT: graded exercise tolerance (cardiac stress test)
H. influenzae: Haemophilus influenzae
H. pylori: Helicobacter pylori
HA: headache
HAA: hepatitis B surface antigen (hepatitis-associated antigen)
HAV: hepatitis A virus
HBcAg: hepatitis B core antigen
Hbg: hemoglobin
HBeAg: hepatitis B e antigen
HBP: high blood pressure
HBsAg: hepatitis B surface antigen
HBV: hepatitis B virus
HC: hydroxycholesterol
HCG: human chorionic gonadotropin
HCL: hairy cell leukemia
HCO_3^-: bicarbonate
$[HCO_3^-]$: bicarbonate concentration
HCT: hematocrit
HCTZ: hydrochlorothiazide
HD: hemodialysis
HDL: high-density lipoprotein
HEENT: head, eyes, ears, nose, and throat
HELLP (preeclampsia with microangiopathic hemolysis, elevated liver function test results, and low platelet count
HFV: high-frequency ventilation
Hgb: hemoglobin
[Hgb]: hemoglobin concentration
H/H: hemoglobin/hematocrit, Henderson-Hesselbach equation
HIAA: 5-hydroxyindoleacetic acid
HIDA: hepatic 2,6-dimethyliminodiacetic acid
HIT: heparin-induced thrombocytopenia
HIV: human immunodeficiency virus
HJR: hepatojugular reflex
HLA: histocompatibility locus antigen
HMG-CoA: 3-hydroxy-3-methylglutaryl coenzyme A
HO: history of
HOB: head of bed

H&P: history and physical examination
HPA: hypothalamic–pituitary–adrenal
hpf: high-power field
HPI: history of the present illness
HPLC: high-pressure liquid chromatography
HPV: human papilloma virus
HR: heart rate
hs: at bedtime (*hora somni*)
HSG: hysterosalpingogram
HSM: hepatosplenomegaly
HSV: herpes simplex virus
5-HT$_3$: 5-hydroxytryptamine
HTLV-III: human T-lymphotropic virus, type III (AIDS agent, HIV)
HTN: hypertension
HUS: hemolytic uremic syndrome
Hx: history
IBW: ideal body weight
IC: inspiratory capacity
ICN: Intensive Care Nursery
ICS: intercostal space
ICSH: interstitial cell-stimulating hormone
ICU: intensive care unit
I&D: incision and drainage
ID: identification, infectious disease
IDDM: insulin-dependent diabetes mellitus
Ig: immunoglobulin
IgG1k: immunoglobulin G1 kappa
IHSS: idiopathic hypertrophic subaortic stenosis
inj: injection
IL: interleukin
IM: intramuscular
IMV: intermittent mandatory ventilation
inf: infusion
INF: intravenous nutritional fluid
Infxn: infection
INH: isoniazid
inhal: inhalation
inj: injection
INR: international normalized ratio
I&O: intake and output
IP$_3$: inositol triphosphate
IPPB: intermittent positive pressure breathing
IPSP: inhibitory postsynaptic potential
iPTH: parathyroid hormone by radioimmunoassay
IPV: inactivated poliomyelitis vaccine
IR: inversion recovery
IRBBB: incomplete right bundle branch block
IRDM: insulin-resistant diabetes mellitus
IRV: inspiratory reserve volume
ISA: intrinsic sympathomimetic activity
IT: intrathecal
ITP: idiopathic thrombocytopenic purpura
IV: intravenous
IVC: intravenous cholangiogram

IVP: intravenous pyelogram
JODM: juvenile-onset diabetes mellitus
JVD: jugular venous distention
K: potassium
KIU: kallikrein inactivation unit
KOR: keep open rate
17-KSG: 17-ketogenic steroids
KUB: kidneys, ureters, bladder
KVO: keep vein open
L: left, lymphocytes
LAD: left axis deviation, left anterior descending
LAE: left atrial enlargement
LAHB: left anterior hemiblock
LAP: left atrial pressure, leukocyte alkaline phosphatase
LBBB: left bundle branch block
LDH: lactate dehydrogenase
LDL: low-density lipoprotein
LE: lupus erythematosus
LH: luteinizing hormone
LHRH: leuteinizing hormone releasing hormone
LIH: left inguinal hernia
liq: liquid
LLL: left lower lobe
LLQ: left lower quadrant
LLSB: left lower sternal border
LMP: last menstrual period
LMWH: low-molecular-weight heparin
LNMP: last normal menstrual period
LOC: loss of consciousness, level of consciousness
LP: lumbar puncture
LPN: licensed practical nurse
LR: lactated Ringer solution
LSB: left sternal border
LSD: lysergic acid diethylamide
HTLV: human T-cell lymphotrophic virus
LUL: left upper lobe
LUQ: left upper quadrant
LV: left ventricle
LVD: left ventricular dysfunction
LVEDP: left ventricular end-diastolic pressure
LVH: left ventricular hypertrophy
M: monocytes
M. pneumoniae: Mycoplasma pneumoniae
MAC: *Mycobacterium avium* complex
MACE: methotrexate, doxorubicin (Adriamycin), cyclophosphamide, epipodophyllotoxin
MAG$_3$: mercaptoacetythiglycine
MAMC: midarm muscle circumference
MAO: monoamine oxidase
MAOI: monoamine oxidase inhibitor
MAP: mean arterial pressure
MAST: military/medical antishock trousers
MAT: multifocal atrial tachycardia
max: maximum

MBC: minimum bactericidal concentration

MBT: maternal blood type

MCDT: mixed connective tissue disease

MCH: mean cell hemoglobin

MCHC: mean cell hemoglobin concentration

MCT: medium-chain triglycerides

MCTD: mixed connective tissue disease

MCV: mean cell volume

MEN: multiple endocrine neoplasia

mEq: milliequivalent

MESNA: 2-mercaptoethane sulfonate sodium

met-dose: metered-dose

Mg: magnesium

MHA-TP: microhemagglutination–*Treponema pallidum*

MHC: major histocompatibility complex

MI: myocardial infarction, mitral insufficiency

MIBG: metaiodobenzyl-guanidine

MIC: minimum inhibitory concentration

min: minimum

MIT: monoiodotyrosine

MLE: midline episiotomy

MMDA: ecstasy

MMEF: maximal midexpiratory flow

mmol: millimole

MMR: measles, mumps, rubella

mo: month

MOPP: mechlorethamine, vincristine (Oncovin), procarbazine, prednisone

6-MP: mercaptopurine

MPF: M phase-promoting factor

MPGN: membrane-proliferative glomerulonephritis

MPTP: analog of meperidine (used by drug addicts)

MRI: magnetic resonance imaging

mRNA: messenger ribonucleic acid

MRS: magnetic resonance spectroscopy

MRSA: methicillin-resistant *Staphylococcus aureus*

MS: mitral stenosis, morphine sulfate, multiple sclerosis, medical student

MSBOS: maximal surgical blood order schedule

MSH: melanocyte-stimulating hormone

MSSA: methicillin-sensitive *Staphylococcus aureus*

MTT: monotetrazolium

MTX: methotrexate

MUGA: multigated (image) acquisition (analysis)

MVA: motor vehicle accident

MVI: multivitamin injection

MVV: maximum voluntary ventilation

MyG: myasthenia gravis

N: nausea

N. gonorrhoeae: *Neisseria gonorrhoeae*

N. meningitidis: *Neisseria meningitidis*

N/A: not applicable

Na: sodium

Na^+/K^+-ATPase: sodium/potassium adenosine triphosphate

NAACP: mnemonic for *N*eoplasm, *A*llergy, *A*ddison disease, *C*ollagen–vascular disease, *P*arasites (causes of eosinophilia)

NAD: no active disease

NAG: narrow-angle glaucoma

NAPA: *N*-acetylated procainamide

NAS: no added sodium

NAVEL: mnemonic for *N*erve, *A*rtery, *V*ein, *E*mpty space, *L*ymphatic

NCV: nerve conduction velocity

NE: norepinephrine

neb: nebulization

NED: no evidence of recurrent disease

NG: nasogastric

NHL: non-Hodgkin lymphoma

NIDDM: non–insulin-dependent diabetes mellitus

NK: natural killer

NKA: no known allergies

NKDA: no known drug allergy

nl: normal

NMR: nuclear magnetic resonance

NPC: nuclear pore complex

NPO: nothing by mouth (*nil per os*)

NRM: no regular medicines

NRTI: nucleoside reverse transcriptase inhibitor

NS: normal saline

NSAID: nonsteroidal antiinflammatory drug

NSCLC: non-small-cell lung cancer

NSILA: nonsuppressible insulin-like activity

NSR: normal sinus rhythm

NT: nasotracheal

NTG: nitroglycerin

OAB: overactive bladder

OB: obstetrics

Obs: observation

OCD: obsessive-compulsive disorder

OCG: oral cholecystogram

7-OCHS: 17-hydroxycorticosteroids

OCP: oral contraceptive pill

OD: overdose, right eye (*oculus dexter*)

oint: ointment

OM: otitis media

OOB: out of bed

ophth: ophthalmic

OPV: oral polio vaccine

OR: operating room

OS: opening snap, left eye (*oculus sinister*)

OSHA: Occupational Safety and Health Administration

OTC: over-the-counter (medications)
OU: both eyes
P-24: HIV core antigen
P. aeruginosa: Pseudomonas aeruginosa
P. mirabilis: Proteus mirabilis
p: para
PA: posteroanterior, pulmonary artery
PAC: premature atrial contraction
PaCO$_2$: arterial partial pressure of carbon dioxide
PAD: diastolic pulmonary artery pressure, public access defibrillator
PAF: paroxysmal atrial fibrillation
PAL: periarterial lymphatic (sheath)
PaO$_2$: arterial partial pressure of oxygen
PAO$_2$: alveolar partial pressure of oxygen
PAOP: pulmonary artery occlusion pressure
PAP: pulmonary artery pressure, prostatic acid phosphatase
PAS: systolic pulmonary artery pressure
PASG: pneumatic antishock garment
PAT: paroxysmal atrial tachycardia
PBM: pharmacy benefit manager
pc: after eating (*post cibum*)
PCA: patient-controlled analgesia
PCI: percutaneous coronary intervention
PCKD: polycystic kidney disease
PCN: penicillin, percutaneous nephrostomy
PCP: *Pneumocystis carinii* pneumonia, phencyclidine
PCR: polymerase chain reaction
PCWP: pulmonary capillary wedge pressure
PDA: patent ductus arteriosus
PDGF: platelet-derived growth factor
PDR: Physicians' Desk Reference
PDS: polydioxanone
PE: pulmonary embolus, physical examination, pleural effusion
PEA: pulseless electrical activity
PEEP: positive end-expiratory pressure
PEG: polyethylene glycol, percutaneous endoscopic gastrostomy
PERRLA: pupils equal, round, reactive to light and accommodation
PERRLADC: pupils equal, round, reactive to light and accommodation directly and consensually
PET: positron emission tomography
PFT: pulmonary function test
PGE$_1$: prostaglandin E$_1$
PI: pulmonic insufficiency (disease)
PICC: peripherally inserted central catheter
PID: pelvic inflammatory disease
PIE: pulmonary infiltrates with eosinophilia
PIH: prolactin-inhibiting hormone
PKU: phenylketonuria
PM: afternoon and night
PMDD: premenstrual dysphoric disorder
PMH: past medical history

PMI: point of maximal impulse
PMN: polymorphonuclear neutrophil
PMNL: polymorphonuclear leukocyte (neutrophil)
PN: parenteral nutrition
PND: paroxysmal nocturnal dyspnea
PNS: peripheral nervous system
PO: by mouth (*per os*)
pod: postoperative day
postop: postoperative, after surgery
PP: pulsus paradoxus, postprandial
P&PD: percussion and postural drainage
PPD: purified protein derivative
PPN: peripheral parenteral nutrition
PR: by rectum
preop: preoperative, before surgery
PRG: pregnancy
PRN: as needed
PRA: plasma renin activity
PRBC: packed red blood cells
PRG: pregnancy
PRN: as often as needed (*pro re nata*)
PS: pulmonic stenosis, partial saturation
PSA: prostate-specific antigen
PSV: pressure support ventilation
PSVT: paroxysmal supraventricular tachycardia
Pt: patient
PT: prothrombin time, physical therapy, posterior tibial
PTCA: percutaneous transluminal coronary angioplasty
PTH: parathyroid hormone
PTHC: percutaneous transhepatic cholangiogram
PTT: partial thromboplastin time
PTU: propylthiouracil
PUD: peptic ulcer disease
PVC: premature ventricular contraction, polyvinyl chloride
PVD: peripheral vascular disease
PVR: peripheral vascular resistance
PWP: pulmonary wedge pressure
PZI: protamine zinc insulin
Q: mathematical symbol for flow
q: every
qd: every day (use not recommended)
q__h: every __ hours
qid: 4 times/day
QNS: quantity not sufficient
qo: every other
qs: quantity sufficient
Qs: volume of blood (portion of cardiac output) shunted past nonventilated alveoli
Qs/Qt: shunt fraction
Qt: total cardiac output
R: right
R/O: rule out
RA: rheumatoid arthritis, right atrium

RAD: right axis deviation
RAE: right atrial enlargement
RAP: right atrial pressure
RBBB: right bundle branch block
RBC: red blood cell (erythrocyte)
RBP: retinol-binding protein
RCC: renal cell carcinoma
RDA: recommended dietary allowance
RDS: respiratory distress syndrome (of
    newborn)
RDW: red cell distribution width
REF: right ventricular ejection fraction
REM: rapid eye movement
RER: rough endoplasmic reticulum
resp: respiratory
RF: rheumatoid factor
% RH: percentage of relative humidity
RIA: radioimmunoassay
RIH: right inguinal hernia
RIND: reversible ischemic neurological
    deficit
RL: Ringer lactate
RLL: right lower lobe
RLQ: right lower quadrant
RME: resting metabolic expenditure
RML: right middle lobe
RMSF: Rocky Mountain spotted fever
RNA: ribonucleic acid
RNase: ribonuclease
RNP: ribonucleoprotein
ROM: range of motion
ROS: review of systems
RPG: retrograde pyelogram
RPR: rapid plasma reagin
rRNA: ribosomal ribonucleic acid
RRR: regular rate and rhythm
RSV: respiratory syncytial virus
RT: radiation therapy, respiratory therapy,
    reverse transcriptase, rubella titer
RTA: renal tubular acidosis
RTC: return to clinic
RTOG: Radiation Therapy Oncology
    Group
RT-PCR: reverse transcription polymer-
    ase chain reaction
RU: resin uptake
RUG: retrograde urethrogram
RUL: right upper lobe
RUQ: right upper quadrant
RV: residual volume
RVEDVI: right ventricular end-diastolic
    volume index
RVH: right ventricular hypertrophy
Rx: treatment
Rxn: reaction
s: without (*sine*)
S: segmented or stab neutrophils
S&A: sugar and acetone
S. aureus: Staphylococcus aureus
S. pyogenes: Streptococcus pyogenes

SA: sinoatrial
SAA: synthetic amino acid
SAE: serious adverse event
SaO$_2$: arterial oxygen saturation
SBE: subacute bacterial endocarditis
SBFT: small bowel follow-through
SBS: short bowel syndrome
SCD: sudden cardiac death
SCr: serum creatinine
segs: segmented cells
SEM: systolic ejection murmur
SER: smooth endoplasmic reticulum
SG: Swan-Ganz, specific gravity
SGA: small for gestational age
SGGT: serum gamma-glutamyl transpepti-
    dase
SGOT: serum glutamic-oxaloacetic trans-
    aminase
SGPT: serum glutamic-pyruvic transam-
    inase
SI: Système International
SIADH: syndrome of inappropriate secre-
    tion of antidiuretic hormone
sig: write on label (*signa*)
SIMV: synchronous intermittent manda-
    tory ventilation
SIRS: systemic inflammatory response
    syndrome
SKSD: streptokinase-streptodornase
SL: sublingual
SLE: systemic lupus erythematosus
SMA: sequential multiple analysis
SMO: slips made out
SMX: sulfamethoxazole
SOAP: mnemonic for *S*ubjective, *O*bjec-
    tive, *A*ssessment, *P*lan
SOB: shortness of breath
SOC: signed on chart
soln: solution
S/P: status post
Sp, sp: species
SPAG: small-particle aerosol generator
SPECT: single-photon emission com-
    puted tomography
SpO$_2$: pulse oximetry reading
SQ: subcutaneous
SR: sustained release
SRP: single recognition particle
SRS-A: slow-reacting substance of ana-
    phylaxis
SSKI: saturated solution of potassium
    iodide
SSRI: selective serotonin reuptake inhibitor
SSS: sick sinus syndrome
stat: immediately (*statim*)
supl: supplement
supp: suppository
susp: suspension
STD: sexually transmitted disease
SVD: spontaneous vaginal delivery

$S\bar{v}O_2$: mixed venous oxygen saturation
SVR: systemic vascular resistance
SVT: supraventricular tachycardia
SWOG: Southwest Oncology Group
Sx: symptom
Sz: seizure
T: one
T_3 RU: triiodothyronine resin uptake
T_3: triiodothyronine
T_4: thyroxine
tabs: tablet(s)
TAH: total abdominal hysterectomy
TB: tuberculosis
TBG: thyroxine-binding globulin, total blood gas
TBLC: term birth, living child
TBW: total body water
T&C: type and cross-match
TCA: tricyclic antidepressant
TC&DB: turn, cough, and deep breathe
TCF: triceps skin fold
TCP: transcutaneous pacer
Td: tetanus-diphtheria toxoid
TD: transdermal
TFT: thyroid function test
6-TG: 6-thioguanine
T&H: type and hold
TIA: transient ischemic attack
TIBC: total iron-binding capacity
tid: 3 times/day
TIG: tetanus immune globulin
TKO: to keep open
TLC: total lung capacity
TMJ: temporomandibular joint
TMP: trimethoprim
TMP-SMX: trimethoprim-sulfamethoxazole
TNFα: tumor necrosis factor alpha
TNM: tumor-nodes-metastases
TNTC: too numerous to count
TO: telephone order
TOPV: trivalent oral polio vaccine
TORCH: toxoplasma, rubella, cytomegalovirus, herpes virus (*O* = other [syphilis])
tox: toxicity
TPA: tissue plasminogen activator
TPN: total peripheral resistance, total parenteral nutrition
TRH: thyrotropin-releasing hormone
tri: trimester
TSH: thyroid-stimulating hormone
TT: thrombin time
TTP: thrombotic thrombocytopenic purpura

TU: tuberculin units
TUR: transurethral resection
TURBT: TUR bladder tumors
TURP: TUR prostate
TV: tidal volume
TVH: total vaginal hysterectomy
Tx: treatment, transplant, transfer
type 2 DM: non-insulin-dependent diabetes mellitus, type 2 diabetes mellitus
UA: urinalysis
UAC: uric acid
UDS: urodynamic studies
UGI: upper gastrointestinal
uln, ULN: upper limit of normal
UPEP: urine protein electrophoresis
URI: upper respiratory tract infection
US: ultrasonography
USP: United States Pharmacopeia
UTI: urinary tract infection
UUN: urinary urea nitrogen
V: vomiting
VAERS: Vaccine Adverse Events Reporting System
VAMP: vincristine, doxorubicin (Adriamycin), methylprednisolone
VAS: visual analog scale
VC: vital capacity
VCUG: voiding cystourethrogram
VDRL: Venereal Disease Research Laboratory
VF: ventricular fibrillation
VLDL: very low density lipoprotein
VMA: vanillylmandelic acid
VO: voice order
VP-16: etoposide
$\dot{V}/\dot{Q}$: ventilation–perfusion
VSS: vital signs stable
VT: ventricular tachycardia
WB: whole blood
WBC: white blood cell, white blood cell count
WD: well developed
WF: white female
WHI: Women's Health Initiative
WHO: World Health Organization
WM: white male
WN: well nourished
wnl, WNL: within normal limits
WPW: Wolff-Parkinson-White
XR: extended release
XRT: x-ray therapy
y: year
YO: years old
ZE: Zollinger-Ellison

"SO YOU WANT TO BE A SCUT MONKEY": AN INTRODUCTION TO CLINICAL MEDICINE*

The transition from the preclinical years to the clinical years of medical school is an important time. Understanding the new responsibilities and the general ground rules can ease this transition. Here we provide a brief introduction to clinical medical training for the new student on the wards.

THE HIERARCHY

Most services have some or all of the following team members.

The Intern

In some programs, the intern is also known as the first-year resident. This person has the day-to-day responsibilities of patient care. This duty, combined with a total lack of seniority, usually serves to keep the intern in the hospital more than the other members of the team and may limit his or her teaching of medical students. Any question you have concerning details in the evaluation of the patient, for example, whether Mrs. Pavona gets a complete blood count this morning or this evening, is usually referred first to the intern.

The Resident

The resident is a member of the house staff who has completed at least 1 year of postgraduate medical education. The most senior resident is typically in charge of the overall conduct of the service and is the person you might ask a question such as "What might cause Mrs. Pavona's white blood cell count to be 142,000?" You might also ask your resident for an appropriate reference on the subject or perhaps to arrange a brief conference on the topic for everyone on the service. A surgical service typically has a chief resident, a physician in the last year of residency who usually runs the day-to-day activities of the service. On medical services the chief resident is usually an appointee of the chair of medicine and primarily has administrative responsibilities often with limited ward duties.

The Attending Physician

The attending physician is also called simply "The Attending," and on nonsurgical services, "the attending." (*Note:* Before we get any more letters—yes, this is a joke!) This physician has completed postgraduate education and has become a member of the teaching faculty. He or she is usually already board-certified in a

---

*Based on a concept initially developed by Epstein A, Frye T (eds.): *So You Want to Be a Toad. College of Medicine, Ohio State University, Columbus, OH.*

specialty but may be newly trained and "board eligible." The attending is morally and legally responsible for the care of all patients whose charts are marked with the attending's name. All major therapeutic decisions made about the care of these patients are ultimately passed by the attending. In addition, this person is responsible for teaching and evaluating house staff and medical students. You might ask this member of the team, "Why are we treating Mrs. Pavona with busulfan?"

The Fellow

The fellow is a physician who has completed his or her postgraduate education and elected to do extra study in one special field, such as nephrology, high-risk obstetrics, or surgical oncology. This person may or may not be an active member of the team and may not be obligated to teach medical students but usually is happy to answer any questions you may ask. You might ask this person to help you read Mrs. Pavona's bone marrow smear.

Physician Extenders

Nurse practitioners and physician assistants are being incorporated into the health care system, including academic medical centers. Their responsibilities vary by service, hospital, and state regulation. These professionals are critical members of the team and excellent resources for both students and patients. You might ask them about Mrs. Pavona's discharge orders.

TEAMWORK

The medical student, in addition to being a member of the medical team, must interact with members of the professional team of nurses, dietitians, pharmacists, social workers, physician assistants, nurse practitioners, and all others who provide direct care for the patient. Good working relations with this group of professionals can make your work go more smoothly; bad relations with them can make your rotation miserable.

Nurses are generally good-tempered but are overworked in most systems. Like most human beings, they respond favorably to polite treatment. Leaving a mess in a patient's room after a floor procedure, standing by idly while a 98-lb licensed practical nurse struggles to move a 350-lb patient onto the chair scale, and obviously listening to three ringing telephones while room call lights flash are acts guaranteed not to please. Do not let anyone talk you into being an acting nurse's aide or ward secretary, but try to be polite and help when you can.

You will occasionally meet a staff member who is having a bad day, and you will be able to do little about it. Returning hostility is unwarranted at these times, and it is best to avoid confrontations except when necessary for the appropriate care of the patient.

When faced with ordering a diet for your first sick patient, you might be confronted with the limitation in your education in nutrition. Fortunately, dietitians are available, and you should never hesitate to call one.

In matters concerning drug interactions, side effects, individualization of dosages, alterations of drug dosing in disease, and equivalence of different brands of the same drug, it never hurts to call the pharmacist. Most academic medical centers have a PharmD resident who follows inpatients on a given floor or service and who will gladly answer any questions and is an excellent resource for additional reference materials.

YOUR HEALTH AND A WORD ON "AGGRESSIVENESS"

In your months of curing disease both day and night, it becomes easy to ignore your own right to keep yourself healthy. With the implementation of the Accreditation Council for Graduate Medical Education (ACGME) guidelines on resident duty hours on July 1, 2004 (www.acgme.org), the numerous bad examples of medical and surgical interns working on 3 hours of sleep a night and eating most of their meals from vending machines have been reduced dramatically. Despite the hit the hospital is taking on sales of candy bars, do not let anyone talk you into believing that you are not entitled to decent meals and sleep, even if the ACGME 80-hour work week rules do not apply to students (yet!). If you offer yourself as a sacrifice, it will be a rare rotation on which you will not become one. On the other hand, try to extend yourself when the need arises. The house staff will appreciate it, and because the house staff usually has significant input into your grade, it may reflect itself in an outstanding grade on the rotation.

You may have the misfortune someday of reading an evaluation that says you were not "aggressive enough." This notion is enigmatic to everyone. Does it mean that the student refused to attempt to start an intravenous line after eight previous failures? Does it mean that the student was not consistently the first to shout out the answer over the mumbling of fellow students on rounds? Whatever constitutes "aggressiveness" must be a dubious virtue at best.

A more appropriate virtue might be **assertiveness in obtaining your education.** Ask **good** questions, read about your patient's illness, review the basics of a procedure before going to the OR, participate actively in your patient's care, take an interest in other patients on the service, and have the house staff show you procedures and review your chartwork. This approach avoids the need for victimizing your patients and comrades, as the definition of *aggression* suggests.

ROUNDS

Rounds are meetings of all members of the service for discussing the care of the patient. Rounds occur daily and are of three kinds.

Morning Rounds

Also known as "work rounds," morning rounds take place anywhere from 6:00 to 9:00 AM on most services and are attended by residents, interns, and students. Morning rounds are the time for discussing what happened to the patient during the night, the progress of the patient's evaluation or therapy or both, the laboratory and radiologic tests to be ordered for the patient, and, last but not least, talking with and evaluating the patient. Know about your patient's most recent laboratory reports and progress—this is a chance for you to look good.

Ideally, differences of opinion and glaring omissions in patient care are politely discussed and resolved at morning rounds. Writing new orders, filling out consultation forms, and making telephone calls related to the patient's care are best done right after morning rounds.

Attending Rounds

Attending rounds vary greatly depending on the service and on the nature of the attending physician. The same people who gathered for morning rounds are at attending rounds, as is the attending. At this meeting, patients are often seen again (especially on the surgical services); significant new laboratory, radiographic, and physical findings are described (often by the student caring for the patient); and new patients are formally presented to the attending (again, often by the medical student).

The most important priority for the student on attending rounds is to **know the patient.** Be prepared to concisely tell the attending what has happened to the patient. Also be ready to give a brief presentation on the patient's illness, especially if it is unusual. The attending will probably not be interested in minor details that do not affect therapeutic decisions. In addition, the attending will probably not wish to hear a litany of normal laboratory values, only the pertinent ones, such as "Mrs. Pavona's platelets are still 350,000/mL in spite of her bone marrow disease." You do not have to tell everything you know on rounds, but you must be prepared to do so.

Disputes among house staff and students usually are bad form on attending rounds. For this reason, the unwritten rule is that any differences of opinion not previously discussed should not be raised initially in the presence of the attending.

Check-out or Evening Rounds

Formal evening rounds on which the patients are seen by the entire team a second time are typically done only on surgical and pediatric services. Other services, such as medicine, often have check-out with the resident on call for the service that evening (sometimes called "card rounds"). Expect to convene for check-out rounds between 3:00 and 7:00 PM on most days.

All new data are presented by the person who collected them (often the student). Orders are again written, laboratory work desired for early the next day is requested, and those on call compile a "scut list" of work to be done that night and a list of patients who need close supervision. To comply with the ACGME directive regarding an 80-hour work week, many services have adopted "night-float" coverage systems. The interns and residents caring for your patients overnight will meet with the team at evening sign-out rounds. These cross-coverage strategies call for clear, concise communication essential during rounds.

BEDSIDE ROUNDS

Bedside rounds are basically the same as other rounds except that tact is at a premium. The first consideration at the bedside must be for the patient. If no one else on the team says "Good morning" and asks how the patient is feeling, do it yourself; this is not a presumptuous act on your part. Keep this encounter brief and then explain to the patient that you will be talking about him or her for a while. Most patients treated this way feel flattered by the attention and listen with interest.

Certain points of a hallway presentation are omitted in the patient's room. The patient's race and sex are usually apparent to all and do not warrant inclusion in your first sentence.

The patient must *never* be called by the name of the disease, eg, Mrs. Pavona is not "a 45-year-old CML (chronic myelogenous leukemia)" but "a 45-year-old *with* CML." The patient's general appearance need not be reiterated. Descriptions of evidence of disease must not be prefaced by words such as *outstanding* or *beautiful*. Mrs. Pavona's massive spleen is not beautiful to her, and it should not be to the physician or student either.

At the bedside, keep both feet on the floor. A foot up on a bed or chair conveys impatience and disinterest to the patient and other members of the team. It is poor form to carry beverages or food into the patient's room.

Although you will probably never be asked to examine a patient during bedside rounds, it is still worthwhile to know how to do so considerately. Bedside examinations are often done by the attending at the time of the initial presentation or by one member of a surgical service on postoperative rounds. First, warn the patient that you are about to examine the wound or affected part. Ask the patient to uncover whatever needs to be exposed rather than boldly removing the patient's clothes yourself. If the patient is unable to do so alone, you may do it, but remember to explain what you are doing. Remove only as much clothing as is necessary, and then promptly cover the patient again. In a ward room, remember to pull the curtain.

Bedside rounds in the intensive care unit call for as much consideration as they do in any other room. That still, naked person on the bed may not be as "out of it" as the resident (or anyone else) believes and may be hearing every word you say. Again, exercise discretion in discussing the patient's illness, plan, prognosis, and personal character as it relates to the disease.

Remember that patient information with which you are entrusted as a health care provider is confidential. There is a time and place to discuss this sensitive information, and public areas such as elevators or cafeterias are not the appropriate location for these discussions.

READING

Time for reading is at a premium on many services, and it is therefore important to use that time effectively. Unless you can remember everything you learned in the first 20 months of medical school, you will probably want to review the basic facts about the disease that brought your patient into the hospital. These facts are most often found in the same core texts that got you through the preclinical years. Unless specifically directed to do so, avoid the temptation to log on to MEDLINE to find all the latest articles on a disease you have not read about for the last 7 months; you do not have the time.

The appropriate time to head for MEDLINE is when a therapeutic dilemma arises and only the most recent literature will adequately advise the team. You may wish to obtain some direction from the attending, the fellow, or the resident before plunging online or into the library on your only Friday night off call this month. Ask the residents and your fellow students which pocket manuals and PDA downloads they found most useful for a given rotation.

THE WRITTEN HISTORY AND PHYSICAL

Much has been written on how to obtain a useful medical history and perform a thorough physical examination, and there is little to add here. Three things worth emphasizing are your own physical findings, your impression, and your own differential diagnosis.

Trust and record your own physical findings, even if other examiners have written things different from those you found. You just may be right, and if not, you have learned something from it. Avoid the temptation to copy another examiner's findings as your own when you are unable to do the examination yourself. Still, it would be an unusually cruel resident who would make you give Mrs. Pavona her fourth rectal examination of the day, and in this circumstance you may write "rectal per resident." *Do not do this routinely just to avoid performing a complete physical examination. Check with the resident first.*

Although not always emphasized in physical diagnosis, your clinical impression is probably the most important part of your write-up. Reasoned interpretation of the medical history and physical examination findings is what separates physicians from the computers touted by the tabloids as their successors. Judgment is learned only by boldly stating your case, even if you are wrong more often than not.

The differential diagnosis, that is, your impression, should include only entities that you consider when evaluating your patient. Avoid including every possible cause of your patient's ailments. List only those that you are seriously considering, and include in your plan what you intend to do to exclude each one. Save the exhaustive list for the time your attending asks for all the causes of a symptom, syndrome, or abnormal laboratory value.

THE PRESENTATION

The object of the presentation is to *briefly* and *concisely* (usually in a few minutes) describe your patient's reason for being in the hospital to all members of the team who do not know the patient and the story. Unlike the write-up, which contains all the data you obtained, the presentation may include only the pertinent positive and negative evidence of a disease and its course in the patient. It is hard to get a feel for what is pertinent until you have seen and done a few presentations yourself.

Practice is important. Try never to read from your write-up, because doing so often produces dull and lengthy presentations. Most attendings will allow you to carry note cards, but this method can also lead to trouble unless content is carefully edited. Presentations are given in the same order as a write-up: identification, chief complaint, history of the present illness, past medical history, family history, psychosocial history, review of systems, physical examination, laboratory and x-ray data, clinical impression, and plan. Only pertinent positives and negatives from the review of systems should be given. These and truly relevant items from other parts of the interview often can be added to the history of the present illness. Finally, the length and content of the presentation vary greatly according to the wishes of the attending and the resident, but you will learn quickly what they do and do not want.

RESPONSIBILITY

Your responsibilities as a student should be clearly defined on the first day of a rotation by either the attending or the resident. Ideally, this enumeration of your duties should also include a list of what you might expect concerning teaching, floor skills, presentations, and all the other things you are paying many thousands of dollars a year to learn.

On some services, you may feel like a glorified unit secretary (clinical rotations are called "clerkships" for good reason!), and you will not be far from wrong. This is *not* what you are going into hock for. The scut work should be divided among the house staff and students.

You will frequently be expected to call for a certain piece of laboratory data or to go review an x-ray with the radiologist. You may then mutter under your breath, "Why waste my time? The report will be on the chart in a day or two!" You will feel less annoyed in this situation if you consider that every piece of data ordered is vital to the care of your patient.

Outpatient clinic experiences are incorporated into many rotations. The same basic rules and skill set necessary for in-patient care can be easily transferred to the outpatient setting. The student's responsibility, again, can be summarized in three words: **know your patient.** The entire service relies to a great extent on a well-informed presentation by the student. The better informed you are, the more time is left for education, and the better your evaluation will be. A major part of becoming a physician is learning responsibility.

ORDERS

Orders are the physician's instructions to nurses and other members of the professional staff concerning the care of the patient. These instructions may include the frequency of assessment of vital signs, administration of medications, respiratory care, laboratory and x-ray studies, and nearly anything else that you can imagine.

There are many formats for writing concise admission, transfer, and postoperative orders. Some rotations may have a precisely fixed set of routine orders, but others leave you and the intern to your own devices. It is important in each case to avoid omitting instructions critical to the care of the patient. Although you will be confronted with a variety of lists and mnemonics, ultimately it is helpful to devise your own system and commit it to memory. Why memorize? Because when you are an intern and it is 3:30 AM, you may overlook something if you try to think it out. One system for writing admission or transfer orders uses the mnemonic "A.A.D.C. VAAN DISSL," which is discussed in Chapter 2.

The word *stat* is the abbreviation for the Latin word *statim,* which means "immediately." When added to any order, it puts the requested study in front of all the routine work waiting to be done. Ideally, a stat order is reserved for the truly urgent situation, but in practice it is often inappropriately used. Most of the blame for this situation rests with physicians who either fail to plan ahead or order stat lab results when routine studies would do.

Student orders usually require a cosignature from a physician, although at some institutions students are allowed to order routine laboratory studies. Do not ask a nurse or pharmacist to act on an unsigned student order; it is **illegal** for them to do so.

The intern is responsible for most orders. The amount of interest shown by the resident and the attending varies greatly, but ideally you will review with the intern the orders for routinely admitted patients. Have the intern show you how to write orders for a few patients, then take the initiative and write the orders yourself and review them with the intern. Unfortunately, this important part of learning basic patient care is becoming increasingly difficult as many medical centers make the transition from paper charts to electronic medical records. Even if your hospital uses computerized orders, take the opportunity to watch the intern or resident entering the orders when you admit patients.

THE DAY

The events of the day and the effective use of time are two of the most distressing enigmas encountered in making the transition from preclinical to clinical education. For example, there are no typical days on surgical services because the operating room schedule prohibits making rounds at a regularly scheduled time every day. The following suggestions will help on any service.

1. Schedule special studies early in the day. The free time after work rounds is usually ideal for this task. Also, call consultants early in the morning. Often they can see your patient on the same day or at least early the next day.
2. Take care of all your business in the radiology department in one trip unless a given problem requires viewing a film promptly. Do *not* make as many separate trips as you have patients.

3. Make a point of knowing when certain services become unavailable, for example, for electrocardiograms, contrast-study scheduling, and blood drawing. Be sure to get these procedures done while it is still possible to do so.

4. Make a daily work or "scut"* list, and write down laboratory results as soon as you obtain them. Few people can keep all the daily data in their heads without making errors.

5. Arrange your travels around the hospital efficiently. If you have patients to see on four different floors, try to take care of all their needs, such as drawing blood, removing sutures, writing progress notes, and calling for consultations, in one trip.

6. Strive to work thoroughly but quickly. If you do not try to get work done early, you never will (this is not to say that you will succeed even if you do try). There is no sin in leaving at 5:00 PM or earlier if your obligations are *completed* and the supervising resident has dismissed you.

A PARTING SHOT

The clinical years are when all the years of premed study in college and the first 2 years of medical school suddenly come together. Trying to tell you adequately about being a clinical clerk is similar to trying to make someone into a swimmer on dry land. The terms for describing new clinical clerks ("scut monkey," "scut boy," "scut dog," "torpedoes") vary from medical center to medical center. These expressions describing the new clinical clerk acknowledge that the transition, a rite of passage, into the next phase of physician training has occurred.

We hope that this "So You Want to Be a Scut Monkey" introduction and the information contained in this book will give you a good start as you enter the "hands-on" phase of becoming a successful and respected physician.

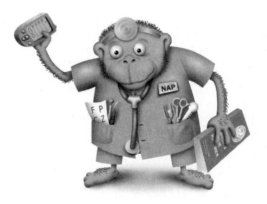

---

*Although the origin of how the word *scut* (real definition: the tail of a hare) entered the medical jargon is obscure, we like to think it represents an acronym for "some common unfinished task" or "some clinically useful training."

HISTORY AND PHYSICAL EXAMINATION

History and Physical Examination
Psychiatric History and Physical
    Examination
Heart Murmurs and Extra Heart Sounds
Blood Pressure Guidelines
Dental Examination

Dermatologic Descriptions
Dermatome and Cutaneous Innervation
Physical Signs, Symptoms, and Eponyms
Example of a Written History and
    Physical Examination

HISTORY AND PHYSICAL EXAMINATION

An example of a complete H&P write-up is on page 20. The details and length of a written H&P can vary with the particular problem and with the service to which the patient is admitted.

History

Identification: Name, age, sex, referring physician, informant (eg, patient, relative, old chart), and reliability of the informant.

Chief Complaint: State, in patient's words, the current problem.

History of the Present Illness (HPI): Define the present illness by quality; quantity; setting; anatomic location and radiation; time course, including when the illness began; whether the complaint is progressing, regressing, or steady; whether the complaint is of constant or intermittent frequency; and aggravating, alleviating, and associated factors. The information should be in chronologic order, including diagnostic tests done before admission. Record related history, including previous treatment for the problem, risk factors, and pertinent negative results. Include family history and psychosocial history pertinent to the chief complaint. Other significant ongoing problems should be included in the HPI in a separate section or paragraph. For instance, if a patient with poorly controlled diabetes mellitus comes to the emergency department because of chest pain, the HPI should first include information regarding the chest pain followed by a detailed history of the diabetes mellitus. If the diabetes mellitus is diet controlled or otherwise well controlled, the history of the diabetes mellitus may be placed in the past medical history.

Past Medical History (PMH): Current medications, including OTC medications, vitamins, and herbal agents; allergies (drug and other, as well as specific allergy manifestations); operations; hospitalizations; blood transfusions, including when and how many units and the type of blood product; trauma; and stable current and past medical problems unrelated to the HPI. **Adult patients:** Ask about diabetes mellitus; HTN; MI; stroke; PUD; asthma; emphysema; thyroid, liver, and kidney disease; bleeding disorders; cancer; TB; hepatitis; and STDs. Also ask about routine health maintenance. The questions for this category depend on the age and sex of the patient but can include last Pap smear and pelvic exam; breast exam; whether the patient does breast self-examinations; date of last mammogram; diphtheria/tetanus immunization; pneumococcal, influenza, and hepatitis B vaccines; stool samples for occult blood; sigmoidoscopy or colonoscopy; cholesterol; HDL cholesterol; functioning smoke alarms on each floor at home; and use of seat belts. **Pediatric patients:** Include prenatal and birth history, feedings, food intolerance, immunization history, hot water heater temperature setting, and use of bicycle helmets.

Family History: Age, status (alive, dead) of blood relatives and medical problems of blood relatives (ask about cancer, especially breast, colon, and prostate; TB, asthma; MI; HTN; thyroid disease; kidney disease; PUD; DM; bleeding disorders; glaucoma, macular degeneration; and depression and alcohol or substance abuse). Write out or use a family tree (see Figure in example of a complete H&P write-up, page 20).

Psychosocial (Social) History: Stressors (financial, significant relationships, work or school, health) and support (family, friends, significant other, clergy); lifestyle risk factors (alcohol, drugs, tobacco, and caffeine use; diet; exercise; exposure to environmental agents; and sexual practices); patient profile (may include marital status and children, sexual orientation; present and past employment; financial support and insurance; education; religion; hobbies; beliefs; living conditions); for veterans include military service history. **Pediatric patients:** Include grade in school and sleep and play habits.

Review of Systems (ROS)

General: Weight loss, weight gain, fatigue, weakness, appetite, fever, chills, night sweats

Skin: Rashes, pruritus, bruising, dryness, skin cancer or other lesions

Head: Trauma, headache, tenderness, dizziness, syncope

Eyes: Vision, changes in visual field, glasses, last prescription change, photophobia, blurring, diplopia, spots or floaters, inflammation, discharge, dry eyes, excessive tearing, history of cataracts or glaucoma

Ears: Hearing changes, tinnitus, pain, discharge, vertigo, history of ear infections

Nose: Sinus problems, epistaxis, obstruction, polyps, changes in or loss of sense of smell

Throat: Bleeding gums; dental history (last checkup, etc); ulcerations or other lesions on tongue, gums, buccal mucosa

Respiratory: Chest pain; dyspnea; cough; amount and color of sputum; hemoptysis; history of pneumonia, influenza and pneumococcal vaccinations, TB exposure and positive PPD

Cardiovascular: Chest pain, orthopnea, trepopnea, dyspnea on exertion, PND, murmurs, claudication, peripheral edema, palpitations

Gastrointestinal: Abdominal pain, dysphagia, heartburn, nausea, vomiting, diarrhea, constipation, hematemesis, indigestion, melena (hematochezia), hemorrhoids, change in stool shape and color, jaundice, fatty food intolerance

Gynecologic: Gravida/para/abortions; age at menarche; last menstrual period (frequency, duration, flow); dysmenorrhea; spotting; menopause; contraceptive method; sexual history, including history of venereal disease, frequency of intercourse, number of partners, sexual orientation and satisfaction, and dyspareunia

Genitourinary: Frequency, urgency, hesitancy; dysuria; hematuria; polyuria; nocturia; incontinence; venereal disease; discharge; sterility; impotence; polyuria; polydipsia; change in urinary stream; and sexual history, including frequency of intercourse, number of partners, sexual orientation and satisfaction, and history of STD

Endocrine: Polyuria, polydipsia, polyphagia, temperature intolerance, glycosuria, hormone therapy, changes in hair or skin texture

Musculoskeletal: Arthralgia, arthritis, trauma, joint swelling, redness, tenderness, limitations in ROM, back pain, musculoskeletal trauma, gout

Peripheral Vascular: Varicose veins, intermittent claudication, history of thrombophlebitis

Hematology: Anemia, bleeding tendency, easy bruising, lymphadenopathy

Neuropsychiatric: Syncope; seizures; weakness; ataxia or coordination problems; alterations in sensations, memory, mood, or sleep pattern, anhedonia, loss of energy, decreased ability to concentrate, change in weight or appetite, family history of depression or suicide; emotional disturbances; drug and alcohol problems

Physical Examination

General: Mood, stage of development, race, and sex. State if patient is in distress or is assuming an unusual position, such as sitting up leaning forward (position often seen in patients with acute exacerbation of COPD or pericarditis). Note if patient appears markedly older or younger than stated age.

Vital Signs: Temperature (note if oral, rectal, axillary or ear), pulse, respirations, BP (may include right arm, left arm, lying, sitting, standing; see page 12), height, weight and BMI (weight in kilograms / [height in meters]^2). Always include BP and heart rate supine and after the patient has been standing 1 min if volume depletion (GI bleeding, pancreatitis, diarrhea, or vomiting) or autonomic insufficiency is suspected, especially if the patient reports dizziness or syncope.

Skin: Rashes, eruptions, scars, tattoos, moles, hair pattern (See pages 13–15 for definitions of dermatologic lesions.)

Lymph Nodes: Location (head and neck, supraclavicular, epitrochlear, axillary, inguinal), size, tenderness, motility, consistency

Head, Eyes, Ears, Nose, and Throat (HEENT)

Head: Size and shape, tenderness, trauma, bruits. **Pediatric patients:** Fontanels, suture lines

Eyes: Conjunctiva; sclera; lids; position of eyes in orbits; pupil size, shape, reactivity; extraocular muscle movements; visual acuity (eg, 20/20); visual fields; fundi (disc color, size, margins, cupping, spontaneous venous pulsations, hemorrhages, exudates, A–V ratio, nicking)

Ears: Hearing test; tenderness, discharge, external canal, tympanic membrane (intact, dull or shiny, bulging, motility, fluid or blood, injected)

Nose: Symmetry; palpation over frontal, maxillary, and ethmoid sinuses; inspection for obstruction, lesions, exudate, inflammation. **Pediatric patients:** Nasal flaring, grunting

Throat: Lips, teeth, gums, tongue, pharynx (lesions, erythema, exudate, tonsillar size, presence of crypts)

Neck: ROM, tenderness, JVD, lymph nodes, thyroid examination, location of larynx, carotid bruits, HJR. Record JVD in relation to the number of centimeters above or below the sternal angle, such as "1 cm above the sternal angle," rather than "no JVD."

Chest: Configuration and symmetry of movement with respiration; intercostal retractions; palpation for tenderness, fremitus, and chest wall expansion; percussion (include diaphragmatic movement between tidal breathing and full inspiration); breath sounds; adventitious sounds (rales, rhonchi, wheezes, rubs). If indicated: vocal fremitus, whispered pectoriloquy, egophony (found with consolidation)

Heart: Rate, inspection, and palpation of precordium for point of maximal impulse, apical impulse, and thrills; auscultation at the apex, LLSB, and right and left second intercostal spaces with diaphragm and apex and LLSB with bell. Also at the apex with bell with patient in the left lateral decubitus position and at the third and fourth intercostal spaces with diaphragm with the patient sitting up, leaning forward, and fully exhaled. (For a description of S_1 and S_2 and where best to hear the heart sounds, see legend for Figure 1–1.)

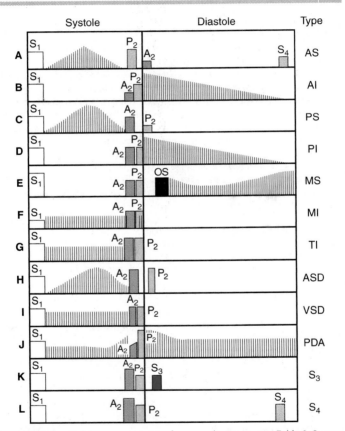

FIGURE 1–1. Graphic representation of common heart murmurs. Table 1–2, page 10, shows abbreviations and descriptions. Height of box indicates intensity of heart sound; hatched lines indicate pattern of murmur. S_1: Occurs at beginning of systole and is closure of the mitral (M_1) and tricuspid (T_1) valves. Normally, T_1 is heard only at the LLSB. S_1 is loudest at the apex. S_2: Occurs at end of systole and is closure of the aortic (A_2) and pulmonic valves (P_2). P_2 is best heard at the L second ICS. S_2 is loudest at R second ICS. The L second ICS is where to listen for splitting of A_2 and P_2. At end inspiration with tidal breathing there is more pronounced splitting of the A_2 and P_2 sounds (they are farther apart than at end expiration). With normal physiology M_1 occurs before T_1; A_2 occurs before P_2.

Breast: Inspection for nipple discharge, inversion, excoriations and fissures, and skin dimpling or flattening of the contour; palpation for masses, tenderness; gynecomastia in men and boys

Abdomen: Shape (scaphoid, flat, distended, obese); examination for scars; auscultation for bowel sounds and bruits; percussion for tympani and masses; liver size (span in midclavicular line); CVA tenderness; palpation for tenderness (if present, check for rebound tenderness); ascites, hepatomegaly, splenomegaly; guarding, inguinal adenopathy

Male Genitalia: Inspection for penile lesions, scrotal swelling, testicles (size, tenderness, masses, varicocele), and hernia; transillumination of testicular masses

Pelvic (Women and Girls): See Chapter 13.

Rectal: Inspection and palpation for hemorrhoids, fissures, skin tags, sphincter tone, masses; presence or absence of stool; test stool for occult blood; in men grade prostate size from small (1+) to massively enlarged (4+); note nodules, tenderness

Musculoskeletal: Amputations, deformities, visible joint swelling, and ROM; palpation of joints for swelling, tenderness, and warmth

Peripheral Vascular: Hair pattern; color change of skin; varicosities; cyanosis; clubbing; palpation of radial, ulnar, brachial, femoral, popliteal, posterior tibial, dorsalis pedis pulses; simultaneous radial pulses; calf tenderness; Homans sign; edema; auscultation for femoral bruits

Neurologic

Mental Status Examination: (If appropriate, see sections "Psychiatric History and Physical," and "Psychiatric Mental Status Examination," page 8.)

Cranial Nerves: There are 12 cranial nerves, the functions of which are as follows:

- **I** Olfactory—Smell
- **II** Optic—Vision, visual fields, and fundi; afferent limb of pupillary response
- **III, IV, VI** Oculomotor, trochlear, abducens—Efferent limb pupillary response, ptosis, volitional eye movements, pursuit eye movements
- **V** Trigeminal—Corneal reflex (afferent), facial sensation; test masseter and temporalis muscle by having patient bite
- **VII** Facial—Raise eyebrows, close eyes tight, show teeth, smile, or whistle, corneal reflex (efferent)
- **VIII** Acoustic—Hearing; test by watch tick, finger rub, Weber–Rinne test (see also page 20) if hearing loss noted on history or gross testing. (Air conduction lasts longer than bone conduction in a healthy person.)
- **IX, X** Glossopharyngeal and vagus—Gag reflex; speech. Palate should move upward in midline
- **XI** Spinal accessory—Shoulder shrug, push head against resistance
- **XII** Hypoglossal—Tongue movement. Test strength by having the patient press tongue against the buccal mucosa on each side while you press a finger against the patient's cheek. Observe for fasciculations.

Motor: Test strength in upper and lower extremities proximally and distally. (Grading system: 5, active motion against full resistance; 4, active motion against some resistance; 3, active motion against gravity; 2, active motion with gravity eliminated; 1, barely detectable motion; 0, no motion or muscular contraction detected)

Cerebellum: Romberg test (see page 19). Heel to shin (should not be with assistance from gravity; instruct a patient sitting with legs dangling to drag the heel of one foot up the shin of the other leg **and not down the shin**), finger to nose, heel-and-toe walking, rapid alternating movements of upper and lower extremities

Sensory: Pain (sharp) or temperature of distal and proximal upper and lower extremities, vibration using either a 128- or 256-Hz tuning fork or position sense of distal parts of upper and lower extremities, and stereognosis or graphesthesia. Identify deficits using dermatome and cutaneous innervation diagrams (Figure 1–2).

FIGURE 1–2. A: Dermatomes and cutaneous innervation patterns, anterior view. (Reproduced, with permission, from: Aminoff MJ et al [eds]: *Clinical Neurology*, 6th ed, McGraw-Hill, 2005.)

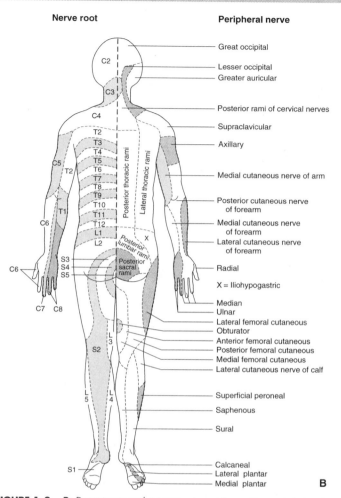

Nerve root

Peripheral nerve

FIGURE 1–2. B: Dermatomes and cutaneous innervation patterns, posterior view. (Reproduced, with permission, from: Aminoff MJ et al [eds]: *Clinical Neurology*, 6th ed, McGraw-Hill, 2005.)

Reflexes: Brachioradialis and biceps C5–6, triceps C7–8, abdominal (upper T8–10, lower T10–12), quadriceps (knee) L3–5, ankle S1–2. (Grading system: 4+, hyperactive with clonus; 3+, brisker than usual; 2+, normal or average; 1+, decreased or less than normal; 0, absent). Check for pathologic reflexes: Babinski sign, Hoffmann sign, snout, others (see pages 15–20). **Pediatric patients:** Moro reflex (startle) and suck reflexes

Database

Laboratory tests, imaging and other available information.

Problem List

(See example, page 23.) Include entry date of problem, date of problem onset, problem number. (In the initial problem list, number the problems in order of their severity. After the initial list is generated, add problems chronologically.) List problem by status: active or inactive.

Assessment

Discussion with a differential diagnosis of each current problem followed by the plan for each problem. The assessment is more than a listing of problems.

Plan

Additional laboratory and diagnostic tests, medical treatment, consults, etc. *Note:* Legibly sign the H&P, and note your title. Record the date and time with each entry.

PSYCHIATRIC HISTORY AND PHYSICAL EXAMINATION

The elements of the psychiatric history and physical are identical to those of the basic H&P. The main difference involves attention to the past psychiatric history and a more detailed mental status examination as described in the following section.

Psychiatric Mental Status Examination

The following factors are evaluated as part of the psychiatric status examination.

- **Appearance:** Gestures, mannerisms, etc
- **Speech:** Coherence, flight of ideas, etc
- **Mood and Affect:** Depression, elation, anger, etc
- **Thought Process:** Blocking, evasion, etc
- **Thought Content:** Worries, hypochondriasis, lack of self-confidence, delusions, hallucinations, etc
- **Motor Activity:** Slow, rapid, purposeful, etc
- **Cognitive Functions:**

    Attention and concentration
    Memory (immediate, recent, and remote recall)
    Calculations
    Abstractions
    Judgment

Folstein Mini-Mental State Examination

Perform a thorough mental status exam on every geriatric patient, patient with AIDS, and patient with suspected dementia. The Mini-Mental State Exam is a quick and simple test, and the results can be followed over time for assessment of progression, improvement, or no changes in the underlying process. The Mini-Mental State Exam (Folstein et al: *J Psychiatr Res* 1975;12:189) is divided into two sections: one assessing orientation, memory, and attention, and the other testing the patient's ability to write a sentence and copy a diagram (usually two pentagons that intersect to form a four-sided figure). Table 1–1 page 9 shows the Mini-Mental State Exam.

HEART MURMURS AND EXTRA HEART SOUNDS

Table 1–2 page 10 and Figure 1–1 page 4 describe the various types of murmurs and extra heart sounds.

TABLE 1–1
The Mini-Mental State Examination

Patient _____

Examiner _____

Date _____

"Mini-Mental State"

Maximum Score	Score	

Orientation

5 — What is the (year) (season) (date) (day) (month)?

5 — Where are we? (state) (county) (town) (hospital) (floor)

Registration

3 — Name 3 objects: 1 second to say each. Then ask the patient all 3 after you have said them. Give 1 point for each correct answer. Then repeat until he learns all 3. Count trials and record.
Trials_____

Attention and Calculation

5 — Serial 7's: One point for each correct. Stop after 5 answers. Alternatively, spell "world" backward.

Recall

3 — Ask for the 3 objects repeated above. Give 1 point for each correct answer.

Language

9 — Point to a pencil, and watch and ask the patient to name it. (2 points)
Repeat the following: "No if's, and's, or but's." (1 point)
Follow a 3-stage command: "Take a paper in your right hand, fold it in half, and put it on the floor." (3 points)
Read and obey the following:
Close your eyes   (1 point)
Write a sentence   (1 point)
Copy design (two intersecting   (1 point)
pentagrams)

_____ Total Score

Assess level of consciousness along the following continuum

Alert   Drowsy   Stupor   Coma

Source: Based on data from: Folstein, Folstein, and McHugh: *J Psychiatr Res* 1975;12:189–198. Used with permission.

TABLE 1–2
Heart Murmurs and Extra Heart Sounds[a]

Type[b]	Description
A. Aortic stenosis (AS)	Heard best at second intercostal space. Systolic (medium-pitched) crescendo–decrescendo murmur with radiation to the carotid arteries. A_2 decreased, ejection click and S_4 often heard at apex. Paradoxical splitting of S_2. Narrow pulse pressure and delayed carotid upstroke and left ventricular hypertrophy (LVH) with lift at apex.
B. Aortic insufficiency (AI)	Heard best at left lower sternal border at third and fourth interspace with patient sitting up, leaning forward and fully exhaled. Diastolic (high-pitched) decrescendo murmur. Often with LVH. Widened pulse pressure, bisferious pulse, Traube sign, Quincke sign, and Corrigan pulse may be seen with chronic aortic insufficiency. S_3 and pulsus alternans often present with acute aortic insufficiency.
C. Pulmonic stenosis (PS)	Heard best at left second intercostal space. Systolic crescendo–decrescendo murmur. Louder with inspiration. Click often present. P_2 delayed and soft if severe. Right ventricular hypertrophy (RVH) with parasternal lift.
D. Pulmonic insufficiency (PI)	Heard best at left second intercostal space. Diastolic decrescendo murmur. Louder with inspiration. RVH usually present.
E. Mitral stenosis (MS)	Localized at the apex. Diastolic (low-pitched rumbling sound) murmur heard best with the bell in the left lateral decubitus position. With increased or decreased S_1. Opening snap (OS) heard best at apex with diaphragm. Increased P_2, right-sided S_4, left-sided S_3 often present. RVH with parasternal lift may be present.
F. Mitral insufficiency (MI)	Heard best at apex. Holosystolic (high-pitched) murmur with radiation to axilla. Soft S1, may be masked by murmur. S_3 and LVH often present. Midsystolic click suggests mitral valve prolapse.

(continued)

TABLE 1-2
Heart Murmurs and Extra Heart Sounds[a] (continued)

Type[b]	Description
G. Tricuspid insufficiency (TI)	Heard best at left lower sternal border. Holosystolic (high-pitched) murmur. Increases with inspiration. Right-sided S_3 often present. Large V wave in jugular venous pulsations.
H. Atrial septal defect (ASD)	Heard best at left upper sternal border. Systolic (medium-pitched) murmur. Fixed splitting of S_2 and RVH, often with left- and right-sided S_4.
I. Ventricular septal defect (VSD)	Heard best at left lower sternal border. Harsh holosystolic (high-pitched) murmur. S_1 and S_2 may be soft.
J. Patent ductus arteriosus (PDA)	Heard best at left first and second intercostal space. Continuous, machinery (medium-pitched) murmur. Increased P_2 and ejection click may be present.
K. Third heart sound (S_3)	Early diastolic sound caused by rapid ventricular filling. Heard best with bell. Left-sided S_3 heard at apex, right-sided S_3 heard at left lower sternal border. Left-sided S_3 seen normally in young people, also pregnancy, thyrotoxicosis, mitral regurgitation, and congestive heart failure.
L. Fourth heart sound (S_4)	Late diastolic sound caused by a noncompliant ventricle. Heard best with bell. Left-sided S_4 heard at apex, right-sided S_4 heard at left lower sternal border. Left-sided S_4 seen with hypertension, aortic stenosis, and myocardial infarction. Right-sided S_4 seen with pulmonic stenosis and pulmonary hypertension.

[a]Refer to Figure 1-1 for graphic representations of murmurs (page 4).
[b]Capital letters preceding type of murmur refer to graphs in Figure 1-1.

BLOOD PRESSURE GUIDELINES

There is a clear association between HTN and coronary artery and cerebrovascular diseases. **Hypertension is defined as systolic BP > 140 mm Hg or diastolic BP > 90 mm Hg in adults.** Measure BP after 5 min of rest with patient seated, feet resting on the floor and arm at heart level. Use the stethoscope bell (the last sounds heard are the Korotkoff sounds, which are low pitched). Take the average of two readings separated by 2 min. Elevated readings on three separate days are required for a diagnosis of HTN. Classification and measurement guidelines for adults are shown in Table 1-3.

TABLE 1–3
Guidelines for Blood Pressure Management in Adults Based on JNC7

CLASSIFICATION OF BLOOD PRESSURE (BP)

Category	SBP (mmHg)		DBP (mmHg)
Normal	<120	and	<80
Prehypertension	120–139	or	80–89
Hypertension, stage 1	140–159	or	90–99
Hypertension, stage 2	≥160	or	≥100

SBP=systolic blood pressure; DBP=diastolic blood pressure

BLOOD PRESSURE MEASUREMENT TECHNIQUES

Method	Notes
In-office	Two readings, 5 min apart, sitting in chair. Confirm elevated reading in contralateral arm
Ambulatory BP monitoring	Indicated for evaluation of "white coat hypertension." Absence of 10–20% BP decrease during sleep may indicate increased cardiovascular disease risk
Patient self-check	Provides information on response to therapy. May help improve adherence to therapy and is useful for evaluating "white coat hypertension."

The National High Blood Pressure Education Program is administered by the National Heart, Lung and Blood Institute (NHLB) at the National Institutes of Health. Copies of the JNC7 Report are available at the NHLB Website at http://www.nhlbi.nih.gov. NIH Publication 03–5233, May 2003. The National High Blood Pressure Education Program is administered by the National Heart, Lung and Blood Institute (NHLB) at the National Institutes of Health. Copies of the JNC7 Report are available at the NHLB Website at http://www.nhlbi.nih.gov. NIH Publication 03–5233, May 2003.

In children 1–10 y old, systolic BP can be calculated as follows: Lower limits (fifth percentile): 70 mm Hg + (child's age in years × 2); typical (fiftieth percentile): 90 mm Hg + (child's age in years × 2).

DENTAL EXAMINATION

The dental examination is an often overlooked part of the general H&P. The patient may have an intraoral problem contributing to the overall medical condition (ie, inability to eat because of a toothache, abscess, or ill-fitting denture in a patient with poorly controlled diabetes) for which a dental consult may be necessary. Loose dentures can compromise manual maintenance of an open airway.

In addition, in an emergency situation in which intubation is necessary, complications can occur if the clinician is unfamiliar with the oral structures.

The patient may be able to give some dental history, including recent toothaches, abscesses, and loose teeth or dentures. Be sure to ask whether the patient is wearing a removable partial denture (partial plate), which should be removed before intubation. Because lost dentures are a chief dental complaint of hospitalized patients, take care not to misplace the removed prosthesis.

Perform a brief dental examination with gloved hand, two tongue blades, and a flashlight. Look for obvious inflammation, erythema, edema, or ulceration of the gingiva (gums) and oral mucosa. Gently tap on any natural teeth to test for sensitivity. Place each tooth between two tongue blades and push gently to check for looseness. This step is especially important for the maxillary anterior teeth, which serve as the fulcrum for the laryngoscope blade. Note abnormal dental findings and request the appropriate consults. Many diseases, including AIDS, STDs, pemphigus, pemphigoid, allergies, uncontrolled diabetes, leukemia, and others, may first manifest themselves in the mouth.

Hospitalized patients often have difficulty cleaning their teeth or dentures. Add this care to the daily orders if indicated. Patients who will be receiving head and neck radiation must be examined and treated for any tooth extractions or dental infections before initiation of radiation therapy. Extractions after radiation to the maxilla and particularly the mandible can lead to osteoradionecrosis, a condition that can be impossible to control.

Eruption of Teeth

The eruption of teeth may be of great concern to new parents. Parents often think something is developmentally wrong with a child if teeth have not appeared by a certain age.

The timing of tooth eruption varies tremendously. Factors contributing to this variation include family history, ethnic background, vitality during fetal development, position of teeth in the arch, size and shape of the dental arch itself, and, in the case of the eruption of permanent teeth, the time at which the primary tooth was lost. Radiographs of the maxilla and mandible show whether the teeth are present. Figure 1–3 on page 14 is a guide to the chronology of tooth eruption. Remember that variations may be greater than 1 y in some cases.

DERMATOLOGIC DESCRIPTIONS

Atrophy: Thinning of the surface of the skin with associated loss of normal markings. Examples: Aging, striae associated with obesity, scleroderma

Bulla: A superficial, well-circumscribed, raised, fluid-filled lesion greater than 1 cm in diameter. Examples: Bullous pemphigoid, pemphigus, dermatitis herpetiformis

Burrow: A subcutaneous linear track made by a parasite. Example: Scabies

Crust: A slightly raised lesion with irregular border and variable color resulting from dried blood, serum, or other exudate. Examples: Scab resulting from an abrasion, impetigo

Ecchymosis: A flat, nonblanching, red-purple-blue lesion that results from extravasation of red blood cells into the skin. Differs from purpura in size; ecchymoses are large purpura lesions. Examples: Trauma, long-term steroid use

Erosion: A depressed lesion resulting from loss of epidermis due to rupture of vesicles or bullae. Example: Rupture of herpes simplex blister

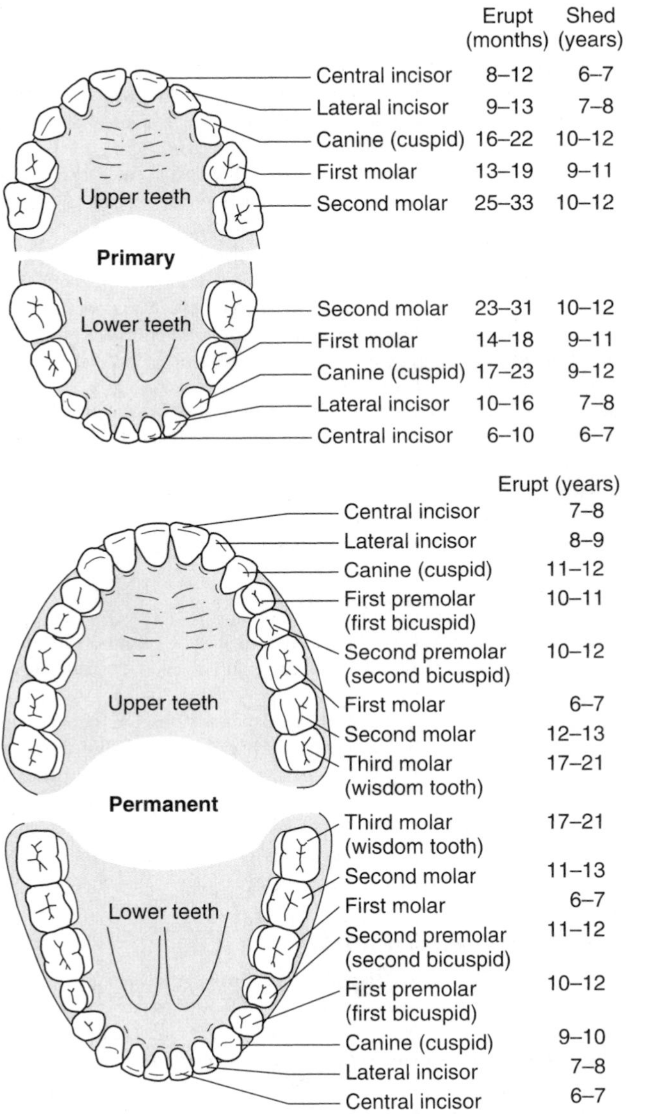

	Erupt (months)	Shed (years)
Central incisor	8–12	6–7
Lateral incisor	9–13	7–8
Canine (cuspid)	16–22	10–12
First molar	13–19	9–11
Second molar	25–33	10–12

Upper teeth

Primary

Lower teeth

	Erupt (months)	Shed (years)
Second molar	23–31	10–12
First molar	14–18	9–11
Canine (cuspid)	17–23	9–12
Lateral incisor	10–16	7–8
Central incisor	6–10	6–7

	Erupt (years)
Central incisor	7–8
Lateral incisor	8–9
Canine (cuspid)	11–12
First premolar (first bicuspid)	10–11
Second premolar (second bicuspid)	10–12
First molar	6–7
Second molar	12–13
Third molar (wisdom tooth)	17–21

Upper teeth

Permanent

Lower teeth

	Erupt (years)
Third molar (wisdom tooth)	17–21
Second molar	11–13
First molar	6–7
Second premolar (second bicuspid)	11–12
First premolar (first bicuspid)	10–12
Canine (cuspid)	9–10
Lateral incisor	7–8
Central incisor	6–7

FIGURE 1–3. Dentition development sequences. There can be wide variation in the age when teeth shed and erupt. (Based on data from: McDonald RE, Avery DR [eds]: *Dentistry for the Child and Adolescent*, Mosby, St. Louis, 1994. Used with permission.)

Excoriation: A linear superficial lesion, which may be covered with dried blood. Early lesions with surrounding erythema. Often self-induced. Example: Scratching associated with pruritus from any cause

Fissure: A deep linear lesion into the dermis. Example: Cracks seen in athlete's foot

Keloid: Irregular, raised lesion resulting from hypertrophied scar tissue. Examples: Often seen with burns; African Americans are more prone to keloid formation than are other people

Lichenification: A thickening of the skin with an increase in skin markings resulting from chronic irritation and rubbing. Example: Atopic dermatitis

Macule: A circumscribed nonpalpable discoloration of the skin less than 1 cm in diameter. Examples: Freckles, rubella, petechiae

Nodule: A solid, palpable, circumscribed lesion larger than a papule and smaller than a tumor. Examples: Erythema nodosum, gouty tophi

Papule: A solid elevated lesion less than 1 cm in diameter. Examples: Acne, warts, insect bites

Patch: A nonpalpable discoloration of the skin with an irregular border, greater than 1 cm in diameter. Example: Vitiligo

Petechiae: Flat, pinhead-sized, nonblanching, red–purple lesions caused by hemorrhage into the skin. Example: Seen in DIC, ITP, SLE, meningococcemia (*Neisseria meningitidis*)

Plaque: A solid, flat, elevated lesion greater than 1 cm in diameter. Examples: Psoriasis, discoid lupus erythematosus, actinic keratosis

Purpura: A condition characterized by flat, nonblanching, red–purple lesions larger than petechiae caused by hemorrhage into the skin. Examples: Henoch–Schönlein purpura, TTP

Pustule: A vesicle filled with purulent fluid. Examples: Acne, impetigo

Scales: Partial separation of the superficial layer of skin. Examples: Psoriasis, dandruff

Scar: Replacement of normal skin with fibrous tissue, often resulting from injury. Examples: Surgical scar, burn

Telangiectasia: Dilatation of capillaries resulting in red, irregular, clustered lines that blanch. Examples: Seen in scleroderma, Osler–Weber–Rendu disease, cirrhosis

Tumor: A solid, palpable, circumscribed lesion greater than 2 cm in diameter. Example: Lipoma

Ulcer: A depressed lesion resulting from loss of epidermis and part of the dermis. Examples: Decubitus ulcers, primary lesion of syphilis, venous stasis ulcer

Vesicle: A superficial, well-circumscribed, raised, fluid-filled lesion that is less than 1 cm in diameter. Examples: Herpes simplex, varicella (chickenpox)

Wheal: Slightly raised, red, irregular, transient lesions secondary to edema of the skin. Examples: Urticaria (hives), allergic reaction to injections or insect bites

DERMATOME AND CUTANEOUS INNERVATION

Figures 1–2 A and B on pages 6 and 7 show dermatome levels and cutaneous innervation distribution useful in the physical examination.

PHYSICAL SIGNS, SYMPTOMS, AND EPONYMS

Allen Test: (See Chapter 13, page 248.)

Apley Test; Apley Grind Test: Determination of meniscal tear in the knee by grinding the joint manually

Argyll Robertson Pupil: Bilaterally small, irregular, unequal pupils that react to accommodation but not to light. Seen with tertiary syphilis

Auspitz Sign: Pinpoint bleeding after removal of a psoriasis scale

Austin Flint Murmur: Late diastolic mitral murmur; associated with aortic insufficiency with a normal mitral valve

Babinski Sign: Extension of the large toe with stimulation of the plantar surface of the foot instead of the normal flexion; indicative of upper motor neuron disease (normal in neonates)

Bainbridge Reflex: Increased heart rate due to increased right atrial pressure

Battle Sign: Ecchymosis behind the ear associated with basilar skull fractures

Beau Lines: Transverse depressions in nails due to previous systemic disease

Beck Triad: JVD, diminished or muffled heart sounds, and decreased BP associated with cardiac tamponade

Bell Palsy: Lower motor neuron lesion of the facial nerve affecting muscles of upper and lower face. Easily distinguished from upper motor lesions, which predominately affect muscles of the lower face because upper motor neurons from each side innervate muscles on both sides of the upper part of the face

Bergman Triad: Altered mental status, petechiae, and dyspnea associated with fat embolus syndrome

Biot Breathing: Abruptly alternating apnea and equally deep breaths (seen with brain injury)

Bisferious Pulse: Double-peaked pulse seen in severe chronic aortic insufficiency

Bitot Spots: Small scleral white patches suggesting vitamin A deficiency

Blumberg Sign: Pain felt in the abdomen when steady constant pressure is quickly released (seen with peritonitis)

Blumer Shelf: Palpable hardness on rectal examination, due to metastatic cancer of the rectouterine pouch (pouch of Douglas) or rectovesical pouch

Bouchard Nodes: Hard, nontender, painless nodules in the dorsolateral aspects of the proximal interphalangeal joints associated with osteoarthritis, caused by hypertrophy of the bone

Branham Sign: Abrupt slowing of the heart rate with compression of the feeding artery (seen with large A–V fistulas)

Brudzinski Sign: Flexion of the neck causing flexion of the hips (seen in meningitis)

Chadwick Sign: Bluish color of cervix and vagina, seen with pregnancy

Chandelier Sign: Extreme pain elicited with movement of the cervix during bimanual pelvic examination (indicates PID)

Charcot Triad: Right upper quadrant pain, fever and chills, and jaundice associated with cholangitis

Cheyne–Stokes Respiration: Repeating cycle of a gradual increase in depth of breathing followed by a gradual decrease to apnea (seen with CNS disorders, uremia, some normal sleep patterns)

Chvostek Sign: Facial spasm elicited by tapping over the facial nerve, indicating hypocalcemia (tetany). May be normal finding in some patients

Corrigan Pulse: Palpable hard pulse immediately followed by sudden collapse (seen in aortic regurgitation)

Cullen Sign: Ecchymosis around the umbilicus associated with severe intraperitoneal bleeding (seen with ruptured ectopic pregnancy and hemorrhagic pancreatitis)

Cushing Triad: HTN, bradycardia, and irregular respiration associated with increased intracranial pressure

Darier Sign: Erythema and edema elicited by stroking of the skin, indicating mastocytosis

Doll Eyes: Conjugated movement of eyes of comatose patients in one direction as head is briskly turned in the other direction. Tests oculocephalic reflex indicating intact brain stem

Drawer Sign: Forward (or backward) movement of the tibia with pressure, indicating laxity or a tear in the anterior (or posterior) cruciate ligament

Dupuytren Contracture: Proliferation of fibrosis tissue of the palmar fascia resulting in contracture of the fourth and/or fifth digits; often bilateral. May be hereditary or seen in patients with chronic alcoholic liver disease or seizures

Duroziez Sign: To-and-fro murmur when stethoscope is pressed over the femoral artery, indicating aortic regurgitation

Electrical Alternans: Beat-to-beat variation in the electrical axis (seen in large pericardial effusions), suggesting impending hemodynamic compromise

Ewart Sign: Dullness to percussion, increased fremitus and bronchial breathing beneath the angle of the left scapula, indicating pericardial effusion

Fong Lesion/Syndrome: Autosomal-dominant anomalies of the nails and patella associated with renal abnormalities

Frank Sign: Fissure of the ear lobe; may be associated with CAD, DM, and HTN

Gibbus: Angular convexity of the spine due to vertebral collapse (associated with osteoporosis or metastasis)

Gregg Triad: Cataracts, heart defects, and deafness with congenital rubella

Grey Turner Sign: Ecchymosis in the flank associated with retroperitoneal hemorrhage

Grocco Sign: Triangular area of paravertebral dullness, opposite side of a pleural effusion

Heberden Nodes: Hard, nontender, painless nodules on the dorsolateral aspects of the distal interphalangeal joints associated with osteoarthritis. Results from hypertrophy of the bone

Hegar Sign: Softening of the distal uterus. Reliable early sign of pregnancy

Hollenhorst Plaque: Cholesterol plaque on retina seen on funduscopic examination (associated with amaurosis fugax)

Hill Sign: Femoral artery pressure 20 mm Hg greater than brachial pressure (seen in severe aortic regurgitation)

Hoffmann Sign/Reflex: Flicking of the volar surface of the distal phalanx causing finger

Homan Sign:

Horner Syndr ing). Fro lung carc

Janeway Lesi with suba

Joffroy Refle ing up (s

Kayser–Fleisc in Wilso

Kehr Sign: L rupture

Kernig Sign: right ang

Koplik Spots: sles)

Korotkoff Sounds: Low-pitched sounds resulting from vibration of the artery, detected when measuring BP with the bell of a stethoscope. The last Korotkoff sound is a more accurate estimate of the true diastolic BP than is diastolic BP measured with the diaphragm.

Kussmaul Respiration: Deep, rapid respiratory pattern (seen in coma or DKA)

Kussmaul Sign: Paradoxical increase in jugular venous pressure on inspiration (seen in constrictive pericarditis, mediastinal tumor, right ventricular infarction, acute cor pulmonale, and congestive heart failure)

Kyphosis: Excessive rounding of the thoracic spinal convexity, associated with aging, especially in women

Lasègue Sign/Straight-Leg-Raising Sign: Pain in the distribution of nerve root when a patient extended in the supine position raises the leg gently; suggests lumbar disk disease.

Levine Sign: Clenched fist over the chest while describing chest pain (associated with angina and AMI)

Lhermitte Sign: Neck flexion results in a "shock sensation" (seen in multiple sclerosis and cervical spine problems)

List: Lateral tilt of the spine; usually associated with herniated disk and muscle spasm

Lordosis: Accentuated normal concavity of the lumbar spine, normal in pregnancy

Louvel Sign: Coughing or sneezing causes pain in the leg with DVT

Marcus Gunn Pupil: Dilation of pupils with swinging flashlight test. Results from unilateral optic nerve disease. Normal pupillary response is elicited when light is directed from the normal eye and a subnormal response when light is quickly directed from the normal eye into the abnormal eye. When light is directed into the abnormal eye, both pupils dilate rather than maintain the previous degree of miosis.

McBurney Point/Sign: Point located one third of the distance from the anterior superior iliac spine to the umbilicus on the right. (Tenderness at the site is associated with acute appendicitis)

McMurray Test: Palpable or audible click on the joint line produced by external rotation of the foot, suggesting medial meniscal injury

Möbius Sign: Inability to maintain convergence, seen in thyrotoxicosis

Moro Reflex (Startle Reflex): Abduction of hips and arms with extension of arms when infant's head and upper body are suddenly dropped several inches while being held. Normal reflex in early infancy

Murphy Sign: Severe pain and inspiratory arrest with palpation of the right upper quadrant during deep inspiration (associated with cholecystitis)

Musset or de Musset Sign: Rhythmic nodding or movement of the head with each heart beat, caused by blood flow back into the heart secondary to aortic insufficiency

Obturator Sign: Hypogastric pain elicited by flexion and internal rotation of the thigh in cases of inflammation of the obturator internus (present with pelvic abscess and appendicitis)

Ortolani Test/Sign: Sign: hip click that suggests congenital hip dislocation. Test: with the infant supine, point the legs toward you and flex the legs to 90 degrees at the hips and knees

Osler Node: Tender, red, raised lesions on the hands or feet (seen with SBE)

Pancoast Syndrome: Carcinoma involving apex of lung, resulting in arm and/or shoulder pain from involvement of brachial plexus and Horner syndrome from involvement of the superior cervical ganglion

Pastia Lines: Linear striations of confluent petechiae in axillary folds and antecubital fossa, seen in scarlet fever

Phalen Test: Prolonged maximum flexion of wrists while opposing dorsum of each hand against each other. A positive test result is pain and tingling in the distribution of the median nerve (seen in carpal tunnel syndrome)

Psoas Sign (Iliopsoas Test): Flexion against resistance or extension of the right hip, producing pain; seen with inflammation of the psoas muscle (present with appendicitis)

Pulsus Alternans: Fluctuation of pulse pressure with every other beat (seen in aortic stenosis and CHF)

Queckenstedt Test: compression of the internal jugular vein during lumbar puncture to determine patency of the subarachnoid space; normal result is immediate increase in CSF pressure

Quincke Sign: Alternating blushing and blanching of the fingernail bed after light compression (seen in chronic aortic regurgitation)

Radovici Sign: Chin contractions caused by scratching of the palm; a frontal release sign

Raynaud Phenomenon/Disease: Pain and tingling in fingers after exposure to cold with characteristic color changes of white to blue and then often red. May be seen with scleroderma and SLE or be idiopathic (Raynaud disease)

Romberg Test: The patient stands with heels and toes together with arms outstretched palms facing up or down or arms at sides. The examiner lightly taps the patient, first with the patient's eyes open and then with the patient's eyes closed. A positive result is the patient's loss of balance. Loss of balance with the eyes open indicates cerebellar dysfunction. Normal balance with eyes open and loss of balance with eyes closed indicate loss of position sense. Used to test position sense and cerebellar function

Roth Spots: Oval retinal hemorrhages with a pale central area occurring in patients with bacterial endocarditis

Rovsing Sign: Pain in the RLQ with deep palpation of the LLQ (seen in acute appendicitis)

Schmorl Node: Degeneration of the intervertebral disk resulting in herniation into the adjacent vertebral body

Scoliosis: Lateral curvature of the spine

Sentinel Loop: A single dilated loop of small or large bowel, usually secondary to localized inflammation such as pancreatitis

Sister Mary Joseph Sign/Node: Metastatic cancer to umbilical lymph node

Stellwag Sign: Infrequent ocular blinking

Tinel Sign: Radiation of an electric shock sensation in the distal distribution of the median nerve elicited by percussion of the flexor surface of the wrist when fully extended (seen in carpal tunnel syndrome)

Traube Sign: Booming or pistol shot sounds heard over the femoral arteries in chronic aortic insufficiency

Trendelenburg Test: Patient shifts weight from one leg to the other while being observed from behind; a pelvic tilt to opposite side suggests hip disease and weakness of the gluteus medius muscle. A normal pelvis does not tilt.

Trousseau Sign: Carpal spasm produced by inflation of a BP cuff above the systolic pressure for 2–3 min, indicates hypocalcemia or migratory thrombophlebitis associated with cancer

Turner Sign: See Grey Turner sign

Virchow Node (Signal or Sentinel Node): A palpable, left supraclavicular lymph node; often first sign of a GI neoplasm, such as pancreatic or gastric carcinoma

von Graefe Sign: Lid lag associated with thyrotoxicosis

Weber–Rinne Test: Weber test: place a 512- or 1024-Hz tuning fork on the middle of the patient's skull to determine if the sound lateralizes. Rinne test: hold the tuning fork against the patient's mastoid process (BC) with the opposite ear covered. The patient indicates when the sound is gone. Then hold the tuning fork next to the ear, and the patient indicates whether the sound is present and when the sound (AC) disappears. Normally AC is better than BC. With sensorineural hearing loss, the Weber test lateralizes to the less affected ear, and AC > BC; with conduction hearing loss, the Weber test lateralizes to the more affected ear, and BC > AC.

Whipple Triad: Hypoglycemia, CNS, and vasomotor symptoms (ie, diaphoresis, syncope); relief of symptoms with glucose (associated with insulinoma)

EXAMPLE OF A WRITTEN HISTORY AND PHYSICAL EXAMINATION

(Adult Admitted to a Medical Service)

- 12/10/06 5:30 PM

Identification: Mr. Robert Jones is a 50-y-old man referred by Dr. Harry Doyle from Whitesburg, Kentucky. The informant is the patient, who seems reliable, and a photocopy of the ER records from Whitesburg Hospital accompanies the patient.

Chief Complaint: "Squeezing chest pain for 10 h, 4 d ago"

HPI: Mr. Jones awoke at 6 AM 3 d ago with squeezing substernal chest pain that felt "like a ton of bricks" sitting on his chest. The chest pain was a 9 on a 10-point scale and decreased in intensity after the trip to the Whitesburg emergency department. The pain radiated to the left side of the neck and left elbow and was associated with dyspnea and diaphoresis. The patient says he experienced no associated nausea. He says the pain seemed to get worse with any movement, and nothing seemed to alleviate it.

Mr. Jones presented to the Whitesburg ER 10 h after the onset of pain and was given 3 NTG tablets SL and 2 mg morphine sulfate. ECG revealed 3-mm ST depression in leads V_1 through V_4. He was admitted to the ICU at Whitesburg Hospital and had an uneventful course. CK increased to 850 U/L at 24 h, and troponin increased to 12.5 ng/mL. He has been taking aspirin 325 mg/d PO, isosorbide dinitrate 20 mg PO q6h, and metoprolol 100 mg PO q12h. He was transferred for possible cardiac catheterization.

Mr. Jones reports having experienced similar chest pain that was less intense and occurred intermittently over the last 3 mo. The pain was precipitated by exercise and relieved with rest. He sought no medical attention in the past. He reports no history of orthopnea, paroxysmal nocturnal dyspnea, dyspnea on exertion, or pedal edema.

(continued)

Mr. Jones has smoked two packs of cigarettes per day for 35 y, reports a 2-y history of HTN, for which he has been taking HCTZ 25 mg/d, and reports no history of hypercholesterolemia or diabetes. He says his BP usually runs 120–130/85 at home. The patient's father died of MI at age 54, and his brother underwent CABG surgery last year at age 48.

PMH

Medications. As above and ranitidine 300 mg PO qhs. Occasional ibuprofen 200 mg 2–3 tabs PO for back pain and acetaminophen 500 mg PO for HA
Vitamins. One-a-day
Herbals. None
Allergies. Penicillin, rash entire body at age 20 y
Surgical Procedures. Appendectomy age 20, Dr. Smith, Whitesburg
Hospitalization. See above.
Trauma. Roof fall in mine accident 10 y ago, injured back. Reports occasional pain, which is relieved with ibuprofen 200 mg 2–3 tabs at a time
Transfusions. None
Illnesses. Reports no asthma, emphysema, thyroid disease, kidney disease, peptic ulcer disease, cancer, bleeding disorders, tuberculosis, or hepatitis. Reports a several-year history of water brash/heartburn and has been on ranitidine for 1 y
Routine Health Maintenance. Last diphtheria/tetanus immunization 3 y ago
Stools for guaiac were negative × 3. Refused sigmoidoscopy. Patient has been seen by Dr. Doyle every 3–4 mo for the last 2 y for HTN.

Family History

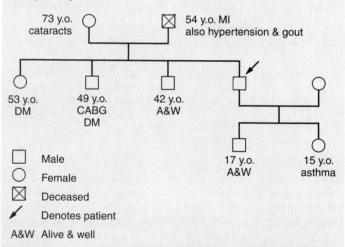

□	Male
○	Female
⊠	Deceased
✒	Denotes patient
A&W	Alive & well

Psychosocial History: Mr. Jones has been married for 25 y and has three children.

Mr. Jones and his family live in a house on 3 acres about 3 miles from Whitesburg. He worked in a coal mine until 10 y ago, when he was injured in a "roof fall." He is currently employed in a local chair factory. He graduated from high school. He is Baptist and attends church regularly. Hobbies include woodworking and gardening. He eats breakfast and supper every day and has a

(continued)

soft drink and crackers for lunch. He currently works 8 h/d Monday through Friday. He reports going to bed every day by 10:00 PM and awakens at 5:30 AM. He drinks one to two cups of coffee per day and reports drinking no alcohol. He says he does not use drugs but smokes as noted earlier. He reports he has never been exposed to environmental toxins. He says he has no financial problems but is concerned about how his illness will affect his income. He has "good" health insurance. He denies any other stressors in his life. His sources of support are his wife, minister, and a sister who lives near the patient.

ROS: Negative unless otherwise noted.

Eyes: Has worn reading glasses since 1995; reports blurred vision for 1 year; last eye appointment 2001. Claims no loss of vision, double vision, or history of cataracts.

Respiratory: Reports cough every morning and has produced one teaspoon of gray sputum for years. Denies hemoptysis or pleuritic chest pain. Last CXR before today was 3 years ago. All other ROS negative.

PHYSICAL EXAMINATION

General: Mr. Jones is a pleasant man lying comfortably supine in bed. He appears to be the stated age.

Vital Signs: Temp 98.6°F orally. Resp 16, HR 88 and regular, BP 110/70 mm Hg left arm supine

Skin: Tattoo left arm, otherwise no lesions

Node: 1×1 left axillary node, nontender and mobile. No other lymphadenopathy

HEENT

Head. Normocephalic, atraumatic, nontender, no lesions

Eyes. Visual acuity 20/40 left and right corrected. External structures normal, without lesions, PERRLA. EOM intact. Visual fields intact. Funduscopic examination discs sharp bilaterally, moderate arteriolar narrowing and A–V nicking

Ears. Hearing intact to watch tick at 3 ft bilaterally. Tympanic membranes intact with good cone of light bilaterally

Nose. Symmetrical. No lesions. Sinuses nontender

Mouth. Several dental fillings, otherwise normal dentition. No lesions

Neck. Full ROM without tenderness. No masses or lymphadenopathy. Carotids +2/4 bilaterally, no bruits. Internal jugular vein visible 2 cm above the sternal angle, patient at 30 degrees

Chest: Symmetrical expansion. Fremitus by palpation bilaterally equal. Diaphragm moves 5.5 cm bilaterally by percussion. Lung fields clear to percussion. Breath sounds normal, except end-inspiratory crackles heard at both bases that do not clear with coughing.

Breast: Normal to inspection and palpation

Heart: No cardiac impulse visible. Apical impulse palpable at the sixth intercostal space 2 cm lateral to the midclavicular line. Normal S_1, physiologically split S_2. S_4 heard at apex. No murmurs, rub, or S_3

(continued)

Abdomen: Flat, no scars. Bowel sounds present. No bruits. Liver 10 cm midclavicular line. No CVA tenderness. No hepatomegaly or splenomegaly by palpation. No tenderness or guarding. No inguinal lymphadenopathy

Genital: Normal circumcised man, both testes descended without masses or tenderness

Rectal: Normal sphincter tone. No external lesions. Prostate smooth without tenderness or nodules. No palpable masses. Stool present, stool for occult blood negative

Musculoskeletal: Lumbar spine decreased flexion to 75 degrees, extension to 5 degrees, decreased rotary and lateral movement. Otherwise full ROM of all joints, no erythema, tenderness, or swelling. No clubbing cyanosis or edema

Peripheral Vascular: Radial, ulnar, brachial, femoral, dorsalis pedis, and posterior tibial pulses +2/4 bilaterally. Popliteal pulses nonpalpable. No femoral bruits

Neurologic: *Cranial nerves*: I through XII intact. *Motor*: +5/5 upper and lower extremity, proximally and distally. *Sensory*: Intact to pinprick upper and lower extremities proximally and distally. Vibratory sense intact in great toes and thumbs bilaterally. Stereognosis intact. *Reflexes*: Biceps, triceps, brachioradialis, quadriceps, and ankles +2/4 bilaterally. Toes down going bilaterally. *Cerebellum*. Romberg sign absent. Intact finger-to-nose and heel-to-shin bilaterally; gait normal–normal heel-and-heel, toe-and-toe, and heel-to-toe gaits. Rapid alternating movements intact upper and lower extremities bilaterally

DATABASE

ECG. HR 80, NSR inverted T waves V_1 through V_5

CXR. Cardiomegaly, otherwise clear

UA. SG 1.020, protein trace otherwise negative

PT, PTT. 12.1, control 11.7, INR 1.1;28, control 27

Chemistry Profile. CK 250 U/L, otherwise normal

Troponin. 4.0 ng/mL

CBC. 6700 WBC; 49% HCT; Hbg 16 g/dL; 43 S, 2 B, 40 L, 5 M, 10 E

PROBLEM LIST

Date Entered	Date of Onset	Problem	Active	Inactive	Date Inactive
12-10-06	9-06	1	Coronary artery disease		
12-10-06	12-10-06	1a	Subendocardial MI—anterior		
12-10-06	2004	2	Hypertension		
12-10-06	1990s	3	Bronchitis		
12-10-06	2004	4	Heartburn/reflux esophagitis		
12-10-06	1996	5	Back injury		
12-10-06	12-10-06	6	Eosinophilia		
12-10-06	2002	7	Blurred vision		
12-10-06	1976	8		Appendicitis	1976

(continued)

ASSESSMENT AND PLAN

Coronary Artery Disease: *Mr. Jones presented with a classic history for MI. The CK and electrocardiogram support the diagnosis. The ST depression without evolving Q waves is consistent with a nontransmural MI. Mr. Jones is at risk of further MI because it was a nontransmural MI, and he needs further evaluation before discharge.*

- Continue aspirin 325 mg/d PO and metoprolol 100 mg q12h.
- Change isosorbide to tid before discharge.
- Monitor by telemetry unit for next 24–48 h.
- Stress test by modified Bruce protocol before discharge.
- Consider cardiac catheterization, especially if further pain occurs or with early positive result of stress test.
- Continue cardiac rehabilitation.

Hypertension: In view of the patient's age, sex, and degree of HTN and the fact that there is no evidence of a secondary cause, the HTN is most likely primary in nature. It is important that BP be well controlled after this infarction. Mr. Jones' BP has been well controlled with HCTZ alone, and he is now also taking metoprolol.

- Continue metoprolol and HCTZ.
- Dietary consult before discharge to instruct patient on low-sodium as well as low-fat diet.
- Continue discussion of other problems as shown earlier.

Chronic Cough with Sputum Production: Most likely chronic bronchitis. Consider bronchiogenic carcinoma; however, CXR is normal except for heart size. Encourage smoking cessation.

Signature: _____

Title: _____

CHARTWORK

How to Write Orders	Preoperative Note
SOAP Note or Daily Progress Note	Operative Note
Discharge Summary/Note	Night of Surgery Note (Postop Note)
On-Service Note	Delivery Note
Off-Service Note	Outpatient Prescription Writing
Bedside Procedure Note	Shorthand for Laboratory Values

HOW TO WRITE ORDERS

Many hospital systems are using online order entry. It is good practice to review the orders in a manual sequence before the order entry is completed by an authorized physician. The following format is useful for writing concise admission, transfer, and postoperative orders. It involves the mnemonic A.A.D.C. VAAN DISSL, which stands for **Admit/Attending, Diagnosis, Condition, Vitals, Activity, Allergies, Nursing procedures, Diet, Ins and outs, Specific medications, Symptomatic medications, and Labs.**

A.A.D.C. VAAN DISSL

Admit: Admitting team, room number

Attending: Name of the attending physician (the person legally responsible for the patient's care) as well as the resident's and intern's names

Diagnosis: List admitting diagnosis or procedure if postop orders.

Condition: Stable, critical, etc

Vitals: Determine frequency of vital signs (temperature, pulse, BP, CVP, PCWP, weight, etc)

Activity: Bedrest, up ad lib, ambulate qid, bathroom privileges, etc

Allergies: Drug reactions and food or environmental allergies (eg, latex, adhesive tape)

Nursing Procedures

Bed Position. Elevate head of bed 30 degrees, etc

Preps. Enemas, scrubs, showers

Respiratory Care. P&PD, TC&DB, etc

Dressing Changes, Wound Care. Change dressing bid, etc

Notify House Officer If. Temperature > 101°F, BP < 90 mm Hg, etc

Diet: NPO, clear liquid, regular, etc

Ins and Outs: All "tubes" a patient may have

Record Daily I&O.

IV Fluids. Specify type and rate.

Drains.

NG Tube, Foley Catheter, ETT, Arterial Lines, Pulmonary Artery Catheter. Specify care desired (eg, NG to low wall suction, Foley to gravity, suction ETT q2h and PRN)

Specific Medications: Diuretic, antibiotics, hormones, etc

Symptomatic Medications: PRN medications (eg, pain medications, laxatives, sleep medications)

2

Labs: Studies such as blood and urine. Times if applicable. Also includes ECGs, radiographs, nuclear scans, consultation requests, etc

SOAP NOTE OR DAILY PROGRESS NOTE

SOAP stands for **Subjective, Objective, Assessment, and Plan.** A sample ICU progress note is reviewed in Chapter 20.

S or **subjective** is how patients say they are feeling that morning. Record their subjective answers to history-related questions. For example, for a patient admitted with chest pain, record the answers to daily follow-up questions: Any further chest pain? If so, how long did it last? Any shortness of breath? How did you sleep last night?

O or **objective** is the place for recording the physical examination and laboratory data. The physical examination should include at least general appearance, vital signs, chest, heart, and abdomen, and any other system in which there is a new complaint or in which there was a finding on admission. Laboratory data may include tests such as the left and right heart catheterization performed the afternoon before or the troponin and CBC drawn the morning the **SOAP** note is being written.

A is the place for recording the **Assessment** of the patient. Evaluate the data, and record any conclusions drawn.

P is where the **Plan** for the day is recorded. Include any new lab tests or medications, changes or additions to previous orders, and discharge or transfer plans.

If the patient has more than one medical problem, address the **Assessment** and **Plan** for each problem separately.

1. List each medical, surgical, and psychiatric problem separately: pneumonia, pancreatitis, CHF, etc.
2. Give each problem a call number: 1, 2, 3 (as on page 23).
3. Retain the number of each problem throughout the hospitalization.
4. When the problem is solved, mark it as such and delete it from the daily progress note.

DISCHARGE SUMMARY/NOTE

At most hospitals a formal discharge note usually is required for any admission longer than 24 h. This note is a framework for the complete dictated note and is a reference, if needed, before the dictated note is transcribed and filed. The following skeleton includes most of the information needed for a discharge note.

Date of Admission: Specify.
Date of Discharge: Specify.
Admitting Diagnosis: List main reason for initial admission.
Discharge Diagnosis: List primary diagnosis and any secondary diagnoses.
Attending Physician and Service Caring for Patient: Provide attending's name and service or practice group.
Referring Physician: Provide name and contact information (eg, address, phone number) if available.
Procedures: Include surgery and any invasive diagnostic procedures (eg, lumbar puncture, arteriogram).
Brief History, Pertinent Physical Findings, and Lab Data: *Briefly* review the main points of the history, physical, and admission lab tests. Do not repeat what is recorded in the admission note; summarize the most important points about the patient's admission.

Hospital Course: Briefly summarize in chronologic order the evaluation, treatment, and progress of the patient during the hospitalization. If the patient has more than one problem during the hospitalization, address each problem separately, and within each problem record the events in chronologic order.

Condition at Discharge: Note whether improved, unchanged, or worse.

Disposition: Record the location to which the patient is discharged (eg, home, another hospital, nursing home). Give the specific address, if available, if the patient is transferred to another medical institution, and note who will be assuming responsibility for the patient.

Discharge Medications: List medications, dosing, and refills.

Discharge Instructions and Follow-up: Note clinic return date, diet instructions, activity restrictions, etc.

Problem List: List active and past medical problems.

ON-SERVICE NOTE

Also known as a "pick-up note," the on-service note is written by a new member of the team taking over the care of a patient who has been on the service for some time. This type of note is more common on medical services. Make the note brief, summarizing the hospital course to date and showing that the patient's care has been reviewed. The following skeleton includes most of the information needed in an on-service note.

Date of Admission: Specify.

Admitting Diagnosis: Specify.

Procedures (with Results) Performed to Date: List.

Hospital Course to Date: Summarize briefly.

Brief Physical Examination: Record findings pertinent to the patient's problems.

Pertinent Lab Data: Summarize key lab tests.

Problem List: Use problem-numbering system as for the SOAP format (page 26).

Assessment: Describe how the patient is progressing and the up-to-date assessment of each problem.

Plan: Outline further testing or therapy planned.

OFF-SERVICE NOTE

If rotating off the service before the patient is discharged, the team member primarily responsible for the patient's care writes an off-service note. The components are identical to those of the on-service note.

BEDSIDE PROCEDURE NOTE

Procedure: Lumbar puncture, thoracentesis, etc

Indications: (eg, R/O meningitis, symptomatic pleural effusion)

Permission: Note risks and benefits explained and indicate the permission is signed and on chart.

Physicians: Note physicians and others present and responsible for the procedure.

Description of Procedure: Indicate type of positioning, prep, anesthesia type and amount (eg, 2 mL 1% lidocaine). Briefly describe technique and instruments used.

Complications: Note any.

Estimated Blood Loss (EBL): Note as "minimal," or, if greater, estimate amount lost.

2

Specimens/Findings Obtained: (eg, opening pressure for LP, CSF appearance, and tubes sent to lab, etc)
Disposition: Describe patient's status after procedure (eg, Patient alert and oriented with no complaints; BP stable).

PREOPERATIVE NOTE

The specific items in the preoperative note depend on institutional guidelines, the nature of the procedure, and the age and health of the patient. For example, an ECG and blood set-up may not be necessary for a 2-year-old being treated for a hernia but are essential for a 70-year-old undergoing aortic valve surgery. The following list includes most of the information needed in a preoperative note.

Preop Diagnosis: Record (eg, "acute appendicitis").
Procedure: Indicate the planned procedure (eg, "exploratory laparotomy").
Labs: Record results of CBC, electrolytes, PT, PTT, urinalysis, etc.
CXR: Note results.
ECG: Note results.
Blood: Follow institutional guidelines for recommended quantities (eg, T&C 2 units PRBC, blood not needed, etc) (see also Chapter 10).
History and Physical: See chart.
Orders: Note any special preop orders, eg, preop colon prep, vaginal douche, prophylactic antibiotics.
Permission: If completed, write "signed and on chart." If not, indicate plans for obtaining informed consent for the procedure. Note briefly risks and benefits explained.

OPERATIVE NOTE

The operative note is written immediately after a surgical procedure to summarize the operation for those who were not present. The note is meant to complement the formal operative summary dictated by the surgeon. The following list includes most of the information needed in an operative note. Hospitals may produce standardized forms for this type of note.

Preop Diagnosis: Record the reason for the operation (eg, "acute appendicitis").
Postop Diagnosis: Record the diagnosis based on the operative findings (eg, "mesenteric lymphadenitis").
Procedure: Specify the operation performed (eg, "exploratory laparotomy").
Surgeons: List the attending physicians, residents, and students who scrubbed on the case, including their titles, eg, MD, CCIV (clinical clerk, fourth year), MSII (second year medical student). It is often helpful to identify the dictating surgeon.
Findings: Briefly note operative findings (eg, "normal appendix with marked lymphadenopathy").
Anesthesia: Specify the type of anesthesia, eg, local, spinal, general, endotracheal.
Fluids: Record the amount and type of fluid administered during the operation, eg, 1500 mL NS, 1 unit PRBC, 500 mL albumin. This information usually is obtained from the anesthesia records.
EBL: Record the estimated blood loss. This information is obtained from the anesthesia or nursing records.
Drains: State location and type of drain, eg, "Jackson–Pratt drain in LUQ," "T-tube in midline."

Specimens: State any samples sent to pathology and the results of examination of any intraoperative frozen sections.

Complications: Note any complications during or after the operation.

Condition: Note where the patient is taken immediately after the operation and the patient's condition (eg, "transferred to the recovery room in stable condition").

NIGHT OF SURGERY NOTE (POSTOP NOTE)

This progress note is written several hours after or the night of surgery.

Procedure: Indicate the operation performed.

Level of Consciousness: Note whether the patient is alert, drowsy, etc.

Vital Signs: Record BP, pulse, respiration.

I&O: Calculate amount of IV fluids, blood, urine output, and other drainage, and attempt to assess fluid balance.

Physical Examination: Examine the chest, heart, abdomen, extremities, and any other part pertinent to the surgery, and record the findings. Examine the dressing for bleeding.

Labs: Review lab results obtained since the operation.

Assessment: Evaluate the postop course thus far (stable, etc).

Plan: Note any changes in orders.

DELIVERY NOTE

Fill in the following: __ -year-old (married or single) G __ now para __, AB __, clinic (note whether patient received prenatal clinic care) patient with EDC __, and prenatal course (specify uncomplicated, or describe any problems). Labor (describe, eg, oxytocin-induced, premature rupture) draped in the usual sterile manner. Under controlled conditions delivered a __ lb __ oz (__ g) viable (specify male or female) infant under __ (specify general, spinal, pudendal, none) anesthesia.

Delivery was by __ (specify SVD with midline episiotomy, or forceps, or cesarean section). Apgar scores were __ at 1 min and __ at 5 min (for Apgar scoring, see Appendix, page 650). Delivery date __; delivery time __. Cord blood sent to lab. Placenta expressed intact with trailing membranes. Lacerations of the __ degree repaired by standard method with good hemostasis and restoration of normal anatomy.

- EBL:
- Maternal blood type (MBT):
- HCT (predelivery and postdelivery):
- Rubella titer:
- RPR test, hepatitis B serology, HIV test, and status of other serology or cultures that can affect a mother's or newborn's health:
- Condition of mother:

OUTPATIENT PRESCRIPTION WRITING

The format for outpatient prescription writing is outlined in the following list and illustrated in Figure 2–1. Controlled substances, such as narcotics, require a DEA number on the prescription. Some states require that the controlled substance be written on a special type of prescription pad (see Chapter 22 for controlled drugs indicated by [C]). For security, the DEA number should never be preprinted on a prescription pad but should be written by hand when the prescription is written.

NICK PAVONA, MD
BENJAMIN FRANKLIN UNIVERSITY MEDICAL CENTER
CHADDS FORD, PA 19317

LICENSE PA MD 685-488-194   DEA NP–3612982

NAME NICK PAVONA, Sr.   AGE 51
ADDRESS Box A-24   DATE 10/24/2006
         Georgetown, MD

> Rx: minoxidil (Rogaine) 2% topical solution
> DISP: 60 mL
> SIG: Apply BID to scalp
>   Brand medically necessary

REFILL   X5
SUBSTITUTION PERMISSIBLE   ☐   *Nick Pavona*   M.D.

TO ENSURE BRAND NAME DISPENSING, PRESCRIBER MUST
SPECIFY "DISPENSE AS WRITTEN" ON THE PRESCRIPTION.*

*This can vary by state; some require that you write "Brand Medically
Necessary" to specify a brand name and not a generic.

FIGURE 2–1. Example of an outpatient prescription. As a safety feature DEA numbers should never be preprinted on a prescription form. The "Dispense as Written" statement can vary by state requirements. This statement requests that the pharmacist fill the prescription as requested and not substitute a generic equivalent.

Elements of an outpatient prescription include:

Patient's Name, Address, and Age: Print clearly where indicated.
Date: State requirements vary, but most prescriptions must be filled within 6 mo.
Rx: Drug name, strength, and type (usually listed as the generic name). Designate "no substitution" if a specific brand name is called for. "Rx" is the abbreviation of the Latin word for "recipe." List the strength of the product (usually in milligrams) and the form (eg, tablet, capsule, suspension, transdermal).
Dispense: Amount of drug (eg, number of capsules) and time period (eg, 1-mo supply, QS [quantity sufficient])
Sig: Short for the Latin "signa," which means "mark through" on patient instructions. Abbreviate the instructions or write them in full. Spelling out directions rather than using abbreviations decreases the likelihood of error. A list of frequently used abbreviations follows; additional abbreviations are on the list at the front of the book.

> ad lib = as much as wanted
> PO = by mouth
> PR = by rectum
> OS = left eye
> OD = right eye
> OU = both eyes
> qd = daily ("qd" is a dangerous abbreviation and **should not be used;** write out "every day" or "Q day"; see "Dangerous Practices," page 32)
> PRN = as needed

$\dot{T}$ = one
$\ddot{T}$ = two
$\dddot{T}$ = three
qhs = every night at bedtime
bid = twice a day
tid = three times a day
q6h = every 6 hours
qid = four times a day. Note that qid and q6h are NOT the same orders: qid means the patient takes the medication four times a day while awake (eg, 8 AM, 12 noon, 6 PM, and 10 PM); q6h means the medication is taken four times a day but by the clock (eg, 6 AM, 12 noon, 6 PM, 12 midnight).

Refills: How many times this prescription can be refilled

Substitution: Whether a generic drug be used instead of the one prescribed

Tips for Safe Prescription Writing

Legibility
1. Take time to write legibly.
2. Print if doing so would make the prescription more legible than handwriting would.
3. Use a typewriter or computer if necessary. Some centers generate prescriptions by computer to eliminate legibility problems.

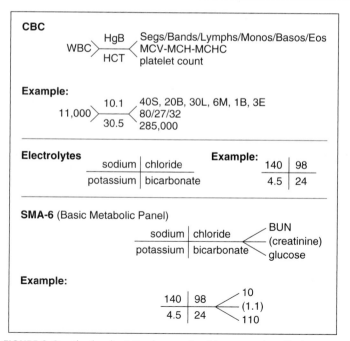

FIGURE 2–2. Shorthand notation for recording laboratory values. The basic metabolic panel is similar to the SMA-6 except that creatinine is also listed.

4. Carefully print the order to avoid misreading. There are many "sound alike" drugs and medications that have similar spellings (eg, Celexa and Celebrex).

Dangerous Prescription Writing Practices

1. **Never** use a trailing zero.
   Correct: 1 mg; Dangerous: 1.0 mg. If the decimal is not seen, a 10-fold overdose can occur.
2. **Never** leave a decimal point "naked." Correct: 0.5 mL; Dangerous: .5 mL. If the decimal point is not seen, a 10-fold overdose can occur.
3. **Never** abbreviate a drug name. The abbreviation can be misunderstood and have multiple meanings.
4. **Never** abbreviate the word "units." The letter *U* can be read as a zero (eg, "6 U regular insulin" can be misread as 60 units). Write the order as "6 units regular insulin."
5. **Never** use "qd" (abbreviation for once a day or every day). When poorly written, the tail of the *q* can make the abbreviation look like "qid," or four times a day. Write out "every day" or "Q day."

SHORTHAND FOR LABORATORY VALUES

The method for recording laboratory values is shown in Figure 2–2, page 31.

DIFFERENTIAL DIAGNOSIS: SYMPTOMS, SIGNS, AND CONDITIONS

Abdominal Distention
Abdominal Pain
Adrenal Mass
Alopecia
Amenorrhea
Anorexia
Anuria
Arthritis
Ascites
Back Pain
Breast Lump
Chest Pain
Chills
Clubbing
Coma
Constipation
Cough
Cyanosis
Delirium
Dementia
Diarrhea
Diplopia
Dizziness
Dysphagia
Dyspnea
Dysuria
Earache
Edema
Epistaxis
Failure to Thrive
Fever
Fever of Unknown Origin (FUO)
Flatulence

Frequency
Galactorrhea
Gynecomastia
Headache
Heartburn (Pyrosis)
Hematemesis, Melenemesis, and Melena
Hematochezia
Hematuria
Hemoptysis
Hepatomegaly
Hiccups (Singultus)
Hirsutism
Impotence (Erectile Dysfunction)
Incontinence (Urinary)
Jaundice
Lymphadenopathy and Splenomegaly
Melena
Nausea and Vomiting
Nystagmus
Oliguria and Anuria
Pleural Effusion
Pruritus
Seizures
Splenomegaly
Syncope
Tremors
Vaginal Bleeding
Vaginal Discharge
Vertigo
Vomiting
Weight Loss
Wheezing

This chapter is a general guide to commonly encountered symptoms and conditions and their frequent causes primarily in adults unless specified. Remember: "There are more uncommon presentations of common diseases than common presentations of uncommon diseases."

ABDOMINAL DISTENTION

Ascites, intestinal obstruction, cysts (ovarian or renal), tumors, hepatosplenomegaly, aortic aneurysm, uterine enlargement (pregnancy), bladder distention, inflammatory mass

ABDOMINAL PAIN

Diffuse: Intestinal angina, early appendicitis, colitis, diabetic ketoacidosis, hereditary angioedema, gastroenteritis, mesenteric thrombosis, mesenteric lymphadenitis, peritonitis, porphyria, sickle cell crisis, uremia, renal colic, renal infarct, pancreatitis

Right Upper Quadrant: Dissecting aneurysm, gallbladder disease (cholecystitis, cholangitis, choledocholithiasis), hepatitis, hepatomegaly, pancreatitis, PUD, pneumonia, pulmonary embolus, pyelonephritis, renal colic, renal infarct, appendicitis (retroperitoneal)

Left Upper Quadrant: Dissecting aneurysm, esophagitis, hiatal hernia, esophageal rupture, gastritis, pancreatitis, PUD, myocardial infarction, pericarditis, pneumonia, pulmonary embolus, pyelonephritis, renal colic, renal infarction, splenic abscess, splenic rupture, splenic infarction

Lower Abdomen: Aortic aneurysm, colitis including inflammatory bowel disease, diverticulitis including Meckel diverticulum, intestinal obstruction, hernia, perforated viscus, pregnancy, ectopic pregnancy, dysmenorrhea, endometriosis, mittelschmerz (ovulation), ovarian cyst or tumor (especially with torsion), PID, renal colic, UTI, rectal hematoma, bladder distention

Right Lower Quadrant: Appendicitis, ectopic pregnancy, ovarian cyst or tumor, salpingitis, mittelschmerz, cholecystitis, perforated duodenal ulcer, Crohn disease

ADRENAL MASS

Adrenal adenoma, adrenal hyperplasia (unilateral or bilateral), adrenal metastasis (solid tumors, lymphoma, leukemia), adrenocortical carcinoma, pheochromocytoma, adrenal myelolipoma, adrenal cyst, adrenal varices, hemorrhage, congenital adrenal hyperplasia, ganglioneuroma, micronodular adrenal disease

ALOPECIA

Male pattern baldness (alopecia, androgenic type in both men and women), trauma and hair pulling, congenital, tinea capitis, bacterial folliculitis, telogen arrest, anagen arrest (chemotherapy, radiation therapy), alopecia areata, discoid lupus

AMENORRHEA

Pregnancy, menopause (physiologic or premature), severe illness, weight loss, stress, excessive athletic training, physiologically delayed puberty, anatomic anomaly (eg, imperforate hymen, uterine agenesis, etc), gonadal dysgenesis (eg, Turner syndrome), hypothalamic and pituitary tumors, virilizing syndromes (eg, polycystic ovaries, idiopathic hirsutism). Amenorrhea is categorized as primary (never had menses) or secondary (cessation of menses).

ANOREXIA

Hepatitis, carcinoma (most types, especially advanced), anorexia nervosa, generalized debilitating diseases, digitalis toxicity, uremia, depression, CHF, pulmonary failure, radiation exposure, chemotherapy

ANURIA

(See Oliguria and Anuria, page 42).

ARTHRITIS

Osteoarthritis, bursitis, tendonitis, connective tissue disease (rheumatoid arthritis, SLE, rheumatic fever, scleroderma, gout, pseudogout, rheumatoid variants [ankylosing spondylitis, psoriatic arthritis, Reiter syndrome]), infection (bacterial, viral, TB, fungal Lyme disease), trauma, sarcoidosis, sickle cell anemia, hemochromatosis, amyloidosis, coagulopathy

ASCITES

(See Chapter 13, page 304, Peritoneal [Abdominal] Paracentesis for more details.) Use the serum albumin to ascitic albumin difference (serum albumin minus ascites albumin) to help differentiate the cause of ascites. If the difference is > 1.1, portal hypertension is present. If the difference is < 1.1, the cause is not portal hypertension). CHF, tricuspid insufficiency, constrictive pericarditis, venous occlusion (including Budd–Chiari syndrome), cirrhosis, pancreatitis, peritonitis (ruptured viscus, TB, bile leak, spontaneous bacterial), tumor (most common ovarian, gastric, uterine, unknown primary, breast, lymphoma), trauma, Meigs syndrome (ovarian fibroma associated with hydrothorax and ascites), myxedema, anasarca (hypoalbuminemia)

BACK PAIN

Herniated disk, spinal stenosis, ankylosing spondylitis, metastatic tumor, multiple myeloma, mechanical back sprain, vertebral body fracture, osteoporosis-induced fracture, infectious processes (diskitis, osteomyelitis, epidural abscess), referred pain (visceral, vascular) including pyelonephritis, colitis and diverticulitis, cancer, endometriosis, abdominal aortic aneurysm, and psychiatric disorder such as malingering, substance abuse, or depression

BREAST LUMP

Cancer, fibroadenoma, fibrocystic breast disease, fat necrosis, gynecomastia (male patients, alcoholic patients)

CHEST PAIN

Deep, Dull, Poorly Localized: Angina, variant angina, unstable angina, AMI, aortic aneurysm, pulmonary embolus, tumor, gallbladder disease, pulmonary HTN

Sharp, Well Localized: Pulmonary embolus, pneumothorax, pleurodynia, pericarditis, atypical MI, hyperventilation, hiatal hernia, esophagitis, esophageal spasm, herpes zoster (pain may precede rash by 2–3 d), aortic aneurysm, breast lesions, various bony and soft-tissue abnormalities (rib fractures, costochondritis, muscle damage), perforated ulcer, acute cholecystitis, pancreatitis

CHILLS

Infection (bacterial with bacteremia, viral, TB, fungal, malaria), neoplasm (Hodgkin disease), drug and transfusion reactions, hypothermia

CLUBBING

Pulmonary causes (bronchiectasis, lung abscesses, tuberculosis, neoplasms, fibrosis), AV malformations, cardiac conditions (congenital cyanotic heart diseases, bacterial endocarditis), GI causes (ulcerative and regional enteritis, cirrhosis), hereditary conditions, thyrotoxicosis

COMA

Use the mnemonic **AEIOU TIPS:** **A**lcohol, **E**ncephalitis (other CNS causes such as epilepsy, hemorrhage, mass), **I**nsulin (hypoglycemia, hyperglycemia), **O**piates (drugs), **U**remia (and other metabolic conditions, eg, hypernatremia, hyponatremia, hypercalcemia, hepatic failure, and thiamine deficiency), **T**rauma, **I**nfection (sepsis), **P**sychiatric causes (catatonia, psychogenic), **S**yncope (or decreased cardiac output, eg, from arrhythmia or aortic stenosis).

CONSTIPATION

Dehydration, lack of exercise, bedrest, medications (narcotics, anticholinergics, antidepressants, calcium channel blockers such as verapamil, diuretics, clonidine, aluminum- or calcium-containing antacids, 5-HT_3-receptor antagonists), laxative abuse, megacolon, spastic colon, chronic suppression of the urge to defecate, fecal impaction (often with paradoxical diarrhea), neoplasm, intestinal obstruction, vascular occlusion of the bowel, inflammatory lesions (diverticulitis, proctitis), hemorrhoids, anal fissures, neurologic disorders (spinal cord lesions or trauma, autonomic insufficiency), depression, diabetes mellitus, porphyria, hypothyroidism, hypercalcemia, hypokalemia, hypomagnesemia

COUGH

Acute: Tracheobronchitis, pneumonia, sinusitis, pulmonary edema, foreign body, toxic inhalation, allergy, pharyngitis (viral or bacterial), asthma, GERD, ACE inhibitors, impacted cerumen or foreign body in ear

Chronic: Bronchitis (smoker), chronic sinusitis, emphysema, cancer (bronchogenic, head and neck, esophageal), TB, interstitial lung disease including sarcoidosis, fungal infection, bronchiectasis, mediastinal lymphadenopathy, thoracic aneurysm, GERD, ACE inhibitors

CYANOSIS

Peripheral: Arterial occlusion and insufficiency, vasospasm and Raynaud disease, venous stasis, venous obstruction

Central: Hypoxia, congenital heart disease (right to left shunt), pulmonary embolus, pseudocyanosis (eg, polycythemia vera), methemoglobinemia

DELIRIUM

Metabolic: Hypoglycemia, hypoxia, hyponatremia, hypernatremia, hypercalcemia, hypercarbia, uremia, hyperthyroidism

Neurologic: Stroke, subdural and epidural hematoma, subarachnoid hemorrhage, postictal state, concussion and contusion, meningitis, encephalitis, brain tumor

Drug- or Toxin-Induced: Lithium intoxication, ethanol, steroids, anticholinergics, sympathomimetics, poisons (eg, mushrooms, carbon monoxide), drugs of abuse including ecstasy (MMDA), gamma hydroxybutyrate (GHB), lysergic acid diethylamide (LSD), phencyclidine (PCP), mescaline

Other: Sepsis, thiamine deficiency, niacin deficiency

DEMENTIA

Chronic CNS Disease: Alzheimer disease, senile dementia, Pick disease, Parkinson disease, chronic demyelinating disease (MS), ALS, brain tumor, normal pressure hydrocephalus, Wilson disease, Huntington disease, lipid storage diseases (eg, Tay–Sachs)

Metabolic: Usually chronic (hypoxia, hypoglycemia, hypocalcemia), hyperammonemia, dialysis, heavy-metal intoxication, pernicious anemia (B_{12} deficiency), niacin and thiamine deficiency (usually chronic alcoholic), post–hepatic coma, medications (barbiturates, phenothiazines, lithium, benzodiazepines, many others)

Infectious: AIDS encephalopathy, brain abscess, chronic meningoencephalitis (eg, fungal, neurosyphilis), encephalitis, Jakob–Creutzfeldt disease

Vascular: Vasculitis, multiple cerebral or cerebellar infarcts

Traumatic: Contusion, hemorrhage, subdural hematoma

Psychiatric: Sensory deprivation, depression (pseudodementia)

DIARRHEA

Acute: Infection (bacterial, viral, fungal, protozoan, parasitic), toxic (food poisoning, chemical), drugs (antibiotics, cholinergic agents, lactulose, magnesium-containing antacids, quinidine, reserpine, guanethidine, metoclopramide, bethanechol, SSRIs, metformin, acarbose, orlistat), appendicitis, diverticular disease, GI bleeding, ischemic colitis, food intolerance, fecal impaction (paradoxical diarrhea), pseudomembranous colitis

Chronic: Postoperative state (gastrectomy, vagotomy, extensive bowel resection, resection of ileocecal valve), Zollinger–Ellison syndrome, regional enteritis, ulcerative colitis, malabsorption, diverticular disease, carcinoma, villous adenoma, gastrinoma, lymphoma of the bowel, functional bowel disorder (irritable colon, mucous colitis), pseudomembranous colitis, endocrine disease (carcinoid, hyperthyroidism, Addison disease), radiation enteritis, drugs, Whipple disease, amyloidosis, AIDS (*Isospora belli, Microsporidia,* and *Cyclospora* are three parasites that can cause diarrhea in HIV patients. Nonparasitic causes include *Salmonella typhimurium, Campylobacter jejuni, Mycobacterium avium-intracellulare,* and cytomegalovirus and idiopathic factors.)

DIPLOPIA

Problems with the third, fourth, or sixth cranial nerve, eg, from vascular disturbances, meningitis, tumor, demyelination, orbital blow-out fracture, hyperthyroidism, ocular myopathy

DIZZINESS

Hyperventilation, depression, hypoglycemia, anemia, volume depletion, hypoxia, trauma, Ménière disease, benign positional vertigo, aminoglycoside toxicity, vestibular neuronitis, MS, brainstem ischemia or stroke, posterior fossa lesions, cerebellar ischemia or stroke, autonomic insufficiency, arrhythmia, aortic stenosis, carotid sinus hypersensitivity, postural tachycardia, subclavian steal, vasovagal reaction, medications including vasodilators, benzodiazepines, and anticonvulsants

DYSPHAGIA

Loss of tongue function, pharyngeal dysfunction (myasthenia gravis), Zenker diverticulum, tumors (bronchogenic, head and neck, and esophageal), stricture, esophageal web, Schatzki ring, lower esophageal sphincter spasm, foreign body, aortic aneurysm, achalasia, scleroderma, diabetic neuropathy, amyloidosis, infection (especially candidiasis), dermatomyositis, polymyositis, MS, brainstem infarction

DYSPNEA

Laryngeal and tracheal infections and foreign bodies, tumors (both intrinsic and extrinsic), COPD, asthma, pneumonia, aspiration, interstitial lung disease, lung carcinoma, atelectasis, pneumothorax, pleural effusion, hemothorax, pulmonary embolus, pulmonary infarction, carbon monoxide poisoning, any cause of pain from respiratory movements, cardiac and noncardiac pulmonary edema, acute coronary syndrome, arrhythmia, aortic stenosis, aortic insufficiency, mitral stenosis, mitral insufficiency, pericardial tamponade, anemia, abdominal distention, myopathies, neuropathies, spinal cord disorders, phrenic nerve and diaphragmatic disorders, GERD, deconditioning, anxiety

DYSURIA

Urethral stricture, stones, blood clot, tumor (bladder, prostate, urethral), prostatic enlargement, infection (urethritis, cystitis, vaginitis, prostatitis), atrophic vaginitis, trauma, bladder spasm, dehydration, urethral syndrome or interstitial cystitis

EARACHE

Otitis media and externa, mastoiditis, serous otitis, otic barotrauma, foreign body, impacted cerumen, referred pain (dental or TMJ)

EDEMA

CHF, constrictive pericarditis, liver disease (cirrhosis), nephrotic syndrome, nephritic syndrome, hypoalbuminemia, malnutrition, myxedema, hemiplegia, volume overload, thrombophlebitis, lymphatic obstruction, medications (nifedipine), venous stasis

EPISTAXIS

Trauma (nose picking, blunt trauma), neoplasm, polyps, foreign body, desiccation, coagulopathy, medications (use of cocaine, nasal sprays), infection (sinusitis), uremia, hypertension (more often a result rather than a cause of epistaxis)

FAILURE TO THRIVE

Environmental: Social deprivation, decreased food intake

Organic: CNS disorder, intestinal malabsorption, cystic fibrosis, parasites, cleft palate, heart failure, endocrine disease, hypercalcemia, Turner syndrome, renal disease, chronic infection, malignant diseases

FEVER

In adults, a morning temperature above 98.8°F (37.2°C) or a night temperature above 99.9°F (37.7°C) is generally defined as a fever. Rectal temperature is generally 1°F (0.6°C) higher and reflects core temperature. Axillary temperature is approximately 1°F (0.6°C) lower than oral temperature. Infection (viral [including HIV and AIDS], bacterial, mycobacterial, fungal, parasitic), neoplasm (lymphoma, leukemia, renal and hepatic carcinoma), connective tissue disease (SLE, vasculitis, rheumatoid arthritis, adult Still disease, temporal arteritis), heat stroke, malignant hyperthermia, thyroid storm, adrenal insufficiency, pulmonary embolus, MI, atrial myxoma, inflammatory bowel disease, factitious factors, drugs (most commonly amphotericin, bleomycin, barbiturates, cephalosporins, methyldopa, penicillins, phenytoin, procainamide, sulfonamides, quinidine, cocaine, LSD, phencyclidine, and amphetamines)

FEVER OF UNKNOWN ORIGIN (FUO)

In adults, defined as a temperature of 101°F (38.3°C) or greater for at least 3 wk and for which a diagnosis is not established after 1 wk of hospitalization. In children, the minimum duration is 2 wk, and the temperature is at least 101.3°F (38.5°C). TB, fungal infection, endocarditis, abscess (especially hepatic), neoplasm (lymphoma, renal cell, hepatoma, preleukemia), atrial myxoma, connective tissue disease, drugs (see Fever), pulmonary embolus, Crohn disease, ulcerative colitis, hypothalamic injury, factitious factors, temporal arteritis in elderly patients

FLATULENCE

Aerophagia, food intolerance, disturbances in bowel motility (diabetes, uremia), lactose intolerance, gallbladder disease, medications including acarbose and orlistat

FREQUENCY

Infection (bladder, prostate), excessive fluid intake, use of diuretics (also coffee, tea, or cola), diabetes mellitus, diabetes insipidus, prostatic obstruction, bladder stones, bladder tumors, pregnancy, psychogenic bladder syndrome, neurogenic bladder, interstitial cystitis

GALACTORRHEA

Hyperprolactinemia, prolonged breast feeding, major stress, pituitary tumors, breast lesions (benign, cancer, inflammatory), idiopathic with menses and after oral contraceptive use

GYNECOMASTIA

Normal (Physiologic):   Newborn, adolescence, aging

Pathologic: Drugs (cimetidine, spironolactone, estrogens, gonadotropins, antiandrogens [bicalutamide, others], marijuana), decreased testosterone (Klinefelter syndrome, testicular failure or absence), increased estrogen production (hermaphroditism, testicular or lung cancer, adrenal and liver diseases)

HEADACHE

Cluster: Severe, sharp, stabbing, usually unilateral clustered every day to every other day, lasting 1/2–2 hrs, classically occur in the early morning (3 AM) over 1–4 mo

Tension: Steady, nonpulsatile bandlike distribution around head, stress-related, increases as day progresses

Migraine: Precipitated by a factor such as menses or a food and preceded by an aura; photophobia, N/V, neurologic complaints, unilateral deep, throbbing severe parietal–temporal pain

Other Types: Benign exertional, benign cough headache, vascular (menstruation, hypertension), ice pick headache, eye strain, acute glaucoma, uveitis, keratitis, sinusitis, dental problems, TMJ disease, trauma, subarachnoid hemorrhage, intracranial mass, carotid or vertebral artery dissection, fever, meningitis, pseudotumor cerebri, trigeminal neuralgia, temporal arteritis (especially in elderly), hypoglycemia, toxin exposure (carbon monoxide poisoning), drugs (vasodilators such as nifedipine [Procardia]), vasculitis

HEARTBURN (PYROSIS)

GERD, esophagitis, hiatal hernia, peptic ulcer, gallbladder disease, medications (eg, alendronate), tumors, scleroderma, food intolerance. Myocardial ischemia can be mistaken for heartburn.

HEMATEMESIS, MELENEMESIS, AND MELENA

Melena: Black tarry stools caused by stomach acid or intestinal bacterial conversion of hemoglobin to the black pigment hematin; suggests blood loss of > 50–100 mL

Hematemesis: Vomiting blood

Melenemesis: Vomiting of material that looks like coffee grounds
    Note: These three conditions suggest a bleeding site in the upper GI tract (ie, proximal to the ligament of Treitz) but can be as distal as the right colon with reflux of blood through the pylorus. Swallowed blood (eg, from epistaxis), esophageal varices, esophagitis, Mallory–Weiss syndrome, hiatal hernia, gastritis, duodenal or gastric ulcer, duodenitis, gastric carcinoma, tumors (small and large bowel), ischemic colitis, and aortoenteric fistula. Bleeding diathesis and anticoagulation can unmask GI tract abnormality. Medications, eg, bismuth-containing mediations and iron supplements can darken stool.

HEMATOCHEZIA

Grossly bloody stool. Massive upper GI bleeding (rapid GI transit), hemorrhoids, anal fissure, diverticular disease, angiodysplasia, polyps, carcinoma, inflammatory bowel disease, ischemic colitis

HEMATURIA (SEE ALSO PAGE 107)

First rule out false-positives: myoglobinuria, hemoglobinuria, porphyria. GU neoplasms (malignant and benign), polycystic kidneys, trauma, infection (urethra, bladder, prostate, etc), stones, glomerulonephritis (primary and secondary such as Wegener granulomatosis, SLE, and polyarteritis nodosa), renal infarction, renal vein thrombosis, enterovesical fistula, sickle cell anemia, vigorous exercise (runner's hematuria), accelerated hypertension, factitious and vaginal and rectal bleeding. Bleeding diathesis and anticoagulation can unmask GU tract abnormalities.

HEMOPTYSIS

Infection (pneumonia, bronchitis, fungal, TB), bronchiectasis, cancer (bronchogenic or metastatic), bronchial adenoma, pulmonary embolus, A–V malformations, Wegener granulomatosis, Goodpasture syndrome, SLE, pulmonary hemosiderosis, foreign body, trauma, bleeding diatheses, excessive anticoagulation (can unmask respiratory tract abnormalities), cardiogenic pulmonary edema, mitral stenosis

HEPATOMEGALY

Right-sided CHF, tricuspid stenosis, hepatitis (viral, alcoholic, drug-induced, autoimmune), fatty liver, tumors (primary and metastatic, lymphoma, chronic myelocytic leukemia, lymphocytic leukemia), amyloid, biliary obstruction, hemochromatosis, chronic granulomatous disease, amyloidosis, infection (schistosomiasis, liver abscess, hydatid cysts), hepatic vein thrombosis, Wolman disease. Riedel lobe is a normal variant, elongated right lobe of the liver with normal total liver volume

HICCUPS (SINGULTUS)

Uremia, electrolyte disorders, diabetes, medications (benzodiazepines, barbiturates, others), emotionally induced (excitement, fright), gastric distention, CNS disorders, psychogenic, thoracic and diaphragmatic disorders (pneumonia, MI, diaphragmatic irritation), alcohol ingestion

HIRSUTISM

Idiopathic, familial, adrenal causes (Cushing disease, congenital adrenal hyperplasia, virilizing adenoma or carcinoma), polycystic ovaries, medications (minoxidil, androgens)

IMPOTENCE (ERECTILE DYSFUNCTION)

Psychogenic, vascular, neurologic (spinal cord injury, radical prostatectomy, rectal surgery, aortic bypass), pelvic radiation, medications (common drugs: antihypertensives, especially thiazide diuretics, beta-blockers and methyldopa; antidepressants especially the SSRIs, anticholinergics; addictive medications: alcohol, narcotics; antipsychotics; antiandrogens: histamine H_2 blockers, finasteride, LHRH analogues, spironolactone, others); history of priapism, Peyronie disease, testicular failure, hyperprolactinemia

INCONTINENCE (URINARY)

Cystitis, dementia and delirium, stroke, prostatic hypertrophy, fecal impaction, peripheral or autonomic neuropathy, medications (diuretics, sedatives, alpha-blockers), diabetes, spinal cord trauma or lesions, MS, childbirth, surgery (prostate, rectal), aging, acute and chronic medical conditions, estrogen deficiency

JAUNDICE

Hepatitis (alcoholic, viral, drug-induced, autoimmune), Gilbert disease, Crigler–Najjar syndrome, Dubin–Johnson syndrome, Wilson disease, drug-induced cholestasis (phenothiazines and estrogen), gallbladder and biliary tract disease (including inflammation, infection, obstruction, and primary and metastatic hepatic tumors), hemolysis, neonatal jaundice, cholestatic jaundice of pregnancy, TPN

LYMPHADENOPATHY AND SPLENOMEGALY

Infection (bacterial, fungal, viral, parasitic, rickettsial), benign neoplasm (histiocytosis), malignant neoplasm (primary lymphoma, metastatic), sarcoid, connective tissue disease (eg, rheumatoid arthritis, SLE, Sjögren syndrome), lipid storage diseases, drugs (eg, phenytoin), HIV and AIDS, splenomegaly without lymphadenopathy (cirrhosis, hereditary spherocytosis, hemoglobinopathies, hairy cell leukemia, histiocytosis X, amyloidosis, Wolman disease)

MELENA

(See Hematemesis, page 40.)

NAUSEA AND VOMITING

Appendicitis, acute cholecystitis, chronic gallbladder disease, PUD, gastritis (especially alcoholic), pancreatitis, gastric distention (diabetic atony, pyloric obstruction), intestinal ischemia, intestinal obstruction, peritonitis, food intolerance, intestinal infection (bacterial, viral, parasitic), acute systemic infections (especially in children), hepatitis, toxins (food poisoning), CNS disorders (tumor, hemorrhagic stroke, hydrocephalus, meningitis; increased intracranial pressure often causes vomiting without nausea), labyrinthitis, Ménière disease, migraine headache, acute coronary syndrome, CHF, endocrine disorders (DKA, adrenal crisis), hypercalcemia, hyperkalemia, hypokalemia, pyelonephritis, nephrolithiasis, uremia, hepatic failure, pregnancy, PID, drugs (opiates, digitalis, chemotherapeutic agents, levodopa, NSAIDs), psychogenic vomiting, porphyria, radiation therapy

NYSTAGMUS

Congenital, vision loss early in life, MS, neoplasms, ocular infarction, toxic or metabolic encephalopathy, alcohol intoxication, thiamine (B_1) deficiency, cerebellar degeneration, medications (anticonvulsants, barbiturates, phenothiazines, lithium, others), encephalitis, vascular brainstem lesions, Arnold–Chiari malformation, nonpathologic (extreme lateral gaze), optikokinetic nystagmus (attempt to fix gaze on a rapidly moving object, eg, a train)

OLIGURIA AND ANURIA

(See also Urinary Indices, page 116.)

    Oliguria is < 500 mL urine/24 h; **anuria** is < 100 mL urine/24 h in adults.

Prerenal: Volume depletion, shock, heart failure, fluids in the third space, renal artery compromise

Renal: Glomerular disease, acute tubular necrosis, bilateral cortical necrosis, interstitial disease (acute and chronic interstitial nephritis, urate or hypercalcemic nephropathy), transfusion reaction, myoglobulinuria, radiographic contrast media (especially in diabetic, dehydrated, and elderly patients and those with multiple myeloma), ESRD, drugs (aminoglycosides, amphotericin B, vancomycin, NSAIDs, cephalosporins, penicillins, and sulfonamides), malignant hypertension, ischemia, emboli, thrombosis, TTP, HUS, and DIC

Postrenal: Bilateral ureteral obstruction, prostatic obstruction, neurogenic bladder

PLEURAL EFFUSION

(See Chapter 13, page 310, Thoracentesis, for more details.)

Transudate: (Pleural to serum protein ratio < 0.5, pleural to serum LDH ratio < 0.6, and pleural LDH < 2/3 the upper limit of normal for serum LDH), CHF, cirrhosis, nephrotic syndrome, peritoneal dialysis

Exudate: (Pleural to serum protein ratio > 0.5, pleural to serum LDH ratio > 0.6, or pleural LDH > 2/3 the upper limit of normal for serum LDH), bacterial or viral pneumonia, pulmonary infarction, TB, rheumatoid arthritis, SLE, malignancy (most common, breast, lung lymphoma, leukemia, ovarian, unknown primary, GI, mesothelioma), pancreatitis, pneumothorax, chest trauma, uremia, peritoneal dialysis

Chylothorax: Traumatic or postoperative complication

Empyema: Bacteria, fungi, TB, trauma, surgery

Hydrothorax: Usually iatrogenic (central venous catheter complication)

PRURITUS

Skin lesions (papulosquamous, vesicobullous, eczematous, contact dermatitis, urticaria, folliculitis, neurotic excoriations, fiberglass dermatitis, infestation [eg, scabies], infection), xerosis (dry skin), especially in winter, liver disease, uremia, diabetes, gout, iron deficiency anemia, multiple myeloma, Hodgkin disease, leukemia, polycythemia vera, systemic mastocytosis, intestinal parasites, drug reactions with or without rash (without rash consider allopurinol, birth control pills, captopril, cephalosporins, cimetidine, clonidine, diuretics, HMG-CoA reductase inhibitors, narcotics, penicillin, phenothiazines, phenytoin), pregnancy, psychosomatic factors, neurologic or circulatory disturbances

SEIZURES

Generalized: Grand mal and petit mal (absence), febrile

Partial Seizures: Partial motor, partial sensory, partial complex (psychomotor or temporal lobe, déjà vu, automatisms)

Causes: Primary or metastatic CNS tumors, trauma, metabolic disorders (eg, hypoglycemia, hypocalcemia, hypomagnesemia, hypophosphatemia, hyponatremia, hypernatremia, acidosis, alkalosis, porphyria, uremia), fever (especially in children), infection (meningitis, encephalitis, abscess), anoxia (arrhythmia, stroke, carbon monoxide poisoning), drugs (alcohol or barbiturate withdrawal, cocaine, amphetamines, ethylene glycol, methanol), lead, collagen–vascular disease (SLE), chronic renal failure, trauma, hypertensive encephalopathy, toxemia of pregnancy, neurodegenerative disorders (eg, Alzheimer disease, Down syndrome, neurofibromatosis, tuberous sclerosis, glycogen or lipid storage diseases), Whipple disease, sickle cell disease, psychogenic factors

SPLENOMEGALY

(See Lymphadenopathy and Splenomegaly, page 42.)

3

SYNCOPE

Vasovagal (simple faint). Orthostatic: volume depletion, sympathectomy (either functional or surgical), diabetes, Shy–Drager syndrome (idiopathic), drugs (eg, TCAs and diuretics). Postprandial in the elderly. Psychiatric: anxiety (hyperventilation), depression, or conversion disorder. Situational: micturition, cough, Valsalva maneuver, or swallowing. Cardiac: arrhythmia (PAT, AF, VT, sinoatrial or atrioventricular block), pacemaker malfunction, aortic stenosis, hypertrophic cardiomyopathy, primary pulmonary hypertension, atrial myxoma, cardiac tamponade, aortic dissection, subclavian steal syndrome, acute coronary syndrome, pregnancy, hypoglycemia, hypoxia, seizure disorder, migraines, subarachnoid hemorrhage, TIA (vertebrobasilar or, rarely, anterior circulation with simultaneous events or 100% stenosis of the carotid artery with a TIA involving the other side). Idiopathic

TREMORS

Resting (Decrease with Movement):   Parkinson disease, Wilson disease, brain tumors (rare), medications (SSRI antidepressants, metoclopramide, phenothiazines [tardive dyskinesia])

Action (Present with Movement):   Benign essential tremor (familial and senile), cerebellar diseases, withdrawal syndromes (alcohol, benzodiazepines, opiates), normal or physiologic (induced by anxiety, fatigue)

Ataxic (Worse at End of Voluntary Movement):   MS, cerebellar diseases

Other: Medication-induced (caffeine [coffee, tea], steroids, valproic acid, bronchodilators), febrile, hypoglycemic, hyperthyroidism, pheochromocytoma

VAGINAL BLEEDING

Normal menstrual period, dysfunctional uterine bleeding (premenopausal bleeding, oral contraceptives, luteal phase defect), anovulatory abnormal uterine bleeding (hypothalamic and pituitary disorders, stress, thyroid and adrenal disease, endometriosis), pregnancy-related (ectopic pregnancy, threatened or spontaneous abortion, retained products of gestation), neoplasia (uterine fibroids; cervical polyps; endometrial, cervical, ovarian, and vulvar carcinoma)

VAGINAL DISCHARGE

Vaginitis due to *Candida albicans, Trichomonas vaginalis, Gardnerella vaginalis, Neisseria gonorrhoeae, Chlamydia trachomatis, Ureaplasma urealyticum, Mycoplasma genitalium,* herpesvirus, chronic cervicitis, tumors, irritants, foreign bodies, estrogen deficiency

VERTIGO

Ménière disease (recurrent vertigo, deafness, tinnitus), labyrinthitis, aminoglycoside toxicity, benign positional vertigo, vestibular neuronitis, brainstem ischemia and infarction, basilar artery migraine, cerebellar infarction, acoustic neuroma, motion sickness, excess of ethanol, quinine, or salicylic acid

VOMITING

(See Nausea and Vomiting page 42.)

WEIGHT LOSS

Normal or Increased Appetite: Diabetes, hyperthyroidism, anxiety, drugs (thyroid), carcinoid, malabsorption (sprue, pancreatic deficiency), parasites

Decreased Appetite: Depression, anorexia nervosa, GI obstruction, carcinoma, liver disease, severe infection, severe cardiopulmonary disease including end-stage COPD, uremia, adrenal insufficiency, hypercalcemia, hypokalemia, intoxication (alcohol, lead), old age, drugs (amphetamines, digitalis), HIV and AIDS

WHEEZING

Large airway difficulty (laryngeal stridor, tracheal stenosis, foreign body, epiglottitis, vocal cord dysfunction), endobronchial tumor, asthma, bronchitis, emphysema, aspiration, pulmonary embolus, anaphylactic reactions, myocardial ischemia with pulmonary edema

LABORATORY DIAGNOSIS: CHEMISTRY, IMMUNOLOGY, SEROLOGY

Principles of Laboratory Testing
ACTH
Albumin
Aldosterone
Alkaline Phosphatase
Alpha-fetoprotein (AFP)
ALT
Ammonia
Amylase
Anti-CCP
ASO Titer
AST
Autoantibodies
Base Excess/Deficit
Beta-Hydroxybutyrate (BHB)
Bicarbonate
Bilirubin
Blood Urea Nitrogen (BUN)
BUN/Creatinine Ratio
C-Peptide
C-Reactive Protein
CA 15-3
CA 19-9
CA-125
Calcitonin
Calcium, Serum
Carbon Dioxide
Carboxyhemoglobin
Carcinoembryonic Antigen (CEA)
Catecholamines, Fractionated Serum
Chloride, Serum
Cholesterol
Clostridium difficile Toxin Assay, Fecal
Cold Agglutinins
Complement (C3, C4, CH_{50})
Cortisol, Serum
Cortrosyn Stimulation Test, 1-Hour ("Short")
Creatine Kinase, Total
Creatinine, Serum
Cryoglobulins
Cytomegalovirus Antibodies
D-Dimer
Dehydroepiandrosterone
Dehydroepiandrosterone Sulfate
Dexamethasone Suppression Test
Erythropoietin

Estradiol, Serum
Estrogen/Progesterone Receptors
Ethanol
Fecal Fat
Fecal Occult Blood Testing (FOBT)
Ferritin
Folate
Follicle-Stimulating Hormone (FSH)
FTA-ABS
Fungal Serologies
Gastrin, Serum
Glucose
Glucose Tolerance Test, Oral
Glutamyl Transferase (GGT)
Glycohemoglobin
Haptoglobin
Helicobacter pylori Antibody Titers
Helicobacter pylori Antigen, Feces
Hepatitis Testing
High-Density Lipoprotein Cholesterol
HLA
Homocysteine, Serum
Human Chorionic Gonadotropin, Serum (HCG)
Human Immunodeficiency Antibody (HIV) Testing
Immunoglobulins, Quantitative
Iron
Iron-Binding Capacity, Total
Lactate Dehydrogenase (LDH)
Lactic Acid
LAP Score
LE Preparation
Lead, Blood
Legionella Antibody
Lipase
Low-Density Lipoprotein Cholesterol
Luteinizing Hormone
Lyme Disease Serology
Magnesium
MHA-TP
β_2-Microglobulin
Monospot
Myoglobin
Natriuretic Peptide, B-Type
Natriuretic Peptide, NT-Pro B-Type
Newborn Screening Panel

(continued)

5'-Nucleotidase	Rocky Mountain Spotted Fever
Oligoclonal Banding, CSF	Antibodies
Osmolality, Serum	Semen Analysis
Oxygen	Sodium, Serum
Parathyroid Hormone	Stool for Occult Blood
Phosphorus	Sweat Chloride
Potassium, Serum	N-Telopeptide (NTx) (Urine and Serum)
Prealbumin	Testosterone
Pregnancy Screening	Thyroglobulin
Progesterone	Thyroid-Stimulating Hormone
Prolactin	Thyroxine, Free (FT_4)
Prostate-Specific Antigen (PSA)	TORCH Battery
Protein Electrophoresis, Serum and	Transferrin
Urine	Triglycerides
Protein, Serum	Triiodothyronine (T_3)
Rapid Plasma Reagin (RPR)	Troponin, Cardiac-Specific
Renin, Plasma	Uric Acid
Renin, Renal Vein	VDRL Test
Retinol-Binding Protein	Vitamin B_{12}
Rheumatoid Factor	Zinc

PRINCIPLES OF LABORATORY TESTING

This chapter outlines commonly ordered blood chemistry, immunology, and serology tests and other common laboratory investigations. Normal values and a guide to the diagnosis of common abnormalities are provided. Additional tests are described in the following chapters: hematology, Chapter 5; urine studies, Chapter 6; microbiology, Chapter 7; and Blood Gases, Chapter 8. Increased or decreased values that are not clinically useful usually are not listed. Because each laboratory has its own set of normal reference intervals, the normal values given should be used only as a guide. Unless specified, values reflect normal levels in adults. The method of collection is included because laboratories have attempted to standardize collection methods; however, be aware that some labs may have other collection methods. Blood specimen tubes are listed in Chapter 13, page 318.

Most laboratories offer AMA-recommended "panel" tests, whereby multiple determinations are performed on a single sample. Although labs may vary, common chemistry panels include the following:

- **AMA Electrolyte Panel:** Sodium, potassium, chloride, CO_2
- **AMA Basic Metabolic Panel:** Calcium, CO_2, chloride, creatinine, glucose, potassium, sodium, BUN
- **AMA Comprehensive Metabolic Panel:** albumin, ALT, AST, total bilirubin, calcium, chloride, CO_2, creatinine, glucose, alkaline phosphatase, potassium, total protein, sodium, BUN
- **AMA Renal Function Panel:** Albumin, calcium, CO_2, chloride, creatinine, glucose, phosphorus serum, potassium, sodium, BUN
- **AMA Hepatic Function Panel:** Total protein, albumin, total bilirubin, direct bilirubin, alkaline phosphate, AST, ALT
- **AMA Lipid Panel:** Cholesterol, HDL, LDL (*calculated from cholesterol and hydroxycholesterol [HC]*), triglycerides

Other Common Panel Tests

Chem-7 Panel/SMA-7: BUN, creatinine, electrolytes (Na, K, Cl, CO_2), glucose

Health Screen-12/SMA-12: Albumin, alkaline phosphatase, AST (SGOT), bilirubin (total), calcium, cholesterol, creatinine, glucose, LDH, phosphate, protein (total), uric acid

Cardiac Enzymes: CK-MB (if total CK > 150 IU/L), troponin

Every reimbursable laboratory test has an associated CPT code used for billing transactions. The CPT (*Current Procedural Terminology*) system was developed by and is a registered trademark of the American Medical Association (AMA). CPT codes have been incorporated as the standard code set for Medicare and Medicaid reimbursement. They also are used in the Health Insurance Portability and Accountability Act (HIPAA) and have been adopted by private insurance carriers and managed care companies.

CPT codes are designated for services that are part of "contemporary medical practice and being performed by many physicians in clinical practice in multiple locations." Each of the codes consists of a five-digit number that is associated with a text descriptor (eg, 82565, Creatinine; blood).

To comply with government regulations as specified by the Centers for Medicare & Medicaid Services (CMS), clinical pathology laboratories require physicians who order tests to provide appropriate *International Classification of Disease, Ninth Revision* (*ICD-9*) diagnosis and procedure codes that in turn indicate which laboratory tests are reimbursable.

ACTH (ADRENOCORTICOTROPIC HORMONE, CORTICOTROPIN)

- 7–10 AM 10–50 pg/mL, PM results are lower • Collection: Lavender top tube

Increased: Addison disease (primary adrenal hypofunction), ectopic ACTH production (small [oat]-cell lung carcinoma, pancreatic islet cell tumors, thymic tumors, renal cell carcinoma, bronchial carcinoid), Cushing disease (pituitary adenoma), congenital adrenal hyperplasia (adrenogenital syndrome)

Decreased: Adrenal adenoma or carcinoma, nodular adrenal hyperplasia, pituitary insufficiency, corticosteroid use

ALBUMIN

- Adult 3.5–5.0 g/dL, child 3.8–5.4 g/dL • Collection: Tiger top tube; part of SMA-12

Decreased: Malnutrition, overhydration, nephrotic syndrome, CF, multiple myeloma, Hodgkin disease, leukemia, metastatic cancer, protein-losing enteropathies, chronic glomerulonephritis, alcoholic cirrhosis, inflammatory bowel disease, collagen–vascular diseases, hyperthyroidism

ALDOSTERONE

- Serum: Supine 3–10 ng/dL early AM, normal sodium intake (3 g sodium/d)
- Upright 5–30 ng/dL; urinary 2–16 mcg/24 h • Collection: Green or lavender top tube

Discontinue antihypertensives and diuretics 2 wk before test. Upright samples should be drawn after 2 h. Primarily used to screen hypertensive patients for possible Conn syndrome (adrenal adenoma producing excess aldosterone)

Increased: Primary hyperaldosteronism, secondary hyperaldosteronism (CHF, sodium depletion, nephrotic syndrome, cirrhosis with ascites, others), upright posture

Decreased: Adrenal insufficiency, panhypopituitarism, supine posture

ALKALINE PHOSPHATASE

• Adult 25–160 IU/L, child 40–400 IU/L (method dependent) • Collection: Tiger top tube; part of SMA-12

A fractionated alkaline phosphatase was formerly used to differentiate the origin of the enzyme in the bone from that in the liver. Replaced by GGT and 5′-nucleotidase measurements

Increased: (Highest levels in biliary obstruction and infiltrative liver disease) Increased calcium deposition in bone (hyperparathyroidism), Paget disease, osteoblastic bone tumors (metastatic or osteogenic sarcoma), osteomalacia, rickets, PRG, childhood, healing fracture, liver disease, eg, biliary obstruction (masses, drug therapy), hyperthyroidism

Decreased: Malnutrition, excess vitamin D ingestion, pernicious anemia, Wilson disease, hypothyroidism, zinc deficiency

ALPHA-FETOPROTEIN (AFP)

• < 6 mg/mL • Third trimester of PRG maximum 550 mg/mL • Collection: Tiger top tube

Increased: Hepatoma (hepatocellular carcinoma), testicular tumor (embryonal carcinoma, malignant teratoma), neural tube defects (in mother's serum [spina bifida, anencephaly, myelomeningocele]), fetal death, multiple gestations, ataxia–telangiectasia, some cases of benign hepatic disease (alcoholic cirrhosis, hepatitis, necrosis)

Decreased: Trisomy 21 (Down syndrome) in maternal serum

ALT (ALANINE AMINOTRANSFERASE)

• 1–45 IU/L, higher in newborns • Collection: Tiger top or red top tube

Increased: Liver disease, liver metastasis, biliary obstruction, pancreatitis, liver congestion (ALT is more elevated than AST in viral hepatitis; AST elevated more than ALT in alcoholic hepatitis)

AMMONIA

• Adult 15–45 mcg/dL (9–27 µmol/L) • Collection: Green top tube, on ice, analyze immediately

Increased: Liver failure, Reye syndrome, inborn errors of metabolism, healthy neonate (normalizes within 48 h of birth)

AMYLASE

• 10–130 U/L (method dependent) • Collection: Tiger top or red top tube

Increased: Acute pancreatitis, pancreatic duct obstruction (stones, stricture, tumor, sphincter spasm secondary to drugs), pancreatic pseudocyst or abscess, alcohol ingestion, mumps, parotiditis, renal disease, macroamylasemia, cholecystitis, peptic ulcer, intestinal obstruction, mesenteric thrombosis, aftermath of surgery

Decreased: Pancreatic destruction (pancreatitis, cystic fibrosis), liver damage (hepatitis, cirrhosis), healthy infant in first year of life

ANTI-CCP (ANTI–CYCLIC CITRULLINATED POLYPEPTIDE ANTIBODIES)

- < 20 EU (ELISA units, assay dependent) • Weak positive: 20–39 EU; moderate positive: 40–59 EU; strong positive: > 60 EU • Collection: Tiger top or red top tube
  Used with RA agglutinin test to diagnose RA. May be positive in early disease, differentiates positive RA test in other diseases

Increased: RA (specificity > 95%, sensitivity 80%), rare false-positives with hepatitis and autoimmune thyroid disease

ASO TITER (ANTISTREPTOLYSIN O/ANTISTREPTOCOCCAL O, STREPTOZYME)

- < 200 IU/mL (Todd units) school-age children • < 100 IU/mL preschool and adults • Varies with lab • Collection: Tiger top tube

Increased: Streptococcal infection (pharyngitis, scarlet fever, rheumatic fever, poststreptococcal glomerulonephritis), RA, other collagen diseases

AST (ASPARTATE AMINOTRANSFERASE)

- 7–42 IU/L • Collection: Tiger top or red top tube; part of SMA-12
  Generally parallels changes in ALT in liver disease

Increased: AMI, liver disease, Reye syndrome, muscle trauma and injection, pancreatitis, intestinal injury or surgery, factitious increase (erythromycin, opiates), burns, cardiac catheterization, brain damage, renal infarction

Decreased: Beriberi (vitamin B_6 deficiency), severe diabetes with ketoacidosis, liver disease, chronic hemodialysis

AUTOANTIBODIES

- Normal = negative • Collection: Tiger top tube

Antinuclear Antibody (ANA, FANA)

Useful screening test in patients with symptoms suggesting collagen–vascular disease, especially if titer is > 1:160. 5% of healthy people can have positive test.

Positive: SLE, drug-induced lupus-like syndromes (eg, from procainamide, hydralazine, isoniazid), scleroderma, MCTD, RA, polymyositis, juvenile RA (5–20%). Low titers are also seen in diseases other than collagen–vascular disease.

Specific Immunofluorescent ANA Patterns

Homogenous. Nonspecific, from antibodies to DNP and native double-stranded DNA. Seen in SLE and a variety of other diseases. Antihistone is consistent with drug-induced lupus.

Speckled. Pattern seen in many connective tissue disorders. From antibodies to ENA, including anti-RNP, anti-Sm, anti-PM-1, and anti-SS. Anti-RNP is positive in MCTD and SLE. Anti-Sm is highly specific for SLE (found in 30% of cases). Anti-SS-A and anti-SS-B are found in Sjögren syndrome and subacute cutaneous lupus.

Peripheral Rim Pattern. From antibodies to native double-stranded DNA and DNP. Seen in SLE

Nucleolar Pattern. From antibodies to nucleolar RNA. Positive in Sjögren syndrome and scleroderma

Anticentromere: CREST syndrome, scleroderma, Raynaud disease

Anti-DNA (Anti–double-stranded DNA): SLE (but negative in drug-induced lupus), chronic active hepatitis, mononucleosis

Antimitochondrial: Primary biliary cirrhosis, autoimmune diseases, eg, SLE

Antineutrophil Cytoplasmic (ANCA)
- **c-ANCA:** Wegener granulomatosis (high titer = 1:80, highly predictive of Wegener granulomatosis)
- **p-ANCA:** Polyarteritis nodosa and other forms of vasculitis, including Churg–Strauss and microscopic polyarteritis
- **x- or atypical ANCA:** Ulcerative colitis

Anti-CCP: Rheumatoid arthritis

Anti-SCL 70: Scleroderma

Antimicrosomal: Hashimoto thyroiditis

Anti–Smooth Muscle: Low titers in a variety of illnesses; high titers (> 1:100) suggestive of chronic active hepatitis

Sjögren Syndrome Antibody (SS-A): Sjögren syndrome, SLE, RA

BASE EXCESS/DEFICIT
- –2 to +2 • See Chapter 8, page 165

BETA-HYDROXYBUTYRATE (BHB)
- 0.2–3.0 mg/dL • Collection: Tiger top or red top tube

Replaces acetoacetate (acetone) in the diagnosis and management of DKA. BHB accounts for about 75% of the ketone bodies in blood; during periods of DKA, BHB increases more than the other two ketoacids (acetoacetate and acetone). BHB is used to assess the severity of DKA and to exclude hyperosmolar nonketotic diabetic coma. It is also useful in the detection of subclinical ketosis and in the management of DKA.

Positive: DKA, starvation, acute alcohol abuse

BICARBONATE ("TOTAL CO₂")
- 23–29 mmol/L • See Carbon Dioxide, page 55

BILIRUBIN
- Total, 0.3–1.0 mg/dL • Direct, < 0.2 mg/dL • Indirect, < 0.8 mg/dL
- Collection: Tiger top tube

Increased Total: Hepatic damage (hepatitis, toxins, cirrhosis), biliary obstruction (stone or tumor), hemolysis, fasting

Increased Direct (Conjugated): Note: Determination of direct bilirubin is usually unnecessary with total bilirubin levels < 1.2 mg/dL; biliary obstruction/cholestasis (gallstone, tumor, stricture), drug-induced cholestasis, Dubin–Johnson and Rotor syndromes

Increased Indirect (Unconjugated): Calculated as total minus direct bilirubin. Hemolytic jaundice caused by any type of hemolytic anemia (eg, transfusion reaction, sickle cell), Gilbert disease, physiologic jaundice of the newborn, Crigler–Najjar syndrome

Bilirubin, Neonatal ("Baby Bilirubin")

• Normal dependent on prematurity and age in days • Critical values usually > 15–20 mg/dL in term infants • Collection: Capillary tube

Increased: Erythroblastosis fetalis, physiologic jaundice (may be due to breast feeding), resorption of hematoma or hemorrhage, obstructive jaundice, others

BLOOD UREA NITROGEN (BUN)

• Birth–1 y: 4–16 mg/dL • 1–40 y 5–20 mg/dL • Gradual slight increase with age • Collection: Tiger top tube
    Less useful measure of GFR than creatinine because BUN is also related to protein metabolism

Increased: Renal failure (including drug-induced from aminoglycosides, NSAIDs), prerenal azotemia (decreased renal perfusion secondary to CHF, shock, volume depletion), postrenal (obstruction), GI bleeding, stress, drugs (especially aminoglycosides)

Decreased: Starvation, liver failure (hepatitis, drugs), PRG, infancy, nephrotic syndrome, overhydration

BUN/CREATININE RATIO (BUN/CR)

• Mean 10, range 6–20; calculation based on serum levels

Increased: Prerenal azotemia (renal hypoperfusion can be due to decreased volume, CHF, cirrhosis/ascites, nephrosis), GI bleed (ratio often > 30), high-protein diet, sepsis/hypermetabolic state, ileal conduit, drugs (steroids, tetracycline)

Decreased: Malnutrition, PRG, low-protein diet, ketoacidosis, hemodialysis, SIADH, drugs

C-PEPTIDE, INSULIN ("CONNECTING PEPTIDE")

• Fasting, 1–5 mg/mL (method dependent) • Collection: Tiger top or red top tube
    Used to differentiate endogenous insulin from exogenous and production/administration; liberated when proinsulin split to insulin; levels reflect endogenous insulin production

Increased: Insulinoma, sulfonylurea ingestion

Decreased: Type 1 diabetes (decreased endogenous insulin), insulin administration (factitious or therapeutic), factitious hypoglycemia

C-REACTIVE PROTEIN (CRP)

• Normal < 0.8 mg/dL • Collection: Tiger top or red top tube
    A nonspecific screen for infectious and inflammatory diseases, correlates with ESR. In the first 24 h, however, ESR may be normal and CRP elevated. CRP returns to normal more quickly than ESR in response to therapy.

Increased: Bacterial infections, inflammatory conditions (acute rheumatic fever, acute RA, MI, unstable angina, transplant rejection, embolus, inflammatory bowel disease), last half of PRG, oral contraceptives, some malignant diseases

CA 15-3

• < 35 U/mL • Collection: Tiger top or red top tube
   Used to detect breast cancer recurrence and monitor therapy. Levels related to stage of disease

Increased: Progressive breast cancer, benign breast disease and liver disease

Decreased: Response to therapy (25% change considered significant)

CA 19-9

• < 37 U/mL • Collection: Tiger top tube
   Primarily used to determine resectability of pancreatic cancer (ie, > 1000 U/mL 95% unresectable)

Increased: GI cancers, eg, pancreas, stomach, liver, colorectal, hepatobiliary, some cases of lung and prostate, pancreatitis

CA-125

• < 35 U/mL • Collection: Tiger top tube
   Not useful screening test for ovarian cancer; best used in conjunction with ultrasonography and physical exam. Rising levels after resection predictive of recurrence

Increased: Ovarian, endometrial, and colon cancer; endometriosis; inflammatory bowel disease; PID; PRG; breast lesions; benign abdominal masses (teratomas)

CALCITONIN (THYROCALCITONIN)

• < 19 pg/mL (method dependent) • Collection: Tiger top tube
   Increased: Medullary carcinoma of the thyroid, C-cell hyperplasia (precursor of medullary carcinoma), small (oat)-cell carcinoma of the lung, newborn state, PRG, chronic renal insufficiency, Zollinger–Ellison syndrome, pernicious anemia

CALCIUM, SERUM

• Infants younger than 1 mo: 7–11.5 mg/dL • 1 mo–1 y: 8.6–11.2 mg/dL
• > 1 y and adults: 8.2–10.2 mg/dL • Ionized: 4.75–5.2 mg/dL • Collection: Tiger top or red top tube; ionized green or red top tube
   For interpretation of total calcium, albumin must be known. If albumin is not normal, corrected calcium is estimated with the following formula. Values for ionized calcium need no special corrections.

   Corrected total Ca = 0.8 (Normal albumin – Measured albumin) + Reported Ca

Increased: (*Note:* Levels > 12 mg/dL may lead to coma and death.) Primary hyperparathyroidism, PTH-secreting tumors, vitamin D excess, metastatic bone tumors, osteoporosis, immobilization, milk–alkali syndrome, Paget disease, idiopathic hypercalcemia of infants, infantile hypophosphatasia, thiazide diuretics, chronic renal failure, sarcoidosis, multiple myeloma

Decreased: (Levels < 7 mg/dL may lead to tetany and death.) Hypoparathyroidism (surgical, idiopathic), pseudohypoparathyroidism, insufficient vitamin D, calcium and phosphorus ingestion (PRG, osteomalacia, rickets), hypomagnesemia, RTA, hypoalbuminemia (cachexia, nephrotic syndrome, CF), chronic renal failure (phosphate retention), acute pancreatitis, factitious condition (low protein and albumin)

CARBON DIOXIDE ("TOTAL CO_2" OR BICARBONATE)

• Adult 23–29 mmol/L, child 20–28 mmol/L • (See Chapter 8 for P_{CO_2} values) • Collection: Tiger top tube; do not expose sample to air

Increased: Compensation for respiratory acidosis (emphysema) and metabolic alkalosis (severe vomiting, primary aldosteronism, volume contraction, Bartter syndrome)

Decreased: Compensation for respiratory alkalosis and metabolic acidosis (starvation, DKA, lactic acidosis, alcoholic ketoacidosis, toxins [methanol, ethylene glycol, paraldehyde], severe diarrhea, renal failure, drugs [salicylates, acetazolamide], dehydration, adrenal insufficiency)

CARBOXYHEMOGLOBIN (CARBON MONOXIDE)

• Nonsmoker < 2% • Smoker < 9% • Toxic > 15% • Collection: Gray or lavender top tube; confirm with lab

Increased: Smokers, smoke inhalation, automobile exhaust inhalation, healthy newborns

CARCINOEMBRYONIC ANTIGEN (CEA)

• Nonsmoker < 3.0 ng/mL • Smoker < 5.0 ng/mL • Collection: Tiger top or red top tube

Not a cancer screening test; used to monitor response to treatment and tumor recurrence in GI tract adenocarcinoma

Increased: Carcinoma (colon, pancreas, lung, stomach), smokers, nonneoplastic liver disease, Crohn disease, ulcerative colitis

CATECHOLAMINES, FRACTIONATED SERUM

• Collection: Green or lavender tube; check with lab

Values vary and depend on the lab and method of assay used. Normal levels shown here are based on an HPLC technique. Patient must be supine in a non-stimulating environment with IV access to obtain sample.

Catecholamine	Plasma (Supine) Levels
Norepinephrine	70–750 pg/mL (SI: 414–435 pmol/L)
Epinephrine	0–100 pg/mL (SI: 0–546 pmol/L)
Dopamine	< 30 pg/mL (SI: 196 pmol/L)

Increased: Pheochromocytoma, neural crest tumors (neuroblastoma); with extra-adrenal pheochromocytoma norepinephrine may be markedly elevated compared with epinephrine

TABLE 4–1
National Cholesterol Education Program New Clinical Guidelines for Cholesterol Testing and Management

STEP 1: Complete lipoprotein profile (mg/dL) after 9- to 12-h fast

<70	Low LDL
70–99	Optimal
100–129	Near optimal/above optimal
130–159	Borderline high
160–189	High
≥190	Very high

STEP 2: Identify presence of clinical atherosclerotic disease that confers high risk for CHD events (CHD risk equivalent):

Clinical CHD or symmptomatic CAD or peripheral arterial disease, TIA, AAA, or diabetes.

STEP 3: Determine presence of major risk factors (other than LDL):

Cigarette smoking; HTN (BP ≥140/90 mm Hg or on BP medications); HDL <40 mg/dL (if ≥60 mg/dL remove one risk factor from count); family history of premature CHD (CHD in male relative <55 y; CHD in female relative <65 y); age (men ≥45 y; women ≥55 y).

STEP 4: If 2+ risk factors (other than LDL) are present without CHD or CHD risk equivalent, assess 10-y (short-term) CHD risk (see Framingham tables @ http://www.nhlbi.nih.gov/guidelines/cholesterol/risk_tbl.htm).

Three levels of 10-y risk: >20%, 10–20%, <10%

STEP 5: Establish LDL goal of therapy, determine need for TLC, determine level for drug consideration.

Risk Category	LDL Goal (mg/dL)	LDL Level to Initiate TLC (mg/dL)	LDL Level to Consider Drug Therapy (mg/dL)
[a]Very high risk (CHD or CHD equivalents) (10-yr risk > 20%)	<70	>70	>70[a]
High risk (CHD or CHD risk equivalents) (10-yr risk >20%)	<100	>100	>100
Moderately high risk 2+ risk factors (10-yr risk 10–20%)	<100	≥100	≥130
Moderate risk 2+ risk factors (10-yr risk < 10%)	<130	≥130	≥160
[b]Low risk 0–1 risk factors (10-yr risk < 10%)	<160	≥160	≥190

[a]Some use LDL-lowering drugs in this category if an LDL cholesterol <70 or 100 mg/dL cannot be achieved by lifestyle changes. Others use drugs that modify triglycerides and HDL, eg, nicotinic acid or fibrate.
[b]Almost all people with 0–1 risk factor have a 10-y risk <10%, thus 10-y risk assessment in people with 0–1 risk factor is not necessary.

(continued)

TABLE 4-1 (continued)

STEP 6: Initiate TLC if LDL is above goal.

TLC diet: Saturated fat <7% of calories, cholesterol <200 mg/d, increased viscous (soluble) fiber (10–25 g/d) and plant stanols/sterols (2 g/d), weight management, and increased physical activity.

STEP 7: Consider adding drug therapy if LDL exceeds levels shown in Step 5 table:

HMG-CoA reductase inhibitors (statins), bile acid sequestrants, nicotinic acid.

STEP 8: Identify metabolic syndrome and treat, if present, after 3 mo of TLC. Metabolic syndrome present if any 3 of the following present:

Risk Factor	Defining Level
Abdominal obesity	Waist circumference[a]
Men	>102 cm (>40 in)
Women	>88 cm (>35 in)
Triglycerides	≥150 mg/dL
HDL cholesterol	
Men	<40 mg/dL
Women	<50 mg/dL
BP	≥130/≥85 mm Hg
Fasting glucose	≥110 mg/dL

[a]Overweight and obesity are associated with insulin resistance and the metabolic syndrome.

Manage metabolic syndrome: control underlying causes (overweight/obesity and physical inactivity); control lipid and non-lipid risk factors if they persist despite these lifestyle therapies; manage HTN, aspirin for CHD prevention; control elevated triglycerides and/or low HDL (as shown in Step 9).

STEP 9: Manage elevated triglycerides (≥150 mg/dL): Primary aim of therapy is to reach LDL goal; intensify weight management, increase physical activity; if triglycerides ≥200 mg/dL after LDL goal is reached, set secondary goal for non-HDL–cholesterol (total HDL) 30 mg/dL higher than LDL goal.

Classification of Serum Triglycerides (mg/dL)	
<150	Normal
150–199	Borderline high
200–499	High
≥500	Very high

(continued)

TABLE 4–1 (continued)

Comparison of LDL Cholesterol and Non-HDL Cholesterol Goals for Three Risk Categories

Risk Category	LDL Goal (mg/dL)	Non-HDL Goal (mg/dL)
CHD and CHD risk equivalent (10-y risk for CHD >20%)	<100	<130
Multiple (2+) risk factors and 10-y risk 20%	<130	<160
0–1 risk factor	<160	<190

- **If triglycerides 200–499 mg/dL after LDL goal is reached, consider adding drug if needed to reach non-HDL goal:** Intensify therapy with LDL-lowering drug, or add nicotinic acid or fibrate to further lower VLDL.

- **If triglycerides ≥500 mg/dL, first lower triglycerides to prevent pancreatitis:** Very-low-fat diet (≤15% of calories from fat), weight management and physical activity, fibrate or nicotinic acid, when triglycerides <500 mg/dL, turn to LDL-lowering therapy.

- **Management of low HDL cholesterol (<40 mg/dL):** First reach LDL goal, then weight management and increase physical activity; if triglycerides 200–499 mg/dL, achieve non-HDL goal. If triglycerides <200 mg/dL (isolated low HDL) in CHD or CHD equivalent, consider nicotinic acid or fibrate.

LDL = low-density lipoprotein; HDL = high-density lipoprotein; CHD = coronary heart disease; CAD = carotid artery disease; AAA = abdominal aortic aneurysm; HTN = hypertension; BP = blood pressure; TLC = therapeutic lifestyle changes; HMG-CoA = hydroxymethylglutaryl coenzyme A.
Based on the Third Report of the Expert Panel on Detection, Evaluation, and Treatment of High Blood Cholesterol in Adults (Adult Treatment Panel or ATP III) (http://www.nhlbi.nih.gov/guidelines/cholesterol) accessed March, 10, 2006, U.S. Department of Health and Human Services, National Institutes of Health, National Heart, Lung, and Blood Institute, Bethesda, MD.

CHLORIDE, SERUM

- 97–107 mEq/L • Collection: Tiger top tube
  Included with electrolytes in most metabolic panels

Increased: Diarrhea, RTA, mineralocorticoid deficiency, hyperalimentation, medications (acetazolamide, ammonium chloride)

Decreased: Vomiting, DM with ketoacidosis, mineralocorticoid excess, renal disease with sodium loss

CHOLESTEROL

- Total • Normal, Table 4–1, page 56; see also Lipid profile, page 77, and Table 4–2, page 59 • Collection: Tiger top or red top tube

TABLE 4–2
Lipoproteins

Frederickson Classification System	Type I (Rare)	Type IIa (Common)	Type IIb (Common)	Type III (Uncommon)	Type IV (Uncommon)	Type V (Uncommon)
Cholesterol	N or slightly ↑	Very ↑	Very ↑	Very ↑	N or slightly ↑	↑
LDL	N	↑	↑	↑	N	N
HDL	N or ↓	N or ↓	N or ↓	N or ↓	N or ↓	N or ↓
Triglycerides	Very ↑	N	↑	Very ↑	Very ↑	↑
Increased lipoproteins	Chylomicrons	LDL	LDL, VLDL	LDL	VLDL	VLDL and chylomicrons
Atherogenesis risk	No increase	Very ↑	↑	↑	No increase	No increase

Increased: Idiopathic hypercholesterolemia, biliary obstruction, nephrosis, hypothyroidism, pancreatic disease (diabetes), PRG, oral contraceptives, hyperlipoproteinemia (types IIb, III, V)

Decreased: Liver disease (eg, hepatitis), hyperthyroidism, malnutrition (cancer, starvation), chronic anemia, steroid therapy, lipoproteinemia, AMI

High-Density Lipoprotein Cholesterol (HDL, HDL-C)

*   Fasting men: 30–70 mg/dL • Women: 30–90 mg/dL
    HDL-C: Best correlation with the development of CAD; decreased HDL-C in men leads to increased risk. Levels < 40 mg/dL associated with increased risk of CAD. Levels > 60 mg/dL associated with decreased risk of CAD

Increased: Estrogen (menstruating women), regular exercise, small ethanol intake, medications (nicotinic acid, gemfibrozil, others)

Decreased: Men, smoking, uremia, obesity, diabetes, liver disease, Tangier disease

Low-Density Lipoprotein Cholesterol (LDL, LDL-C)

*   50–190 mg/dL
    Elevated levels correlate with CAD risk.

Increased: Excess dietary saturated fats, hyperlipoproteinemia, biliary cirrhosis, endocrine disease (diabetes, hypothyroidism)

Decreased: Malabsorption, severe liver disease, abetalipoproteinemia

CLOSTRIDIUM DIFFICILE TOXIN ASSAY, FECAL

*   Normal = negative

Positive: > 90% of cases of pseudomembranous colitis; 30–40% of antibiotic-associated colitis, and 6–10% of antibiotic-associated diarrhea. False-positive in some healthy adults and neonates

COLD AGGLUTININS

*   < 1:32 • Collection: Lavender or blue top tube
    Most frequently used to screen for atypical pneumonia

Increased: Atypical pneumonia (mycoplasmal pneumonia), other viral infections (especially mononucleosis, measles, mumps), cirrhosis, parasitic infections, Waldenström macroglobulinemia, lymphoma and leukemia, multiple myeloma

COMPLEMENT

*   Collection: Tiger or red top tube
    Complement describes a series of sequentially reacting serum proteins that participate in pathogenic processes and cause inflammatory injury.

Complement C3

*   85–155 mg/dL (method dependent)
    Decreased level suggests activation of the classical or alternative pathway or both.

Increased: RA (variable finding), rheumatic fever, various neoplasms (GI, prostate, others), acute viral hepatitis, MI, PRG, amyloidosis

Decreased: SLE, glomerulonephritis (poststreptococcal and membranoproliferative), sepsis, SBE, chronic active hepatitis, malnutrition, DIC, gram-negative sepsis

Complement C4

- 20–50 mg/dL (method dependent)

Increased: RA (variable finding), neoplasia (GI, lung, others)

Decreased: SLE, chronic active hepatitis, cirrhosis, glomerulonephritis, hereditary angioedema (test of choice)

Complement CH$_{50}$ (Total)

- 33–61 mg/mL (method dependent)
  Tests of complement deficiency in the classical pathway

Increased: Acute-phase reactants (eg, tissue injury, infections)

Decreased: Hereditary complement deficiencies

CORTISOL, SERUM

- 8 AM, 5.0–23.0 mg/dL • 4 PM, 3.0–15.0 mg/dL (method dependent) • Collection: Green or red top tube

Increased: Adrenal adenoma, adrenal carcinoma, Cushing disease, nonpituitary ACTH-producing tumor, steroid therapy, oral contraceptives

Decreased: Primary adrenal insufficiency (Addison disease), congenital adrenal hyperplasia, Waterhouse–Friderichsen syndrome, ACTH deficiency

CORTROSYN STIMULATION TEST, 1-HOUR ("SHORT")

- Collection: Red top tube
  Used to diagnose adrenal insufficiency. Cortrosyn, an ACTH analogue, is given (0.25 mg IM or IV in adults). Blood is collected for serum cortisol measurement 60 min later. Consider obtaining informed consent for this chemically invasive procedure.

Normal response: Serum cortisol increase > 20 mcg/dL 60 min after Cortrosyn is given.

Abnormal response: Serum cortisol < 20 mcg/dL 60 min after Cortrosyn administration; primary adrenal insufficiency (Addison disease), pituitary insufficiency (insufficient stimulation of the adrenal glands by pituitary ACTH), or chronic suppression by exogenous steroids

CREATINE KINASE, TOTAL (CK)

- 25–145 mU/mL • Collection: Tiger top tube
  Used in suspected MI or muscle diseases. Heart, skeletal muscle, and brain have high levels.

Increased: Muscle damage (AMI, myocarditis, muscular dystrophy, muscle trauma [including injections], aftermath of surgery), brain infarction, defibrillation, cardiac catheterization and surgery, rhabdomyolysis, polymyositis, hypothyroidism

CPK Isoenzymes

MB: (Normal < 6%, heart origin) increased in AMI (begins in 2–12 h, peaks at 12–40 h, returns to normal in 24–72 h); troponin is marker of choice for AMI; pericarditis with myocarditis, rhabdomyolysis, crush injury, Duchenne muscular dystrophy, polymyositis, malignant hyperthermia, cardiac surgery

MM: (Normal 94–100%, skeletal muscle origin) increased in crush injury, malignant hyperthermia, seizures, IM injections

BB: (Normal 0%, brain origin) brain injury (CVA, trauma), metastatic neoplasms (eg, prostate), malignant hyperthermia, colonic infarction

CREATININE, SERUM (SCR)

• Men: < 1.2 mg/dL • Women: < 1.1 mg/dL • Children 0.5–0.8 mg/dL • Collection: Tiger or red top tube

   A clinically useful estimate of GFR. In general, SCr doubles with each 50% reduction in GFR. Creatine clearance based on urinary collection is considered the most accurate method (see Chapter 6).

Increased: Renal failure (prerenal, renal, or postrenal obstruction or medication-induced [aminoglycosides, NSAIDs, others]), gigantism, acromegaly, ingestion of red meat, false-positive with DKA

Decreased: PRG, decreased muscle mass, severe liver disease

CRYOGLOBULINS (CRYOCRIT)

• < 0.4% (negative if qualitative) • Collection: prewarmed red top tube; contact lab before collecting; transport at body temperature

   Cryoglobulins are abnormal proteins that precipitate out of serum at low temperatures. Cryocrit (quantitative) is preferred over qualitative method. Request analysis of positive results for immunoglobulin class and light-chain type.

Monoclonal: Multiple myeloma, Waldenström macroglobulinemia, lymphoma, CLL

Mixed Polyclonal or Mixed Monoclonal: Infectious diseases (viral, bacterial, parasitic), eg, SBE or malaria; SLE; RA; essential cryoglobulinemia; lymphoproliferative diseases; sarcoidosis; chronic liver disease (cirrhosis)

CYTOMEGALOVIRUS (CMV) ANTIBODIES

• IgM < 1:8, IgG < 1:16 • Collection: Tiger top tube

   Used in neonates (CMV is the most common intrauterine infection), post-transfusion CMV infection, screening of organ donors and recipients. Most adults have detectable titers. In neonates, CMV Ab titer may be passive from mother. CMV PCR viral load may be more useful in neonates and in diagnosing active CMV infection in adults.

Increased: Serial measurements 10–14 d apart with a 4× increase in titers or a single IgM > 1:8 suggest acute infection. Universally increased titers in AIDS. IgM most useful in neonatal infections, but many false-positives; less likely to be positive owing to maternal CMV antibodies. With IgM half-life of 1 month, takes 2–3 months to see drop.

D-DIMER (SEE ALSO CHAPTER 5, PAGE 102)

• Negative • Collection: Sky blue top tube

   D-Dimers are proteins released with fibrinolytic breakdown of fibrin; used to evaluate suspected DVT and PE; level returns to normal if clot stabilized (ie, treated with heparin) and not undergoing any further fibrin deposition or plasmin activation

Increased: DVT, PE, MI, CVA, sickle cell crisis, cancer, renal failure, CHF, life-threatening infections

DEHYDROEPIANDROSTERONE (DHEA)

• Men: 2.0–13.0 ng/mL • Premenopausal women: 1.0–11.0 ng/mL • Post-menopausal: 0.5–5.0 ng/mL (method dependent) • Collection: Red top tube

Increased: Anovulation, polycystic ovaries, adrenal hyperplasia, adrenal tumors

Decreased: Menopause

DEHYDROEPIANDROSTERONE SULFATE (DHEAS)

• Men: 30–300 mcg/dL • Women: 40–200 mcg/dL • Collection: Tiger top tube

Increased: Hyperprolactinemia, adrenal hyperplasia, adrenal tumor, polycystic ovaries, lipoid ovarian tumors

Decreased: Menopause

DEXAMETHASONE SUPPRESSION TEST

Used to confirm or exclude the diagnosis of Cushing syndrome (increased serum cortisol)

Overnight Test: The "rapid" screening version. Patient takes 1 mg of dexamethasone PO at 11 PM and fasts overnight; draw red top tube at 8 AM for serum cortisol. Consider sleeping pill hs for anxious or stressed patients. If 8 AM cortisol is < 3 mcg/dL, the pituitary–adrenal axis suppresses normally, which excludes Cushing syndrome. An 8 AM serum cortisol ≥ 3 mcg/dL is abnormal. Result should be interpreted cautiously; many false-positives (obesity, major anxiety/depression, severe stress, exogenous estrogen or anticonvulsant therapy, pregnancy, alcoholism). Use 24-h urine collection for urinary free cortisol and creatinine as a screen for Cushing syndrome in these patients (see Chapter 6).

Two-Day Low-Dose Dexamethasone Suppression Test: Day 1, draw a baseline serum cortisol (red top tube) and collect 24-h urine for free cortisol and creatinine. At 6 AM day 2, give 0.5 mg of dexamethasone PO q6h × 8 doses. On day 3, collect another 24-h urine for urinary free cortisol excretion and creatinine. On days 3 and 4 draw red top tube at 8 AM. Normal: suppression (cortisol < 5 mcg/dL) by day 4 or urinary free cortisol < 10% of baseline; this result excludes Cushing syndrome. Failure to suppress serum cortisol and/or urinary free cortisol increases the likelihood of Cushing syndrome; false-positives with rapid dexamethasone metabolizers, anticonvulsant therapy, severe depression or stress, alcoholism.

High-Dose Dexamethasone Suppression Test: Similar to the low-dose test except that 2 mg of dexamethasone is given PO q6h × 8 doses; serum cortisol is not drawn. If urinary free cortisol < 90% of baseline, suppressible pituitary adenoma is likely, otherwise a nonpituitary cause of Cushing syndrome should be sought.

ERYTHROPOIETIN (EPO)

- 4–16 mU/mL • Collection: Tiger top or red top tube
  EPO is a renal hormone that stimulates RBC production.

Increased: PRG, secondary polycythemia (eg, high altitude, COPD), tumors (renal cell carcinoma, cerebellar hemangioblastoma, hepatoma, others), PCKD, anemias with bone marrow unresponsiveness (eg, aplastic anemia, iron deficiency)

Decreased: Bilateral nephrectomy, anemia of chronic disease (ie, renal failure, nephrotic syndrome), primary polycythemia (*Note:* Determination of EPO levels before administration of recombinant EPO for renal failure is not usually necessary.)

ESTRADIOL, SERUM

- Collection: Tiger top or red top tube
  Serial measurements useful in evaluation of fetal well-being, especially in high-risk PRG; amenorrhea; and gynecomastia in male patients

Female Patients	**Normal Value**
Follicular phase	25–75 pg/mL
Midcycle peak	200–600 pg/mL
Luteal phase	100–300 pg/mL
Pregnancy	
1st trimester	1–5 ng/mL
2nd trimester	5–15 ng/mL
3rd trimester	10–40 ng/mL
Postmenopause	5–25 pg/mL
Oral contraceptives	<50 pg/mL
Male Patients	
Prepubertal	2–8 pg/mL
Adult	10–60 pg/mL

ESTROGEN/PROGESTERONE RECEPTORS

Determined with fresh surgical breast cancer specimens. Presence of the receptors (ER-positive, PR-positive) is associated with improved outcome and increased likelihood of responding to endocrine therapy (eg, tamoxifen); 50–75% of breast cancers are estrogen-receptor-positive.

ETHANOL (BLOOD ALCOHOL)

- 0 mg/dL • Collection: Tiger top or red top tube; do not use alcohol to clean venipuncture site, use povidone-iodine
  Physiologic changes can vary with degree of alcohol tolerance of an individual.

- < 50 mg/dL: Limited muscular incoordination
- 50–100 mg/dL: Pronounced incoordination
- 100–150 mg/dL: Mood and personality changes; intoxication over the legal limit in most states
- 150–400 mg/dL: Nausea, vomiting, marked ataxia, amnesia, dysarthria
- > 400 mg/dL: Coma, respiratory insufficiency and death

FECAL FAT

• Quantitative 2–6 g/d on an 80–100 g/d fat diet • 72-h collection time (refrigerate sample) • Random sample Sudan III or IV stain, < 60 droplets fat/hpf

Aids in diagnosis of malabsorption, steatorrhea. Most fat normally absorbed in small bowel

Increased: Pancreatic dysfunction (chronic pancreatitis, CF, Shwachman–Diamond syndrome), diarrhea with or without fat malabsorption (any diarrhea state alters fat absorption), regional enteritis (Crohn disease), celiac disease

FECAL OCCULT BLOOD TEST (FOBT)

• Normal: Negative • Collection: Diet free of exogenous peroxidases (fish, horseradish, turnips), no vitamin C or medicines that irritate GI tract (eg, NSAIDS). Patient collects 2–3 consecutive stool specimens and uses a wooden stick to place sample on assay card. Rectal exam sample may also be used.

Annual FOBT reduces colorectal cancer deaths 15–33%. Test based on detecting stool peroxidase activity. Hemoccult II test entails use of guaiac-impregnated paper and developer to detect oxidation of a colorless indicator to a colored (blue) one in the presence of hemoglobin pseudoperoxidase. More sensitive assays are immunochemical tests such as HemSelect (HS) and FlexSure (FS) in which anti-human hemoglobin antibodies are used to detect stool human hemoglobin.

Positive: Colon or rectal polyps or cancer, hemorrhoids, anal fissures, esophageal or gastric cancer, peptic ulcers, ulcerative colitis, Crohn disease, GERD, esophageal varices, vascular ectasia

False-Positive: Recent dental procedure with bleeding gums, eating red meat within 3 days of test, fish, turnips, horseradish, or drugs such as colchicines and oxidizing drugs (eg, iodine and boric acid)

False-Negative: High doses of vitamin C

FERRITIN

• Men: 20–500 ng/mL • Women: 20–200 ng/mL • Collection: Tiger top or red tube

Ferritin is the major storage protein for iron and is most useful in anemia work-up; used to differentiate iron deficiency from anemia of chronic disease. An acute phase reactant

Increased: Iron excess (hemochromatosis, hemosiderosis), porphyria, sideroblastic anemia, malignancies (leukemia, Hodgkin disease), type 2 DM, postpartum state, chronic inflammation (eg, RA), hyperthyroidism

Decreased: Iron deficiency (earliest and most sensitive test before RBC morphologic change)

FOLATE (FOLIC ACID)

• Serum > 3.5 mcg/L • RBC folate • 270–600 ng/mL • Collection: Lavender top tube

Serum folate fluctuates with diet. RBC levels are indicative of tissue stores. Vitamin B_{12} deficiency can impede the ability of RBCs to take up folate despite normal serum folate level.

Increased: Folic acid administration

Decreased: Malnutrition/malabsorption (folic acid deficiency), massive cellular growth (cancer) or cell turnover, ongoing hemolysis, medications (trimethoprim, some anticonvulsants, oral contraceptives), vitamin B_{12} deficiency (low RBC levels), PRG

FOLLICLE-STIMULATING HORMONE (FSH)

• Men: < 13 IU/L • Women: nonmidcycle < 20 IU/L, midcycle surge < 40 IU/L; midcycle peak should be 2 × basal level • Postmenopausal 40–160 IU/L • Collection: Tiger top or red top tube

Used in work-up of impotence, male infertility, and female amenorrhea

Increased: (Hypergonadotropic > 40 IU/L) postmenopausal, surgical/chemical castration, gonadal failure, gonadotropin-secreting pituitary adenoma

Decreased: (Hypogonadotropic < 5 IU/L) prepubertal, hypothalamic and pituitary dysfunction, PRG

FTA-ABS (FLUORESCENT TREPONEMAL ANTIBODY ABSORBED)

• Normal = nonreactive • Collection: Tiger top tube

Test of choice to confirm syphilis after positive RPR. Can be negative in early primary syphilis and remain positive after treatment

Positive: Syphilis, other treponemal infections (yaws, pinta, bejel); false-positive (Lyme disease, leprosy, malaria), PRG, other diseases with increased ANA or immunoglobulins

FUNGAL SEROLOGIES

• Negative or no bands identified • Collection: Tiger top or red top tube

A screen for fungal antibodies; used to detect antibodies to *Histoplasma capsulatum, Blastomyces dermatitidis, Aspergillus* species, *Candida* species, and *Coccidioides immitis.* Serum clinical utility limited; best for testing CSF for *Coccidioides*

GASTRIN, SERUM

• Fasting < 100 pg/mL • Postprandial 95–140 pg/mL • Collection: Tiger top tube, immediately transport to lab and freeze serum

Make sure patient is not taking H_2 blockers or antacids.

Increased: Zollinger–Ellison syndrome, medications (antacids, H_2 blockers, proton-pump inhibitors [PPIs]) pyloric stenosis, pernicious anemia, atrophic gastritis, ulcerative colitis, renal insufficiency, steroid and calcium administration

Decreased: Vagotomy and antrectomy

GLUCOSE

• Fasting, < 110 mg/dL • Collection: Tiger top or red top tube

American Diabetes Association Diagnostic Criterion for Diabetes: normal fasting < 100 mg/dL, impaired fasting 100–125 mg/dL on more than one occasion or any random level > 200 mg/dL when associated with symptoms such as polyuria, polydipsia, polyphagia, and weight loss.

Increased: DM (types 1 and 2), Cushing syndrome, acromegaly, increased epinephrine (eg, injection, pheochromocytoma, stress, burns), acute and chronic pancreatitis, ACTH administration, spurious cause (sample from site above IV containing dextrose), advanced age, pancreatic glucagonoma, drugs (glucocorticoids, thiazide diuretics)

Decreased: Pancreatic disorders (islet cell tumors), extrapancreatic tumors (carcinoma of adrenal gland, stomach), hepatic disease (hepatitis, cirrhosis, tumors), endocrine disorders (early diabetes, hypothyroidism, hypopituitarism), functional disorders (after gastrectomy), pediatric problems (prematurity, infant of diabetic mother, ketotic hypoglycemia, enzyme diseases), exogenous insulin, oral hypoglycemic agents, malnutrition, sepsis

GLUCOSE TOLERANCE TEST (GTT), ORAL (OGTT)

A fasting glucose level $\geq$ 126 mg/dL or a random glucose > 200 mg/dL (11.1 mmol/L) is the threshold for diagnosis of DM; confirmation on a subsequent day precludes the need for glucose challenge. GTT is not necessary for diagnosis of DM and may be useful in gestational DM. Unreliable in the presence of severe infection, prolonged fasting, or after insulin injection. After an 8–12 h overnight fast (water only), a fasting blood glucose sample is drawn, and the patient ingests a 75-g oral glucose load, usually by drinking "glucola" (100 g for gestational DM screening, 1.75 mg/kg ideal body weight in children up to 75 g). Glucose drawn 30 min, 1, 2 and 3 h after glucose load.

Interpretation of GTT

Normal glucose tolerance: Glucose < 140 mg/dL 2 h after glucose load
   Impaired fasting glucose: Fasting glucose > 110 mg/dL and < 126 mg/dL risk factor for future diabetes

Impaired glucose tolerance: Glucose 140–199 mg/dL 2 h after glucose load
   Diabetes: Glucose > 200 mg/dL 2 h after glucose load

Gestational Diabetes: OTT usually done at about 28 wk with any two of the following glucose levels diagnostic: fasting > 105 mg/dL, 1-h > 190 mg/dL, 2-h > 165 mg/dL, or 3-h > 145 mg/dL

GLUTAMYL TRANSFERASE (GGT)

• Men: 9–50 U/L • Women: 8–40 U/L • Collection: Tiger top tube
   Parallels changes in serum alkaline phosphatase and 5′-nucleotidase in liver disease. Sensitive indicator of alcoholic liver disease

Increased: Liver disease (hepatitis, cirrhosis, obstructive jaundice), pancreatitis

GLYCOHEMOGLOBIN (GHB, GLYCATED HEMOGLOBIN, GLYCOHEMOGLOBIN, HBA₁c, HBA₁ HEMOGLOBIN A₁c, GLYCOSYLATED HEMOGLOBIN)

• Interpretation: Nondiabetic < 6%, near normal 6–7% • Excellent glucose control < 7% • Good control 7–8% • Fair control 8–9% • Poor control > 10%
• Collection: Lavender top tube
   Mean plasma glucose is equal to $(HbA_{1c} \times 35.6) - 77.3$. Useful in long-term monitoring control of blood sugar in diabetic patients; reflects levels over preceding 3–4 mo; not used to diagnose DM

Increased: DM (uncontrolled), lead intoxication

Decreased: Chronic renal failure, hemolytic anemia, PRG, chronic blood loss

HAPTOGLOBIN

- 40–180 mg/dL • Collection: Tiger top or red top tube

Increased: Obstructive liver disease, any cause of increased ESR (inflammation, collagen–vascular diseases)

Decreased: Any type of hemolysis (eg, transfusion reaction), liver disease, anemia, oral contraceptives, childhood and infancy

HELICOBACTER PYLORI ANTIBODY TITERS

- IgG < 0.17 = negative

Most patients with gastritis and ulcer disease have chronic *H. pylori* infection that should be controlled. Positive in 35–50% of patients without symptoms (increases with age). Use in dyspepsia controversial. Methods to test for *H. pylori:* noninvasive (serology, ^{13}C or ^{14}C urea breath test one of the most accurate noninvasive tests currently available, fecal assay [see below]) and invasive ("gold standard" gastric mucosal biopsy and *Campylobacter*-like organism test). The IgG subclass is found in all patient populations; occasionally only IgA antibodies can be detected. Serology most useful in newly diagnosed *H. pylori* infection or monitoring response to therapy. IgG levels decrease slowly after treatment and can remain elevated after infection clears.

Positive: Active or recent *H. pylori* infection, some asymptomatic carriers

HELICOBACTER PYLORI ANTIGEN, FECES

- Collection: 5 g of stool in a screw-capped, plastic container. Submit promptly to lab. Watery, diarrheal specimens or stool in transport media, swabs, or preservatives cannot be tested.

Uses: diagnosis of *H. pylori* and monitoring *H. pylori* clearing after therapy. Persons without symptoms should not be tested.

Positive: *H. pylori* antigen present in the stool

Negative: Absence of detectable antigen; does not exclude the possibility of infection by *H. pylori*

HEPATITIS TESTING

Recommended hepatitis panel tests based on clinical settings are shown in Table 4–3, page 69 and pattern interpretation in Table 4–4, page 71. Profile patterns of hepatitis A and B are shown in Figures 4–1, page 71 and 4–2, page 72.

- Hepatitis tests • Collection: Tiger top tube

Hepatitis A

Anti-HAV Ab: Total antibody to hepatitis A virus; confirms previous exposure to hepatitis A virus, elevated for life

Anti-HAV IgM: IgM antibody to hepatitis A virus; indicative of recent infection with hepatitis A virus; declines typically 1–6 mo after symptoms

TABLE 4–3
Hepatitis Panel Testing to Guide the Ordering of Hepatitis Profiles for Given Clinical Settings

Clinical Setting	Test	Purpose
SCREENING TESTS		
Pregnancy	HBsAg[a]	All expectant mothers should be screened during third trimester
High-risk patients on admission (homosexuals, dialysis patients)	HBsAg	To screen for chronic or active infection
Percutaneous inoculation		
Donor	HBsAg	To test patient's blood (esp. dialysis and HIV patients) for infectivity with hepatitis B and C if a health care worker is exposed
	Anti-HBc IgM	
	Anti-Hep C	
Victim	HBsAg	To test exposed health care worker for immunity or chronic infection
	Anti-HBc	
	Anti-Hep C	
Pre-HBV vaccine	Anti-HBc	To determine if a high-risk individual is infected or has antibodies to HBV
	Anti-HBs	
Screening blood	HBsAg	Used by blood banks to screen donors for hepatitis B and C
	Anti-HBc	
	Anti-Hep C	
DIAGNOSTIC TESTS		
Differential diagnosis of acute jaundice, hepatitis, or fulminant liver failure	HBsAg	To differentiate HBV, HAV, and hepatitis C in an acutely jaundiced patient with hepatitis of fulminant liver failure
	Anti-HBc IgM	
	Anti-HAV IgM	
	Anti-Hep C	
Chronic hepatitis	HBsAg	To diagnose HBV infection: if positive for HBsAg to determine infectivity
	HBeAg	If HBsAg patient worsens or is very ill, to diagnose concomitant infection with hepatitis delta virus
	Anti-HBe	
	Anti-HDV (total + IgM)	

(continued)

TABLE 4–3 (continued)

Clinical Setting	Test	Purpose
MONITORING		
Infant follow-up	HBsAg Anti-HBc Anti-HBs	To monitor the success of vaccination and passive immunization for perinatal transmission of HBV 12–15 mo after birth
Postvaccination screening	Anti-HBs	To ensure immunity has been achieved after vaccination (CDC recommends "titer" determination, but usually qualitative assay is adequate)
Sexual contact	HBsAg Anti-HBc Anti-Hep C	To monitor sexual partners of a patient with chronic HBV or hepatitis C

ᵃSee Abbreviations list on page xiii for definition of abbreviations.

Hepatitis B

HBsAg: Hepatitis B surface antigen. Earliest marker of HBV infection; indicates chronic or acute infection. Used by blood banks to screen donors; vaccination does not affect this test

Anti-HBc-Total: IgG and IgM antibody to hepatitis B core antigen; confirms either previous exposure to hepatitis B virus (HBV) or ongoing infection. Used by blood banks to screen donors

Anti-HBc IgM: IgM antibody to hepatitis B core antigen. Early and best indicator of acute infection with hepatitis B

HBeAg: Hepatitis Be antigen; indicates infectivity. Order only when evaluating for chronic HBV infection

HBV-DNA: Most sensitive and specific early evaluation of hepatitis B; may be detectable when all other markers are negative

Anti-HBe: Antibody to hepatitis Be antigen; associated with resolution of active inflammation

Anti-HBs: Antibody to hepatitis B surface antigen; indicates immunity and clinical recovery from infection or previous immunization with hepatitis B vaccine. Use to assess effectiveness of vaccine; request titer levels

Anti-HDV: Total antibody to delta hepatitis; confirms previous exposure. Use with known acute or chronic HBV infection

Anti-HDV IgM: IgM antibody to delta hepatitis; indicates recent infection. Use in known acute or chronic HBV infection

TABLE 4–4
Interpretation of Viral Hepatitis Serologic Testing Patterns

Anti-HAV (IgM)	HBsAg	Anti-HBc (IgM)	Anti-HBc (Total)	Anti-C (ELISA)	Interpretation
+	−	−	−	−	Acute hepatitis A
+	+	−	+	−	Acute hepatitis A in hepatitis B carrier
−	+	−	+	−	Chronic hepatitis B[a]
−	−	+	+	−	Acute hepatitis B
−	+	+	+	−	Acute hepatitis B
−	−	−	+	−	Past hepatitis B infection
−	−	−	−	+	Hepatitis C[b]
−	−	−	−	−	Early hepatitis C or other cause (other virus, toxin)

[a]Patients with chronic hepatitis B (either active hepatitis or carrier state) should have HBeAg and anti-HBe checked to determine activity of infection and relative infectivity. Anti-HBs is used to determine response to hepatitis B vaccination.
[b]Anti-C often takes 3–6 mo before being positive. PCR may allow earlier detection.

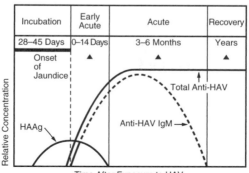

FIGURE 4–1. Hepatitis A diagnostic profile. See individual tests in text. (Based on data from Abbott Laboratories, Diagnostic Division, North Chicago, Illinois. Used with permission.)

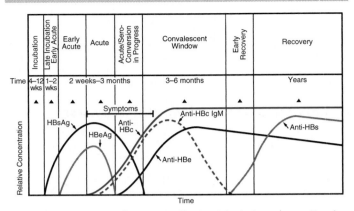

FIGURE 4–2. Hepatitis B diagnostic profile. See individual tests in text. (Based on data from Abbott Laboratories, Diagnostic Division, North Chicago, Illinois. Used with permission.)

Hepatitis C

Anti-HCV: Antibody against hepatitis C. Indicative of active viral replication and infectivity. Used by blood banks to screen donors. Many false-positives

HCV-RNA: Nucleic acid probe detection of current HCV infection

HIGH-DENSITY LIPOPROTEIN CHOLESTEROL

• See Cholesterol, page 58.

HLA (HUMAN LEUKOCYTE ANTIGENS; HLA TYPING)

• Collection: Green top tube
   Used to identify a group of antigens on the cell surface that are the primary determinants of histocompatibility; useful in assessing transplantation compatibility. Some HLA antigens are associated with specific diseases but are not diagnostic of these diseases.

HLA-B27: Ankylosing spondylitis, psoriatic arthritis, Reiter syndrome, juvenile RA

HLA-DR4/HLA DR2: Chronic Lyme disease arthritis

HLA-DRw2: MS

HLA-B8: Addison disease, juvenile-onset diabetes, Graves disease, gluten enteropathy

HOMOCYSTEINE, SERUM

• Normal fasting 5–15 µmol/L • Fasting target < 10 µmol/L
   An independent risk factor for CAD and atherosclerosis. Moderate, intermediate, and severe hyperhomocysteinemia refer to concentrations 16–30, 31–100, and > 100 µmol/L, respectively. May be useful for screening high-risk patients

and recommendation of strategies for obtaining target of < 10 μmol/L (ie, dietary, lifestyle changes, vitamin supplementation)

Increased: Vitamin B_{12}, B_6, and folate deficiency, renal failure, medications (nicotinic acid, theophylline, methotrexate, levodopa, anticonvulsants) advanced age, hypothyroidism, impaired kidney function, SLE, certain medications, disorders of methionine metabolism and in nonfasting state

HUMAN CHORIONIC GONADOTROPIN, SERUM (HCG)

• Normal, < 3.0 mIU/mL • 10 d after conception > 3 mIU/mL • 30 d, 100–5000 mIU/mL • 10 wk, 50,000–140,000 mIU/mL • > 16 wk, 10,000–50,000 mIU/mL • Thereafter levels slowly decline • Collection: Tiger top tube

Increased: PRG, some testicular tumors (nonseminomatous germ cell tumors, but not seminoma), trophoblastic disease (hydatidiform mole, choriocarcinoma levels usually > 100,000 mIU/mL)

HUMAN IMMUNODEFICIENCY VIRUS (HIV) TESTING

See Figure 4–3, CDC guidelines. Any HIV-positive person > 13 y with a CD4+ T-cell level < 200/mL or an HIV-positive patient with a CDC-defined indicator condition (eg, pulmonary candidiasis, disseminated histoplasmosis, HIV wasting, Kaposi sarcoma, TB, various lymphomas, PCP, and others) is considered to have AIDS. Confidentiality in HIV testing is regulated by law. Most states

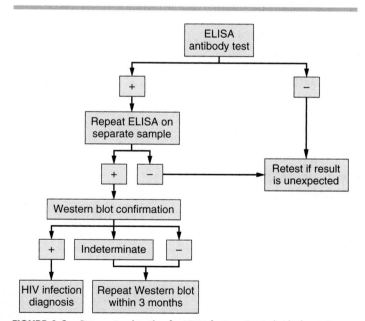

FIGURE 4–3. Diagnostic algorithm for HIV infection. See individual tests in text. (Based on data from GlaxoSmithKline, Research Triangle Park, North Carolina. Used with permission.)

require consent for HIV testing. Release of HIV information by phone is likewise prohibited in most states. This information is normally released only in writing to the ordering attending physician on a confidential basis.

HIV Antibody

• Normal = negative • Collection: Tiger top tube

Recognize both HIV-1 and HIV-2 antibodies. Uses: diagnosis of AIDS and blood screening for transfusion. Antibodies develop 1–4 mo after infection.

HIV Antibody, ELISA

• Normal = negative

Initial screen to detect HIV antibody; positive test is repeated or confirmed by Western blot.

Positive: AIDS, asymptomatic HIV infection, if indeterminate, repeat in 1 mo or perform PCR for HIV-1 DNA or RNA

False-Positive: Autoimmune or connective tissue diseases, hyperbilirubinemia, HLA antibodies, flu vaccine within 3 mo, hemophilia, rheumatoid factor, alcoholic hepatitis, dialysis patients

False-Negative: Acute seroconversion (first 3–4 wk of HIV infection), advanced AIDS, autoimmune disease, renal failure and hemodialysis, cystic fibrosis, multiple PRGs or transfusions, liver disease, injectable drug use, vaccination

HIV PCR, DNA

• Normal = negative

Performed on peripheral blood mononuclear cells, most sensitive assay for diagnosing infection; preferred test to diagnose HIV in children < 18 mo

HIV PCR, RNA

• Normal = undetectable

Quantifies "viral load." Establishes diagnosis before antibody production or when HIV antibody is indeterminate. Obtained at baseline, an important piece of information for modifying HIV therapy (see below, HIV Plasma Viral Load). Not recommended for children < 18 mo

HIV Plasma Viral Load Test (PVL test)

• Interpretation: viral load < 500 HIV RNA copies/mL, low; viral load < 40,000 HIV RNA copies/mL, high. Use same assay for serial plasma viral load testing. Best predictor of progression to AIDS and death among HIV-infected persons. Used as a baseline and for initiation or modification of HIV therapy but not for diagnosis. Initiation of antiretroviral drug therapy is usually recommended when the PVL is 10,000 to 30,000 copies/mL or when CD4+ counts are < 350–500/mm^3 ($0.35–0.50 \times 10^9$/L). PVL levels usually show a 1- to 2-log reduction within 4–6 wk after therapy is started; goal is no detectable virus in 16–24 wk. The methods are

  • **PCR** most common; results reported as copies/mL of plasma.
  • **bDNA** (branched-chain DNA assay) reported as units/mL of plasma.
  • **NASBA** (nucleic acid sequence–based amplification) infrequently used; reported units/mL of plasma.

Increased: Acute HIV infection, clinical AIDS, disease progression, drug resistance

Decreased: Response to therapy, remission

HIV Western Blot

• Normal = negative
   The reference procedure for confirming the presence or absence of HIV antibody.

IMMUNOGLOBULINS, QUANTITATIVE

• **IgG:** 65–1500 mg/dL • **IgM:** 40–345 mg/dL • **IgA:** 76–390 mg/dL • **IgE:** 0–380 IU/mL • **IgD:** 0–8 mg/dL • Collection: Tiger top or red top
   Used to evaluate immunodeficiency diseases; during replacement therapy, to evaluate humoral immunity

Increased: Multiple myeloma (myeloma immunoglobulin increased, other immunoglobulins decreased); Waldenström macroglobulinemia (IgM increased, others decreased); lymphoma; carcinoma; bacterial infection; liver disease; sarcoidosis; amyloidosis; myeloproliferative disorders; IgE increased in allergic states

Decreased: Hereditary immunodeficiency, leukemia, lymphoma, nephrotic syndrome, protein-losing enteropathy, malnutrition, transient hypogammaglobulinemia of infancy

IRON

• Men: 55–160 mcg/dL • Women: 40–155 mcg/dL • Collection: Tiger top or red top tube

Increased: Hemochromatosis, hemosiderosis caused by excessive iron intake, excess destruction or decreased production of erythrocytes, liver necrosis

Decreased: Iron deficiency anemia, nephrosis (loss of iron-binding proteins), normochromic anemia of chronic diseases and infections

IRON-BINDING CAPACITY, TOTAL (TIBC)

• 250–400 mg/dL • Collection: Tiger top or red top tube
   Normal iron/TIBC ratio: 20–50%. Decreased ratio (< 10%) diagnostic of iron deficiency anemia. Increased ratio in hemochromatosis

Increased: Acute and chronic blood loss, iron deficiency anemia, hepatitis, oral contraceptives

Decreased: Anemia of chronic diseases, cirrhosis, nephrosis/uremia, hemochromatosis, iron therapy overload, hemolytic anemia, aplastic anemia, thalassemia, megaloblastic anemia

LACTATE DEHYDROGENASE (LD, LDH)

• Adults < 230 U/L • Higher in childhood • Collection: Tiger top or red top tube; avoid hemolysis, which can increase LDH

Increased: AMI, cardiac surgery, prosthetic valve, hepatitis, pernicious anemia, malignant tumors, PE, hemolysis (anemias or factitious), renal infarction, muscle injury, megaloblastic anemia, liver disease

LDH Isoenzymes (LDH 1 to LDH 5)

Normal ratio LDH 1/LDH 2 < 0.6–0.7. Ratio > 1 (also called "flipped"), suspect recent MI (can also be seen in pernicious or hemolytic anemia). With AMI, LDH begins to rise 12–48 h after MI, peaks at 3–6 d, and returns to normal at 8–14 d. LDH 5 is > LDH 4 in liver disease. (*Note:* Troponin is considered marker of choice for AMI.)

LACTIC ACID (LACTATE)

• 4.5–19.8 mg/dL • Collection: Gray top tube on ice
    Suspect lactic acidosis with elevated anion gap in the absence of other causes (renal failure, ethanol or methanol ingestion).

Increased: Lactic acidosis due to hypoxia, hemorrhage, shock, sepsis, cirrhosis, exercise, ethanol, DKA, regional ischemia (extremity, bowel) spurious factors (prolonged use of a tourniquet)

LAP SCORE (LEUKOCYTE ALKALINE PHOSPHATASE SCORE/STAIN)

• 50–150 • Collection: Fingerstick blood sample directly on slide; smear and air dry
    Differential diagnosis of CML versus leukemoid reaction; evaluation of polycythemia vera, myelofibrosis with myeloid metaplasia, and paroxysmal nocturnal hemoglobinuria

Increased: Leukemoid reaction, acute inflammation, Hodgkin disease, PRG, liver disease, polycythemia vera

Decreased: CML, nephrotic syndrome

LE (LUPUS ERYTHEMATOSUS) PREPARATION

• Normal = no cells seen

Positive: SLE, scleroderma, RA, drug-induced lupus (procainamide, others)

LEAD, BLOOD

• Adult < 70 mcg/dL • Child < 20 mg/dL • Collection: Lavender, navy, or green top tube; lab-specific
    Neurologic findings at 15 mg/dL in children and 30 mg/dL in adults; severe symptoms (lethargy, ataxia, coma) > 60 mg/dL

Increased: Lead poisoning, occupational exposure

LEGIONELLA ANTIBODY

• Normal: < 1:32 titers • Collection: Tiger top or red top tube
    Obtain two serum samples: acute (within 2 wk of onset) and convalescent (at least 3 wk after onset of fever). A fourfold rise in titers or a single titer of 1:256 is diagnostic.

Increased: Legionella infection; false-positives with *Bacteroides fragilis, Francisella tularensis, Mycoplasma pneumoniae*

LIPASE

• < 52 U/L (method dependent) • Collection: Tiger top tube

Increased: Acute or chronic pancreatitis, pseudocyst, pancreatic duct obstruction (stone, stricture, tumor, drug-induced spasm), fat embolus syndrome, renal failure, dialysis, usually normal in mumps, malignant gastric tumor, intestinal perforation, diabetes (usually in DKA only)

LIPID PROFILE/LIPOPROTEIN PROFILE/LIPOPROTEIN ANALYSIS

• See also Cholesterol, page 58, and Triglycerides, page 88.

Usually includes cholesterol, HDL cholesterol, LDL cholesterol (calculated), triglycerides. Initial screening for cardiac risk includes total cholesterol, LDL, and HDL as outlined in Table 4–1. The main blood lipids, ie, cholesterol and triglycerides, are carried by lipoproteins. Lipoproteins are classified by density (least dense to most dense):

- **Chylomicrons** least dense, rise to surface of unspun serum; normally found only after a fatty meal is eaten (a **"lipemic specimen"** refers to the presence of these chylomicrons)
- **VLDL** mainly of triglycerides. With triglycerides < 400 mg/dL, the ratio of cholesterol to triglycerides is 1:5 in VLDL.
- **LDL** carries most cholesterol in fasting state.
- **HDL** densest and consists of mostly apoproteins and cholesterol

LOW-DENSITY LIPOPROTEIN-CHOLESTEROL (LDL, LDL-C)

• See Cholesterol, page 58.

LUTEINIZING HORMONE, SERUM (LH)

• Men: 1–13 IU/L • Women (follicular or luteal): 6–30 IU/L midcycle peak increases two- to threefold over follicular or luteal, postmenopausal > 12–55 IU/L
• Collection: Tiger top or red top tube

Increased: (Hypergonadotropic > 40 IU/L) postmenopause, surgical or radiation castration, ovarian or testicular failure, polycystic ovaries

Decreased: (Hypogonadotropic < 40 IU/L prepubertal) hypothalamic or pituitary dysfunction, Kallmann syndrome, LHRH analogue therapy

LYME DISEASE SEROLOGY

• Normal varies with lab assay, ELISA < 1:8 • Western blot nonreactive

Most useful for comparing acute and convalescent serum levels for relative titers. IgM antibody detectable 2–4 wk after onset of rash; IgG rises in 4–6 wk and peaks up to 6 mo after infection and may stay elevated for months to years.

Positive: Infection with *Borrelia burgdorferi,* syphilis, and other rickettsial diseases. Confirm positive with Western blot with multiple bands of identity

Negative: After antibiotic therapy or during first few weeks of disease

MAGNESIUM

• 1.3–2.1 mg/dL • Collection: Tiger top or red top tube

Increased: Renal failure, hypothyroidism, magnesium-containing antacids, Addison disease, diabetic coma, severe dehydration, lithium intoxication

Decreased: Malabsorption, steatorrhea, alcoholism and cirrhosis, hyperthyroidism, aldosteronism, diuretics, acute pancreatitis, hyperparathyroidism, hyperalimentation, NG suctioning, chronic dialysis, renal tubular acidosis, drugs (cisplatin, amphotericin B, aminoglycosides), hungry bone syndrome, hypophosphatemia, intracellular shifts with respiratory or metabolic acidosis

MHA-TP (MICROHEMAGGLUTINATION, *TREPONEMA PALLIDUM*)

• Normal < 1:160 • Collection: Tiger top tube

Confirmatory test for syphilis, similar to FTA-ABS. Once positive, remains so; do not use to judge treatment effect. False-positives: other treponemal infections (eg, pinta, yaws), mononucleosis, SLE

β_2-MICROGLOBULIN

• 0.07–0.18 mcg/dL • Collection: Tiger top or red top tube

A portion of the class I MHC antigen; useful marker for following progression of HIV and B-cell malignancies (eg, multiple myeloma); levels < 4 mcg/d/L good prognosis in multiple myeloma

Increased: HIV infection, especially during periods of exacerbation, lymphoid malignant diseases, renal diseases (diabetic nephropathy, pyelonephritis, ATN, nephrotoxicity from medications), transplant rejection, inflammatory conditions

Decreased: Treatment of HIV with AZT (zidovudine)

MONOSPOT

• Normal = negative • Collection: Tiger top or red top tube

Positive: Mononucleosis, rarely in leukemia, serum sickness, Burkitt lymphoma, viral hepatitis, RA

MYOGLOBIN

• 30–90 ng/mL • Collection: Tiger top tube

Increased: Skeletal muscle injury (crush, injection, surgical procedure), delirium tremens, rhabdomyolysis (burns, seizures, sepsis, hypokalemia, others), AMI (6–12 h after)

NATRIURETIC PEPTIDE, B-TYPE (BNP)

• < 100 pg/mL normal • Collection: Lavender top tube on ice

BNP released by the ventricular myocardium secondary to volume and pressure overload. BNP increases sodium and water excretion. CHF severity correlates with BNP level (< 100 pg/mL rules out CHF, 100–400 pg/mL is borderline, > 400 pg/mL is highly suggestive of CHF). BNP used to differentiate CHF and other causes of dyspnea (eg, COPD).

Increased: CHF/left ventricular dysfunction. *Note:* cross-reacts with IV nesiritide (Natrecor)

NATRIURETIC PEPTIDE, NT-PRO B-TYPE, PLASMA

• Normal: < 200 pg/mL • Collection: lavender top tube

With ventricular volume expansion and/or pressure overload, Pro BNP is cleaved to release "active" BNP (see above), and the "inactive" N-terminal (NT) called NT-Pro BNP. Both BNP and NT-Pro BNP are markers of atrial and ventricular distension. Levels < 200 pg/mL exclude CHF, 200–400 pg/mL indicates compensated CHF, 400–2,000 pg/mL suggests moderate CHF, and > 2000 is consistent with moderate to severe CHF. NT-Pro-BNP advantages over BNP: greater stability, longer half-life, not cross-reactive with recombinant BNP (nesiritide, Natrecor). May provide more prognostic information than traditional risk factors

4

Increased: CHF/left ventricular dysfunction

NEWBORN SCREENING PANEL

Newborn screening varies by state law and is used to evaluate for a variety of inherited conditions: Phenylalanine (phenylketonuria); leucine (branched-chain ketonuria); galactose-1-phosphate uridyl transferase (galactosemia); methionine (homocystinuria); thyroxine, TSH (hypothyroidism); hemoglobin electrophoresis (sickle cell); biotinidase (biotinidase deficiency)

5'-NUCLEOTIDASE

• 2–15 U/L • Collection: Tiger top or red top tube
  Uses: work-up of increased alkaline phosphatase and biliary obstruction

Increased: Obstructive or cholestatic liver disease, liver metastasis, biliary cirrhosis

OLIGOCLONAL BANDING, CSF

• Normal = negative • Collection: Tiger top or red top tube and simultaneous CSF sample collected in a plain tube by LP
  Performed simultaneously on CSF and serum samples when MS is suspected. Agarose gel electrophoresis reveals multiple bands in the IgG region not seen in the serum with a positive test. Oligoclonal banding is present in as many as 90% of patients with MS. Occasionally seen in other CNS inflammatory conditions and CNS syphilis

OSMOLALITY, SERUM

• 278–298 mOsm/kg • Collection: Tiger top tube
  A rough estimation of osmolality is [2(Na) + BUN/2.8 + glucose/18]. Measured value is usually less than calculated value. If measured value is 15 mOsm/kg less than calculated, consider methanol, ethanol, or ethylene glycol ingestion or another unmeasured substance.

Increased: Hyperglycemia; ethanol, methanol, mannitol, or ethylene glycol ingestion; increased sodium because of water loss (diabetes, hypercalcemia, diuresis)

Decreased: Low serum sodium, diuretics, Addison disease, SIADH (seen in bronchogenic carcinoma, hypothyroidism), iatrogenic causes (poor fluid balance)

OXYGEN

• See Chapter 8, Table 8–1, page 164.

PARATHYROID HORMONE (PTH) INTACT

• 10–60 pg/mL (method dependent) • Collection: red top tube on ice; submit to lab immediately

The upper limit of the reference range may be lower in regions of the world with more daily hours of sunshine. If renal function is normal and serum calcium is elevated, an intact PTH concentration of > 50 pg/mL strongly suggests primary hyperparathyroidism.

Increased: Primary hyperparathyroidism, secondary hyperparathyroidism (eg, hypocalcemia states such as chronic renal failure)

Decreased: Hypoparathyroidism, hypercalcemia not due to hyperparathyroidism

PHOSPHORUS

• Adult 2.5–4.5 mg/dL • Child 4.0–6.0 mg/dL • Collection: Tiger top or red top tube

Increased: Hypoparathyroidism (surgical, pseudohypoparathyroidism), excess vitamin D, secondary hyperparathyroidism, renal failure, bone disease (healing fractures), Addison disease, childhood, factitious increase (hemolysis of specimen)

Decreased: Hyperparathyroidism, alcoholism, diabetes, hyperalimentation, acidosis, alkalosis, gout, salicylate poisoning, IV steroid, glucose or insulin administration, hypokalemia, hypomagnesemia, diuretics, vitamin D deficiency, phosphate-binding antacids

POTASSIUM, SERUM

• 3.5–5 mEq/L • Collection: Tiger top or red top tube

Increased: Factitious increase (hemolysis of specimen, thrombocytosis), renal failure, Addison disease, acidosis, spironolactone, triamterene, ACE inhibitors, dehydration, hemolysis, massive tissue damage, excess intake (oral or IV), potassium-containing medications

Decreased: Diuretics, decreased intake, vomiting, NG suctioning, villous adenoma, diarrhea, Zollinger–Ellison syndrome, chronic pyelonephritis, RTA, metabolic alkalosis (primary aldosteronism, Cushing syndrome)

PREALBUMIN

• See Chapter 11.

PREGNANCY SCREENING

• Normal blood values based on gestational age, others based on chromosomal analysis. First-trimester screen offers advantages over second-trimester screen. Negative results reduce maternal anxiety. Positive results allow women to take advantage of first-trimester chorionic villus sampling (CVS) at 10–12 wk or second-trimester amniocentesis (≥15 weeks). American College of Obstetricians and Gynecologists recommends all women > 35 y at delivery be offered CVS or amniocentesis (diagnoses 99.9% of screened chromosomal abnormalities).

First Trimester Screening ("combined screening")

Maternal serum beta-HCG, PAPP-A (pregnancy associated plasma protein-A, with ultrasound-determined nuchal transparency)

Done at 11–13 wk. Screen of low-risk pregnant women (< 35 y) for Down syndrome and trisomy 18 (detects ~ 85% of cases of Down syndrome and ~ 97% of trisomy 18). Measures free beta-HCG and PAPP-A in combination with ultrasound assessment of fetal nuchal translucency (measure of fluid in the fetal neck).

Second Trimester Screening

("Quadruple screening") Maternal serum AFP, HCG, estriol, and inhibin A

Done at 15–21 wk of PRG to detect open neural tube defects, Down syndrome, and trisomy 18 (detects ~ 80% of open neural tube defects, ~ 85% of cases of Down syndrome, ~ 60% of cases of trisomy 18)

Chorionic Villus Sampling (CVS)

Performed at 10–12 wk of PRG; placental tissue removed percutaneously and studied for chromosomal analysis (~ 1% risk of complications such as miscarriage)

Amniocentesis

Performed at 13–14 wk of PRG (early amniocentesis) or at 15 wk and later (traditional amniocentesis). Chromosomal analysis is performed on the fetal skin cells in the amniotic fluid. Risk similar to CVS

PROGESTERONE

- Collection: Tiger top tube
  Used to confirm ovulation and corpus luteum function

Sample Collection	Normal Value (women)
Follicular phase	<1 ng/mL
Luteal phase	5–20 ng/mL
Pregnancy	
1st trimester	10–30 ng/mL
2nd trimester	50–100 ng/mL
3rd trimester	100–400 ng/mL
Postmenopause	<1 ng/mL

PROLACTIN

- Men: 1–20 ng/mL • Women: 1–25 ng/mL • Collection: Tiger top or red top tube
  Used in work-up of infertility, impotence, hirsutism, amenorrhea, and pituitary neoplasm

Increased: PRG, nursing after PRG, prolactinoma, hypothalamic tumors, sarcoidosis or granulomatous disease of the hypothalamus, hypothyroidism, renal failure, Addison disease, phenothiazines, haloperidol

PROSTATE-SPECIFIC ANTIGEN (PSA)

- < 4 ng/dL (some consider < 2.5 ng/dL normal)
  Most useful as a measure of response to therapy of prostate cancer; approved for screening for prostate cancer

Increased: Prostate cancer (levels > 10/dL increase likelihood of spread), acute prostatitis, BPH, prostatic infarction, prostate surgery (after biopsy, resection levels are elevated for 4–6 wk), vigorous prostatic massage (routine rectal exam does not elevate levels), rarely after ejaculation (some suggest refraining from sexual activity for 24–48 h before test)

Decreased: Radical prostatectomy (should be "undetectable" or < 0.2 ng/dL), response to therapy for prostatic carcinoma (radiation or hormonal therapy), response to antibiotics in acute bacterial prostatitis

PSA Velocity/PSA Doubling Time

A rate of rise in PSA of > 0.75 ng/dL/y (velocity) is suggestive of prostate cancer on the basis of at least three separate assays 6 mo apart. Increased PSA doubling time < 3 mo before diagnosis or < 10 mo after treatment (radiation or surgery) suggests a poor prognosis.

PSA Free and Total

Prostate cancer tends to be associated with lower free PSA levels in proportion to total PSA; free/total PSA can improve the specificity of PSA in the range of total PSA from 2.0–10.0 ng/mL. Ratio free/total < 10% indicates > 50% chance of positive biopsy; > 25%, 8–10% risk of positive biopsy. Some recommend prostate biopsy only if the free PSA percentage is low; others use the ratio to guide further biopsy after an initial negative biopsy.

PROTEIN ELECTROPHORESIS, SERUM AND URINE (SERUM PROTEIN ELECTROPHORESIS, SPEP) (URINE PROTEIN ELECTROPHORESIS, UPEP)

Qualitative analysis of serum proteins is used in the work-up of hypoglobulinemia, macroglobulinemia, α_1-antitrypsin deficiency, collagen disease, liver disease, and myeloma and occasionally in nutritional assessment. Serum electrophoresis yields five bands (Figure 4–4, page 83, and Table 4–5, page 84). If monoclonal gammopathy or a low globulin fraction is detected, quantitative immunoglobulin tests should be ordered. Urine protein electrophoresis can be used to evaluate proteinuria and to detect Bence Jones protein (light chain), which is associated with myeloma, Waldenström macroglobulinemia, and Fanconi syndrome.

PROTEIN, SERUM

- 6.0–8.0 g/dL • See also Serum Protein Electrophoresis, above. • Collection: Tiger top or red top tube

Increased: Multiple myeloma, Waldenström macroglobulinemia, benign monoclonal gammopathy, lymphoma, chronic inflammatory disease, sarcoidosis, viral illnesses

Decreased: Malnutrition, inflammatory bowel disease, Hodgkin disease, leukemia, any cause of decreased albumin

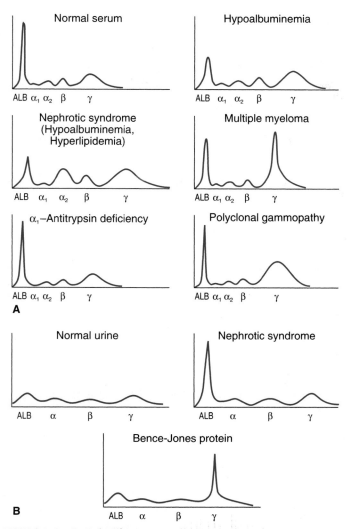

FIGURE 4-4. Examples of (**A**) serum and (**B**) urine electrophoresis patterns, See also Table 4-5, page 84. (Courtesy of Dr. Steven Haist.)

RAPID PLASMA REAGIN (RPR) TEST FOR SYPHILIS

• Normal: nonreactive • Collection: Tiger top or red top tube

Has replaced VDRL as the screening test for syphilis (*T. pallidum*). Confirm positive with a specific treponemal test (fluorescent treponemal antibody-absorbed (FTA-ABS) or microhemagglutination assay (TP-MHA). Not for testing CSF

TABLE 4–5
Normal Serum Protein Components and Fractions as Determined by Electrophoresis, Along with Associated Conditions[a]

Protein Fraction	Percentage of Total Protein	Constituents	Increased	Decreased
Albumin	52–68	Albumin	Dehydration (only known cause)	Nephrosis, malnutrition, chronic liver disease
Alpha-1 (α_1) globulin	2.4–4.4	Thyroxine-binding globulin, antitrypsin, lipoproteins, glycoprotein, transcortin	Inflammation, neoplasia	Nephrosis, α_1-antitrypsin deficiency (emphysema related)
Alpha-2 (α_2) globulin	6.1–10.1	Haptoglobin, glycoprotein, macroglobulin, ceruloplasmin	Inflammation, infection, neoplasia, cirrhosis	Severe liver disease, acute hemolytic anemia
Beta (β) globulin	8.5–14.5	Transferrin, glycoprotein, lipoprotein	Cirrhosis, obstructive jaundice	Nephrosis
Gamma (γ) globulins (immunoglobulins)	10–21	IgA, IgG, IgM, IgD, IgE	Infections, collagen-vascular diseases, leukemia, myeloma	Agammaglobulinemia, hypogammaglobulinemia, nephrosis

[a](See also Figure 4–4, page 83)

Positive: Syphilis; false-positives: other infections, pregnancy, drug addiction, collagen–vascular disease

RENIN, PLASMA (PLASMA RENIN ACTIVITY [PRA])

• Adults, normal-sodium diet, upright 1–6 ng/mL/h (position and method dependent • Collection: Lavender top tube, send to lab on ice

Used in work-up of HTN with hypokalemia. Values highly dependent on salt intake and position. Stop diuretics, estrogens for 2–4 wk before testing.

Increased: Medications (ACE inhibitors, diuretics, oral contraceptives, estrogens), PRG, dehydration, renal artery stenosis, adrenal insufficiency, chronic hypokalemia, upright posture, salt-restricted diet, edematous conditions (CHF, nephrotic syndrome), secondary hyperaldosteronism

Decreased: Primary aldosteronism (renin will not increase with relative volume depletion, upright posture)

RENIN, RENAL VEIN

• Normal L & R should be equal

A ratio of > 1.5 (affected/unaffected) suggestive of renovascular hypertension

RETINOL-BINDING PROTEIN (RBP)

• Adults 3–6 mg/dL • Children 1.5–3.0 mg/dL • Collection: Tiger top or red top tube

Decreased: Malnutrition, vitamin A deficiency, intestinal malabsorption of fats, chronic liver disease

Increased: Advanced chronic renal disease

RHEUMATOID FACTOR (RF, RA LATEX TEST)

• < 15 IU kit or > 1:40 • Collection: Tiger top or red top tube

RF is an IgM autoantibody; may be negative early in the disease; a positive/elevated RF suggests more severe disease. Can be done on serum or synovial fluid. Initial work-up should include both RF and anti-CCP.

Increased: RA (present in 80%); juvenile RA usually negative for RF, False-positives: other collagen–vascular diseases (lupus erythematosus, scleroderma, Sjögren syndrome) hepatitis, cirrhosis of the liver, lymphomas, and other infections (endocarditis, tuberculosis, viral infections, chronic infections, hepatitis, chronic hepatic disease, syphilis); 1–2% of healthy persons and > 20% of healthy persons > 65 y

Decreased: Anti-TNF-alpha therapy

ROCKY MOUNTAIN SPOTTED FEVER ANTIBODIES (RMSF)

• Normal: < 4× increase in paired acute and convalescent sera • IgG < 1:64 • IgM < 1:8 • Collection: Tiger top tube or red top acute and convalescent

The diagnosis of RMSF is made with acute and convalescent titers that show a 4× increase or a single convalescent titer > 1:64 in the clinical setting of RMSF. Occasional false-positives in late PRG

SEMEN ANALYSIS

- Volume 2–5 mL • Sperm count > 20–40×10^6/mL • Motility $> 60\%$
- Forward migration • Morphology $> 60\%$ normal

    Collect after 48–72 h abstinence, analyze in 1–2 h. May not be valid after a recent illness or high fever. Verify abnormal by serial tests.

Decreased: After vasectomy (should be 0 sperm after 3 mo), varicocele, primary testicular failure (ie, Klinefelter syndrome), secondary testicular failure (chemotherapy, radiation, infections), varicocele, aftermath of recent illness, congenital obstruction of the vas, retrograde ejaculation, endocrine causes (eg, hyperprolactinemia, low testosterone)

SODIUM, SERUM

- 136–145 mmol/L • Collection: Tiger top or red top tube

Increased: Associated with low total body sodium (glycosuria, mannitol, or lactulose use, urea, excess sweating), normal total body sodium (diabetes insipidus [central and nephrogenic], respiratory losses, and sweating), and increased total body sodium (administration of hypertonic sodium bicarbonate, Cushing syndrome, hyperaldosteronism)

Decreased: Associated with excess total body sodium and water (nephrotic syndrome, CHF, cirrhosis, renal failure), excess body water (SIADH [small-cell lung cancer; pulmonary disease including TB, lung cancer, pneumonia; CNS disease including trauma, tumors, and infections; perioperative stress; drugs including SSRIs and ACE inhibitors; and aftermath of colonoscopy], hypothyroidism, adrenal insufficiency, psychogenic polydipsia, beer potomania), decreased total body water and sodium (diuretic use, RTA, use of mannitol or urea, mineralocorticoid deficiency, cerebral salt wasting, vomiting, diarrhea, pancreatitis), and pseudohyponatremia (hyperlipidemia, hyperglycemia, multiple myeloma)

STOOL FOR OCCULT BLOOD

See Fecal Occult Blood Test (FOBT), Hemoccult Test

SWEAT CHLORIDE

- 5–40 mEq/L • Collection: 100–200 mg sweat on filter paper after electrical stimulation of sweating by pilocarpine iontophoresis on an extremity

Increased: CF (not valid on children < 3 wk); Addison disease, meconium ileus, and renal failure can occasionally raise levels.

N-TELOPEPTIDE (NTX) (URINE AND SERUM)
Urine

- Healthy women: Premenopausal 19–63 nM BCE/mM creatinine; Postmenopausal 26–124 nM BCE/mM creatinine • Healthy men: 21–83 nM BCE/mM creatinine

Serum

- Premenopausal women: 6.2–19.0 nM BCE • Men > 25 y: 5.4–24.2 nM BCE

    N-Telopeptides of type I collagen (NTx) are end products of bone resorption and allow monitoring of bone metabolism. Reported as nanomolar bone collagen equivalents per liter (nM BCE/L). In urine, values are corrected per milli-molars of creatinine per liter (mM creatinine/L). Serum NTx provides a quantitative measurement of bone resorption. A baseline NTx level is obtained before antiresorptive therapy (ie, bisphosphonate) with periodic testing until decrease in NTx achieved

Increased: Osteoporosis, Paget disease, primary hyperparathyroidism, bony metastasis

Decreased: Response to bisphosphonate therapy (decrease of 30–40% from baseline after 3 mo of therapy is typical of bisphosphonate therapy)

TESTOSTERONE
• Men: free 10–150 pg/mL, total 100–1100 ng/dL • Women and girls: See following table

Age (y)	Normal Value (women and girls)
1–11	< 75 mg/dL
12–18	< 120 mg/dL
> 18	< 75 mg/dL
Postmenopausal	< 50 mg/dL

Increased: Adrenogenital syndrome, ovarian stromal hyperthecosis, polycystic ovaries, menopause, ovarian tumors

Decreased: Hypogonadism, hypopituitarism, Klinefelter syndrome, male andropause

THYROGLOBULIN
• < 33 ng/mL • Collection: Tiger top or red top tube
  Useful for following nonmedullary thyroid carcinoma

Increased: Differentiated thyroid carcinoma (papillary, follicular), Graves disease, nontoxic goiter

Decreased: Hypothyroidism, testosterone, steroids, phenytoin

THYROID-STIMULATING HORMONE (TSH)
• 0.4–4.8 mIU/L • Collection: Tiger top or red top tube
  Best screen test for thyroid dysfunction; useful for monitoring thyroid replacement therapy and confirming TSH suppression in patients with thyroid cancer taking thyroxine therapy

Increased: Primary hypothyroidism, values > 5–7 mIU/L suggest borderline or subclinical primary hypothyroidism

Decreased: Primary hyperthyroidism, in secondary and tertiary hypothyroidism TSH levels can be decreased or normal (these cases make up less than 1% of all cases of hypothyroidism)

THYROXINE, FREE (FT$_4$)

- Normal: 0.8–1.7 ng/dL • Collection: Tiger top or red top tube

Confirms thyroid dysfunction after abnormal TSH. FT$_4$ and TSH provide the best assessment of thyroid function in abnormal serum TBG levels or binding characteristics (eg, PRG, medication with estrogens, androgens, phenytoin, or salicylates). FT$_4$ misleading with abnormal binding proteins or major illnesses that cause "euthyroid sick syndrome." Heparin, circulating free fatty acids, and antithyroxine autoantibodies can also cause aberrant results.

Increased: Hyperthyroidism or exogenous thyroxine administration

Decreased: Hypothyroidism

TORCH BATTERY

- Normal = negative • Collection: Tiger top tube

Serial determinations best (acute and convalescent titers); based on serologic evidence of exposure to toxoplasmosis, rubella, CMV, and herpesviruses

TRANSFERRIN

- 210–360 mg/dL • Collection: Tiger top or red top tube, avoid hemolysis

Used in work–up of anemia; transferrin levels can also be assessed by total iron-binding capacity.

Increased: Acute and chronic blood loss, iron deficiency, hemolysis, oral contraceptives, PRG, viral hepatitis

Decreased: Anemia of chronic disease, cirrhosis, nephrosis, hemochromatosis, malignant diseases

TRIGLYCERIDES

- Recommended value: < 150 mg/dL; borderline high: 150–199 mg/dL; high 200–499 mg/dL; very high > 500 mg/dL • Collection: Red top tube (*Note:* Tiger top tubes contain a silicone serum separator gel [SST] that interferes with triglycerides) • Fasting required

Increased: Nonfasting specimen hypothyroidism, liver diseases, poorly controlled DM, alcoholism, pancreatitis, AMI, nephrotic syndrome, familial disorders, medications (oral contraceptives, estrogens, beta-blockers, cholestyramine)

Decreased: Malnutrition, malabsorption, hyperthyroidism, Tangier disease, medications (nicotinic acid, clofibrate, gemfibrozil), congenital abetalipoproteinemia

TRIIODOTHYRONINE (T$_3$)

- 80–200 ng/dL • Collection: Red top tube

Used when hyperthyroidism suspected but T$_4$ is normal (T$_3$ thyrotoxicosis); not used to diagnose hypothyroidism

Increased: Hyperthyroidism, T$_3$ thyrotoxicosis, PRG, exogenous T$_4$, any cause of increased TBG, eg, oral estrogen or PRG

Decreased: Hypothyroidism and euthyroid sick state, any cause of decreased TBG

TROPONIN, CARDIAC-SPECIFIC

• Troponin I (TI) < 0.35 ng/mL • Troponin T (TT) < 0.2 mcg/L (method dependent)

Used to diagnose AMI; increases rapidly 3–12 h after MI, peak at 24 h, and may stay elevated for several days (TI 5–7 d, TT up to 14 d). Serial testing recommended. More cardiac-specific than CK-MB

Positive: Myocardial damage, including MI, myocarditis (false-positive: renal failure)

4

URIC ACID (URATE)

• Men: 3.4–8 mg/dL • Women: 2.4–6 mg/dL • Collection: Tiger top or red top tube

Increase associated with increased catabolism, nucleoprotein synthesis, or decreased renal clearing of uric acid (ie, thiazide diuretics, renal failure)

Increased: Gout, renal failure, destruction of massive amounts of nucleoproteins (leukemia, anemia, chemotherapy, toxemia of PRG), drugs (especially diuretics), lactic acidosis, hypothyroidism, PCKD, parathyroid diseases

Decreased: Uricosuric drugs (salicylates, probenecid, allopurinol), Wilson disease, Fanconi syndrome

VDRL TEST (VENEREAL DISEASE RESEARCH LABORATORY)

VDRL is now approved only for testing CSF for syphilis. RPR (see page 83) is the standard screening test.

VITAMIN B$_{12}$ (EXTRINSIC FACTOR, CYANOCOBALAMIN)

• Normal 200–700 pg/mL • Collection: Red top tube

Increased: Excessive intake, myeloproliferative disorders

Decreased: Inadequate intake (especially strict vegetarians), malabsorption, hyperthyroidism, PRG

ZINC

• 60–130 mcg/dL • Collection: Check with lab; special collection to limit contamination

Increased: Metal fume fever

Decreased: Pernicious anemia, inadequate dietary intake (parenteral nutrition, alcoholism), malabsorption, increased needs (PRG, severe burns, wound healing), acrodermatitis enteropathica, dwarfism, hepatic disease

LABORATORY DIAGNOSIS: CLINICAL HEMATOLOGY

Blood Collection
Blood Smears: Wright Stain
Normal CBC Values
Normal CBC Variations
Hematocrit
The Left Shift
Reticulocyte Count

CBC Diagnostics
Lymphocyte Subsets
RBC Morphology Differential Diagnosis
WBC Morphology Differential
  Diagnosis
Coagulation and Other Hematologic
  Tests

5

BLOOD COLLECTION

Venipuncture is discussed in detail in Chapter 13, page 316. The best CBC sample is venous blood drawn with a 22-gauge or larger needle. For a routine CBC, venous blood must be placed in a special hematology lab tube, usually a purple top tube, containing an anticoagulant (EDTA) with which the blood must be mixed gently. Blood for a CBC should be fresh, < 3 h old. Most samples for coagulation studies are submitted in a blue top (citrate) tube. (See page 318 for detailed description of blood collection tubes.) If a **capillary fingerstick** or **heelstick** (see page 280) is used, the hematocrit may be falsely low. If the finger has to be "milked," sludging of the RBCs can create a falsely high hematocrit. Wright staining can also be done and viewed as outlined in the next section.

BLOOD SMEARS: WRIGHT STAIN

Most clinical labs perform automated cell counts. The formal blood smear and Wright stain can provide a manual differential leukocyte count for the evaluation of anemia and other conditions. The slide is usually available for review by students and house staff. The main benefit is to allow identification of abnormal cells and other subtleties that may not be detected with automated systems (Figure 5–1).

Viewing the Film: The Differential WBC

1. Examine the smear in an area where the red cells approximate one another but do not overlap.
2. If the film is too thin or if a rough-edged spreader is used, as many as 50% of the WBCs may accumulate in the edges and tail (see Figure 5–1).
3. WBCs are *not* randomly dispersed even in a well-made smear. Polys and monos predominate at the margins and tail, and lymphs are prevalent in the middle of the film. To overcome this problem, use the "high dry" or oil immersion objective and count cells in a strip running the entire length of the film. Avoid the lateral edges of the film.
4. If fewer than 200 cells are counted in a strip, count another strip until at least 200 are seen. The special white cell counter found in most labs is

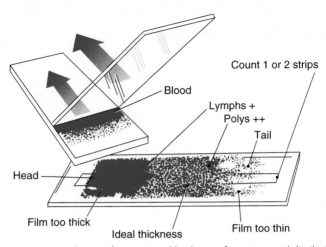

FIGURE 5-1. Technique of preparing a blood smear for staining and distribution of white blood cells on the standard smear.

ideal for this purpose. In patients receiving chemotherapy, the total count may be so small that only a 25–50 cell differential is possible.

5. In smears of blood from patients with very high white counts, such as those with leukemia, count the cells in any well-spread area where the different cell types are easy to identify. Table 5–1 shows the correlation between the number of cells in a smear and the estimated white cell count. Estimate the platelet count by averaging the number of platelets seen in 10 hpf (under oil immersion) and multiplying by 20,000.

NORMAL CBC VALUES

A CBC panel generally includes WBC count, RBC count, Hgb, HCT, MCH, MCHC, MCV, RDW, and usually platelets. The differential is usually ordered separately. Normal CBC, differential, and platelet values are outlined in Tables 5–2 and 5–3.

TABLE 5-1
Estimate of WBC Based on Cells Counted in a Blood Smear

WBC/hpf (high dry or 40×)	Estimated WBC (per mm³)
2–4	4000–7000
4–6	7000–10,000
6–10	10,000–13,000
10–20	13,000–18,000

WBC = white blood cells; hpf = high-power field.

TABLE 5-2
Normal CBC for Selected Age Ranges

Age	WBC Count (cells/mm³) [SI: 10⁹/L]	RBC Count (10⁶/μL) [SI: 10¹²/L]	Hemoglobin (g/dL) [SI: g/L]	Hematocrit (%)	MCH (pg) [SI: pg]	MCHC (g/dL) [SI: g/L]ᵃ	MCV (μm³) [SI: fL]	RDW
Adult ♂	4500–11,000 [4.5–11.0]	4.73–5.49 [4.73–5.49]	14.40–16.60 [144–166]	42.9–49.1	27–31	33–37	76–100	11.5–14.5
Adult ♀	As above	4.15–4.87	12.2–14.7	37.9–43.9	As above	As above	As above	As above
11–15 y	4500–13,500	4.8	13.4	39	28	34	82	
6–10 y	5000–14,500	4.7	12.9	37.5	27	34	80	
4–6 y	5500–15,500	4.6	12.6	37.0	27	34	80	
2–4 y	6000–17,000	4.5	12.5	35.5	25	32	77	
4 mo–2 y	6000–17,500	4.6	11.2	35.0	25	33	77	
1 wk–4 mo	5500–18,000	4.7±0.9	14.0±3.3	42.0±7.0	30	33	90	
24 h–1 wk	5000–21,000	5.1	18.3±4.0	52.5	36	35	103	
First day	9400–34,000	5.1±1.0	19.5±5.0	54.0±10.0	38	36	106	

ᵃTo convert standard reference value to SI units, multiply by 10.
WBC = white blood cell; RBC = red blood cell; MCH = mean cell hemoglobin; MCHC = mean cell hemoglobin concentration; MCV = mean cell volume; RDW = red cell distribution width.

5

TABLE 5–3
Normal CBC for Selected Age Ranges

Age	Platelet Count [10³/μL] [SI: 10⁹/L]	Lymphocytes, Total (% WBC count)	Neutrophils, Band (% WBC count)	Neutrophils, Segmented (% WBC count)	Eosinophils (% WBC count)	Basophils (% WBC count)	Monocytes (% WBC count)
Adult ♂	238±49	34	3.0	56	2.7	0.5	4.0
Adult ♀	270±58	As above	As above	As above	As above	As above	As above
11–15 y	282±63	38	3.0	51	2.4	0.6	4.3
6–10 y	351±85	39	3.0	50	2.4	0.6	4.2
4–6 y	357±70	42	3.0	39	2.8	0.6	5.0
2–4 y	357±70	59	3.0	30	2.6	0.5	5.0
4 mo–2 y	As above	61	3.1	28	2.6	0.4	4.8
1 wk–4 mo	As above	56	4.5	30	2.8	0.5	6.5
24 h–1 wk	240–380	24–41	6.8–9.2	39–52	2.4–4.1	0.5	5.8–9.1
First day	As above	24	10.2	58	2.0	0.6	5.8

CBC = complete blood count; WBC = white blood cell.

NORMAL CBC VARIATIONS

Hbg and HCT are highest at birth (20 g/100 mL and 60%, respectively). The values fall steeply to a minimum at 3 mo (9.5 g/100 mL and 32%). Then they slowly rise to near adult levels at puberty; thereafter both values are higher in men. A normal decrease occurs in pregnancy. The number of WBCs is highest at birth (mean of 25,000/mm³) and slowly falls to adult levels by puberty. Lymphs predominate (as much as 60% from the second week of life until age 5–7 y, when polys begin to predominate).

HEMATOCRIT

Because plasma and red cells are lost in equal amounts in acute bleeding, the HCT does not immediately reflect the loss, sometimes not for 2–3 h. In anemia, the red cell indices and reticulocyte count should be checked.

THE LEFT SHIFT

The degree of nuclear lobulation of PMNs indicates cell age. A predominance of immature cells with only one or two nuclear lobes separated by a thick chromatin band is called a **"shift to the left."** Conversely, a predominance of cells with four nuclear lobes is called a **"shift to the right."** (For historical information, left and right designations come from the formerly used manual lab counters, in which the keys for entering stabs were located on the left of the keyboard.) As a rule, 55–80% of PMNs have two to four lobes. More than 20 five-lobed cells/100 WBCs suggests megaloblastic anemia, a six- or seven-lobed poly being diagnostic.

"Bands" or **"stabs,"** the more immature forms of PMNs (the more mature are called **"segs"**), are identified by the fact that the connections between ends or lobes of a nucleus are greater than one-half the width of the hypothetical round nucleus. In bands or stabs, the connection between the lobes of the nucleus is by a thick band; in segs, by a thin filament. A band is defined as a connecting strip wide enough to reveal two distinct margins with nuclear material in between. A filament is so narrow that no intervening nuclear material is present.

For practical purposes, **a left shift is present in the CBC when > 10–12% bands are seen or when the total PMN count (segs plus bands) is > 80.**

Left Shift: Bacterial infection, toxemia, hemorrhage, myeloproliferative disorders

Right Shift: Liver disease, megaloblastic anemia, iron deficiency anemia, glucocorticoid use, stress reaction

RETICULOCYTE COUNT

- Collection: Lavender top tube

The reticulocyte count is not a part of a routine CBC. The reticulocyte count is used in the initial work-up of anemia and in monitoring the effect of hematinic or erythropoietin therapy, monitoring recovery from myelosuppression, or monitoring engraftment after bone marrow transplantation. Reticulocytes are juvenile RBCs with remnants of cytoplasmic basophilic RNA. The presence of these cells is suggested by basophilia of the RBC cytoplasm on Wright stain **(polychromasia);** however, confirmation requires a special reticulocyte stain. The result is reported as a percentage. Use the following equation to calculate the **corrected reticulocyte count** for interpretation of the results

$$\text{Corrected reticulocyte count} = \frac{\text{Reported count} \times \text{Patient's HCT}}{\text{Normal HCT}}$$

This corrected count is an excellent indicator of erythropoietic activity. The **normal corrected reticulocyte count = < 1.5%.**

Normal bone marrow responds to a decrease in erythrocytes (shown by a decreased HCT) with an increase in the production of reticulocytes. A low reticulocyte count with anemia suggests a chronic disease, a deficiency disease, marrow replacement, or marrow failure.

CBC DIAGNOSTICS

• See Tables 5–2, page 93, and 5–3, page 94, for age- and sex-specific normal ranges. Beyond the total WBC count, identification of the specific white cell alteration may aid in the differential diagnosis.

White Cells (Leukocytes)

• See Table 5–2, page 93.

Increased: Infection, inflammatory process (rheumatoid arthritis, allergy) leukemia, severe stress (physical and emotional), postoperative state (physiologic stress), severe tissue damage (eg, burns), steroids

Decreased: Bone marrow failure (aplastic anemia, infection, tumor, fibrosis, radiation damage), cytotoxic agent or medication (eg, chloramphenicol, linezolid, chemotherapeutic agents), collagen–vascular disease such as lupus, liver or spleen disease, vitamin B_{12} or folate deficiency

Basophils • 0–1%
Increased: Chronic myeloid leukemia, aftermath of splenectomy, polycythemia, Hodgkin disease, and, rarely, recovery from infection or hypothyroidism

Decreased: Acute rheumatic fever, pregnancy, aftermath of radiation therapy, steroid therapy, thyrotoxicosis, stress

Eosinophils • 1–3%
Increased: Allergy, parasites, skin disease, malignancy, drugs, asthma, Addison disease, collagen–vascular disease (mnemonic **NAACP: N**eoplasm, **A**llergy/asthma, **A**ddison disease, **C**ollagen–vascular disease, **P**arasites), and pulmonary disease, including Löffler syndrome and PIE

Decreased: Steroids, ACTH, aftermath of stress (infection, trauma, burns), Cushing syndrome

Lymphocytes ("Lymphs") • 24–44% • See also Lymphocyte Subsets, page 98
Increased: Viral infection (AIDS, measles, rubella, mumps, whooping cough, smallpox, chickenpox, influenza, hepatitis, infectious mononucleosis), acute infectious lymphocytosis in children, acute and chronic lymphocytic leukemia

Decreased: (Normal in 22% of population) Stress, burns, trauma, uremia, some viral infections, HIV and AIDS, bone marrow suppression after chemotherapy, steroids, MS

Atypical Lymphocytes • > 20%: Infectious mononucleosis, CMV infection, infectious hepatitis, toxoplasmosis, malignancy • < 20%: Viral infections (mumps, rubeola, varicella), rickettsial infections, TB

Monocytes ("Monos") • 3–7%
Increased: Bacterial infection (TB, SBE, brucellosis, typhoid, recovery from acute infection), protozoan infection, infectious mononucleosis, leukemia, Hodgkin disease, ulcerative colitis, regional enteritis
Decreased: Lymphocytic leukemia, aplastic anemia, steroid use

PMNs (Polymorphonuclear Neutrophils, Neutrophils, "Polys") • 40–76% • See also The Left Shift, page 95.
Increased
Physiologic (Normal): Severe exercise, last months of pregnancy, labor, surgery, newborn state, steroid therapy
Pathologic: Bacterial infection, noninfective tissue damage (MI, pulmonary infarction, pancreatitis, crush or injury, burn injury), metabolic disorder (eclampsia, DKA, uremia, acute gout), leukemia
Decreased: Pancytopenia, aplastic anemia, PMN depression (a mild decrease is referred to as **neutropenia**; a severe decrease is called **agranulocytosis**), marrow damage (x-rays, poisoning with benzene, antitumor drugs), severe overwhelming infection (disseminated TB, septicemia), acute malaria, severe osteomyelitis, infectious mononucleosis, atypical pneumonia, some viral infections, marrow obliteration (osteosclerosis, myelofibrosis, malignant infiltrate), drugs (more than 70, including chloramphenicol, phenylbutazone, chlorpromazine, quinine), vitamin B_{12} and folate deficiencies, hypoadrenalism, hypopituitarism, dialysis, familial decrease, idiopathic causes

Red Cells

An automated device such as a Coulter Counter is used to measure red cell number, mean corpuscular volume (MCV), and hemoglobin concentration. The hematocrit and other parameters are calculated from those values.

Hematocrit

• Men 40–54%; women 37–47%
Calculated from MCV and red cell number; the percentage volume of red cells in a given volume of blood
Increased: Primary polycythemia (polycythemia vera), secondary polycythemia (reduced fluid intake or excess fluid loss), congenital or acquired heart and lung disease, high altitude, heavy smoking, tumors (renal cell carcinoma, hepatoma)
Decreased: Megaloblastic anemia (folate or B_{12} deficiency); iron deficiency anemia; sickle cell anemia or other hemoglobinopathy; acute or chronic blood loss; sideroblastic anemia, hemolysis; anemia due to chronic disease, dilution, alcohol, or drugs

MCH (Mean Cellular [Corpuscular] Hemoglobin) • 27–31 pg (SI: pg)
The amount of hemoglobin in the average red cell. Calculated as

$$MCH = \frac{Hemoglobin\ (g/L)}{RBC\ (10^6/\mu L)}$$

Increased: Macrocytosis (megaloblastic anemia, high reticulocyte count)
Decreased: Microcytosis (iron deficiency, sideroblastic anemia, thalassemia)

MCHC (Mean Cellular [Corpuscular] Hemoglobin Concentration) • 33–37 g/dL (SI: 330–370 g/L)

The average concentration of Hbg in a given volume of red cells. Calculated as

$$MCHC = \frac{\text{Hemoglobin (g / dL)}}{\text{Hematocrit}}$$

Increased: Very severe, prolonged dehydration; spherocytosis

Decreased: Iron deficiency anemia, overhydration, thalassemia, sideroblastic anemia

MCV (Mean Cell [Corpuscular] Volume) • 78–98 μm^3 (SI: fL)

The average volume of red blood cells; measured directly with the automated cell counter

Increased/Macrocytosis: Megaloblastic anemia (B_{12}, folate deficiency), macrocytic (normoblastic) anemia, reticulocytosis, myelodysplasia, Down syndrome, chronic liver disease, treatment of AIDS with AZT, chronic alcoholism, cytotoxic chemotherapy, radiation therapy, phenytoin (Dilantin) use, hypothyroidism, newborn state

Decreased/Microcytosis: Iron deficiency, thalassemia, some cases of lead poisoning or polycythemia

Normal: Anemia of chronic disease, acute blood loss, primary bone marrow failure

RDW (Red Cell Distribution Width) • 11.5–14.5%

RDW is a measure of the degree of **anisocytosis** (variation in RBC size) and is determined with an automated counter.

Increased: Many types of anemia (iron deficiency, pernicious, folate deficiency, thalassemia), liver disease

Platelets

• 150,000–450,000 μL

Platelet counts may be normal in number but abnormal in function, as occurs in aspirin therapy. Abnormalities of platelet function are assessed by bleeding time and platelet aggregation studies.

Increased: Sudden exercise, trauma, fracture, aftermath of asphyxia, aftermath of surgery (especially splenectomy), acute hemorrhage, myeloproliferative disorders, leukemia, aftermath of childbirth, carcinoma, cirrhosis, iron deficiency

Decreased: DIC, ITP, TTP, HUS, congenital disease, marrow suppressants (chemotherapy, alcohol, radiation), burns, snake and insect bites, leukemia, aplastic anemia, hypersplenism, infectious mononucleosis, viral infection, cirrhosis, massive transfusion, HELLP syndrome (a severe form of preeclampsia with microangiopathic hemolysis, elevated liver function test results, and low platelet count), preeclampsia and eclampsia, prosthetic heart valve, more than 30 drugs (NSAIDs, anticonvulsants, aspirin, thiazides, others)

LYMPHOCYTE SUBSETS

Specific monoclonal antibodies are used to identify specific T and B cells. Lymphocyte subsets are useful in the diagnosis of AIDS and various types of leukemia and lymphoma. The designation **CD (clusters of differentiation)** has replaced the older antibody designations. Results are most reliably reported as an absolute number of cells/μL rather than as a percentage. A CD4/CD8 ratio < 1 is seen in AIDS. Absolute CD4 count is used to determine when to initiate therapy with antiretroviral agents or to administer prophylaxis of certain infections, eg, PCP. The CDC considers an HIV-positive patient to have AIDS if the CD4 count < 200.

Normal Lymphocyte Subsets

- Total lymphocytes 660–4600/μL
- T cells 644–2201 μL (60–88%)
- B cells 82–392 μL (3–20%)
- Helper/inducer T cells (CD4) 493–1191 μL (34–67%)
- Suppressor/cytotoxic T cells (CD8) 182–785 μL (10–42%)
- CD4/CD8 ratio > 1

RBC MORPHOLOGY DIFFERENTIAL DIAGNOSIS

The following are erythrocyte abnormalities and the associated conditions. General terms include **poikilocytosis** (irregular RBC shape such as sickle or burr) and **anisocytosis** (irregular RBC size such as microcytes and macrocytes).

Basophilic Stippling: Lead or heavy-metal poisoning, thalassemia, severe anemia
Burr Cells (Acanthocytes): Severe liver disease; high levels of bile, fatty acids, or toxins
Heinz Bodies: Drug-induced hemolysis
Helmet Cells: Microangiopathic hemolysis (TTP, HUS, HELLP syndrome), hemolytic transfusion reaction, transplant rejection
Howell–Jolly Bodies: Asplenia
Nucleated RBCs: Severe bone marrow stress (eg, hemorrhage, hemolysis, hypoxia), marrow replacement by tumor, extramedullary hematopoiesis
Polychromasia: A bluish red cell on routine Wright stain suggests reticulocytes
Sickling: Sickle cell anemia
Schistocytes: DIC, microangiopathic anemia, severe burns, drug effect (CSA, tacrolimus, ticlopidine, others)
Spherocytes: Hereditary spherocytosis, immune hemolysis, severe burns, ABO transfusion reaction
Target Cells (Leptocytes): Thalassemia, hemoglobinopathies, liver disease, any hypochromic anemia, aftermath of splenectomy

WBC MORPHOLOGY DIFFERENTIAL DIAGNOSIS

The following are conditions associated with changes in the normal morphology of WBCs.

Auer Rods: AML
Döhle Inclusion Bodies: Severe infection, burns, malignancy, pregnancy
Hypersegmentation: Megaloblastic anemia
Toxic Granulation: Severe illness (sepsis, burn, high fever)

COAGULATION AND OTHER HEMATOLOGIC TESTS

The coagulation cascade is shown in Figure 5–2, page 100. A variety of coagulation-related and other blood tests follow.

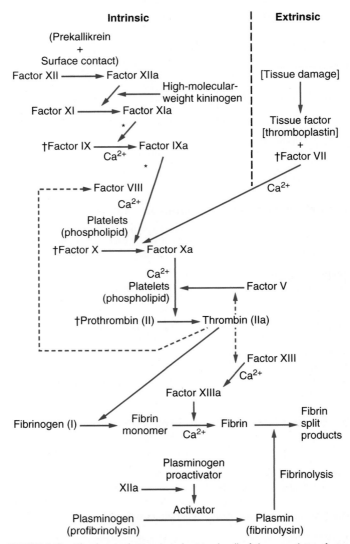

FIGURE 5–2. Blood coagulation cascade. Nearly all of the coagulation factors apparently exist as inactive proenzymes (Roman numerals) that when activated (Roman numeral + a) activate the next proenzyme in the sequence. * = Heparin acts to inhibit. † = Plasma content decreased by coumarin.

Anti-Xa Test (anti–factor Xa, anti–activated factor X)

•Anti-Xa heparin units per milliliter of plasma • Collection: Blue top tube

Used to monitor heparin therapy when the PTT cannot be used (ie, patient with lupus anticoagulant). Only test for monitoring low-molecular-weight (LMW) heparin (eg, Lovenox)

Therapeutic: LMW heparin: 0.5–1.0 anti-Xa units/mL

Prophylaxis: LMW heparin: 0.2–0.4 anti-Xa units/mL

Activated Clotting Time (ACT)

• 114–186 s • Collection: Black top tube from instrument manufacturer

A bedside test used in the operating room, dialysis unit, or other facility to document neutralization of heparin (ie, after CABG, heparin is reversed) or monitoring of antithrombin inhibitors (bivalirudin)

Increased: Heparin, some platelet disorders, severe clotting factor deficiency

Antithrombin III (AT-III)

• 17–30 mg/dL or 80–120% of control value • Collection: Blue top tube, patient must be off heparin for 6 h

Used in evaluation of thrombosis

Decreased: Autosomal-dominant familial AT-III deficiency, PE, severe liver disease, late pregnancy, oral contraceptives, nephrotic syndrome (lost in urine with resulting increase in factor II and X activity), DIC, heparin therapy (> 3 d)

Increased: Warfarin (Coumadin), after MI

Bleeding Time

• Duke, Ivy < 6 min; Template < 10 min • Collection: A bedside test performed by technicians. After a small incision is made, the wound is wicked with filter paper every 30 s until the fluid is clear.

In vivo test of hemostasis, platelet function, local tissue factors, and clotting factors. Nonsteroidal medications should be stopped 5–7 d before the test, because these agents can affect platelet function.

Increased: Thrombocytopenia, von Willebrand disease, defective platelet function, drugs such as NSAIDs, uremia

Coombs Test, Direct (Direct Antiglobulin Test)

• Normal = negative • Collection: Purple top tube

Patient's erythrocytes; test for the presence of antibody on the patient's cells and for the screening for autoimmune hemolytic anemia

Positive: Autoimmune hemolytic anemia, hemolytic transfusion reaction, some drug sensitizations (methyldopa, levodopa, cephalosporins, penicillin, quinidine), hemolytic disease of the newborn (erythroblastosis fetalis)

Coombs Test, Indirect (Indirect Antiglobulin Test/ Autoantibody Test)

• Normal = negative • Collection: Purple top tube

Patient's serum; check for cross-match before blood transfusion. Test for antibodies against red cell antigens in the patient's serum.

Positive: Isoimmunization from previous transfusion, autoimmune hemolytic anemia, incompatible blood or medications (eg, methyldopa)

Factor V (Leiden) Mutation

• Normal = negative • Collection: Lavender or blue top tube

Factor V Leiden **(activated protein C [APC] resistance)** is the most common hereditary blood coagulation disorder in the United States (5–7%). Heterozygotes have thrombosis risk **(thrombophilia)** three to eight times that of the general population. The risk among homozygotes is 140 times that of the general population. A PCR and reverse dot blot genetic test.

Positive: Factor V mutation

Fibrin D-Dimers (See also Chapter 4, page 62)

• Negative or < 0.25 mcg/mL • Collection: Blue, green, or purple top tube
  Evidence of fibrin formation, fibrin cross-linking, and fibrinolysis

Increased: DIC, thromboembolic disease (PE, arterial or venous thrombosis)

Fibrin Degradation Products (FDP), Fibrin Split Products (FSP)

• < 10 mcg/mL • Collection: Blue top tube
  Generally replaced by the fibrin D-dimer as a screen for DIC

Increased: DIC (usually > 40 mcg/mL), any thromboembolic condition (DVT, MI, PE), hepatic dysfunction

Fibrinogen

• 123–370 mg/dL (SI: 1.23–3.7 g/L) • (Panic levels < 100 or > 500) • Collection: Blue top tube
  Most useful in management of DIC and congenital hypofibrinogenemia

Increased: Inflammatory reaction, oral contraceptives, pregnancy, cancer (kidney, stomach, breast)

Decreased: DIC (sepsis, amniotic fluid embolism, abruptio placentae), surgery (prostate, open heart), neoplastic and hematologic conditions, acute severe bleeding, burns, venomous snake bite, congenital disorder

Mixing Studies (Circulating Anticoagulant Screen)

• Collection: Blue top tube
  Used to evaluate prolonged PT or PTT. Normal plasma is mixed with patient plasma, and the abnormal clotting time is measured again in the mix. If the clotting time corrects, a factor deficiency exists. Assay for factors VIII, IX, XI, and XII to identify the specific factor (note: warfarin may also give this result). If the clotting time does not correct, an inhibitor is present (ie, lupus anticoagulant [associated with thrombosis and habitual abortion], heparin, argatroban, high-dose danaparoid, specific factor inhibitor). Prolonged **RVVT (Russell viper venom time)** is used to diagnose lupus anticoagulant. (RVV activates factor X.)

Partial Thromboplastin Time (Activated Partial Thromboplastin Time, PTT, aPTT)

• 27–38 s • Collection: Blue top tube
  Used to evaluate the intrinsic coagulation system (see Figure 5–2, page 100). Most often used to monitor heparin therapy

Increased: Heparin, defect in the **intrinsic coagulation system** (except factors VII and XIII), prolonged application of tourniquet before drawing of sample, hemophilia A and B, von Willebrand disease (sometimes normal), lupus antico-agulant (antiphospholipid antibody), DIC

Prothrombin Time (PT)

• 11.5–13.5 s (INR, normal = 0.8–1.4) • Collection: Blue top tube

Used to evaluate the **extrinsic coagulation system** (see Figure 5–2, page 100), which includes factors I, II, V, VII, and X. The use of **INR** instead of patient/control ratio to guide warfarin therapy is now the standard. **INR provides a more standardized result; measures the control against a WHO standard reagent.** Therapeutic INR is 2–3 for DVT, PE, TIAs, and atrial fibrillation. Mechanical heart valves require an INR of 2.5–3.5 (see also Chapter 22, Table 22–10, page 644). Not affected by heparin

Increased: Drugs (warfarin), vitamin K deficiency, fat malabsorption, liver disease, prolonged application of tourniquet before drawing of sample, DIC, massive transfusion

Sedimentation Rate (Erythrocyte Sedimentation Rate, ESR)

• Collection: Lavender top tube

A nonspecific test; high sensitivity and low specificity. Most useful in serial measurement to follow the course of disease (eg, polymyalgia rheumatica or temporal arteritis)

Wintrobe Scale: • Men, 0–9 mm/h; women, 0–20 mm/h

Increased: Any type of infection, inflammation, rheumatic fever, endocarditis, neoplasm, AMI, multiple myeloma

Thrombin Time

• 10–14 s • Collection: Blue top tube

Measure of conversion of fibrinogen to fibrin and fibrin polymerization. Used to detect the presence of heparin and hypofibrinogenemia

Increased: Systemic heparin, DIC, fibrinogen deficiency, congenitally abnormal fibrinogen molecules

LABORATORY DIAGNOSIS: URINE STUDIES

Urinalysis Procedure
Urinalysis, Normal Values
Differential Diagnosis for Routine
    Urinalysis
Urine Sediment
Spot or Random Urine Studies

Creatinine Clearance
24-Hour Urine Studies
Other Urine Studies
Urinary Indices in Renal Failure
Urine Output
Urine Protein Electrophoresis

URINALYSIS PROCEDURE

For routine urinalysis, a fresh (less than 1-h old), clean-catch urine sample is acceptable. If the analysis cannot be performed immediately, refrigerate the sample. (When urine stands at room temperature for a long time, casts and red cells undergo lysis, and the urine becomes alkalinized with precipitation of salts.) See Chapter 13, Urinary Tract Procedures, page 312, for sample collection.

1. Pour 5–10 mL of well-mixed urine into a centrifuge tube.
2. Check for appearance (color, turbidity, odor). If a urine sample looks grossly cloudy, it is sometimes advisable to examine an unspun sample. If you use an unspun sample, make a note that you have done so. In general, a spun sample is more desirable for routine urinalysis.
3. Spin the capped sample at 3000 rpm (450g) for 3–5 min.
4. While the sample is in the centrifuge, use the dipstick (eg, Chemstrip) supplied by your lab to perform the dipstick evaluation on the remaining sample. Read the results according to the color chart on the bottle. Allow the correct amount of time before reading the test (usually 1–2 min) to avoid false results. **Chemstrip 10** provides 10 tests (specific gravity, pH, leukocytes, nitrite, protein, glucose, ketone, urobilinogen, bilirubin, and blood.) Other strips may provide less.) Agents that color the urine (phenazopyridine [Pyridium]) may interfere with the reading. Dipstick specific gravity (SG) measurement is possible, but a refractometer also can be used to determine SG.
5. Decant and discard the supernatant. Mix the remaining sediment by flicking it with a finger and pouring or pipetting one or two drops onto a microscope slide. Cover with a coverslip.
6. Examine 10 low-power fields (10× objective) for epithelial cells, casts, crystals, and mucus. Casts are usually reported as number per low-power field and tend to collect around the periphery of the coverslip.
7. Examine several high-power fields (40× objective) for epithelial cells, crystals, RBCs, WBCs, bacteria, and parasites (trichomonads). RBCs, WBCs, and bacteria are usually reported as number per high-power field. The following two reporting systems are commonly used:

System One	System Two
Rare = < 2/field	Trace = < $1/4$ of field
Occasional = 3–5/field	1+ = $1/4$ of field
Frequent = 5–9/field	2+ = $1/2$ of field
Many = "large number"/field	3+ = $3/4$ of field
TNTC = too numerous to count	4+ = field is full

URINALYSIS, NORMAL VALUES

1. *Appearance:* "Dark yellow or amber in color and clear"
2. *Specific Gravity*
   a. Neonates: 1.012
   b. Infants: 1.002–1.006
   c. Children and Adults: 1.001–1.035 (typical with normal fluid intake 1.016–1.022)
3. *pH*
   a. Neonates: 5–7
   b. Children and Adults: 4.6–8.0
4. *Negative for:* Bilirubin, blood, acetone, glucose, protein, nitrite, leukocyte esterase, reducing substances
5. *Trace:* Urobilinogen
6. *RBC:* Male 0–3/hpf, female 0–5/hpf
7. *WBC:* 0–4/hpf
8. *Epithelial Cells:* Occasional
9. *Hyaline Casts:* Occasional
10. *Bacteria:* None
11. *Crystals:* Some limited crystals based on urine pH (see following section)

DIFFERENTIAL DIAGNOSIS FOR ROUTINE URINALYSIS

Appearance

Colorless: Diabetes insipidus, diuretics, excess fluid intake
Dark: Acute intermittent porphyria, advanced malignant melanoma
Cloudy: UTI (pyuria), amorphous phosphate salts (normal in alkaline urine or urine left standing at room temperature. Adding a small amount of acid to the sample will confirm), blood, mucus, bilirubin
Pink/Red:
Heme(+). Blood, Hbg, sepsis, dialysis, myoglobin
Heme(–). Food coloring, beets, sulfa drugs, nitrofurantoin, salicylates
Orange/Yellow: Dehydration, phenazopyridine (Pyridium), rifampin, bile pigments
Brown/Black: Myoglobin, bile pigments, melanin, cascara, iron, nitrofurantoin, alkaptonuria
Green/Blue: Urinary bile pigments, indigo carmine, methylene blue
Foamy: Proteinuria, bile salts

Bilirubin

Limited utility on dipstick

Positive: (Only conjugated bilirubin appears in urine) Obstructive jaundice (intra-hepatic and extrahepatic), hepatitis. False-positive with stool contamination

Blood (Hematuria)

If the dipstick is positive for blood, but no red cells are seen, free Hbg may be present (transfusion reaction, from lysis of RBCs if pH is < 5 or > 8) or myoglobin is present (crush injury, burn, or tissue ischemia).

Positive: Stones, trauma, tumors (benign and malignant, anywhere in the urinary tract), BPH, urethral stricture, coagulopathy, infection, menses (contamination), polycystic kidneys, interstitial nephritis, hemolytic anemia, transfusion reaction, instrumentation (eg, Foley catheter)

Glucose

Glucose oxidase technique in most kits is specific for glucose and does not react with lactose, fructose, or galactose; therefore screen infant urine with another assay such as Clinitest.

Positive: DM, pancreatitis, pancreatic carcinoma, pheochromocytoma, Cushing disease, shock, burns, pain, steroids, hyperthyroidism, renal tubular disease, iatrogenic causes; false-positive: uncapped dipstick container bottle after several days, specimen contamination with liquid bleach

Ketones

Used primarily to detect acetone and acetoacetic acid and not β-hydroxybutyric acid

Positive: Starvation, high-fat diet, DKA, vomiting, diarrhea, hyperthyroidism, PRG, febrile state (especially in children), aspirin overdose; false-positive: some Parkinson medications, cystinuria, stimulant laxative (such as Ex-Lax)

Leukocyte Esterase

Used to detect 5 WBCs/hpf or lysed WBCs. Combined with the nitrite test, leukocyte esterase has a positive predictive value of 74% for UTI if both tests are positive and a negative predictive value of > 97% if both tests are negative. May not be reliable in children with UTI

Positive: UTI (false-positive: vaginal/fecal contamination; pediatric urine bag collection)

Nitrite

Many bacteria convert nitrates to nitrite. (See earlier, Leukocyte Esterase, and see Chapter 7)

Positive: Infection (negative test does not exclude infection because some organisms [*Streptococcus faecalis,* other gram-positive cocci], do not produce nitrite, and urine must be in the bladder for several hours to allow the nitrite reaction to take place)

Odor

Limited utility: strong ammonia smell suggests UTI; asparagus consumption

pH

Acidic: High-protein (meat) diet, ammonium chloride, mandelic acid and other medications, acidosis (due to ketoacidosis [starvation, diabetic], COPD)

Basic: UTI, RTA, diet (high-vegetable diet, milk, immediately after meals), sodium bicarbonate therapy, vomiting, metabolic alkalosis

Protein

Proteinuria on dipstick should be quantified with 24-h urine studies. Normal protein excretion is < 150 mg/24 h or 10 mg/100 mL in a spot specimen (*dipstick approximations:* Negative, 0–50; trace, 50–150; 1+, 150–300; 2+, 300–1000; 3+, 1–3; 4+, > 3 gm/L). Bence Jones globulins (plasma cell myeloma, macroglobulinemia; lymphoma may be missed on dipstick and determined on urine protein electrophoresis).

Positive: Pyelonephritis, glomerulonephritis, glomerular sclerosis (diabetes), nephrotic syndrome, myeloma, postural causes, preeclampsia, inflammation and malignant diseases of lower urinary tract, functional causes (fever, stress, heavy exercise), malignant hypertension, CHF

Reducing Substances

Positive: Glucose, fructose, galactose, false-positives (eg, vitamin C, salicylates, antibiotics)

Specific Gravity

Corresponds with osmolarity except with osmotic diuresis (high glucose). Random value 1.003–1.030. Value > 1.022 after 12 h food/fluids fast suggests normal renal concentrating ability. **Isosthenuria** (SG fixed at 1.010 regardless of intake) suggests renal tubular dysfunction.

Increased: Volume depletion, CHF, adrenal insufficiency, DM, SIADH, increased proteins (nephrosis), newborn state; if markedly increased (1.040–1.050), artifact or recent administration of radiographic contrast media

Decreased: Diabetes insipidus, pyelonephritis, glomerulonephritis, water load with normal renal function (note effective management in kidney stone patients, hydrate to keep SG very low)

Urobilinogen

Limited utility on dipstick (*Note:* Urobilinogen is colorless)

Positive: Hemolysis, cirrhosis, CHF with hepatic congestion, hepatitis, hyperthyroidism, suppression of intestinal flora with antibiotics

URINE SEDIMENT

Many labs no longer do microscopic examinations unless requested or if there is an abnormal dipstick test result.

Figure 6–1 is a diagram of materials found in urine sediments.

Red Blood Cells (RBCs): Trauma, pyelonephritis, genitourinary TB, cystitis, prostatitis, stones, tumors (malignant and benign), coagulopathy, and any cause of blood on dipstick test (see Differential Diagnosis for Routine Urinalysis, Blood, page 107)

White Blood Cells (WBCs): Infection anywhere in the urinary tract, TB, renal tumors, acute glomerulonephritis, radiation, interstitial nephritis (analgesic abuse)

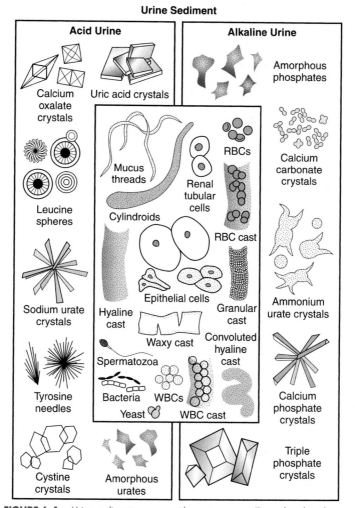

FIGURE 6-1. Urine sediment as seen with a microscope. (Reproduced, with permission, from: Greene MG [ed]: *The Harriet Lane Handbook: A Manual for Pediatric House Officers*, 12th ed., Year Book Medical Publishers, Chicago, IL, 1991.)

Epithelial Cells: ATN, necrotizing papillitis. (Most epithelial cells are from an otherwise unremarkable urethra.)

Parasites: *Trichomonas vaginalis, Schistosoma haematobium* infection

Yeast: *Candida albicans* infection (especially in diabetic or immunosuppressed patients or if a vaginal yeast infection is present)

Spermatozoa: Normal in men immediately after intercourse or nocturnal emission

Crystals
• Normal

Acidic urine: Calcium oxalate (small, square crystals with a central cross; octa-hedrons), uric acid (rhomboids, hexagons, squares)

Alkaline urine: Calcium carbonate/phosphate, triple phosphate (struvite, magne-sium ammonium phosphate associated with urea-splitting UTI and possi-ble stone formation [coffin lids])

• Abnormal

Any: Cystine (colorless hexagons), sulfonamide, leucine (bicycle wheels), tyrosine, cholesterol

Excessive: Calcium oxalate (excess vitamin C or spinach, ileitis, ethylene glycol poisoning, urolithiasis), uric acid (gout, leukemia, tumor lysis during chemotherapy), triple phosphate (urea splitting UTI and with "infection" stone formation), indinavir (crystals in patients on HIV therapy)

Contaminants: Cotton threads, hair, wood fibers, amorphous substances (all usually unimportant); "dirty urine" may suggest enterovesical fistula

Mucus: Large amounts of mucus suggest urethral disease (normal from ileal conduit or continent urinary diversion that uses bowel) or enterovesical fistula.

Glitter Cells: WBCs lysed in hypotonic solution

Casts: Localizes some or all of the disease process to the kidney itself

> *Hyaline Casts.* Acceptable unless "numerous," benign hypertension, neph-rotic syndrome, after exercise
> *RBC Casts.* Acute glomerulonephritis, lupus nephritis, SBE, Goodpasture disease, aftermath of streptococcal infection (poststreptococcal glomerulo-nephritis), vasculitis, malignant hypertension
> *WBC Casts.* Pyelonephritis, acute interstitial nephritis, glomerulonephritis
> *Epithelial (Tubular) Casts.* Tubular damage, nephrotoxin, virus
> *Granular Casts.* Breakdown of cellular casts, leads to waxy casts; "dirty brown granular casts" typical for ATN
> *Waxy Casts.* All cellular casts can become waxy casts. Severe chronic renal disease, amyloidosis
> *Fatty Casts.* Nephrotic syndrome, DM, damaged renal tubular epithelial cells
> *Broad Casts.* Chronic renal disease

SPOT OR RANDOM URINE STUDIES

A spot urine, which is often ordered to aid in the diagnosis of various conditions, is done with only a small sample (10–20 mL) of urine.

Spot Urine for β₂-Microglobulin

• < 1 mg/24 h or 0–160 g/L (keep sample refrigerated) • A marker of renal tubu-lar injury

Increased: Diseases of the proximal tubule (ATN, interstitial nephritis, pyelo-nephritis), viral diseases, drug-induced nephropathy (aminoglycosides), diabe-tes, trauma, sepsis, HIV, lymphoproliferative and lymphodestructive diseases (multiple myeloma, plasmacytoma)

Spot Urine for Cytology

Used as an adjunct in the diagnosis of urothelial cancers (primarily transitional cell carcinoma of the bladder, kidney and ureter); limited or no role for renal cell carcinoma. Use a 3-h postvoid and not an AM sample.

Spot Urine for Electrolytes

Utility is limited because of variations in daily fluid and salt intake; not useful if a diuretic has been taken.

1. **Sodium < 10 mEq/L:** Volume depletion, hyponatremic states, prerenal azotemia (eg, CHF, shock), hepatorenal syndrome, glucocorticoid excess
2. **Sodium > 20 mEq/L:** SIADH, ATN (usually > 40 mEq/L), postobstructive diuresis, high salt intake, Addison disease, hypothyroidism, interstitial nephritis
3. **Chloride < 10 mEq/L:** Chloride-sensitive metabolic alkalosis (vomiting, excessive diuretic use), volume depletion
4. **Potassium < 10 mEq/L:** Hypokalemia, potassium depletion, extrarenal loss

Spot Urine for Erythrocyte Morphology

The morphology of red cells in a urine sample positive for blood may indicate of the nature of the hematuria. **Eumorphic red cells** are seen in postrenal, non-glomerular bleeding. **Dysmorphic red cells** are associated with glomerular causes of bleeding. Labs vary, but > 90% dysmorphic erythrocytes with asymptomatic hematuria indicates a renal glomerular source of bleeding, especially if associated with proteinuria or casts (eg, IgA nephropathy, poststreptococcal glomerular disease, sickle cell disease or trait). If there are 90% eumorphic erythrocytes or even "mixed" results (10–90% eumorphic erythrocytes), a postrenal cause of hematuria requires urologic evaluation (eg, hypercalciuria, urolithiasis, cystitis, trauma, tumors, hemangioma, exercise induced, BPH).

Spot Urine for Microalbumin

Normal < 30 mcg albumin/mg creatinine (timed collection < 20 mcg/min)

Used to determine whether a diabetic patient is at risk of nephropathy or cardiovascular disease. Perform two or three separate determinations over 6 mo to confirm; spot urine preferred. Diabetic patients with a level of 30–300 mcg often need an ACE inhibitor or angiotensin receptor blocker. Six percent of the healthy population has microalbuminuria. The following are the ranges for microalbuminuria recommended by the American Diabetes Association:

Category	Spot Collection (mcg/mg Cr)	24-h Collection (mg/24 h)	Timed Collection (mcg/min)
Normoalbuminuria	< 30	< 30	< 20
Microalbuminuria	30–299	30–299	20–199
Macroalbuminuria	≥ 300	≥ 300	≥ 200

Reproduced, with permission, from the American Diabetes Association, *Diabetes Care* 2004;27:S15–S35.

Spot Urine for Myoglobin

• Qualitative negative

Positive: Skeletal muscle conditions (crush injury, electrical burns, carbon monoxide poisoning, delirium tremens, surgical procedures, malignant hyperthermia), polymyositis

Spot Urine for Osmolality

• 75–300 mOsm/kg, varies with water intake
   Patients with normal renal function should concentrate > 800 mOsm/kg after 14-h fluid restriction; < 400 mOsm/kg is a sign of renal impairment.

Increased: Dehydration, SIADH, adrenal insufficiency, glycosuria, high-protein diet

Decreased: Excessive fluid intake, diabetes insipidus, acute renal failure, medications (acetohexamide, glyburide, lithium)

Spot Urine for Protein

• Normal < 10 mg/dL (0.1 g/L) or < 20 mg/dL (0.2 g/L) for a sample taken in the early AM
   See page 108 for the differential diagnosis of protein in the urine.

CREATININE CLEARANCE

Normal
• *Men.* Total creatinine 1–2 g/24 h; clearance 85–125 mL/min/1.73 m^2
• *Women.* Total creatinine 0.8–1.8 g/24 h; clearance 75–115 mL/min 1.73 m^2
• *Children.* Total creatinine (> 3 y) 12–30 mg/kg/24 h; clearance 70–140 mL/min/1.73 m^2 (1.17–2.33 mL/s/1.73 m^2)

Decreased: Decreased creatinine clearance results in an increase in serum creatinine usually secondary to renal insufficiency. See Chapter 4, page 60, for differential diagnosis of increased serum creatinine.

Increased: Early DM, PRG

Methods for Determination of Creatinine Clearance (CrCl)

CrCl is a sensitive indicator of early renal insufficiency. Clearances are ordered for evaluation of patients with suspected renal disease and monitoring of patients taking nephrotoxic medications (eg, gentamicin). CrCl decreases with age; CrCl of 10–20 mL/min indicates severe renal failure and usually the need for dialysis.

1. **Formal 24-h Urinary Collection for Creatinine Clearance.** Order a concurrent SCr and a 24-h urine creatinine. A shorter time interval can be used (eg, 12 h), but the formula must be corrected for this change; a 24-h sample is less prone to collection error.

Example: The following are calculations of (a) CrCl from a 24-h urine sample with a volume of 1000 mL, (b) a urine creatinine of 108 mg/100 mL, and (c) a SCr of 1 mg/100 mL (1 mg/dL).

$$\text{Clearance} = \frac{\text{Urine creatinine} \times \text{Total urine volume}}{\text{Plasma creatinine} \times \text{Time}}$$

$$\text{Clearance} = \frac{(108 \text{ mg} / 100 \text{ mL}) (1000 \text{ mL})}{(1 \text{ mg} / 100 \text{ mL}) (1440 \text{ min})} = 75 \text{ mL} / \text{min}$$

To determine whether there is a valid, full 24-h collection, the sample should contain 18–25 mg/kg/24 h of creatinine for men or 12–20 mg/kg/24 h for women. If the patient is an adult (150 lb = body surface area of 1.73 m²), clearance is not routinely adjusted for body size. Adjustment must be made for pediatric patients.

If the values in the previous example are for a 10-year-old boy weighing 70 lb (1.1 m²), the clearance is:

$$75 \text{ mL} / \text{min} \times \frac{1.73 \text{ m}^2}{1.1 \text{ m}^2} = 118 \text{ mL} / \text{min}$$

2. **Estimated Creatinine Clearance.** Online calculators for adults and children are available at: www.nkdep.nih.gov/professionals/gfr_calculators (Accessed May 29, 2006)

Adults:

- **Modification of Diet in Renal Disease (MDRD) equation** (*Ann Intern Med* 1999;130:137–147). *The equation does not require weight; results normalized to 1.73²* BSA, an accepted adult average BSA.

$$\text{GFR} = 186 \times [\text{SCr}]^{-1.154} \times [\text{age}]^{-0.203}$$
$$\times [0.742 \text{ if patient is female or} \times 1.21 \text{ if African American}]$$

Cockcroft-Gault equation:

$$\text{CrCl estimate} = \frac{(140 - \text{age}) \times \text{wt (kg) (if female,} \times 0.85)}{\text{Cr} \times 72}$$

Children: Use the Schwartz equation:

$$\text{GFR(mL/min/1.73}^2) = \text{k (Height)} / \text{Serum creatinine}$$

where k is a constant (0.33, premature infants; 0.45, term infants to 1 y; 0.55, children to 13 y; 0.65, male adolescents; 0.55, female adolescents), height is in centimeters, and SCr is in mg/dL.

24-HOUR URINE STUDIES

Many diseases, most of them endocrine, can be diagnosed with assays of 24-h urine samples.

Calcium, Urine

Normal: On a calcium-free diet < 150 mg/24 h, average-calcium diet (600–800 mg/24 h) 100–250 mg/24 h

Increased: Hyperparathyroidism, hyperthyroidism, hypervitaminosis D, distal RTA (type I), sarcoidosis, immobilization, osteolytic lesions (bony metastasis, multiple myeloma), Paget disease, glucocorticoid excess, immobilization, furosemide

Decreased: Medications (thiazide diuretics, estrogens, oral contraceptives), hypothyroidism, renal failure, steatorrhea, rickets, osteomalacia

Catecholamines, Fractionated

Used to evaluate neuroendocrine tumors, including pheochromocytoma and neuroblastoma. Avoid caffeine and methyldopa (Aldomet) before test.

Normal: Values are variable and depend on the assay method used. Norepinephrine 15–80 mg/24 h, epinephrine 0–20 mg/24 h, dopamine 65–400 mg/24 h

Increased: Pheochromocytoma, neuroblastoma, epinephrine administration, presence of drugs (methyldopa, tetracyclines cause false increases)

Cortisol, Free

Used to evaluate adrenal cortical hyperfunction, screening test of choice for Cushing syndrome

Normal: 10–110 mg/24 h
 Increased: Cushing syndrome (adrenal hyperfunction), stress during collection, oral contraceptives, PRG

Creatinine

• See pages 62 and 112.

Cysteine

Used to detect cystinuria, homocystinuria, monitor response to therapy

Normal: 40–60 mg/g creatinine

Increased: Heterozygotes < 300 mg/g creatinine; homozygotes > 250 mg/g creatinine

5-HIAA (5-Hydroxyindoleacetic Acid)

5-HIAA is a serotonin metabolite useful in the diagnosis of carcinoid syndrome.

Normal: 2–8 mg /24-h urine collection

Increased: Carcinoid tumors (except rectal), certain foods (banana, pineapple, tomato, walnuts, avocado), phenothiazine derivatives

Metanephrines

Used to detect metabolic products of epinephrine and norepinephrine, primary screening test for pheochromocytoma

Normal: < 1.3 mg/24 h for adults, but variable in children

Increased: Pheochromocytoma, neuroblastoma (neural crest tumors), false-positive with drugs (phenobarbital, guanethidine, hydrocortisone, MAO inhibitors)

Protein

• See also Urine Protein Electrophoresis, page 82.

Normal: < 150 mg/24 h

Increased: Nephrotic syndrome usually associated with > 3.5 g/1.73 m^2/24 h

17-Ketogenic Steroids (17-KGS, Corticosteroids)

Overall adrenal function test, largely replaced by serum or urine cortisol levels

Normal: Men 5–24 mg/24 h; women 4–15 mg/24 h

Increased: Adrenal hyperplasia (Cushing syndrome), adrenogenital syndrome

Decreased: Panhypopituitarism, Addison disease, acute steroid withdrawal

17-Ketosteroids, Total (17-KS)

Used to measure DHEA, androstenedione (adrenal androgens); largely replaced by assay of individual elements

Normal: Men 8–20 mg/24 h; women 6–15 mg/dL. *Note:* Low values in prepubertal children

Increased: Adrenal cortex abnormalities (hyperplasia [Cushing disease], adenoma, carcinoma, adrenogenital syndrome), severe stress, ACTH or pituitary tumor, testicular interstitial tumor and arrhenoblastoma (both produce testosterone)

Decreased: Panhypopituitarism, Addison disease, castration in men

Vanillylmandelic Acid (VMA)

VMA is the urinary product of both epinephrine and norepinephrine; good screening test for pheochromocytoma, also used to diagnose and follow up neuroblastoma and ganglioneuroma

Normal: < 7–9 mg/24 h

Increased: Pheochromocytoma, other neural crest tumors (ganglioneuroma, neuroblastoma), factitious causes (chocolate, coffee, tea, methyldopa)

OTHER URINE STUDIES
Drug Abuse Screen

• Normal = negative

Test for common drugs of abuse, often used for employment screening for critical jobs. Assay varies by facility and may include tests for amphetamines, barbiturates, benzodiazepines, marijuana (cannabinoid metabolites), cocaine metabolites, opiates, phencyclidine.

Xylose Tolerance Test (D-Xylose Absorption Test)

• 5 g xylose in 5-h urine specimen after 25-g oral dose of xylose or 1.2 g after 5-g oral dose • Collection: Patient is on NPO status after midnight except for water

• After 8 AM void, 25 g of D-xylose (or 5 g if GI irritation is a concern) is dissolved in 250 mL water • Patient drinks an additional 750 mL water, and urine is collected for the next 5 h.

Used to assess proximal bowel function; differentiates malabsorption due to pancreatic insufficiency and that due to intestinal problems

Decreased: Celiac disease (nontropical sprue, gluten-sensitive enteropathy), false decrease with renal disease

URINARY INDICES IN RENAL FAILURE

Use Table 6–1 to differentiate the causes (renal or prerenal) of oliguria. (See also Oliguria and Anuria, page 42.)

TABLE 6–1
Urinary Indices Useful in the Differential Diagnosis of Oliguria

Index	Prerenal	Renal (ATN)[a]
Urine osmolality	>500	<350
Urinary sodium	<20	>40
Urine/serum creatinine	>40	<20
Urine/serum osmolarity	>1.2	<1.2
Fractional excreted sodium[b]	<1	>1
Renal failure index (RFI)[c]	<1	>1

[a]Acute tubular necrosis (intrinsic renal failure).

[b]Fractional excreted sodium: $\dfrac{\text{Urine /Serum sodium}}{\text{Urine /Serum creatinine}} \times 100$

[c]Renal failure index: $\dfrac{\text{Urine sodium} \times \text{Serum creatinine}}{\text{Urine creatinine}}$

URINE OUTPUT

Although clinical situations vary greatly, the usual, minimal acceptable urine output for an adult is 0.5–1.0 mL/kg/h (daily volume normally 750–2000 mL/d).

URINE PROTEIN ELECTROPHORESIS

See Protein Electrophoresis, Serum and Urine, page 82, and Figure 4–5, page 83.

CLINICAL MICROBIOLOGY

General Principles of Clinical
    Microbiology
Microbiology Techniques
    Acid-Fast Stain
    Blood Culture
    Darkfield Examination
    Giemsa Stain
    Gonorrhea Smear and Culture
    Gram Stain and Common
        Pathogens
    India Ink Preparation
    KOH Preparation
    Lyme Disease Testing
    Malaria Smear
    Molecular Microbiology
    Nasal Culture
    Pinworm Preparation
    Sputum Culture
Stool Culture
Stool Leukocyte Stain
Stool for Ova and Parasites
Syphilis Testing
Throat Culture
Tzanck Smear
Urine Culture
Vaginal Wet Preparation
Viral Cultures and Serology
Differential Diagnosis of Common
    Infections and Empiric Therapy
Common Clinical Applications
Bioterrorism
Subacute Bacterial Endocarditis
    Prophylaxis
Isolation Protocols

GENERAL PRINCIPLES OF CLINICAL MICROBIOLOGY

Some of the most common tests performed on patients are the procurement of tissue or body fluids for direct detection of pathogenic organisms to prove or disprove the presence of infection. The results of these tests are critical in guiding the selection of antibiotics for targeted therapy. The following clinical microbiology principles must be considered.

Severity or Degree of Risk: There is a difference between an otherwise healthy patient with a complaint of dysuria consistent with a UTI versus a patient with neutropenia and a high fever. The first needs a simple urinalysis with a routine bacterial culture. The second needs a "pan" culture (as in the prefix "pan-," meaning "all" or "every"), which includes a pair of blood cultures, urinalysis with culture and sensitivity, sputum sample if a productive cough is present), and a chest x-ray to rule out pneumonia. The second patient also needs prompt treatment with empiric broad-spectrum antibiotics because she is at high risk of septicemia and death.

Broad Coverage with Empiric Antibiotics: Initiation of antibiotics that broadly *cover* a newly recognized infection in a timely and appropriate manner often is lifesaving. Selecting the wrong antibiotic, the wrong dose, an improper route, or delaying treatment, however, can increase morbidity and mortality.

Timing: Whenever feasible, specimens should be obtained and cultures performed before antibiotics are started. However, antibiotics should never be delayed in the face of a possible life-threatening infection, such as meningitis. After the culture data become available, antibiotic therapy can be narrowed or "de-escalated" to the antibiogram of the recovered organism.

Source Control: Collections of pus and infected fluids such as abscesses and empyema *must be drained if at all possible.* Failure to drain pockets of infection can compromise the outcome. The classic example is necrotizing fasciitis, which is a **surgical emergency.** Without surgery, mortality approaches 100%.

True Infection versus Contamination and Colonization: True infection is almost always accompanied by inflammation, usually marked by the presence of neutrophils in clinical specimens (absent in neutropenia) and clinical signs and symptoms. The presence of a large number of epithelial cells in a sample or the growth of normal skin flora often signifies contamination and colonization secondary to improper collection of specimens, although there are exceptions.

Antimicrobial Resistance: Drug resistance is a serious problem in modern medicine. In the past medicine stayed ahead of antimicrobial resistance with the development of new antibiotics to overcome new resistance patterns. Now, as vancomycin-resistant enterococci spread throughout the health care system and new clones of methicillin-resistant *Staphylococcus aureus* become more prevalent, antibiotic resistance is minimized only through proper antibiotic stewardship. To this end the CDC has launched a 12-step program for preventing antimicrobial resistance in hospitals.

CDC Campaign to Prevent Antimicrobial Resistance in Healthcare Settings: 12 Steps to Prevent Antimicrobial Resistance Among Hospitalized Adults

PREVENT INFECTION

Step 1. Vaccinate: Give influenza/pneumococcal vaccine to at-risk patients before discharge; get influenza vaccine annually.

Step 2. Get the Catheters Out: Use catheters only when essential; use the correct catheter; use proper insertion and catheter-care protocols; remove catheters when they are no longer essential.

DIAGNOSE AND TREAT INFECTION EFFECTIVELY

Step 3. Target the Pathogen: Obtain cultures; target empiric therapy to likely pathogens and local antibiogram; target definitive therapy to known pathogens and antimicrobial susceptibility test results.

Step 4. Access the Experts: Consult infectious diseases experts about patients with serious infections.

USE ANTIMICROBIALS WISELY

Step 5. Practice Antimicrobial Control: Engage in local antimicrobial control efforts.

Step 6. Use Local Data: Know your antibiogram; know your patient population.

Step 7. Treat Infection, Not Contamination: Use proper antisepsis for blood and other cultures; culture the blood, not the skin or catheter hub; use proper methods to obtain and process all cultures.

Step 8. Treat Infection, Not Colonization: Treat pneumonia, not the tracheal aspirate. Treat bacteremia, not the catheter tip or hub. Treat UTI, not the indwelling catheter.

(continued)

Step 9. Know When to Say "No" to Vanco: Treat infection, not contaminants or colonization. Fever in a patient with an IV catheter is not a routine indication for vancomycin.

Step 10. Stop Antimicrobial Treatment: When infection is cured; when cultures are negative and infection is unlikely; when infection is not diagnosed.

PREVENT TRANSMISSION

Step 11. Isolate the Pathogen: Use standard infection control precautions. Contain infectious body fluids (follow airborne, droplet, and contact precautions). When in doubt, consult infection control experts.

Step 12. Break the Chain of Contagion: Stay home when you are sick. Keep your hands clean. Set an example.

(Adapted from http://www.cdc.gov/drugresistance/healthcare/ha/12steps_HA.htm. Accessed July 3, 2006.)

7

MICROBIOLOGY TECHNIQUES

Acid-Fast Stain (AFB Smear, Kinyoun Stain)

Clinical microbiology labs can perform a "modified" acid-fast stain for organisms that are weakly acid-fast staining (eg, *Nocardia* spp.). Acid-fast bacilli (AFB) stain red to bright pink against the light blue background (*Mycobacterium tuberculosis* [TB], *Mycobacterium scrofulaceum, M. avium-intracellulare,* and others). These organisms have a beaded rod appearance under oil immersion and must be cultured on specialized media. Rapid-growing AFB include *Mycobacterium abscessus, Mycobacterium chelonae,* and *Mycobacterium fortuitum* and can usually be cultured in fewer than 7 d. Most other AFB (*M. tuberculosis, M. avium* complex, *Mycobacterium kansasii, Mycobacterium marinum*) take at least 7–10 d to grow. *Mycobacterium gordonae* is thought to be nonpathogenic.

Blood Culture

Peripheral cultures are always preferred over cultures drawn through a catheter. All bloodstream catheters become colonized over time, which causes a high rate of false-positive cultures. To help distinguish contamination from true bacteremia, always draw culture specimens in pairs with at least one and preferably both specimens drawn from peripheral blood.

Procedure

1. Review the technique of venipuncture (see Chapter 13). Clean and disinfect the skin first with alcohol and then with chlorhexidine to reduce skin flora contamination. Do not touch the site after cleaning or before needle entry. If the needle is touched or you need to re-enter the vein, discard the needle and start again.

2. Culture technique varies from institution to institution. Use a closed vacuum collection system that incorporates the collection bottle (eg, BacTec). Keep the collection bottle below the site to prevent reflux. An aerobic bottle and an anaerobic bottle constitute a "set" drawn from the same venipuncture site.

3. The volume of blood drawn influences results, with a 3% increase in sensitivity per each additional milliliter of blood obtained. Collect 10 mL of blood per culture for adults. Usually two or three sets of blood cultures are

drawn at intervals of 30–60 min. However, if antibiotics are being started immediately, it is acceptable to draw the cultures closer together.

4. Special tubes and culture technique are required for mycobacteria and fungi. Centrifugation–lysis (isolator) systems are used to culture *M. avium-intracellulare, M. tuberculosis,* and dimorphic fungi such as *Histoplasma capsulatum.* Also perform an acid-fast smear. Contact your laboratory for specific instructions and special tubes.

Interpretation: Preliminary blood culture results are usually available in 12–48 h and should not be formally reported as negative before 4 d.

- A single blood culture that is positive for one of the following organisms usually suggests contamination; on rare occasions these agents are the causative pathogen: *Staphylococcus epidermidis, Staphylococcus hominis, Bacillus* spp., and *Corynebacterium diphtheriae* (and other diphtheroids).
- Negative results do not exclude bacteremia, and false-positives can result from contamination. Gram-negative organisms, fungi, and anaerobes are considered pathogenic until proven otherwise.
- The presence of yeast in the blood necessitates treatment with a systemic antifungal agent and repeated blood cultures to document clearance. An ophthalmologic exam to rule out endophthalmitis is mandatory. Yeast usually enters the blood through central line infection, PICC line infection, or a GI source. Removal of the catheter with subsequent blood cultures to document the clearance of fungemia is usually mandatory.
- The most common cause of culture-negative infective endocarditis is previous antibiotic therapy. However, a variety of fastidious and difficult to culture pathogens can cause infective endocarditis. The classic group is the so-called **HACEK** organisms (slow-growing gram-negative bacteria in the oropharynx): *H*aemophilus parainfluenzae and *aphrophilus, A*ctinobacillus, *C*ardiobacterium, *E*ikenella (called the "fight bite bug" after the hand soft-tissue infection sometimes contracted by a person who strikes another person in the mouth), and *K*ingella. Other causes of culture-negative infective endocarditis are *Bartonella* spp., *Coxiella burnetii* (the agent of Q fever), brucellosis, psittacosis, and the causative organism of Whipple disease, ***Tropheryma whippleii.*** If a fastidious organism is suspected, the microbiology lab should be informed and cultures held for 4 wk. Special culture media can also be ordered.

Darkfield Examination

Used to identify *Treponema pallidum,* the organism that causes syphilis. Rectal and oral lesions cannot be examined with this technique because of the presence of nonpathogenic spirochetes.

Giemsa Stain

Used to identify intracellular organisms such as chlamydiae and *Plasmodium* (malaria) and other parasites

Gonorrhea Smear and Culture

Neisseria gonorrhoeae can be cultured from many sites, including female genital tract (endocervix the preferred site), male urethra, urine, anorectum, throat, and synovial fluid. The specimen is plated on selective **(Thayer–Martin** or **Transgrow)** medium. Because of the high incidence of coinfection with *Chlamydia* and *T. pallidum* (syphilis), *Chlamydia* cultures and syphilis serology should also be performed, especially in women and girls with genital GC infections.

1. In men and boys with a urethral discharge, insert a **calcium alginate swab** (Calgiswab) into the urethra to collect the specimen, and then plate it.
2. Because anorectal stains may contain nonpathogenic *Neisseria* spp., avoid fecal contact. Apply the swab only to anal crypts.

The GC smear (see Chapter 13, page 299) has a low sensitivity (< 50% in female endocervical smear) but is reliable (> 95%) in male patients with urethral discharge. A rapid EIA **(gonococcal antigen assay [Gonozyme])** can be used to diagnose cervical or urethral GC (not throat or anus) infections in less than 1 h. DNA probe testing **(Gen-Probe)** is becoming widespread for rapid diagnosis.

Gram Stain and Common Pathogens

A Gram stain is essential for differentiating gram-positive from gram-negative bacteria. The morphologic features of the organism also are determined by observation of a Gram stain. The procedure can be applied to blood, sputum, peritoneal fluid:

1. Smear the specimen onto a glass slide in a thin layer. If time permits, allow it to air-dry. The specimen also can be fixed under low heat, usually with a Bunsen burner. Heat the slide until it is warm, not hot, when touched to the back of your hand.
2. Timing for the stain is not critical, but allow at least 10 s for each set of reagents.
3. Apply the crystal violet (Gram stain), rinse with tap water, apply iodine solution, and rinse with water.
4. Decolorize carefully with acetone–alcohol solution until the blue color is barely visible in the runoff. (Be careful; most Gram stains are ruined in this step.)
5. Counterstain with a few drops of safranin, rinse the slide with water, and blot it dry with lint-free bibulous or filter paper.
6. Use the high dry and oil immersion lenses on the microscope to examine the slide. If the Gram stain is satisfactory, any polys on the slide are pink with light blue nuclei. On a Gram stain of sputum, an excessive number of epithelial cells (> 25/hpf) means the sample contains more spit than sputum. **Gram-positive organisms stain dark blue to purple; gram-negative organisms stain red.**

Common Pathogens: Initial lab reports identify the Gram stain characteristics of the organisms. Complete identification requires culture of the organism. The lab algorithms for gram-positive and gram-negative organisms are shown in Figures 7–1 and 7–2, pages 122–123. Gram stain characteristics of clinically important bacteria are shown in Table 7–1, page 124.

India Ink Preparation

India ink is used primarily on CSF to identify fungal organisms (especially cryptococci).

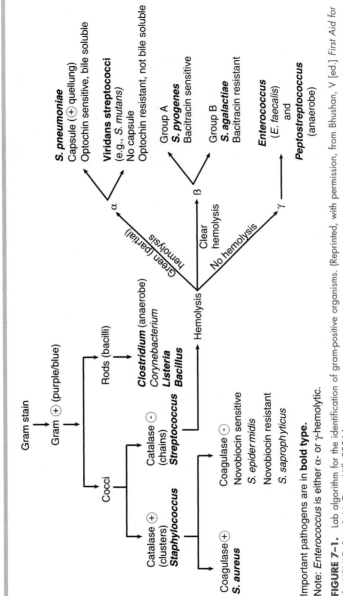

Important pathogens are in **bold type**.

Note: *Enterococcus* is either α- or γ-hemolytic.

FIGURE 7-1. Lab algorithm for the identification of gram-positive organisms. (Reprinted, with permission, from Bhushan, V [ed.] *First Aid for the USMLE, Step 1*, McGraw-Hill, 2006.)

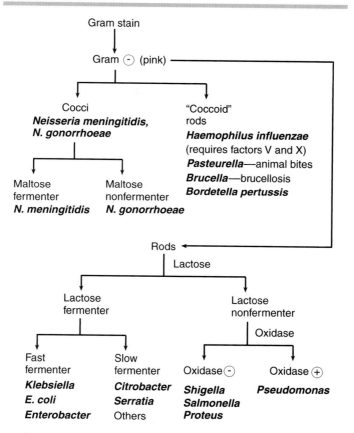

Important pathogens are in **bold type.**

FIGURE 7–2. Lab algorithm for the identification of gram-negative organisms. (Reprinted, with permission, from Bhushan, V [ed.] *First Aid for the USMLE, Step 1,* McGraw-Hill, 2006.)

KOH Preparation

KOH (potassium hydroxide) preps are used to diagnose fungal infections and are often a bedside procedure. Vaginal KOH preps are discussed in Chapter 13, page 299.

1. Apply the specimen (vaginal secretion, sputum, hair, skin scrapings) to a slide. Obtain skin scrapings of a lesion by gentle scraping with a no. 15 scalpel blade (see page 245 for description).
2. Add 1 or 2 gtt of 10% KOH solution and mix. Gentle heating (optional) may accelerate dissolution of the keratin. A fishy odor from a vaginal prep suggests the presence of *Gardnerella vaginalis* (see page 299).
3. Put a coverslip over the specimen, and examine for branching hyphae and blastospores, which indicate the presence of a fungus. KOH should destroy

TABLE 7-1
Gram Stain Characteristics and Key Features
of Common Organisms

Gram Staining Pattern and Organisms	Identifying Key Features
Gram-Positive Cocci	
Enterococcus spp. (*E. faecalis*) (Note: These are equivalent group D *Streptococcus*)	Pairs, chains; catalase-negative
Peptostreptococcus spp.	Anaerobic
Staphylococcus spp.	Clusters; catalase-positive
Staphylococcus aureus	Clusters; catalase-positive; coagulase-positive; beta-hemolytic; yellow pigment
Staphylococcus epidermidis	Clusters; catalase-positive; coagulase-negative; skin flora
Staphylococcus saprophyticus	Clusters; catalase-positive; coagulase-negative
Streptococcus spp.	Pairs, chains, catalase-negative
Streptococcus agalactiae (group B)	Pairs, chains; catalase-negative; vaginal flora
Streptococcus bovis (group D *Enterococcus*)	Pairs, chains; catalase-negative
Streptococcus faecalis (group D *Enterococcus*)	Pairs, chains; catalase-negative
Streptococcus pneumoniae (*Pneumococcus*, group B)	Pairs, lancet-shaped; alpha-hemolytic; optochin-sensitive
Streptococcus pyogenes (group A)	Beta-hemolytic
Streptococcus viridans	Pairs, chains; catalase-negative; alpha-hemolytic, optochin-resistant
Gram-Negative Cocci	
Acinetobacter spp.	Filamentous, branching pattern
Moraxella (Branhamella) catarrhalis	Diplococci in pairs
Neisseria gonorrhoeae (gonococcus)	Diplococci in pairs, often intracellular; ferments glucose but not maltose
Neisseria meningitidis (meningococcus)	Diplococci in pairs; ferments glucose and maltose
Veillonella spp.	Anaerobic
Gram-Positive Bacilli	
Actinomyces	Branching, beaded, rods; anaerobic
Bacilli anthracis (anthrax)	Spore-forming rod
Clostridium spp. (*C. difficile, C. botulinum, C. tetani*)	Large, with spores; anaerobic

(continued)

**TABLE 7–1
(Continued)**

Gram Staining Pattern and Organisms	Identifying Key Features
Corynebacterium spp. (*C. Diphtheriae*)	Small, pleomorphic diphtheroid; skin flora
Eubacterium spp.	Anaerobic
Lactobacillus spp.	Common vaginal bacterium; anaerobic
Listeria monocytogenes	Beta-hemolytic
Mycobacterium spp. (limited staining)	Only rapidly growing species gram stain (*M. abscessus, M. chelonae, M. fortuitum*)
Nocardia	Beaded, branched rods; partially acid-fast-staining
Propionibacterium acne	Small, pleomorphic diphtheroid; anaerobic
Gram-Negative Bacilli	
Acinetobacter spp.	Lactose-negative, oxidase-negative
Aeromonas hydrophilia	Lactose-negative (usually) oxidase-positive
Bacteroides fragilis	Anaerobic
Bordetella pertussis	Coccoid rod
Brucella (brucellosis)	Coccoid rod
Citrobacter spp.	Lactose-positive (usually)
Enterobacter spp.	Lactose-positive (usually)
Escherichia coli	Lactose-positive
Fusobacterium spp.	Long, pointed shape; anaerobic
Haemophilus ducreyi	Gram-negative bacilli
Haemophilus influenzae	Coccoid rod, requires chocolate agar to support growth
Klebsiella spp.	Lactose-positive
Legionella pneumophila	Stains poorly, use silver stain and special medium
Morganella morganii	Lactose-negative, oxidase-negative
Proteus mirabilis	Lactose-negative, oxidase-negative, indole-negative
Proteus vulgaris	Lactose-negative, oxidase-negative, indole-positive
Providencia spp.	Lactose-negative, oxidase-negative
Pseudomonas aeruginosa	Lactose-negative, oxidase-positive blue-green pigment
Salmonella spp.	Lactose-negative, oxidase-negative
Serratia spp.	Lactose-negative, oxidase-negative
Serratia marcenscens	Lactose-negative, oxidase-negative, red pigment

(continued)

7

TABLE 7–1
(Continued)

Gram Staining Pattern and Organisms	Identifying Key Features
Shigella spp.	Lactose-negative, oxidase-negative
Stenotrophomonas (Xanthomonas) maltophilia	Lactose-negative, oxidase-negative
Vibrio chloerae (cholera)	Gram-negative bacilli
Yersinia enterocolitica	Gram-negative bacilli
Yersinia pestis (bubonic plague)	Gram-negative bacilli

ªOrganisms are aerobic unless otherwise specified.

7

most elements other than fungus. If dense keratin and debris are present, allow the slide to sit for several hours and then repeat the microscopic examination. Lowering the substage condenser provides better contrast between organisms and background.

Lyme Disease Testing (See Also Chapter 4)

Order **only when there is real clinical suspicion** and not to screen patients with vague, nonspecific complaints but no exposure to the tick vector (*Ixodes dammini* in the eastern United States and *Ixodes pacificus* in the western United States).

The EIA is a screening test and is highly sensitive. If the EIA result is positive or indeterminate, a Western blot is used to confirm or to disprove Lyme disease. The Western blot is performed in two parts: an IgM assay (positive if 2 of 3 bands are positive) and an IgG assay (positive if 5 of 10 bands are positive).

Malaria Smear

Travelers with fever who have recently returned from regions where malaria is endemic need to have malaria ruled out because certain forms can be rapidly fatal. Prophylaxis is never 100%, and breakthrough infections occur.

The reference standard for malaria diagnosis is serial examination of sets of thick and thin blood smears. A single set of smears is *never* adequate for ruling out malaria.

1. Perform smears every 12 h until the diagnosis is made or excluded. A rapid dipstick test also can be performed. The thin smears are used to identify the species of malaria, which is used to guide treatment.
2. Report confirmed cases of malaria to the CDC. The reporting form is available at http://www.cdc.gov/malaria/clinicians.htm#case (accessed July 5, 2006)

Molecular Microbiology

Molecular techniques are used to identify many bacterial and viral organisms without culturing. Many tests rely on DNA probes to identify the pathogens (eg, Gen-Probe). The following microbes are commonly identified from clinical specimens (ie, swab, serum, tissue). Availability varies by clinical facility. Common microorganisms identifiable with a PCR/DNA probe are *Chlamydia trachomatis, Borrelia burgdorferi* (Lyme disease), HIV, *Mycoplasma pneumoniae, M. tuberculosis, N. gonorrhoeae*, hepatitis B, and HPV. Other probes are under development.

Nasal Culture

Obtain the specimen from deep in the nasopharynx and not the anterior nares. Do not let the swab touch the skin. Curved swabs are available through most pathology labs. If resistance is met in one nares, try the other side and do not force. Gently rotate the swab and attempt to rest there for 20 s. Place the swab in the provided tube (eg, Culturette). Cultures of nasopharyngeal specimens are useful in identifying *S. aureus* and *Neisseria meningitidis* infections and carriers. Normal nasal flora include *S. epidermidis, S. aureus, Streptococcus pneumoniae, Haemophilus influenzae,* and several others.

Pinworm Preparation (Cellophane Tape Test)

Used to identify infestation with *Enterobius vermicularis.* Wrap a 3-in piece of *clear* cellophane (eg, Scotch) tape around a glass slide (sticky side out). Touch the slide to the patient's perianal skin in four quadrants and examine it under a microscope to find pinworm eggs. The best sample is collected either in the early morning before bathing or several hours after retiring.

Sputum Culture

(See Pulmonary Infections, page 154)

Stool Culture

(See Infectious Diarrhea, page 155)

Stool Leukocyte Stain

(See Infectious Diarrhea, page 155)

Stool for Ova and Parasites

If a patient has toxic diarrhea, consider the possibility of parasitic disease, and order a stool for "ova and parasites." Protozoa (*Blastocystis, Giardia,* and amebae such as *Entamoeba histolytica*) cannot be cultured and are identified when mature, mobile organisms or cysts are found at microscopic examination of freshly passed feces. Immunosuppressed (eg, HIV-positive) persons may have infection with *Cryptosporidium,* microsporidia, and *Isospora belli. Strongyloides* often causes GI symptoms in persons with normal immune function.

Ova of parasites such as nematodes (*Ascaris, Strongyloides*), cestodes (*Taenia, Hymenolepis*), and trematodes (Schistosoma) are frequently identified in the stool.

Syphilis Testing

(See Chapter 4)

Throat Culture

Used to differentiate viral from bacterial (usually group A beta-hemolytic streptococci, eg, *Streptococcus pyogenes*) pharyngitis.

1. Obtain the sample with a tongue blade and a good light source.
2. **Do not attempt a culture if epiglottitis (croup) is suspected** (stridor, drooling).

3. Use the culture swab and try to touch only the involved area, not the oral mucosa or tongue. If the patient is uncooperative, use an archlike swath that touches both the tonsillar areas and the posterior pharynx.
4. If *N. gonorrhoeae* infection is suspected, use Thayer–Martin medium.
5. Culture diphtheria (*C. diphtheriae*, which has a characteristic pseudomembrane) on special medium and notify the lab.

Throat cultures take 24–48 h for completion. An office-based rapid antigen assay also can be performed. Because the sensitivity of this test is only about 80%, the culture provides a "backup" in the case of a false-negative result. Such a small delay in the start of antibiotics does not increase the risk of development of rheumatic fever.

Normal flora on routine throat culture can include alpha-hemolytic streptococci, nonhemolytic *Staphylococcus*, saprophytic *Neisseria* spp., *Haemophilus*, *Klebsiella*, *Candida*, and diphtheroids.

7

Tzanck Smear

Named after Arnault Tzanck. Used in the diagnosis of herpesvirus infections (ie, herpes zoster or simplex).

1. Clean a cutaneous vesicle (not a pustule or crusted lesion) with alcohol, allow it to air dry, and gently unroof it with a no. 15 scalpel blade.
2. Scrape the base of the vesicle with the blade, and place the material on a glass slide. After the specimen air dries, stain the slide with Wright or Giemsa stain. Use high power and oil immersion to identify multinucleated giant cells (epithelial cells infected with herpesviruses). The presence of these cells strongly suggests viral infection; culture is necessary to identify the specific virus.

Urine Culture

(See page 141)

Vaginal Wet Preparation

(See Chapter 13, page 299)

Viral Cultures and Serology

The laboratory provides the proper collection container for the specific virus. Common pathogenic viruses cultured include **herpes simplex** (from genital vesicles, throat), **CMV** (from urine or throat), **varicella-zoster** (from skin vesicles in children with chickenpox and adults with shingles), and enterovirus (rectal swab, throat). For serologic testing, obtain an **acute specimen (titer)** as early as possible in the course of the illness, and take a **convalescent specimen (titer)** 2–4 wk later. A convalescent titer fourfold greater than the acute titer indicates active infection (see Chapter 4 for selected viral antibody titers). With the development of PCR techniques, biopsies performed on older lesions may yield useful information when cultures are negative.

DIFFERENTIAL DIAGNOSIS OF COMMON INFECTIONS AND EMPIRIC THERAPY

The pathogens causing common infectious diseases are outlined in Table 7–2 along with empiric therapeutic recommendations. The antimicrobial drug of choice for the management of infection is usually the most active drug against

(*Text continues on page 141.*)

TABLE 7-2
Organisms That Cause Common Infectious Diseases with Recommended Empiric Therapy[a]

Site/Condition	Common Uncommon but Important	Common Empiric Therapy (Modify based on clinical factors such as Gram stain)
BONES AND JOINTS		
Osteomyelitis	*Staphylococcus aureus* *Enterobacteriaceae* If nail puncture: *Pseudomonas* spp.	Oxacillin, nafcillin
Joint, septic arthritis	*S. aureus* Group A strep *Enterobacteriaceae* Gonococci	Oxacillin; ceftriaxone if gonococci
Joint, prosthetic	*S. aureus, S. epididymis, Streptococcus* spp.	Vancomycin plus ciprofloxacin
BREAST		
Mastitis, postpartum	*S. aureus*	Cefazolin, nafcillin, oxacillin
BRONCHITIS	In adolescent/young patient: *Mycoplasma pneumoniae* Respiratory viruses In chronic adult infection: *Streptococcus pneumoniae, Haemophilus influenzae, Moraxella catarrhalis Chlamydia pneumoniae*	Treatment controversial because most infections are viral; treat if febrile, associated with sinusitis, positive sputum culture in patients with COPD, or if duration >7 days; doxycycline, erythromycin, azithromycin, clarithromycin

(continued)

TABLE 7-2
(Continued)

Site/Condition	Common Uncommon but Important	Common Empiric Therapy (Modify based on clinical factors such as Gram stain)
CERVICITIS (nongonococcal)	*Chlamydia, Mycoplasma hominis,* *Ureaplasma,* others	Azithromycin single dose, doxycycline (evaluate and treat partner)
CHANCROID	*Haemophilus ducreyi*	Ceftriaxone or azithromycin as single dose
CHLAMYDIA Urethritis, cervicitis, conjunctivitis, proctitis	*Chlamydia trachomatis*	Azithromycin, doxycycline (amoxicillin if pregnant)
Neonatal ophthalmia, pneumonia		Erythromycin
Lymphogranuloma venereum	*C. trachomatis* (specific serotypes, L1, L2, L3)	Doxycycline
DIVERTICULITIS (no perforation or peritonitis)	Enterobacteriaceae, enterococci, bacteroids	TMP–SMX, ciprofloxacin plus metronidazole
EAR Acute mastoiditis	*S. pneumoniae* Group A strep *S. aureus*	Amoxicillin, ampicillin/clavulanic acid, cefuroxime
Chronic mastoiditis	Polymicrobial: Anaerobes Enterobacteriaceae Rarely: *Mycobacterium tuberculosis*	Ticarcillin/clavulanic acid, imipenem

(continued)

TABLE 7-2
(Continued)

Site/Condition	Common Uncommon but Important	Common Empiric Therapy (Modify based on clinical factors such as Gram stain)
EAR (continued)		
Otitis externa	*Pseudomonas* spp. Enterobacteriaceae In diabetic or malignant otitis: *Pseudomonas* spp.	Topical agents such as Cortisporin otic, TobraDex Malignant otitis externa: acute aminoglycoside, plus ceftazidime, imipenem, or piperacillin
Otitis media	*S. pneumoniae, H. influenzae,* *M. catarrhalis,* viral causes *S. aureus,* group A strep In nasal intubation: Enterobacteriaceae, *Pseudomonas* spp.	Amoxicillin, ampicillin/clavulanic acid, cefuroxime
EMPYEMA	*S. pneumoniae, S. aureus*	Cefotaxime, ceftriaxone
ENDOCARDITIS		
Native valve	*S. viridans* *S. pneumoniae* Enterococci *S. bovis*	Parenteral: penicillin or ampicillin or oxacillin or nafcil- lin plus gentamicin; vancomycin plus gentamicin
IV drug use	*S. aureus* *Pseudomonas* spp.	Nafcillin plus gentamicin

(continued)

131

TABLE 7-2
(Continued)

Site/Condition	Common Uncommon but Important	Common Empiric Therapy (Modify based on clinical factors such as Gram stain)
ENDOCARDITIS (continued)		
Prosthetic valve	If early (<6 mo after implantation) S. epidermidis S. aureus Enterobacteriaceae If late (>6 mo after implantation) S. viridans Enterococci S. epidermidis S. aureus	Vancomycin plus rifampin plus gentamicin
EPIGLOTTITIS	H. influenzae S. pneumoniae S. aureus Group A strep	Ceftriaxone, cefotaxime, cefuroxime ampicillin/sulbactam, or TMP–SMX
GALLBLADDER		
Cholecystitis	Acute: E. coli, Klebsiella, Enterococcus Chronic obstruction: anaerobes, coliforms, Clostridium	
Cholangitis	E. coli, Klebsiella, Enterococcus	Ampicillin plus gentamicin w/wo metronidazole, imipenem

(continued)

132

TABLE 7-2
(Continued)

Site/Condition	Common Uncommon but Important	Common Empiric Therapy (Modify based on clinical factors such as Gram stain)
GASTROENTERITIS		
Afebrile, no gross blood or WBC in stool	Virus, mild bacterial form	Supportive care only
Febrile, gross blood, WBC in stool	Enteropathogenic *E. coli* *Shigella* *Salmonella* *Campylobacter* *Vibrio* *C. difficile* *Listeria monocytogenes*	Empiric treatment pending cultures: ciprofloxacin, levofloxacin
GRANULOMA INGUINALE	*Calymmatobacterium granulomatis*	Doxycycline, TMP–SMX
GONORRHEA (urethra, cervix, rectum, pharynx)	*Neisseria gonorrhoeae*	Cefixime, ciprofloxacin, ofloxacin, ceftriaxone all as single dose; treat also for chlamydia
MENINGITIS (Empiric therapy before cultures)		
Neonate	Group B streptococci, *E. coli, L. monocytogenes*	Ampicillin plus cefotaxime
Infant 1–3 mo	*S. pneumoniae* *N. meningitidis*	

(continued)

7

133

TABLE 7-2
(Continued)

Site/Condition	Common Uncommon but Important	Common Empiric Therapy (Modify based on clinical factors such as Gram stain)
MENINGITIS (continued)		
Child/adult, community acquired	*S. pneumoniae* *N. meningitidis, H. influenzae*	Vancomycin plus ceftriaxone
Postoperative or traumatic	*S. epidermitis, S. aureus, S. pneumoniae, Pseudomonas*	Vancomycin plus ceftazidime
Immunosuppressed (ie, steroids)	Gram-negative bacilli; *L. monocytogenes*	Ampicillin plus ceftazidime
History of alcohol abuse	*S. pneumoniae, L. monocytogenes* *Pseudomonas* spp. *H. influenzae*	Ampicillin plus ceftriaxone or cefotaxime plus vancomycin
HIV infection	*Cryptococcus*	Amphotericin B (acutely), fluconazole
NOCARDIOSIS	*Nocardia asteroides*	Sulfisoxazole, TMP-SMX
PELVIC INFLAMMATORY DISEASE	Gonococci Enterobacteriaceae *Bacteroides* spp. *Chlamydia* Enterococci *M. hominis*	Ofloxacin and metronidazole or ceftriaxone (single dose) plus doxycycline; parenteral cefotetan or cefoxitin plus doxycycline

(continued)

134

TABLE 7-2
(Continued)

Site/Condition	Common Uncommon but Important	Common Empiric Therapy (Modify based on clinical factors such as Gram stain)
PERITONITIS		
Primary (spontaneous)	*S. pneumoniae* Enterobacteriaceae	Cefotaxime or ceftriaxone
Secondary (to bowel perforation, etc.)	Enterobacteriaceae, *Bacteroides* spp. Enterococci *Pseudomonas* spp.	Suspect small bowel: piperacillin, mezlocillin, meropenem, cefoxitin Suspect large bowel: clindamycin plus aminoglycosides
Peritoneal, dialysis-related	*S. epidermidis* *S. aureus* Enterobacteriaceae *Candida*	Based on culture
PHARYNGITIS	Respiratory virus Gonococci *C. diphtheria* Epstein–Barr virus (infectious mono); spirochetes, anaerobes	Exudative (group A strep): benzathine penicillin G, erythromycin, loracarbef, azithromycin

(continued)

TABLE 7-2
(Continued)

Site/Condition	Common Uncommon but Important	Common Empiric Therapy (Modify based on clinical factors such as Gram stain)
PNEUMONIA		
Neonate	Viral (CMV, herpes), bacterial (group B strep, L. monocytogenes, coliforms, S. aureus, Chlamydia)	Ampicillin or nafcillin plus gentamicin
Infants (1–24 mo)	Most viral such as RSV; S. pneumoniae, Chlamydia, Mycoplasma	Cefuroxime; if critically ill, cefotaxime, ceftriaxone plus cloxacillin
Child (3 mo–5 y)	As above	Erythromycin, clarithromycin; if critically ill, cefuroxime plus erythromycin
Child (5–18 y)	Mycoplasma, respiratory viruses, S. pneumoniae, C. pneumoniae	Clarithromycin, azithromycin; erythromycin
Adult community-acquired	M. pneumoniae, C. pneumoniae, S. pneumoniae Smokers: as above plus M. catarrhalis, H. influenzae	Clarithromycin, azithromycin If hospitalized, third-generation cephalosporin plus azithromycin
Adult community-acquired aspiration	S. pneumoniae and flora, including anaerobes (eg, Fuso-bacterium, Bacteroides spp.) Enterobacteriaceae	
Adult community-acquired or ventilator-associated	S. pneumoniae, coliforms, Pseudomonas, Legionella	Imipenem, meropenem
HIV-associated	Pneumocystis Others, as above TB, fungi	Pneumocystis: TMP–SMX; may require steroids

(continued)

TABLE 7-2
(Continued)

Site/Condition	Common Uncommon but Important	Common Empiric Therapy (Modify based on clinical factors such as Gram stain)
SINUSITIS	S. pneumoniae H. influenzae M. catarrhalis Anaerobes	Acute: TMP-SMX ampicillin, amoxicillin/clavulanic acid, clarithromycin

	In nosocomial, nasal intubations, etc.:
	  S. aureus
	  Pseudomonas spp.
	  Enterobacteriaceae	

SKIN/SOFT TISSUE		
Acne	Propionibacterium acne	Tetracycline, minocycline, topical clindamycin
Acne rosacea	Possible skin mite	Topical: metronidazole, doxycycline
Burns	S. aureus, Enterobacteriaceae, Pseudomonas, Proteus	Topical: silver sulfadiazine Sepsis: Aztreonam or tobramycin plus cefoperazone, ceftazidime or piperacillin
Bite (human and animal)	Herpes simplex virus, Providencia, Serratia, Candida Anaerobes P. multiloculada	Ampicillin/sulbactam IV or amoxicillin/clavulanic acid PO
Cellulitis	Streptococcus spp. (group A, B, C, G) Anaerobic	Diabetic: nafcillin, oxacillin with or without penicillin; if anaerobic, high-dose penicillin G, cefoxitin, cefotetan

(continued)

137

TABLE 7-2
(Continued)

Site/Condition	Common Uncommon but Important	Common Empiric Therapy (Modify based on clinical factors such as Gram stain)
SKIN/SOFT TISSUE *(continued)*		
Decubitus	Group A strep (*S. pyogenes*) Anaerobes, *S. aureus*, Enterobacteria Polymicrobial anaerobic	If acutely ill: imipenem, meropenem, ticarcillin/ clavulanic acid
Erysipelas	Group A strep (*S. pyogenes*)	Nafcillin, oxacillin, dicloxacillin, cefazolin
Impetigo	Group A strep *S. aureus*	Penicillin, erythromycin, oxacillin or nafcillin if *S. aureus*
Tinea capitis (scalp) "ringworm"	Fungus: *Trichophyton* spp., *Microsporum* spp.	Terbinafine, itraconazole, fluconazole
Tinea corporis (body)	Fungus: *Trichophyton* spp., *Epidermophyton*	Topical: ciclopirox, clotrimazole, econazole, ketocona- zole, miconazole, terconazole, others Itraconazole, fluconazole, terbinafine
Tinea unguium	Various fungi	Itraconazole, fluconazole, terbinafine
SYPHILIS (less than 1 y duration)	*Treponema pallidum*	Benzathine penicillin G one dose, doxycycline, tetracycline, ceftriaxone
TUBERCULOSIS		
Pulmonary, HIV (–)	*Mycobacterium tuberculosis*	INH, rifampin ethambutol plus pyrazinamide at least 6 mo (+/– pyridoxine)
TB exposure, PPD (–)		Children <5 INH ×3 mo (+/– pyridoxine), repeat PPD in 3 mo, others observe INH 6–12 mo (+/– pyroxine)
Prophylaxis in high-risk patients (diabetics, IV drug users, immunosuppressed, etc.)		
PPD + conversion		INH 6–12 mo (+/– pyridoxine)

(continued)

138

TABLE 7-2
(Continued)

Site/Condition	Common Uncommon but Important	Common Empiric Therapy (Modify based on clinical factors such as Gram stain)
ULCER DISEASE (duodenal or gastric, not NSAID related)	*Helicobacter pylori*	Omeprazole plus amoxicillin plus clarithromycin
URINARY TRACT INFECTION		
Cystitis	Enterobacteriaceae (*E. coli* most common) *Staphylococcus saprophyticus* (young female) *Candida*	Quinolone, TMP–SMX *Candida:* fluconazole or amphotericin B bladder irrigation
Urethritis	Gonococci, *C. trachomatis*, *Trichomonas* Herpesvirus *Ureaplasma urealyticum*	Ceftriaxone, cefixime, ciprofloxacin, ofloxacin (all one dose) plus azithromycin (single dose) or doxycycline (treat partner)
Prostatitis, acute <35 y	*C. trachomatis* Gonococci Coliforms *Cryptococcus* (AIDS)	Ofloxacin
Prostatitis, acute >35 y	Coliforms	Quinolone, TMP–SMX; if acutely ill gentamicin/ampicillin IV

(continued)

139

TABLE 7-2
(Continued)

Site/Condition	Common Uncommon but Important	Common Empiric Therapy (Modify based on clinical factors such as Gram stain)
URINARY TRACT INFECTION (continued)		
Prostatitis, chronic bacterial	Coliforms, enterococci, *Pseudomonas*	Long-term ciprofloxacin or ofloxacin
Pyelonephritis	Enterobacteriaceae (*E. coli*) Enterococci *Pseudomonas* spp.	If acutely ill, gentamicin/ampicillin IV; quinolone, TMP–SMX
VAGINA		
Candidiasis	*C. albicans* *C. glabrata, C. tropicalis*	Fluconazole, itraconazole
Trichomonas	*Trichomonas vaginalis*	Metronidazole (treat partner)
Vaginosis, bacterial	Polymicrobial (*Gardnerella vaginalis, Bacteroides, M. hominis*)	Metronidazole (PO or vaginal gel); clindamycin, PO or intravaginally

ªAll antimicrobial therapy should be based on complete clinical data, including results of Gram stains and cultures. See also Tables 7–3 (Viral), page 142, 7–4 (HIV), page 146, 7–5 (Fungal), page 148, 7–6 (Parasitic), page 150, and 7–7 (Tick-Borne), page 152.
Note: These guidelines are based on agents commonly involved in adult infections. Actual anti-microbial treatment should be guided by microbiologic studies interpreted in the clinical setting.
INH = isoniazid; TMP–SMX = trimethoprim–sulfamethoxazole.

(*Text continued from page 128.*)

the pathogenic organism or the least toxic alternative. The choice of drugs is modified by the site of infection, clinical status (allergy, renal disease, pregnancy, etc), and susceptibility testing.

Tables 7–2 through 7–7 provide empiric treatment guidelines for common infectious diseases, including bacterial, viral, HIV, fungal, parasitic, and tickborne diseases. Additional resources include *The Sanford Guide to Antimicrobial Therapy* (www.sanfordguide.com) and the Johns Hopkins *ABX Guide* (www.hopkins-abxguide.org).

COMMON CLINICAL APPLICATIONS
Urinary Tract Infection (UTI)

Sample Collection
- A "midstream" or "clean catch" urine sample (see Chapter 13) gives about 85% accurate results for women and girls and uncircumcised men and boys but can be contaminated, as are specimens from long-term Foley catheters.
- The best urine is obtained through a recently placed Foley catheter or from a "straight cath" to minimize contamination (see Chapter 13). Suprapubic needle aspiration is the most accurate method of obtaining urine but is almost never done in adults because of risks. Any growth in urine obtained with these in-and-out techniques is considered positive.
- **Never** collect urine directly from a urostomy bag; it will be grossly contaminated. The presence of a urostomy (ie, ileal conduit) necessitates that a catheter be placed to collect the specimen.
- If a urine specimen cannot be taken to the lab within 60 min, refrigerate it.
- Differentiating a true urinary tract infection from contamination or simple colonization can be challenging. Pyuria plus bacteriuria usually equals UTI. In general, if an infection is present, inflammatory cells (except in neutropenia) should be detectable in the urine. UA is used to detect inflammatory WBCs and should be ordered with the culture. The presence of epithelial cells suggests contamination; urinary diversion with a bowel segment is an exception.

Urinalysis: (See also Chapter 6)
The leukocyte esterase test is used to detect the granules in neutrophils (not lymphocytes) and is a marker for pyuria. The number of WBCs found is probably the most dependable marker for true pyuria. Enterobacteriaceae (gram-negative rods such as *Escherichia coli, Klebsiella,* and *Proteus*) reduce nitrate to nitrite. If the urine nitrite test is positive, > 10,000 gram-negative rods are likely present. Gram-positive cocci do not convert nitrate to nitrite, so a negative nitrite test does not help rule out UTI.

Gram stain is not routinely done on urine samples but should be performed if the patient is acutely ill and septic. Identification of either gram-positive cocci or gram-negative cocci can be used to guide initial antibiotic therapy. If the urine Gram stain reveals cocci in chains, infection with an *Enterococcus* species is likely.

Urine Culture: A colony count < 10,000 is insignificant, as is the presence of mixed organisms. A colony count > 100,000 is indicative of true infection. Counts of 10,000–100,000 must be interpreted, usually in conjunction with the UA results and the clinical situation. The presence of more than three organisms usually indicates contamination unless the process is chronic, a GI fistula is

(*Text continues on page 154.*)

TABLE 7–3
Pathogens and Drugs of Choice for Treating Common Viral Infections[a]

Viral Infection	Drug of Choice	Adult Dosage
CMV		
Retinitis, colitis, esophagitis	Ganciclovir (*Cytovene*)[b]	5 mg/kg IV q12h × 14–21d, 5 mg/kg/d IV or 6 mg/kg IV 5×/wk or 1 g PO tid
	(*Vitrasert*[b]) implants or foscarnet (*Foscavir*)	4.5 mg intraocularly q 5–8 mo
		60 mg/kg IV q8h or 90 mg/kg IV q1–2 h × 14–21 d followed by 90–120 mg/kg/d IV
	or cidofovir (*Vistide*)	5 mg/kg/wk IV × 2 wk, then 5 mg/kg IV q2 wk
	or fomivirsen (*Vitravene*)	330 mcg intravitreally q2 wk × 2 then 1/mo
EBV		
Infectious mononucleosis	None	
HAV	None, but gamma globulin within 2 wk of exposure may limit infection	0.2 mL/kg IM × 1
HBV		
Chronic hepatitis	Lamivudine (*Epivir HBV*)	100 mg PO 1×/d × 1–3 y
	Interferon alfa-2b (*Intron A*)	5 million units/d or 10 million units 3×/wk SC or IM × 4 mo

(continued)

142

7

TABLE 7-3
(Continued)

Viral Infection	Drug of Choice	Adult Dosage
HCV		
Chronic hepatitis	Interferon alfa-2b plus ribavirin (*Rebetron*)	3 million units 3×/wk SC plus ribavirin 1000–1200 mg/d PO × 2 mo
	Interferon alfa-2b (*Intron A*)	3 million units SC or IM 3×/wk × 12–24 mo
	Interferon alfa-2a (*Roferon-A*)	3 million units SC or IM 3×/wk × 12–24 mo
	Interferon alfacon-1 (*Infergen*)	9 mcg 3×/wk × 6 mo
HIV		
(See Table 7–4, page 146)		
HSV		
Orolabial herpes in the immunocompetent with multiple recurrences	Penciclovir (*Denavir*)	1% cream applied q2h while awake × 4 d
Genital herpes		
First occurrence	Acyclovir (*Zovirax*)	400 mg PO tid or 200 mg PO 5×/d × 7–10 d
	or famciclovir (*Famvir*)	250 mg PO tid × 5–10 d
	or valacyclovir (*Valtrex*)	1 g PO bid × 7–10 d
Recurrence	Acyclovir (*Zovirax*)	400 mg PO tid × 5 d
	or famciclovir (*Famvir*)	125 mg PO bid × 5 d
	or valacyclovir (*Valtrex*)	500 mg PO bid × 5 d

(continued)

TABLE 7-3
(Continued)

Viral Infection	Drug of Choice	Adult Dosage
Genital herpes (continued)		
Chronic suppression	Acyclovir (Zovirax)	400 mg PO bid
	or famciclovir (Famvir)	500–1000 mg PO 1×/d
	or valacyclovir (Valtrex)	250 mg PO bid
Mucocutaneous in the immunocompromised	Acyclovir (Zovirax) or acyclovir (Zovirax)	5 mg/kg IV q8h × 7–14 d
		400 mg PO 5×/d × 7–14 d
Encephalitis	Acyclovir (Zovirax)	10–15 mg/kg IV q8h × 14–21 d
Neonatal	Acyclovir (Zovirax)	20 mg/kg IV q8h × 14–21 d
Acyclovir-resistant	Foscarnet (Foscavir)	40 mg/kg IV q8h × 14–21 d
Keratoconjunctivitis	Trifluridine (Viroptic)	1 drop 1% solution topically, q2h, up to 9 gtt/d × 10 d
INFLUENZA A VIRUS	Rimantadine (Flumadine)	200 mg PO 1×/d or 100 mg PO bid × 5 d
	Amantadine (Symmetrel)	100 mg PO bid × 5 d
INFLUENZA A AND B VIRUS	Zanamivir (Relenza)	10 mg bid × 5d by inhaler
	Oseltamivir (Tamiflu)	75 mg PO bid × 5 d
MEASLES		
Children	None (immunize, See Chapter 22)	
Adults	None or ribavirin	20–35 mg/kg/d × 7 d

(continued)

TABLE 7-3
(Continued)

Viral Infection	Drug of Choice	Adult Dosage
PAPILLOMA VIRUS (HPV)		
Anogenital warts	Podofilox or podophyllin	Topical application (see Chapter 22)
	Interferon alfa-2b (*Intron A*)	1 million units intralesional 3×/wk × 3 wk
	Imiquimod, 5% cream (*Aldara*)	Apply 3/wk h, remove 6–10 h later up to 16 wk
RSV		
Bronchiolitis	Ribavirin (*Virazole*)	Aerosol treatment 1218 h/d × 3–7 d
VZV		
Exposure prophylaxis in the immuno-compromised (HIV, steroids, etc.)	Varicella zoster immune globulin	See package insert
Varicella (>12 y old)	Acyclovir (*Zovirax*)	20 mg/kg (800 mg max) PO qid × 5 d
Herpes zoster	Valacyclovir (*Valtrex*)	1 g PO tid × 7 d
	or famciclovir (*Famvir*)	500 mg PO tid × 7 d
	or acyclovir (*Zovirax*)	800 mg PO 5x/d × 7–10 d
Varicella or zoster in the immunocompromised	Acyclovir (*Zovirax*)	10 mg/kg IV q8h × 7 d
Acyclovir-resistant	Foscarnet (*Foscavir*)	40 mg/kg IV q8h × 10 d

aBased on Guidelines from the CDC published in MMWR and the Medical Letter Vol. 41 December 3, 1999.
bThe generic drug name appears in regular type; the trade name appears in parentheses afterward in italics.
CMV = cytomegalovirus; EBV = Epstein–Barr virus; HAV = hepatitis A virus; HBV = hepatitis B virus; HCV = hepatitis C virus; HIV = human immunodeficiency virus; HPV = human papilloma virus; HSV = herpes simplex virus; RSV = respiratory syncytial virus; VZV = varicella-zoster virus.

7

TABLE 7-4
Antiretroviral Regimens Recommended for Management of HIV-1 Infection in Antiretroviral-Naïve Patients

Regimen	Drugs	No. of Pills
Preferred Regimens		
NNRTI-based	**Efavirenz + (lamivudine or emtricitabine) + (zidovudine or tenofovir DF) (AII)**—(note: efavirenz is not recommended for use in the first trimester of pregnancy or in women with high pregnancy potential[a])	2–3
PI-based	**Lopinavir/ritonavir (coformulation) + (lamivudine or emtricitabine) + zidovudine (AII)**	6–7
Alternative Regimens		
NNRTI-based	**Efavirenz** + (lamivudine or emtricitabine) + (abacavir or didanosine or stavudine) **(BII)**—(note: efavirenz is not recommended for use in the first trimester of pregnancy or in women with high pregnancy potential[a])	2–4
	Nevirapine + (lamivudine or emtricitabine) + (zidovudine or stavudine or didanosine or abacavir or tenofovir) **(BII)**—[note: high incidence (11%) of symptomatic hepatic events was observed in women with pre-nevirapine CD4-T cell counts >240 cells/mm³ and men with CD4-T cell counts >400 cells/mm³ (6.3%). Nevirapine should not be initiated in these patients unless the benefit clearly outweighs the risk.]	3–6
PI-based	**Atazanavir** + (lamivudine or emtricitabine) + (zidovudine or stavudine or abacavir or didanosine) or (tenofovir + ritonavir 100 mg/d) **(BII)**	3–6
	Fosamprenavir (lamivudine or emtricitabine) + (zidovudine or stavudine or abacavir or tenofovir or didanosine) **(BII)**	5–8
	Fosamprenavir/ritonavir[b] + (lamivudine or emtricitabine) + (zidovudine or stavudine or abacavir or tenofovir or didanosine) **(BII)**	5–8

(continued)

146

TABLE 7–4
(Continued)

Regimen	Drugs	No. of Pills
	Indinavir/ritonavir[b] + (lamivudine or emtricitabine) + (zidovudine or stavudine or abacavir or tenofovir or didanosine) **(BII)**	7–12
	Lopinavir/ritonavir + (lamivudine or emtricitabine) + (stavudine or abacavir or tenofovir or didanosine) **(BII)**	5–8
	Nelfinavir + (lamivudine or emtricitabine) + (zidovudine or stavudine or abacavir or tenofovir or didanosine) **(CII)**	5–8
	Saquinavir (sgc, hgc, or tablets)[c]/**ritonavir**[b] + (lamivudine or emtricitabine) + (zidovudine or stavudine or abacavir or tenofovir or didanosine) **(BII)**	7–15
3 NRTI-based	**Abacavir** + zidovudine + lamivudine—only when a preferred or an alternative NNRTI- or PI-based regimen cannot or should not be used **(CII)**	2

[a]Women with child-bearing potential implies women who want to conceive or those who are not using effective contraception.
[b]Low-dose (100–400 mg) ritonavir per day.
[c]sgc = soft gel capsule; hgc = hard gel capsule.
AII = Strong recommendation with the clinical trial results; BII = Moderate recommendation with clinical trial results; CII = Optional recommendation with clinical trials results; NRTI = two nucleoside/nucleotide reverse transcriptase inhibitors; NNRTI = either a nonnucleoside reverse transcriptase inhibitor or a ritonavir-boosted or unboosted protease inhibitor; PI = protease inhibitor.
http://aidsinfo.nih.gov/contentfiles/adultandadolescentGL.pdf (accessed July 3, 2006)

TABLE 7-5
Systemic Drugs for Managing Fungal Infections

Infection	Drug of Choice	Alternatives
ASPERGILLOSIS	Amphotericin B or itraconazole	Amphotericin B lipid complex, amphotericin cholesteryl complex liposomal amphotericin B
BLASTOMYCOSIS	Itraconazole or amphotericin B	Fluconazole
CANDIDIASIS		
Oral (thrush)	Fluconazole or itraconazole	Nystatin lozenge or swish and swallow
Stomatitis, esophagitis, vaginitis in AIDS	Fluconazole or itraconazole	Parenteral or oral amphotericin B
Systemic	Amphotericin B or fluconazole	
Cystitis/vaginitis	See Table 7–2, page 129	
COCCIDIOIDOMYCOSIS		
Pulmonary (otherwise healthy)	No drug usually recommended	
Pulmonary (high risk)	Itraconazole or fluconazole	Amphotericin B
CRYPTOCOCCOSIS		
In non-AIDS patient	Amphotericin B or fluconazole	Amphotericin B fluconazole
Meningitis (HIV/AIDS)	Amphotericin B plus 5-flucytosine; then long-term suppression with fluconazole	Amphotericin B lipid complex

(continued)

TABLE 7-5
(Continued)

Infection	Drug of Choice	Alternatives
HISTOPLASMOSIS		
Pulmonary, disseminated		
Otherwise healthy	Moderate disease: itraconazole	Severe: amphotericin B
HIV/AIDS	Amphotericin B, followed by itraconazole suppression	Itraconazole
MUCORMYCOSIS	Amphotericin B	No dependable alternative
PARACOCCIDIOIDOMYCOSIS	Itraconazole	Amphotericin B
SPOROTRICHOSIS		
Cutaneous	Itraconazole	Potassium iodide 1–5 mL tid
Systemic	Itraconazole	Amphotericin B

TABLE 7–6
Drugs for Treating Selected Parasitic Infections

Infection	Drug
Amebiasis (*Entamoeba histolytica*)	
Asymptomatic	Iodoquinol or paramomycin
Mild to moderate intestinal disease	Metronidazole or tinidazole
Severe intestinal disease, hepatic abscess	Metronidazole or tinidazole
Ascariasis (*Ascaris lumbricoides*, roundworm)	Albendazole, mebendazole or pyrantel pamoate
Cryptosporidiosis (*Cryptosporidium*)	Paromomycin
Cutaneous larva migrans (creeping eruption, dog and cat hookworm)	Albendazole, thiabendazole or ivermectin
Cyclospora infection	Trimethoprim–sulfamethoxazole
Enterobius vermicularis (pinworm)	Pyrantel pamoate, mebendazole or albendazole
Filariasis (*Wuchereria bancrofti*, *Brugia malayi*, *Loa loa*)	Diethylcarbamazine
Giardiasis (*Giardia lamblia*)	Metronidazole
Hookworm infection (*Ancylostoma duodenale*, *Necator americanus*)	Albendazole, mebendazole, or pyrantel pamoate
Isosporiasis (*Isospora belli*)	Trimethoprim–sulfamethoxazole
Lice (*Pediculus humanus*, *P. capitis*, *Phthirus pubis*)	1% permethrin (topical) or 0.5% malathion
Malaria (*Plasmodium falciparum*, *P. ovale*, *P. vivax*, and *P. malariae*)	
Chloroquine-resistant *P. falciparum*	Quinine sulfate plus doxycycline, tetracycline, clindamycin or pyrimethamine–sulfadoxine (oral)
Chloroquine-resistant *P. vivax*	Quinine sulfate plus doxycycline, or pyrimethamine–sulfadoxine (oral)
All *Plasmodium* except chloroquine-resistant *P. falciparum*	Chloroquine phosphate (oral)
All *Plasmodium* (parenteral)	Quinine gluconate or quinine dihydrochloride
Prevention of relapses: *P. vivax*, and *P. ovale* only	Primaquine phosphate

(continued)

TABLE 7–6
(Continued)

Infection	Drug
Malaria, prevention	
Chloroquine-sensitive areas	Chloroquine phosphate
Chloroquine-resistant areas	Mefloquine or doxycycline
Mites, see Scabies	
Pinworm, see *Enterobius*	
Pneumocystis carinii **pneumonia**	Trimethoprim–sulfamethoxazole Alternative: TMP-dapsone, clindamycin-primaquine, pentamidine; mild disease oral, moderate to severe IV plus steroids
Primary and secondary prophylaxis	Trimethoprim–sulfamethoxazole
Roundworm, see Ascariasis	
Scabies (*Sarcoptes scabiei*)	5% Permethrin topically Alternatives: ivermectin, 10% crotamiton
Strongyloidiasis (*Strongyloides stercoralis*)	Ivermectin
Tapeworm infection	
Adult (intestinal stage)	
Diphyllobothrium latum (fish), *Taenia saginata* (beef), *Taenia solium* (pork), *Dipylidium caninum* (dog), *Hymenolepis nana* (dwarf tapeworm)	Praziquantel
Larval (tissue stage)	
Echinococcus granulosus (hydatid cyst)	Albendazole
Cysticercus cellulosae (cysticercosis)	Albendazole or praziquantel
Toxoplasmosis (*Toxoplasma gondii*)	Pyrimethamine plus sulfadiazine
Trichinosis (*Trichinella spiralis*)	Steroids for severe symptoms plus mebendazole
Trichomoniasis (*Trichomonas vaginalis*)	Metronidazole or tinidazole
Hairworm infection (*Trichostrongylus colubriformis*)	Pyrantel pamoate
Trypanosomiasis (*Trypanosoma cruzi*, Chagas disease)	Benznidazole
Trichuriasis (*Trichuris trichiuria*, whipworm)	Mebendazole or albendazole
Visceral larva migrans, toxocariasis (*Toxocara canis*)	Albendazole or mebendazole

7

TABLE 7-7
Guide to Common Tick-Borne Diseases

	Rocky Mountain Spotted Fever	Human Granulocytic Ehrlichiosis	Lyme Disease	Babesiosis
Causative Agent	*Rickettsia rickettsii* (bacterium)	*Ehrlichia* spp. (bacterium)	*Borrelia burgdorferi* (bacterium)	*Babesia microti* (protozoan)
Season	Mostly spring, summer	Peaks in summer, may be seen year-round	Mostly spring, but year-round	Mostly spring/summer
Vector Habits	*American Dog Tick* Found in high grass and low shrubs, fields	*Deer Tick* (black-legged) Found in woodlands, old fields, landscaping with significant ground cover vegetation	Same as for the deer tick	Same as for the deer tick
	Lone Star Tick Found in woodlands, forest edge, and old fields			

(continued)

TABLE 7-7
(Continued)

	Rocky Mountain Spotted Fever	Human Granulocytic Ehrlichiosis	Lyme Disease	Babesiosis
Classical Clinical Presentation	Sudden moderate to high fever, severe headache, maculopapular rash (with planer/palmer presentation)	Fever, headache, constitutional symptoms	EM rash, constitutional symptoms, arthritis, cardiovascular and nervous system involvement	Fever, hemolytic anemia, constitutional symptoms
Incubation Period	2–14 d	1–30 d	3–30 d	1–52 wk
Diagnosis	Clinical serology	Clinical serology	Clinical serology, culture	Thick and thin blood smears
Treatment	Adults—doxycycline Children/pregnant women—chloramphenicol	Adults—tetracyclines Children/pregnant women—consult specialist	Doxycycline, amoxicillin, cefuroxime for 14–21 d	Clindamycin/quinine

EM = erythema multiforme.

(Text continued from page 141.)

present, or the patient has undergone certain types of urinary diversion. Routine cultures are insufficient for detection of *N. gonorrhoeae* and *Chlamydia*.

Pulmonary Infection

Sputum Culture and Stain: An early morning sample is preferred because such samples are more likely to be from the lower airway. A Gram stain can be used to guide therapy; if bacteria can be seen on the Gram stain, they must number > 10,000 and are probably significant. As with Gram stain of any clinical specimen, a **high neutrophil to epithelial cell ratio** suggests a less contaminated specimen. The presence of > 25 epithelial cells/hpf suggests that the specimen is more spit than sputum and is useless.

Steps to improve the quality of the sputum collection include:

1. Careful instructions to the patient to produce a deep sample. If the patient cannot mobilize the secretions, P&PD along with nebulizer treatments may help, as may nasotracheal suctioning with a specimen trap.
2. Most labs do not accept anaerobic sputum cultures (critical in the diagnosis of aspiration pneumonia and lung abscesses) unless obtained by transtracheal aspiration or endobronchial endoscopic collection and submitted in special anaerobic transport media.
3. PCP is diagnosed with expectorated sputum about 10% of the time. Therefore a technique such as open lung biopsy or endobronchial lavage must be used. Specialized stains for identifying *Pneumocystis carinii* include methenamine silver, Giemsa, and toluidine blue.

Pulmonary Viral Culture: Viral cultures are performed on both nasopharyngeal washes and bronchoscopy specimens. The viral culture medium must be refrigerated. After the specimen is collected, the medium should be transported to the microbiology lab without delay. Specific cultures should be ordered on the basis of the clinical situation. Examples include herpes simplex virus, varicella-zoster virus, CMV, and other viruses such as enteroviruses.

Rapid Influenza Test: Use a nasal swab to detect both influenza A and influenza B; useful when influenza is circulating in the community.

Pulmonary TB

1. Place all patients with possible pulmonary TB in respiratory isolation.
2. Evaluate patients with suspected TB with serial **sputum acid-fast bacterial smears and culture.** Obtain three sputum samples on three separate days. Early morning sputum collection is preferred because the specimen is more likely to be from the lower airway. Prepare an AFB smear to detect acid-fast bacilli (see page 119). If the smear is positive, continue respiratory isolation. Monitor culture results; forward positive cultures to the reference lab for antimycobacterial susceptibility testing.
3. If a patient with possible TB is immunosuppressed and the clinical condition is worsening, consider early bronchoscopy and chest CT to better evaluate the lung parenchyma.
4. Verify that the mycobacteria recovered are in the *M. tuberculosis* complex. Techniques are as follows:

   - Culture on special growth media, nucleic acid probes, and nucleic acid amplification methods such as PCR. Send all isolates for drug susceptibility testing so proper therapy can be given.

- Because skin testing for TB may not be helpful, order a blood test (T-SPOT.TB or QunatiFERON-TB Gold) to detect serum levels of gamma-interferon in response to specific TB antigens.
- Promptly report confirmed cases of TB to the local public health authorities so that antituberculosis medications can be prescribed. The public health department can also set up direct observed therapy (DOT) to ensure compliance with treatment.

CNS Infection

(See also Lumbar Puncture, Chapter 13)

1. Obtain a head CT before LP if any of the following is true: focal neurologic signs are present, a seizure has occurred, optic papilledema is present, the patient's age > 60 y, HIV-1–positive or immunocompromised state is present, a change in mental status has occurred.
2. Measure opening pressure. A high opening pressure (> 25 cm water) suggests possible brain herniation and risk of death.
3. Order routine tests: cell count, protein, glucose, Gram stain, and bacterial culture.
4. Order PCR for the following viruses: herpes simplex, varicella-zoster, and West Nile. Order viral culture for CMV and enterovirus.
5. Order a CSF cryptococcal antigen test and an India ink stain to directly visualize the cryptococcal organism.
6. Order AFB smear and culture, syphilis testing by VDRL, and a fungal smear and culture if the patient has identifying risk factors on H&P and when sufficient clinical suspicion exists.
7. Because cryptococcal meningitis can be life threatening in HIV/AIDS patients, obtain CSF opening pressure because cryptococci can impede the flow of CSF with severe consequences (severe headache, cranial nerve deficits, seizure disorder, and brainstem herniation).

Skin and Soft Tissue Infection

The spectrum of skin and soft-tissue infections runs the gamut from routine uncomplicated infections such as cellulitis of an extremity to life-threatening emergencies such as necrotizing fasciitis. Two basic questions need to be addressed.

1. Is there a collection (eg, abscess) in the region of the infection that has to be drained? If doubt exists, imaging of the infected area can depict pockets of infection and provide guidance on drainage. Such drainage procedures yield material for Gram stain, culture, and sensitivity testing. Fungal staining with culture and acid-fast smears with culture should also be ordered.
2. Are contiguous structures already involved or at risk if the infection spreads? Examples of contiguous spread are orbital cellulitis leading to CNS infection and diabetic foot ulcer or sacral decubitus ulcer causing osteomyelitis.

Infectious Diarrhea

Stool Culture: A fresh stool sample is cultured for diagnosis of the cause of diarrhea and identification of disease carriers. Most common pathogens *Salmonella* species, *Shigella,* and *E. coli* 0.157 can be grown on standard media. *Yersinia* and *Campylobacter* require a special culture medium.

Stool Leukocyte Stain (Fecal Leukocytes, Löffler Methylene Blue Stain):
The presence of WBCs signifies inflammation in the bowel. Stain differentiates treatable diarrhea (ie, bacterial) from other causes. Used to detect causes of Crohn disease, ulcerative colitis, TB, and amebic infection as well, but many causes of severe diarrhea are viral. The positive predictive value of a bacterial pathogen as a cause of diarrhea is 70%.

Clostridia difficile: Clinical course can be quite variable, ranging from simple diarrhea of short duration to cases of fulminant pseudomembranous colitis, which can be rapidly fatal. The classic triad of fever, leukocytosis, and diarrhea always suggests the possibility of *C. difficile* colitis. Risk factors for acquisition include antibiotic exposure (clindamycin and cephalosporins most common), certain chemotherapies, advanced age, increasing severity of illness, and anything that disturbs bowel motility, including surgery and medicines. Most labs use ELISA to test for the presence of organisms by detecting antigen (see Chapter 4). The organism must be present if the antigen is present. Two toxins, designated A and B, are routinely sought.

Stool for Ova and Parasites: (See page 127)

HIV-1 Testing and Screening

(See also Chapter 4)
The bases of routine HIV-1 testing are the EIA screening test, which is used to detect antibody to the HIV virus, and the confirmatory Western blot.

If the screening test for HIV is positive, Western blot testing is performed to confirm true infection. HIV antibodies usually appear 4–16 wk after initial infection occurs. The ability to detect the antibody in the serum of a patient is called **seroconversion.**

Testing for HIV-1 in Acute Retroviral Syndrome: New infection with HIV often manifests as a protean mononucleosis-like illness that has been designated **acute retroviral syndrome** (estimated incidence 20–90% in different series). The syndrome occurs 1–6 wk after infection and is marked by fever, lymphadenopathy, myalgia, and pharyngitis (nonexudative, unlike the pharyngitis that occurs with mononucleosis). Maculopapular viral exanthema, usually on the trunk, occurs in about 50% of patients. **The most important factor in the diagnosis of acute retroviral syndrome is to have a high index of clinical suspicion.** Because of its protean nature, the diagnosis is missed in many cases.

Testing for acute retroviral syndrome and new asymptomatic HIV-1 infection can be problematic. HIV-1 seroconversion (when specific antibodies become detectable in the serum and can be used for diagnostic purposes) usually occurs 4–16 wk after new infection. HIV-1 P24 antigen appears in the serum usually in the first 2 wk of new infection and remains detectable until the host generates sufficient anti-P24 antibody to neutralize the antigen.

The P24 assay has been replaced by plasma HIV-1 RNA PCR viral detection assays. A high viral load (> 100,000 viral copies/mL) in the appropriate clinical setting with an exposure history is highly specific and sensitive for the diagnosis of a new HIV infection. The viral load is almost always > 100,000 copies/mL and often > 1 million copies/mL. A low viral load (< 50,000 viral copies/mL) is probably a false-positive result. Because of its extremely high sensitivity, PCR testing is susceptible to lab contamination.

HIV-1 and Pregnancy: Decreasing the incidence of vertical transmission of HIV-1 from mother to infant is an issue of paramount importance. The use of

highly active antiretroviral therapy (HAART) in conjunction with scheduled cesarean section and abstinence from breast feeding has led to a drop in vertical transmission rates from 25% to < 2%. The decision to initiate HAART in a pregnant woman is a complex decision requiring discussion and careful assessment of risk to both mother and fetus. Administer HAART to a pregnant woman if she meets the standard criteria for starting HAART, such as a CD4 T-cell count of 200–350 CD4 T cells/mL, a high viral load (> 55,000 viral copies/mL), and the presence of an AIDS-defining illness. Other, more specific criteria include a viral load greater than 1000 copies/mL. Some infectious disease specialists recommend delaying HAART until the 10th–12th week of pregnancy to avoid the early organogenesis period of gestation. Consider resistance testing to detect viral resistance.

Baseline Tests after New Diagnosis of HIV and Referral to HIV Specialist:
The tests used for most of the major clinical decisions regarding HIV-1 therapy are HIV-1 RNA viral load and CD4 T-cell count. The results are used in decisions about when to initiate HAART, when to change HAART in the face of virologic failure (viral load no longer suppressed), and when to give prophylaxis to prevent opportunistic infections such as PCP, cerebral toxoplasmosis, and disseminated *M. avium-intracellulare* infection.

1. Order a series of routine tests such as a comprehensive metabolic panel and a CBC to assess the patient's basic organ function.
2. Order a fasting lipid panel because of the risk of adverse lipid effects during treatment with certain classes of HAART, such as protease inhibitors.
3. If a patient has an allergy to TMP–SMX and will need prophylaxis or develops an allergy during prophylaxis and may be given dapsone, order a G6PD assay to rule out G6PD deficiency, especially if the patient is of Mediterranean or African origin or descent.
4. Review the initial treatment in Table 7–4, page 146. HIV guidelines are available online at: www.aidsinfo.nih.gov/guidelines

Hepatitis

(See also Chapter 4, page 68)

Hepatitis A Testing: Acute hepatitis A is diagnosed when anti–hepatitis A IgM antibodies are present. These antibodies appear soon after the initial infection and persist for approximately 4 mo.

Anti–hepatitis A IgG titer increases slowly, reaching its peak approximately 4 mo after infection, and then persists for many years.

Hepatitis B Testing: The incubation period of hepatitis B is about 12 wk. Hepatitis B surface antigen (HbsAg) usually appears in the first 10 wk after exposure. If HbsAg remains elevated much beyond the first 6 mo, then the diagnosis of chronic hepatitis B is made.

Hepatitis C Testing: HCV **screening** for both surveillance of the blood supply and routine clinical screening is by detection of anti-HCV antibody. The anti-HCV EIA, however, does not show whether the patient has had previous infection and cleared it (about 15% of patients) or if the patient has active infection. Because the EIA was designed with high sensitivity to screen for disease (ie, to protect the blood supply) false-positive tests are not uncommon. False-positive results are most common in screening of low-risk patients. It is extremely important to realize that anti-HCV antibody does not appear in a newly infected patient until at least 8–10 wk after the infective event.

The recombinant immunoblot assay (RIBA) was designed to help stratify the **risk of true infection.** RIBA results are categorized as negative (no antigen detected), indeterminate (one antigen detected), or positive (two or more antigens detected). The clinical utility of RIBA is somewhat limited. If the EIA is positive in a low-risk patient and the RT-PCR for HCV RNA is negative, a negative RIBA makes the possibility of infection extremely remote. A better approach may be to repeat the HCV RNA RT-PCR and to test aminotransferases in 6 mo.

Confirmatory testing is best performed with HCV RT-PCR of clinical specimens. HCV RNA testing is broken down into two categories:

- *Qualitative testing,* which has a lower threshold for detecting virus and is useful for confirming infection.
- *Quantification* of the viral load, which is more appropriate for monitoring response to therapy.

Genotyping of HCV is performed if treatment is being considered, because some specific genotypes of the virus are more susceptible to therapy than are others. Most of the HCV-infected patients in North America have genotype 1, which is much less likely to clear with the standard intense treatment with ribavirin and pegylated interferon, which has to be given for 48 wk.

BIOTERRORISM

Recognizing unusual patterns in disease presentation, detecting such events, and having a high clinical index of suspicion are critical. Certain situations or patterns should prompt contacting public health officials or the CDC. Examples are:

- Any disease or suspected disease on the Category A, B or C list:
    Category A: Anthrax, smallpox, botulism, viral hemorrhagic fever, tularemia, plague
    Category B (lower mortality than A): Q fever, typhus, melioidosis (or glanders), psittacosis, brucellosis, spread of toxins (eg, Ricin)
    Category C (emerging pathogens with bioweapon potential): multiple-drug-resistant TB, Nipah virus, others.
- A case of disease or cluster of cases in the wrong season, such as an outbreak of "influenza" that occurs in the summer.
- Appearance of an infectious disease in the wrong region, such as a case of coccidioidomycosis in the northeastern United States.
- Fulminant progression of a usually benign infection in a healthy host.
- An infectious disease occurring without the presence of its mandatory vector.

Contact information and additional resources:

- CCDC, www.bt.cdc.gov
- CDC Emergency Response Hotline (24/7) (770) 488-7100
- CDC Botulism Hotline (404) 639-2206; after hours (404) 639-2206

SUBACUTE BACTERIAL ENDOCARDITIS PROPHYLAXIS

The most recent SBE guidelines were released by the American Heart Association in 1997 (*JAMA* 1997;277:1794) and also in 2005 (*Med Lett* 2005;47:59). The guidelines specify which patients are at high, moderate, or low risk of bacteremia and indicate which procedures are more likely to be associated with bacterial endocarditis. **SBE prophylaxis is recommended only for patients who are at high or moderate risk.** See Tables 7–8, page 159, and 7–9, page 160, for regimens.

TABLE 7–8
SBE Prophylaxis for Oral, Respiratory, or Esophageal Procedures[a]

Prophylaxis	Agent	Regimen[b]
Standard prophylaxis	Amoxicillin	Adults: 2 g; children: 50 mg/kg PO 1 h before procedure
Unable to take oral medications	Ampicillin	Adults: 2 g IM or IV; children: 50 mg/kg or IV 30 min before procedure
Allergic to penicillin	Clindamycin or	Adults: 600 mg; children: 20 mg/kg PO 1 h before procedure
	Cephalexin or cefadroxil	Adults: 2 g; children; 50 mg/kg PO 1 h before procedure
	Azithromycin or clarithromycin	Adults: 500 mg; children: 15 mg/kg PO 1 h before procedure Adults: 600 mg; children: 20 mg/kg IV 30 min before procedure
Penicillin allergic and unable to take oral medications	Clindamycin or cefazolin	Adults: 600 mg or 1 g; children: 25 mg/kg IM or IV 30 min before procedure

[a]See text page 158 for recommended risk groups.
[b]Total children's dose should not exceed adult dose.

High Risk: Prosthetic cardiac valves, history of bacterial endocarditis, complex cyanotic congenital heart disease, surgically constructed systemic pulmonary shunt

Moderate Risk: Congenital cardiac malformations other than those in the high- and low-risk groups, acquired valvular disease (eg, rheumatic heart disease), hypertrophic cardiomyopathy, mitral valve prolapse with regurgitation or thickened leaflets

Low Risk: Isolated ASD secundum; repair of AV septal defect or PDA; previous CABG; mitral valve prolapse without regurgitation; innocent heart murmurs; previous Kawasaki disease or rheumatic fever without valve dysfunction; pacemaker or implanted defibrillator

ISOLATION PROTOCOLS

The following category names vary somewhat from institution to institution, but the general principles are applicable in most circumstances. Contact your infection control department with specific questions or if you are unsure of the proper procedure.

Standard Precautions: For *all* patients:

- Wash hands before and after patient care, including before and after using gloves in **all circumstances!**

TABLE 7–9
SBE Prophylaxis for GU/GI (Excluding Esophageal) Procedures[a]

Patient	Agents	Regimen
High-risk	Ampicillin + gentamicin	Adults: ampicillin 2 g IM/IV + gentamicin 1.5 mg/kg (max 120 mg) within 30 min of procedure; 6 h later, ampicillin 1 g IM/IV or amoxicillin 1 g PO Children: ampicillin 50 mg/kg IM or IV (2 g max) + gentamicin 1.5 mg/kg within 30 min of procedure; 6 h later, ampicillin 25 mg/kg IM/IV or amoxicillin 25 mg/kg PO
High-risk allergic to ampicillin/amoxicillin	Vancomycin + gentamicin	Adults: vancomycin 1 g IV over 1–2 h + gentamicin 1.5 mg/kg IV/IM (120 mg max); dose within 30 min of starting procedure Children: vancomycin 20 mg/kg IV over 1–2 h + gentamicin 1.5 mg/kg IV/IM; complete dose within 30 min of starting procedure
Moderate-risk	Amoxicillin or ampicillin	Adults: amoxicillin 2 g PO 1 h before procedure, or ampicillin 2 g IM/IV within 30 min of starting procedure Children: amoxicillin 50 mg/kg PO 1 h before procedure, or ampicillin 50 mg/kg IM/IV within 30 min of starting procedure
Moderate-risk allergic to ampicillin/amoxicillin	Vancomycin	Adults: vancomycin 1 g IV over 1–2 h complete infusion within 30 min of starting procedure Children: vancomycin 20 mg/kg IV over 1–2 h; complete infusion within 30 min of starting procedure

[a]See text page 158 for recommended risk groups.
Total children's dose should not exceed adult dose.

- Put on gloves before contact with nonintact skin, mucous membranes, body secretions, excretions, or fluids, and blood.
- Wear mask and eye protection to protect the mucous membranes of the eyes, nose, and mouth.
- Wear a gown during procedures and activities that are likely to generate sprays or splashes of either body fluids or blood. Remove a soiled gown immediately and place it in the proper receptacle, then wash your hands.

Strict Precautions: For special contagious conditions; essentially *airborne precautions in combination with contact precautions* (herpes zoster, chickenpox disseminated or present in an immunocompromised host, smallpox either suspected or confirmed, suspected or confirmed avian influenza, severe acute respiratory syndrome [SARS], any suspected or confirmed case of viral hemorrhagic fever):

- Wear N95 mask, gown, and gloves.
- Place the patient in a *negative*-pressure room so that air is always moving **into** the room, thereby confining any contagion to the room.

Airborne Precautions: For airborne diseases (eg, suspected or confirmed TB and rubeola):

- Wear N95 mask when entering the patient's room. (No mask is required for people entering the room who are immune to the disease.)
- Maintain patient's room at negative pressure.

Contact Precautions: For numerous conditions (eg, influenza [also requires droplet precautions], RSV, drainage of large abscess, lice and scabies, acute diarrhea of a probable infectious nature, *C. difficile* infection, infection with drug-resistant bacteria [vancomycin-resistant enterococci, methicillin-resistant *S. aureus, vancomycin-intermediate-resistant S. aureus, vancomycin-resistant S. aureus*], and herpes zoster outbreak in an immunocompetent patient)

- Wear gown and gloves.

Droplet Precautions: (Influenza [also requires contact precautions], rubella, mumps, pertussis, diphtheria, meningococcal diseases including meningitis, scarlet fever in infants and small children, parvovirus B19, invasive disease secondary to *H. influenzae* infection and mycoplasmal pneumonia)

- Wear a standard surgical mask and gloves.

BLOOD GASES AND ACID–BASE DISORDERS

Blood Gas Basics
Normal Blood Gas Values
Venous Blood Gases
Capillary Blood Gases
General Principles of Blood Gas
    Determinations
Acid–Base Disorders: Definition
Mixed Acid–Base Disorders
Interpretation of Blood Gases
Metabolic Acidosis: Diagnosis and
    Treatment

Metabolic Alkalosis: Diagnosis and
    Treatment
Respiratory Acidosis: Diagnosis and
    Treatment
Respiratory Alkalosis: Diagnosis and
    Treatment
Hypoxia
Sample Acid–Base Problems

BLOOD GAS BASICS

Blood gases provide information concerning the oxygenation, ventilatory, and acid-base status of the patient. Blood gas results are usually given as pH, Po_2, Pco_2, $[HCO_3^-]$, base excess or deficit (base difference), and O_2 saturation. This test gives information on acid–base homeostasis (pH, Pco_2, $[HCO_3^-]$, and base difference) and on blood oxygenation (Po_2, O_2 saturation). Arterial blood gases (ABG) are most commonly measured; venous, mixed venous, and capillary blood gases are measured less frequently. Indications for blood gas determinations are as follows (*Respir Care* 2001;46:498–505):

- To determine a patient's ventilatory ($Paco_2$), acid–base (pH and $Paco_2$), and oxygenation and O_2-carrying capacity (Pao_2 and O_2Hb)
- To quantitate the response to therapeutic intervention (eg, supplemental O_2 administration, mechanical ventilation) or diagnostic evaluation (eg, exercise desaturation)
- Monitoring the severity and progression of documented disease processes (eg, COPD)

NORMAL BLOOD GAS VALUES

Normal values for blood gas analysis are given in Table 8–1, page 164, and capillary blood gases are discussed in a following section. Mixed venous blood gases are reviewed in Chapter 20. **The bicarbonate concentration ($[HCO_3^-]$) from the blood gas is a calculated value and should not be used in interpretation of blood gases; the $[HCO_3^-]$ from a concurrent chemistry panel should be used.** *Note:* The HCO_3^- values on the chemistry panel and those calculated from the blood gases should be about the same. A major discrepancy (> 10% difference) means one or more of the three values is in error (pH, Pco_2, or $[HCO_3^-]$). The most common cause of discrepancies is drawing the blood gas and chemistry panel samples at different times. ABGs and chemistry panels $[HCO_3^-]$ should be obtained at the same time for the most accurate interpretation.

TABLE 8-1
Normal Blood Gas Values

Measurement	Arterial Blood	Mixed Venous Blood[a]	Venous Blood
pH (range)	7.40 (7.37–7.44)	7.36 (7.31–7.41)	7.36 (7.31–7.41)
PO_2 (mm Hg) [decreases with age]	80–100	35–40	30–50
PCO_2 (mm Hg)	36–44	41–51	40–52
O_2 saturation (%) [decreases with age]	>95	60–80	60–85
HCO_3^- (mEq/L)	22–26	22–26	22–28
Base difference (deficit/excess)	–2 to +2	–2 to +2	–2 to +2

[a]Obtained from the right atrium, usually through a pulmonary artery catheter.

8

VENOUS BLOOD GASES

There is little difference between arterial and venous pH and $[HCO_3^-]$ (except in severe CHF and shock). Venous blood gas levels may occasionally be used to assess acid–base status, but venous O_2 levels are significantly less than arterial values (see Table 8–1).

CAPILLARY BLOOD GASES

A CBG is obtained from a highly vascularized capillary bed. CBG is often used for pediatric patients because obtaining the sample is easier (through the heel) and less traumatic (no risk of arterial thrombosis, hemorrhage) than obtaining an ABG sample. (See Chapter 13, page 280, Heelstick.)

When interpreting a CBG, apply the following rules:

- **pH:** Same as arterial or slightly lower (Normal = 7.35–7.40)
- **PCO_2:** Same as arterial or slightly higher (Normal = 40–45 mm Hg)
- **PO_2:** Lower than arterial (Normal = 45–60 mm Hg)
- **O_2 saturation:** > 70% is acceptable. Saturation is probably more useful than PO_2 itself in interpretation of a CBG.

GENERAL PRINCIPLES OF BLOOD GAS DETERMINATIONS

Interpretation of O_2 values is discussed on page 172

1. The blood gas analyzers in most labs measure pH and PCO_2 as well as PO_2. $[HCO_3^-]$ and base difference are calculated with the **Henderson–Hasselbalch equation:**

$$pH = pK_a + \frac{\log[HCO_3^-] \text{ in mmol / L}}{0.03 \times PCO_2 \text{ in mm Hg}}$$

or the **Henderson equation:**

$$[H^+] \text{ in mmol} / L = \frac{24 \times Pco_2 \text{ in mm Hg}}{[HCO_3^-] \text{ in mmol} / L}$$

2. For a rough estimate of $[H^+]$, $[H^+] = (7.80 - pH) \times 100$, or add 1 mEq/L to 40 mEq for every 0.01 below 7.40 and subtract 1 mEq/L from 40 mEq for every 0.01 above 7.40 (accurate for pH 7.25–7.48); 40 mEq/L = $[H^+]$ at the normal pH of 7.40. pH is a log scale; for every change of 0.3 in pH from 7.40 the $[H^+]$ doubles or halves. For pH 7.10, $[H^+] = 2 \times 40$, or 80 nmol/L, and for pH 7.70, $[H^+] = \frac{1}{2}$ 40, or 20 nmol/L.

3. The calculated $[HCO_3^-]$ should be within 2 mEq/L of the $[HCO_3^-]$ of a venous measurement drawn at the same time. If not, an error has been made in collection or in determination of the values, and both samples should be recollected.

4. Two additional relationships derived from the Henderson–Hasselbalch equation should be committed to memory. These two rules are helpful in interpreting blood gas results, particularly in defining a simple versus a mixed blood gas disorder:

Rule I: A change in Pco_2 up or down 10 mm Hg is associated with an increase or decrease in pH of 0.08 units. As Pco_2 decreases, pH increases; as the Pco_2 increases, pH decreases.

Rule II: A pH change of 0.15 is equivalent to a base change of 10 mEq/L. A decrease in base (ie, $[HCO_3^-]$) is termed a **base deficit,** and an increase in base is termed a **base excess.**

ACID–BASE DISORDERS: DEFINITION

1. Acid–base disorders are common clinical problems. **Acidemia** is a pH < 7.37, and **alkalemia** is a pH > 7.44. **Acidosis and alkalosis** are used to describe the process by which pH changes. The primary causes of acid–base disturbances are abnormalities in the respiratory, metabolic, and renal systems. As the Henderson–Hasselbalch equation shows, a respiratory disturbance leading to an abnormal Pco_2 alters the pH, and similarly a metabolic disturbance altering $[HCO_3^-]$ changes the pH.

2. Any primary disturbance in acid–base homeostasis invokes a **normal compensatory response.** A primary metabolic disorder leads to respiratory compensation, and a primary respiratory disorder leads to an acute metabolic response due to the buffering capacity of body fluids *and* chronic compensation (1–2 d) due to alterations in renal function.

3. The degree of compensation can be expressed in terms of the degree of primary acid–base disturbance. Table 8–2, page 166, lists the major categories of primary acid–base disorders, the primary abnormality, the secondary compensatory response, and the expected compensation based on the primary abnormality. These changes are defined graphically in Figure 8–1, page 167.

MIXED ACID–BASE DISORDERS

1. Most acid–base disorders result from a single primary disturbance of the normal physiologic compensatory response (called **simple acid–base disorders**). In some cases (eg, serious illness), two or more primary disorders

TABLE 8–2
Simple Acid-Base Disturbances

Acid–Base Disorder	Primary Abnormality	Expected Compensation	Expected Degree of Compensation
Metabolic acidosis	$\downarrow\downarrow\downarrow[HCO_3^-]$	$\downarrow\downarrow Pco_2$	$Pco_2 = (1.5 \times [HCO_3^-]) + 8$
Metabolic alkalosis	$\uparrow\uparrow\uparrow[HCO_3^-]$	$\uparrow\uparrow Pco_2$	$\uparrow$ in $Pco_2 = \Delta\,[HCO_3^-] \times 0.6$
Acute respiratory acidosis	$\uparrow\uparrow\uparrow Pco_2$	$\uparrow[HCO_3^-]$	$\uparrow$ in $[HCO_3^-] = \Delta\,Pco_2/10$
Chronic respiratory acidosis	$\uparrow\uparrow\uparrow Pco_2$	$\uparrow\uparrow[HCO_3^-]$	$\uparrow$ in $[HCO_3^-] = 4 \times \Delta\,Pco_2/10$
Acute respiratory alkalosis	$\downarrow\downarrow\downarrow Pco_2$	$\downarrow[HCO_3^-]$	$\downarrow$ in $[HCO_3^-] = 2 \times \Delta\,Pco_2/10$
Chronic respiratory alkalosis	$\downarrow\downarrow\downarrow Pco_2$	$\downarrow\downarrow[HCO_3^-]$	$\downarrow$ in $[HCO_3^-] = 5 \times \Delta\,Pco_2/10$

8

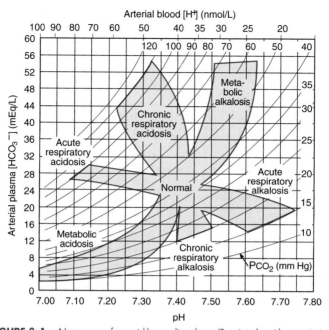

FIGURE 8–1. Nomogram for acid–base disorders. (Reprinted, with permission, from: Cogan MG: *Fluid and Electrolytes,* Originally published by Appleton & Lange, Copyright © 1991 by the McGraw-Hill Companies, Inc.)

may occur simultaneously, resulting in a **mixed acid–base disorder.** The net effect of mixed disorders can be additive (eg, metabolic acidosis and respiratory acidosis) and result in extreme alteration of pH. Or, the effects can be opposite (eg, metabolic acidosis and respiratory alkalosis) and nullify somewhat the effect of the other on pH.

2. To determine the presence of a mixed acid–base disorder with a blood gas value, follow the six steps in the Interpretation of Blood Gases (see next section). Alterations in either $[HCO_3^-]$ or P_{CO_2} that differ from expected compensation levels indicate a second process. Two of the examples given in the following section illustrate the strategies used in identifying a mixed acid–base disorder.

INTERPRETATION OF BLOOD GASES

Use a consistent, stepwise approach to interpretation of blood gases. (See Figure 8–1, page 167.)

Step 1: Determine whether the numbers fit.

$$[H^+] = \frac{24 \times P_{CO_2}}{[HCO_3^-]}$$

The right side of the equation should be within about 10% of the left side. If the numbers do not fit, obtain another ABG and chemistry panel for $[HCO_3^-]$.

Example. pH 7.25, PCO_2 48 mm Hg, $[HCO_3^-]$ 29 mEq/L.

$$56 = 24 \times \frac{48}{29}$$
$$56 \neq 40$$

This blood gas cannot be interpreted, and samples for ABG and $[HCO_3^-]$ must be recollected. The most common reason for the numbers not fitting is that the ABG and the chemistry panel $[HCO_3^-]$ were obtained at different times.

Step 2:   Next, determine whether acidemia (pH < 7.37) or alkalemia (pH > 7.44) is present.

Step 3:   Identify the primary disturbance as metabolic or respiratory. For example, if acidemia is present, is the PCO_2 > 44 mm Hg (respiratory acidosis), or is the $[HCO_3^-]$ < 22 mEq/L (metabolic acidosis)? In other words, identify which component, respiratory or metabolic, is altered in the same direction as the pH abnormality. If both components act in the same direction—eg, both respiratory (PCO_2 > 44 mm Hg) and metabolic $[HCO_3^-]$ < 22 mEq/L) acidosis are present—then this is a **mixed acid–base problem** (see Step 4). The primary disturbance is the one that varies the most from normal. That is, with a $[HCO_3^-]$ of 6 mEq/L and PCO_2 of 50 mm Hg, the primary disturbance would be metabolic acidosis; the $[HCO_3^-]$ is only 25% of normal, whereas the increase in PCO_2 is only 25% above normal.

Step 4:   After identifying the primary disturbance, use the equations in Table 8–2, page 166, to calculate the expected compensatory response. If the difference between the actual value and the calculated value is great, a mixed acid–base disturbance is present.

Step 5:   Calculate the anion gap:

$$\text{Anion gap} = [Na^+] - ([Cl^-] + [HCO_3^-])$$

A normal anion gap is 8–12 mEq/L. If the anion gap is increased, proceed to Step 6.

Step 6: If the anion gap is elevated, compare the changes from normal between the anion gap and $[HCO_3^-]$. If the change in anion gap is similar to the change in $[HCO_3^-]$ from normal, gap acidosis is present and there is **no** metabolic alkalosis **or** nongap metabolic acidosis. If the change in anion gap is greater than the change in $[HCO_3^-]$ from normal, metabolic alkalosis is present in addition to gap metabolic acidosis. If the change in the anion gap is less than the change in $[HCO_3^-]$ from normal, nongap metabolic acidosis is present in addition to gap metabolic acidosis. (See Examples 5, 6, and 7, pages 176–177.)

Finally, be sure the interpretation of the blood gas is consistent with the clinical setting.

METABOLIC ACIDOSIS: DIAGNOSIS AND TREATMENT

Metabolic acidosis represents an increase in acid in body fluids reflected by a decrease in $[HCO_3^-]$ and a compensatory decrease in PCO_2.

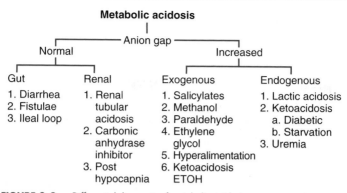

FIGURE 8–2. Differential diagnosis of metabolic acidosis.

Differential Diagnosis

The diagnosis of metabolic acidosis (Figure 8–2, page 169) can be classified as anion gap or non–anion gap acidosis. The **anion gap** (Normal range, 8–12 mEq/L) is calculated as:

$$\text{Anion gap} = [Na^+] - ([Cl^-] + [HCO_3^-])$$

Anion Gap Acidosis: Anion gap > 12 mEq/L; caused by a decrease in $[HCO_3^-]$ balanced by an increase in an unmeasured acid ion from either endogenous production or exogenous ingestion (**normochloremic acidosis**).

Non–Anion Gap Acidosis: Anion gap = 8–12 mEq/L; caused by a decrease in $[HCO_3^-]$ balanced by an increase in chloride (**hyperchloremic acidosis**). Renal tubular acidosis is a type of nongap acidosis that can be associated with a variety of pathologic conditions (Table 8–3, page 170). The anion gap is helpful in identifying metabolic gap acidosis, nongap acidosis, and mixed metabolic gap and nongap acidosis. If an elevated anion gap is present, a closer look at the anion gap and $[HCO_3^-]$ helps differentiate (a) pure metabolic gap acidosis, (b) metabolic nongap acidosis, (c) mixed metabolic gap and nongap acidosis, and (d) metabolic gap acidosis and metabolic alkalosis.

Treatment of Metabolic Acidosis

1. Correct the underlying disorder (eg, control diarrhea).
2. Bicarbonate therapy is reserved for severe metabolic gap acidosis. If the pH < 7.20, correct to above 7.20 with sodium bicarbonate. The total replacement dose of HCO_3^- can be calculated as follows:

$$HCO_3^- \text{ needed in mmol} = \frac{\text{Base deficit (mmol)} \times \text{Patient's weight (kg)}}{4}$$

3. Replace with **one-half the total amount of bicarbonate over 8–12 h** and reevaluate. Be aware of sodium and volume overload during replacement.

TABLE 8-3
Renal Tubular Acidosis: Diagnosis and Management

Clinical Condition	Renal Defect	GFR	Serum [HCO₃⁻] (mmol/L)	Serum [K+] (mmol/L)	Minimal Urine pH	Associated Disease States	Treatment
Normal	None	N	24–28	3.5–5	4.8–5.2	None	N/A
Proximal RTA (type II RTA)	Proximal H+ secretion	N	15–18	↓	<5.5	Drugs, Fanconi syndrome, various genetic disorders, dysproteinemic states, secondary hyperparathyroidism, toxins (heavy metals), tubulointerstitial diseases, nephrotic syndrome, paroxysmal nocturnal hemoglobinuria	NaHCO₃ or KHCO₃ (10–15 mmol/kg/d), thiazide diuretics
Classic distal RTA (type I RTA)	Distal H+ secretion	N	20–30	↓	>5.5	Various genetic disorders, autoimmune diseases, nephrocalcinosis, drugs, toxins, tubulointerstitial diseases, hepatic cirrhosis, empty sella syndrome	NaHCO₃ (1–3 mmol/kg/d)
Buffer deficiency (type III RTA)	Distal NH₃ delivery	↓	15–18	N	<5.5	Chronic renal insufficiency, renal osteodystrophy, severe hypophosphatemia	NaHCO₃ (1–3 mmol/kg/d)
Generalized distal RTA (type IV RTA)	Distal Na+ reabsorption, K+ secretion, and H+ secretion	↓	24–28	↑	<5.5	Primary mineralocorticoid deficiency (eg, Addison disease), hyporeninemic hypoaldosteronism, diabetes mellitus, tubulointerstitial diseases, nephrosclerosis, drugs), salt-wasting mineralocorticoid-resistant hyperkalemia	Fludrocortisone (0.1–0.5 mg/d) dietary K+ restriction, NaHCO₃ (1–3 mmol/kg/d) furosemide (40–160 mg/d)

A normal or isotonic bicarbonate drip is made with 3 amp $NaHCO_3$ (50 mEq $NaHCO_3$/amp) in 1 L D_5W.

METABOLIC ALKALOSIS: DIAGNOSIS AND TREATMENT

Metabolic alkalosis represents an increase in $[HCO_3^-]$ with a compensatory rise in Pco_2.

Differential Diagnosis

In two basic categories of diseases the kidneys retain HCO_3^- (Figure 8–3). They can be differentiated in terms of response to treatment with sodium chloride and also by the urinary $[Cl–]$ as determined by ordering a "spot," or "random" urine for chloride (U_{Cl}).

Chloride-Sensitive (Responsive) Metabolic Alkalosis: The initial problem is a sustained loss of chloride out of proportion to the loss of sodium (either by renal or GI losses). This chloride depletion results in renal sodium conservation leading to a corresponding reabsorption of HCO_3^- by the kidney. In this category of metabolic alkalosis, the urinary $[Cl–]$ is < 10 mEq/L, and the disorders respond to treatment with intravenous NaCl.

Chloride-Insensitive (Resistant) Metabolic Alkalosis: The pathogenesis in this category is direct stimulation of the kidneys to retain HCO_3^- irrespective of electrolyte intake and losses. The urinary $[Cl–]$ > 10 mEq/L, and these disorders do not respond to NaCl administration.

Treatment of Metabolic Alkalosis

Correct the underlying disorder.
1. **Chloride-responsive**
   a. Replace volume with NaCl if depleted.
   b. Correct hypokalemia if present.
   c. NH_4Cl and HCl should be reserved for extreme cases.

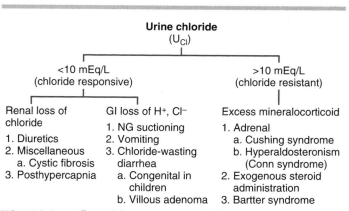

Urine chloride
(U_{Cl})

<10 mEq/L (chloride responsive)		>10 mEq/L (chloride resistant)
Renal loss of chloride	**GI loss of H+, Cl–**	**Excess mineralocorticoid**
1. Diuretics	1. NG suctioning	1. Adrenal
2. Miscellaneous	2. Vomiting	a. Cushing syndrome
a. Cystic fibrosis	3. Chloride-wasting diarrhea	b. Hyperaldosteronism (Conn syndrome)
3. Posthypercapnia	a. Congenital in children	2. Exogenous steroid administration
	b. Villous adenoma	3. Bartter syndrome

FIGURE 8–3. Differential diagnosis of metabolic alkalosis.

   2. Chloride-resistant
      a. Correct the underlying problem, such as stopping exogenous steroids.

RESPIRATORY ACIDOSIS: DIAGNOSIS AND TREATMENT

Respiratory acidosis is a primary rise in PCO_2 with a compensatory rise in plasma $[HCO_3^-]$. Increased PCO_2 occurs in clinical situations in which decreased alveolar ventilation occurs.

Differential Diagnosis

Neuromuscular Abnormalities with Ventilatory Failure: Muscular dystrophy, myasthenia gravis, Guillain–Barré syndrome, hypophosphatemia

Central Nervous System: Drugs (sedatives, analgesics, tranquilizers, ethanol), CVA, central sleep apnea, spinal cord injury (cervical)

Airway Obstruction: Chronic (COPD), acute (asthma), upper airway obstruction, obstructive sleep apnea

Thoracic–Pulmonary Disorders: Bony thoracic cage (flail chest, kyphoscoliosis), parenchymal lesions (pneumothorax, severe pulmonary edema, severe pneumonia), large pleural effusions, scleroderma, marked obesity (pickwickian syndrome)

Treatment of Respiratory Acidosis

Improve Ventilation: Intubate patient and initiate mechanical ventilation, increase ventilator rate, reverse narcotic sedation with naloxone (Narcan), etc.

RESPIRATORY ALKALOSIS: DIAGNOSIS AND TREATMENT

Respiratory alkalosis is a primary fall in PCO_2 with a compensatory decrease in plasma $[HCO_3^-]$. Respiratory alkalosis occurs with increased alveolar ventilation.

Differential Diagnosis

Central Stimulation: Anxiety, hyperventilation syndrome, pain, head trauma or CVA with central neurogenic hyperventilation, tumors, salicylate overdose (often mixed metabolic gap acidosis and respiratory alkalosis), fever, early sepsis

Peripheral Stimulation: PE, CHF (mild), interstitial lung disease, pneumonia, altitude, hypoxemia of any cause (see later, Hypoxia)

Miscellaneous: Hepatic insufficiency, PRG, progesterone, hyperthyroidism, iatrogenic mechanical overventilation

Treatment of Respiratory Alkalosis

Correct the underlying disorder.

Hyperventilation Syndrome: Best controlled by having the patient rebreathe into a paper bag to increase PCO_2, decrease ventilator rate, increase amount of dead space with ventilator, or manage underlying cause.

HYPOXIA

The second type of information gained from a blood gas level, in addition to acid–base results, is oxygenation. Results usually are given as PO_2 and O_2 satu-

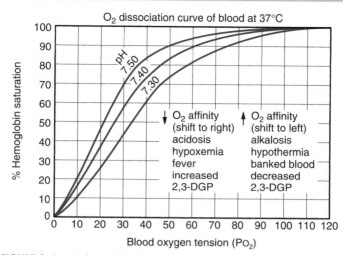

FIGURE 8–4. Oxyhemoglobin dissociation curve.

ration (see Table 8–1, page 164, for normal values). These two parameters are related to each other.

Oxygen saturation at any given PO_2 is influenced by temperature, pH, and the level of 2,3-diphosphoglycerate (2,3-DPG) as shown in Figure 8–4, page 173.

Oxygenation can also be determined noninvasively with pulse oximetry. **Pulse oximetry** is used to measure pulse rate and SaO_2 and can reduce the need for ABG measurements. The transcutaneous technique (detector placed on the finger, toe, top of the ear, earlobe of adults and the foot, palm, great toe, or thumb of children) is sensitive in the detection of arterial desaturation only. The technology is based on the different red and infrared light absorption characteristics of oxygenated and deoxygenated hemoglobin. The technique may be less accurate in cases of poor perfusion, motion, sensor exposure to ambient light, skin pigmentation (usually at saturations < 80% only), use of IV contrast agents, and the presence of abnormal hemoglobins (carboxy hemoglobin, methemoglobin). Normal pulse oximetry readings should be 95–99% in a healthy person on room air and can vary slightly according to age, state of fitness, and altitude. Anemia, elevated bilirubin, and sickle cell disease do not affect readings.

Hypoxia Differential Diagnosis

$\dot{V}/\dot{Q}$ *Abnormalities:* COPD (emphysema, chronic bronchitis, asthma), atelectasis, pneumonia, PE, ARDS, pneumothorax, pneumoconiosis, CF, obstructed airway

Alveolar Hypoventilation: Skeletal abnormalities, neuromuscular disorders, pickwickian syndrome, sleep apnea

Decreased Pulmonary Diffusing Capacity: Pneumoconiosis, pulmonary edema, drug-induced pulmonary fibrosis (bleomycin), collagen–vascular diseases

Right-to-Left Shunt: Congenital heart disease (eg, tetralogy of Fallot, transposition of the great arteries)

SAMPLE ACID–BASE PROBLEMS

In each of these examples, use the technique for blood gas interpretation on page 167 to identify the acid–base disorder.

Example 1

A patient with COPD has a blood gas of pH 7.34, P_{CO_2} 55 mm Hg, and $[HCO_3^-]$ 29 mEq/L.

Step 1:

$$46 = 24 \times \frac{55}{29}$$
$$46 \approx 45$$

The numbers fit because the difference between the calculated and observed values is < 10%.

Step 2: pH < 7.37, acidemia.

Step 3: P_{CO_2} > 44 mm Hg, and $[HCO_3^-]$ is not < 22 mEq/L, respiratory acidosis.

Step 4: Normal compensation for chronic (COPD) respiratory acidosis (from Table 8–2, page 166).

$$\Delta[HCO_3^-] = 4 \times \Delta\,(P_{CO_2}\,/10) = 4 \times \frac{15}{10} = 6$$

Expected $[HCO_3^-]$ is 24 mEq/L + 6 = 30, which is close to the measured $[HCO_3^-]$ of 29 mEq/L, simple respiratory acidosis. This patient has chronic respiratory acidosis due to hypoventilation (simple acid–base disorder).

Example 2

Immediately after cardiac arrest a patient has pH 7.25, P_{CO_2} 28 mm Hg, and $[HCO_3^-]$ 12 mEq/L.

Step 1:

$$56 = 24 \times \frac{28}{12}$$
$$56 = 56$$

The numbers fit.

Step 2: pH < 7.37, acidemia.

Step 3: $[HCO_3^-]$ is < 22 mEq/L and P_{CO_2} is **not** > 44 mm Hg, metabolic acidosis.

Step 4: (See Table 8–2, page 166)

$$P_{CO_2} = (1.5 \times [HCO_3^-] + 8) = (1.5 \times 12) + 8 = 26$$

The expected P_{CO_2} of 26 mm Hg is very similar to the measured value of 28 mm Hg, so this condition is simple metabolic acidosis. The patient has lactic acidosis following cardiopulmonary arrest (simple acid–base disorder).

Example 3

A young man with a fever of 103.2°F and a fruity odor on his breath has a blood gas of pH 7.36, P_{CO_2} 9 mm Hg, and $[HCO_3^-]$ 5 mEq/L.

Step 1:

$$45 = \frac{24}{5} \times 9$$
$$43 \approx 45$$

The numbers fit.

Step 2: pH < 7.37 indicates acidemia.

Step 3: $[HCO_3^-]$ < 22 mEq/L and P_{CO_2} is **not** > 44 mm Hg, thus metabolic acidosis is present.

Step 4: The expected compensation in P_{CO_2} can be calculated as follows (see Table 8–2, page 166):

$$P_{CO_2} = (1.5 \times [HCO_3^-]) + 8 \pm 2$$
$$= (1.5 \times 5) + 8 \pm 2$$
$$= 17.5 \pm 2$$

The expected P_{CO_2} is 17.5 mm Hg, but the reading is 9 mm Hg, indicating a second process, respiratory alkalosis. This patient has metabolic acidosis due to DKA and concomitant respiratory alkalosis possibly due to early sepsis and fever (mixed acid–base disorder).

Example 4

A 30-year-old woman who is 30 wk PRG presents with nausea and vomiting. Blood gas analysis reveals pH 7.55, P_{CO_2} 25 mm Hg, and $[HCO_3^-]$ 22 mEq/L.

Step 1:

$$28 = 24 \times \frac{25}{22}$$
$$28 \approx 27$$

The numbers fit.

Step 2: pH < 7.44 indicates alkalemia.

Step 3: P_{CO_2} < 36 mm Hg, and $[HCO_3^-]$ is **not** > 26 mEq/L, thus respiratory alkalosis is present.

Step 4: The expected compensation for chronic respiratory alkalosis (ie, pregnancy) is calculated from Table 8–2, page 166:

$$\Delta[HCO_3^-] = 5 \times \Delta P_{CO_2} / 10$$
$$= 5 \times \frac{15}{10} = 7.5$$

The calculated $[HCO_3^-]$ is 24 – 7.5, or 16–17 mEq, but the actual $[HCO_3^-]$ is 22 mEq/L, indicating relative secondary metabolic alkalosis ($[HCO_3^-]$ is higher than expected). This patient has respiratory alkalosis due to pregnancy and relative secondary metabolic alkalosis due to vomiting.

Example 5

A 19-year-old patient with diabetes has an anion gap of 29 mEq/L and a $[HCO_3^-]$ of 6 mEq/L.

Step 1:

$$29 \text{ mmol/L actual gap}$$
$$\underline{-10} \text{ mmol/L normal gap}$$
$$19 \text{ mmol/L expected change in } [HCO_3^-]$$

Step 2:

$$24 \text{ mmol/L normal } [HCO_3^-]$$
$$\underline{-19} \text{ mmol/L expected change in } [HCO_3^-]$$
$$5 \text{ mmol/L expected change in } [HCO_3^-]$$

Actual $[HCO_3^-]$ is 6 mEq/L, close to the expected $[HCO_3^-]$ of 5 mEq/L. Thus pure metabolic gap acidosis is present, most likely from DKA.

Example 6

A 21-year-old patient with diabetes presents with nausea, vomiting, and abdominal pain. The anion gap is 23 mEq/L, and the $[HCO_3^-]$ is 18 mEq/L.

Step 1:

$$23 \text{ mmol/L actual gap}$$
$$\underline{-10} \text{ mmol/L normal gap}$$
$$13 \text{ mmol/L expected change in } [HCO_3^-] \text{ from normal}$$

Step 2:

$$24 \text{ mmol/L normal } [HCO_3^-]$$
$$\underline{-13} \text{ mmol/L expected change in } [HCO_3^-]$$
$$11 \text{ mmol/L expected change in } [HCO_3^-]$$

The $[HCO_3^-]$ is 18 mEq/L and not the 11 mEq/L expected from pure metabolic gap acidosis. Because the actual $[HCO_3^-]$ is higher than expected, this condition is mixed metabolic gap acidosis and metabolic alkalosis. The patient has metabolic gap acidosis from DKA and metabolic alkalosis from vomiting.

Example 7

A 55-year-old patient who drinks a fifth of whiskey per day has a 2-wk history of diarrhea. The anion gap is 17 mEq/L, and the $[HCO_3^-]$ is 10 mEq/L.

Step 1:

$$17 \text{ mmol/L actual gap}$$
$$\underline{-10} \text{ mmol/L normal gap}$$
$$7 \text{ mmol/L expected change in } [HCO_3^-] \text{ from normal}$$

Step 2:

$$24 \text{ mmol/L normal } [HCO_3^-]$$
$$\underline{-7} \text{ mmol/L expected change in } [HCO_3^-]$$
$$17 \text{ mmol/L expected change in } [HCO_3^-]$$

Actual $[HCO_3^-]$ is 10 mEq/L and not the expected 17 mEq/L of pure metabolic gap acidosis. Because the actual $[HCO_3^-]$ is lower than expected, mixed metabolic gap acidosis and metabolic nongap acidosis must be present. The patient has metabolic nongap acidosis from diarrhea and metabolic gap acidosis from alcoholic ketoacidosis.

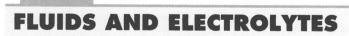

FLUIDS AND ELECTROLYTES

Principles of Fluids and Electrolytes
Composition of Parenteral Fluids
Composition of Body Fluids
Ordering IV Fluids

Determining an IV Rate
Electrolyte Abnormalities: Diagnosis
  and Treatment

PRINCIPLES OF FLUIDS AND ELECTROLYTES
Fluid Compartments
Example: 70-kg man (1 L = 1 kg)

Total Body Water: 42,000 mL (60% of BW)
- Intracellular: 28,000 mL (40% of BW)
- Extracellular: 14,000 mL (20% of BW)
- Plasma: 3500 mL (5% of BW)
- Interstitial: 10,500 mL (15% of BW in a 70-kg man)

Total Blood Volume
Total blood volume = 5600 mL (8% of BW in a 70-kg man)

Red Blood Cell Mass
• Man, 20–36 mL/kg ($1.15–1.21$ L/m^2) • Woman, 19–31 mL/kg ($0.95–1.0$ L/m^2)

Water Balance
• 70-kg man

The minimum obligate water requirement to maintain homeostasis (if temperature and renal-concentrating ability are normal and solute [urea, salt] excretion is minimal) is about 800 mL/d, which would yield 500 mL of urine.

"Normal" Intake: 2500 mL/d (about 35 mL/kg/d baseline)
- Oral liquids: 1500 mL
- Oral solids: 700 mL
- Metabolic (endogenous): 300 mL

"Normal" Output: 1400–2300 mL/d
- Urine: 800–1500 mL
- Stool: 250 mL
- Insensible loss: 600–900 mL (lungs and skin). (With fever, each degree above 98.6°F [37°C] adds 2.5 mL/kg/d to insensible losses; insensible losses are decreased if a patient is undergoing mechanical ventilation; free water gain can occur from humidified ventilation.)

Baseline Fluid Requirement

Afebrile 70-kg Adult: 35 mL/kg/24 h

If Not a 70-kg Adult: Calculate the water requirement according to the following kg method:

- For the first 10 kg of body weight: 100 mL/kg/d *plus*
- For the second 10 kg of body weight: 50 mL/kg/d *plus*
- For the weight above 20 kg: 20 mL/kg/d

Electrolyte Requirements

- 70-kg adult, unless otherwise specified

Sodium (as NaCl):   80–120 mEq/d (children, 3–4 mEq/kg/24 h)

Chloride: 80–120 mEq/d as NaCl

Potassium: 50–100 mEq/d (children, 2–3 mEq/kg/24 h). In the absence of hypokalemia and with normal renal function, most of this K is excreted in the urine. Of the total amount of K, 98% is intracellular, and 2% is extracellular.

     If the serum K level is normal, about 4.5 mEq/L, the total extracellular pool of $K^+ = 4.5 \times 14$ L $= 63$ mEq. K is easily interchanged between intracellular and extracellular stores under conditions such as acidemia or alkalemia. K demands increase with diuresis and building of new body tissues (anabolic states).

Calcium: 1–3 g/d, most of which is secreted by the GI tract. Routine administration is not needed in the absence of specific indications.

Magnesium: 20 mEq/d. Routine administration is not needed in the absence of specific indications, such as parenteral hyperalimentation, massive diuresis, ethanol abuse (frequently needed), or preeclampsia.

Glucose Requirements

- 100–200 g/d (65–75 g/d/m²). During starvation, caloric needs are supplied by body fat and protein; most protein comes from the skeletal muscles. Every gram of nitrogen in the urine represents 6.25 g of protein broken down. The **protein-sparing effect** is one of the goals of basic IV therapy. Administration of at least 100 g/d of glucose reduces protein loss more than one half. Almost all IV fluid solutions supply glucose as dextrose (pure dextrorotatory glucose). Pediatric patients need about 100–200 mg/kg/h.

COMPOSITION OF PARENTERAL FLUIDS

Parenteral fluids are generally classified according to molecular weight and oncotic pressure. Colloids have a molecular weight > 8000 and have high oncotic pressure. Crystalloids have a molecular weight < 8000 and have low oncotic pressure.

Colloids

- Albumin (see Table 10–2, page 198)
- Blood products (eg, RBCs, single-donor plasma) (see Chapter 10, page 200)
- Plasma protein fraction (Plasmanate) (see Chapter 22)
- Synthetic colloids (hetastarch [Hespan], dextran) (see Chapter 22)

Crystalloids

Table 9–1, page 182, describes common crystalloid parenteral fluids.

COMPOSITION OF BODY FLUIDS

Table 9–2, page 183, gives the average daily production and amount of some of the major electrolytes present in various body fluids.

ORDERING IV FLUIDS

One of the most difficult tasks to master is choosing appropriate IV therapy for a patient. The patient's underlying illness, vital signs, serum electrolytes, and a host of other variables must be considered. The following are general guidelines for IV therapy. Specific requirements for each patient can vary tremendously from these guidelines.

Maintenance Fluids

The following amounts provide the minimum requirements for routine daily needs:

1. **70-kg Man:** 5% dextrose in one-fourth concentration normal saline (D_5 ¼ NS) with 20 mEq/L KCl at 125 mL/h. (This infusion delivers about 3 L/d of free water.)
2. **Other Adult Patients:** Also use D_5 ¼ NS with 20 mEq/L KCl. Determine the 24-h water requirement with the "kg method" (page 180) and divide by 24 h to determine the hourly rate.
3. **Pediatric Patients:** Use the same solution as for adults, but determine the daily fluid requirements by either of the following methods:
   a. *Kg Method:* (page 180)
   b. *Meter Squared Method:* Maintenance fluids are 1500 mL/m²/d. Divide by 24 to get the flow rate per hour. To calculate the surface area, use the "rule of sixes" nomogram (Table 9–3, page 183). Formal body surface area charts are in the Appendix.

Specific Replacement Fluids

Fluids are used to replace excessive, nonphysiologic losses.

Gastric Loss (Nasogastric Tube, Emesis): D_5 ½ NS with 20 mEq/L KCl

Diarrhea: D_5LR with 15 mEq/L KCl. Use body weight as a replacement guide (about 1 L for each 1 kg, or 2.2 lb, lost).

Bile Loss: D_5LR with 25 mEq/L (½ amp) of sodium bicarbonate milliliter for milliliter

Pancreatic Loss: D_5LR with 50 mEq/L (1 amp) HCO_3^- milliliter for milliliter

Burn Patients: Use the Parkland or the Rule of Nines formula:
   Parkland Formula.

$$\text{Total fluid required during the first 24 h} = (\% \text{ body burn}) \times (\text{body weight in kg}) \times 4 \text{ mL}$$

Replace with LR over 24 h. Use

- One half of the total over first 8 h (from time of burn)

TABLE 9–1
Composition of Commonly Used Crystalloids

Fluid	Glucose (g/L)	Electrolytes (mEq/L)[a]							kcal/L
		Na+	Cl-	K+	Ca2+	HCO3-	Mg2+	HPO4^2-	
D5W (5% dextrose in water)	50	—	—	—	—	—	—	—	170
D10W (10% dextrose in water)	100	—	—	—	—	—	—	—	340
D20W (20% dextrose in water)	200	—	—	—	—	—	—	—	680
D50W (50% dextrose in water)	500	—	—	—	—	—	—	—	1700
1/2 NS (0.45% NaCl)	—	77	77	—	—	—	—	—	—
3% NS	—	513	513	—	—	—	—	—	—
NS (0.9% NaCl)	—	154	154	—	—	—	—	—	—
D5 1/4 NS (0.22% NaCl)	50	38	38	—	—	—	—	—	170
D5 1/2NS (0.45% NaCl)	50	77	77	—	—	—	—	—	170
D5NS (0.9% NaCl)	50	154	154	—	—	—	—	—	170
D5LR (5% dextrose in lactated Ringer)	50	130	110	4	3	27	—	—	180
Lactated Ringer	—	130	110	4	3	27	—	—	<10
Ionosol MB	50	25	22	20	—	23	3	3	170
Normosol M	50	40	40	13	—	16	3	—	170

[a]HCO3 is administered in these solutions as lactate that is converted to bicarbonate.

TABLE 9–2
Composition and Daily Production of Body Fluids

	Electrolytes (mEq/L)				
Fluid	Na$^+$	Cl$^-$	K$^+$	HCO$_3^-$	Average Daily Production^a (mL)
Sweat	50	40	5	0	Varies
Saliva	60	15	26	50	1500
Gastric juice	60–100	100	10	0	1500–2500
Duodenal fluid	130	90	5	0–10	300–2000
Bile	145	100	5	15	100–800
Pancreatic juice	140	75	5	115	100–800
Ileal fluid	140	100	2–8	30	100–9000
Diarrhea	120	90	25	45	—

^{a}In adults.

- One fourth of the total over second 8 h
- One fourth of the total over third 8 h

Rule of Nines. Used for estimating percentage of body burned in adults. Figure 9–1, page 184, shows the calculations for body burn area in adults and children. This system is also useful for determining ongoing fluid losses from a burn until it is healed or grafted.

TABLE 9–3
"Rule of Sixes" Nomogram for Calculating Fluids in Children^a

Weight (lb)	Body Surface Area (m^2)
3	0.1
6	0.2
12	0.3
18	0.4
24	0.5
30	0.6
36	0.7
42	0.8
48	0.9
60^b	1.0

^{a}Over 100 lb, treat as an adult.
^{b}After 60 lb, add 0.1 for each additional 10 lb.

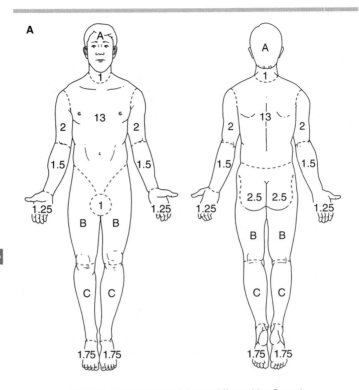

Relative Percentages of Areas Affected by Growth

Area	Age		
	10	15	Adult
A = half of head	5.5	4.5	3.5
B = half of one thigh	4.25	4.5	4.75
C = half of one leg	3	3.25	3.5

FIGURE 9–1. Tables and graphics for estimating extent of burns in adults (**A**) and children (**B**). For adults, another way of estimating percentage of the body surface burned is the rule of nines: Each arm is 9%, each leg is 9%, the head is 9%, the anterior aspect of the body is 9%, the posterior aspect of the body is 9%, and the perineum is 1%. (From: Current Surgical Diagnosis and Treatment, 12th ed., Doherty, GM [editor]. McGraw-Hill, 2006. Used with permission.)

B

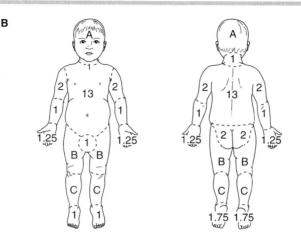

Relative Percentages of Areas Affected by Growth

Area	Age		
	0	1	5
A = half of head	9.5	8.5	6.5
B = half of one thigh	2.75	3.25	4
C = half of one leg	2.5	2.5	2.75

FIGURE 9–1. Continued.

Fluid losses can be estimated as

Loss in mL = (25 × % body burn) × m² body surface area

DETERMINING AN IV RATE

Most IV infusions are regulated with infusion pumps. If a mechanical infusion device is not immediately available, use the following formulas to determine the infusion rate.

For a MAXI Drip Chamber: Use 10 gtt/mL; thus
- 10 gtt/min = 60 mL/h or
- 16 gtt/min = 100 mL/h

For a MINI Drip Chamber: Use 60 gtt/mL; thus
- 60 gtt/min = 60 mL/h or
- 100 gtt/min = 100 mL/h

ELECTROLYTE ABNORMALITIES: DIAGNOSIS AND TREATMENT

In all of the following situations, the primary goal is to correct the underlying condition. Unless specified, all dosages are for adults. (See Chapter 4 for the differential diagnosis of laboratory findings.)

- **Pseudohyperkalemia.** Due to leukocytosis, thrombocytosis, hemolysis, poor venipuncture technique (prolonged tourniquet time)
- **Inadequate Excretion.** Renal failure, volume depletion, medications that block K^+ excretion (eg, spironolactone, triamterene), hypoaldosteronism (due to adrenal disorders and hyporeninemic states [such as type IV RTA], NSAIDs, ACE inhibitors), long-standing use of heparin, digitalis toxicity, sickle cell disease, renal transplantation
- **Redistribution.** Tissue damage, acidosis (a 0.1 decrease in pH increases serum K^+ approximately 0.5–1.0 mEq/L because of extracellular shift of K^+), beta-blockers, decreased insulin, succinylcholine
- **Excess Administration.** K-containing salt substitutes, oral replacement, K^+ in IV fluids

Symptoms: Weakness, flaccid paralysis, confusion

Signs
- Hyperactive deep tendon reflexes, decreased motor strength
- ECG changes such as peaked T waves, wide QRS, loss of P wave, sine wave, asystole
- K^+ = 7–8 mEq/L ventricular fibrillation risk: 5%
- K^+ = 10 mEq/L ventricular fibrillation risk: 90%

Treatment
- Monitor patient with ECG if symptoms are present or if K^+ > 6.5 mEq/L; discontinue all K^+ intake, including IV fluids; order a repeat stat K^+ to confirm.
- **Rapid correction.** These steps only protect the heart from K^+ shifts; total body K^+ must be reduced with one of the treatments described in Slow Correction.

    Calcium chloride, 500 mg, slow IV push (only protects heart from effects of hyperkalemia)
    Alkalinize with 50 mEq (1 amp) Na bicarbonate (causes intracellular K^+ shift)
    50 mL $D_{50}W$, IV push, with 10–15 units regular insulin, IV push (causes intracellular K shift)

- **Slow Correction**
    Sodium polystyrene sulfonate (Kayexalate) 20–60 g orally with 100–200 mL of sorbitol, or 40 g Kayexalate with 40 g sorbitol in 100 mL water as enema. Repeat doses qid as needed.
    Dialysis (hemodialysis or peritoneal dialysis)

- **Correct Underlying Cause.** For example, stop K-sparing diuretics, ACE inhibitors, mineralocorticoid replacement for hypokalemia

Hypokalemia
• K^+ < 3.6 mEq/L

Mechanisms: Due to inadequate intake, loss, or intracellular shifts

- **Inadequate Intake.** Oral or IV
- **GI Tract Loss.** (Urinary chloride usually < 10 mEq/d; chloride-responsive alkalosis) vomiting, diarrhea, excess sweating, villous adenoma, fistula
- **Renal Loss.** Diuretics and other medications (amphotericin, high-dose penicillins, aminoglycosides, cisplatin), diuresis other than with diuretics (osmotic, eg, hyperglycemia or ethanol induced), vomiting (from meta-

bolic alkalosis due to volume depletion), renal tubular disease (distal or proximal RTA, Bartter syndrome (due to increased renin and aldosterone levels), hypomagnesemia, ingestion of natural licorice, mineralocorticoid excess (primary and secondary hyperaldosteronism, Cushing syndrome, steroid use), and ureterosigmoidostomy

- **Redistribution (Intracellular Shifts).** Metabolic alkalosis (each 0.1 increase in pH lowers serum K^+ approximately 0.5–1.0 mEq/L; due to intracellular shift of K^+), insulin administration, beta-adrenergic agents, familial periodic paralysis and therapy for megaloblastic anemia

Symptoms
- Muscle weakness, cramps, tetany
- Polyuria, polydipsia

Signs
- Decreased motor strength, orthostatic hypotension, ileus, ECG changes, such as flattening of T waves, U wave becoming obvious (U wave is the upward deflection after the T wave.)

Treatment: Therapy depends on the cause.
- History of HTN, GI symptoms, or use of certain medications suggests the diagnosis.
- A 24-h urine for K^+ may be helpful if the diagnosis is unclear. Level < 20 mEq/d suggests extrarenal loss or redistribution, > 20 mEq/d suggests renal losses.
- A serum K^+ level of 2 mEq/L represents a deficit of about 300 mEq in a 70-kg adult. To change K^+ from 3 mEq/L to 4 mEq/L it takes about 100 mEq of K^+ in a 70-kg adult.
- Control underlying cause.
- Hypokalemia potentiates the cardiac toxicity of digitalis. In the setting of digoxin use, hypokalemia should be aggressively treated.
- Treat hypomagnesemia if present. It is difficult to correct hypokalemia in the presence of hypomagnesemia.
- **Rapid Correction.** Give KCl IV. Monitor heart with replacement > 20 mEq/h. IV K^+ can be painful and damaging to veins.

    Patient < 40 kg: 0.25 mEq/kg/h × 2 h
    Patient > 40 kg: 10–20 mEq/h × 2 h
    Severe (< 2 mEq/L): Maximum 40 mEq/h IV in adults. In all cases check a stat K^+ after each 2–4 h of replacement.

- **Slow Correction.** Give KCl orally (see Table 22–8, page 642) for K^+ supplements).

    Adults: 20–40 mEq two to three times a day (bid or tid)
    Children: 1–2 mEq/kg/d in divided doses

Hypercalcemia

- Ca^{2+} > 10.2 mg/dL

Mechanisms
- **Parathyroid-Related.** Hyperparathyroidism with secondary bone resorption
- **Malignancy-Related.** Solid tumors with metastasis (breast, ovary, lung, kidney); paraneoplastic syndromes (squamous cell, renal cell, transitional cell carcinomas, lymphoma, and myeloma)

- **Vitamin-D–Related.** Vitamin D intoxication, sarcoidosis, other granulomatous disease
- **High Bone Turnover.** Hyperthyroidism, Paget disease, immobilization, vitamin A intoxication
- **Renal Failure.** Secondary hyperparathyroidism, aluminum intoxication
- **Other.** Thiazide diuretics, milk–alkali syndrome, familial hypocalciuric hypercalcemia, exogenous intake

Symptoms
- Stones (renal colic), bones (osteitis fibrosa), moans (constipation), and groans (neuropsychiatric symptoms—confusion) as well as polyuria, polydipsia, fatigue, anorexia, nausea, vomiting

Signs
- HTN, hyporeflexia, mental status changes
- Shortening of the QT interval on the ECG

Treatment: Usually emergency treatment if symptoms are not present and Ca^{2+} > 13 mEq/L

Use saline diuresis: D_5NS at 250–500 mL/h
Give furosemide (Lasix) 20–80 mg or more IV (saline and furosemide correct most cases).
Euvolemia or hypervolemia must be maintained. Hypovolemia results in Ca reabsorption.

- **Other Second-Line Therapies**

Calcitonin 2–8 IU/kg IV or SQ q6–12h if diuresis has not worked after 2–3 h
Pamidronate 60 mg IV over 24 h (one dose only)
Gallium nitrate 200 mg/m^2 IV infusion over 24 h for 5 d
Plicamycin 25 mcg/kg IV over 2–3 h (use as last resort; very potent)
Corticosteroids. Hydrocortisone 50–75 mg IV q6h
Hemodialysis

- **Chronic Therapy**

Correct underlying condition, discontinue contributing medications (eg, thiazides).
Oral medications (prednisone 30 mg PO bid or phosphorus/K/Na supplement [Neutra-Phos] 250–500 mg PO qid) can be effective chronic therapy for diseases such as breast cancer and sarcoidosis.

Hypocalcemia

• Ca^{2+} < 8.4 mg/dL

Mechanisms: Decreased albumin can result in decreased total Ca (see page 54).

- **PTH.** Responsible for the immediate regulation of Ca levels
- **Critical Illness.** Sepsis and other ICU-related conditions can cause decreased Ca because of the decrease in albumin that often occurs in critically ill patients; ionized Ca may be normal.
- **PTH Deficiency.** Acquired (surgical excision or injury, infiltrative diseases such as amyloidosis and hemochromatosis, irradiation), hereditary hypoparathyroidism (pseudohypoparathyroidism), hypomagnesemia

- **Vitamin D Deficiency.** Chronic renal failure, liver disease, use of phenytoin or phenobarbital, malnutrition, malabsorption (chronic pancreatitis, aftermath of gastrectomy)
- **Other.** Hyperphosphatemia, acute pancreatitis, osteoblastic metastasis, medullary carcinoma of thyroid, massive transfusion

Symptoms
- Hypertension, peripheral and perioral paresthesia, abdominal pain and cramps, lethargy, irritability in infants

Signs
- Hyperactive DTRs, carpopedal spasm (Trousseau sign, see page 19)
- Presence of Chvostek sign (see page 16) (facial nerve twitch, present in as many as 25% of healthy adults)
- Generalized seizures, tetany, laryngospasm
- Prolonged QT interval on ECG

Treatment
- **Acute Symptomatic**

  100–200 mg of elemental Ca IV over 10 min in 50–100 mL of D_5W followed by an infusion containing 1–2 mg/kg/h over 6–12 h. 10% Ca gluconate contains 93 mg of elemental Ca. 10% Ca chloride contains 272 mg of elemental Ca. Check magnesium levels and replace if low.

- **Chronic**

  For renal insufficiency, use vitamin D along with oral Ca supplements (see the following lists) and phosphate-binding antacids (eg, Phospho gel, AlternaGEL).
  Ca supplements:

  Ca carbonate (eg, Os-Cal) 650 mg PO qid (28% Ca)
  Ca citrate (eg, Citracal) 950-mg tablets (21% Ca)
  Ca gluconate 500- or 1000-mg tablets (9% Ca)
  Ca glubionate (eg, Neo-Calglucon) syrup 115 mg/5 mL (6.4% Ca)
  Ca lactate 325- or 650-mg tablets (13% Ca)

Hypermagnesemia
- $Mg^{2+} > 2.1$ mEq/L

Mechanisms
- **Excess Administration.** Management of preeclampsia with magnesium sulfate
- **Renal Insufficiency.** Exacerbated by ingestion of magnesium-containing antacids
- **Others.** Rhabdomyolysis, adrenal insufficiency

Symptoms and Signs
- 3–5 mEq/L: Nausea, vomiting, hypotension, decreased reflexes
- 7–10 mEq/L: Hyporeflexia, weakness, drowsiness, quadraparesis
- > 12 mEq/L: Coma, bradycardia, respiratory failure

Treatment: Clinical hypermagnesemia necessitating therapy is infrequently encountered in patients with normal renal function.

- Ca gluconate: 10 mL of 10% solution (93 mg elemental Ca) over 10–20 min in 50–100 mL of D_5W given IV to reverse symptoms (useful in patients being treated for eclampsia).
- Stop magnesium-containing medications (hypermagnesemia is common in renal failure patients taking magnesium-containing antacids).
- Insulin and glucose as for hyperkalemia. Furosemide and saline diuresis
- Dialysis

Hypomagnesemia

• $Mg^{2+} < 1.5$ mEq/L

Mechanisms

- **Decreased Intake or Absorption.** Malabsorption, chronic GI losses, deficient intake (alcoholics), TPN without adequate supplementation
- **Increased Loss.** Diuretics, other medications (gentamicin, cisplatin, amphotericin B, others), RTA, DM (especially DKA), alcoholism, hyperaldosteronism, excessive lactation
- **Other.** Acute pancreatitis, hypoalbuminemia, vitamin D therapy

Symptoms

- Weakness, muscle twitches, asterixis, vertigo
- Symptoms of hypocalcemia and hypokalemia (hypomagnesemia may cause hypocalcemia and hypokalemia)

Signs

- Tachycardia, tremor, hyperactive reflexes, tetany, seizures
- ECG may show prolongation of PR, QT, and QRS intervals as well as ventricular ectopy and sinus tachycardia

Treatment

- **Severe: Tetany or Seizures.** Monitor patient with ECG in ICU. 2 g magnesium sulfate in D_5W infused over 10–20 min. Follow with magnesium sulfate: 1 g/h for 3–4 h, watch for DTRs and monitor levels. Repeat replacement if necessary. These patients often have hypokalemic and hypophosphatemic and should be given supplements. Hypocalcemia may also result from hypomagnesemia.
- **Moderate.** $Mg^{2+} < 1.0$ mEq/L but asymptomatic: Magnesium sulfate: 1 g/h for 3–4 h, monitor levels, and repeat replacement if necessary.
- **Mild.** Magnesium oxide: 1 g/d PO (available over the counter in 140-mg capsules and in 400- and 420-mg tablets). May cause diarrhea.

Hyperphosphatemia

• $PO_4^{3-} > 4.5$ mg/dL

Mechanisms

- **Increased Intake and Absorption.** Iatrogenic, abuse of laxatives or enemas containing phosphorus, vitamin D, granulomatous disease
- **Decreased Excretion** (Most Common Cause). Renal failure, hypoparathyroidism, adrenal insufficiency, hyperthyroidism, acromegaly, sickle cell anemia
- **Redistribution and Cellular Release.** Rhabdomyolysis, acidosis, chemotherapy-induced tumor lysis, hemolysis, plasma cell dyscrasia

Symptoms and Signs: Mostly related to tetany as a result of hypocalcemia (see page 190) caused by the hyperphosphatemia or metastatic calcification (deposition of calcium phosphate in various soft tissues)

Treatment
- Low-phosphate diet
- Phosphate binders such as aluminum hydroxide gel (eg, Amphojel) or aluminum carbonate gel (eg, Basaljel) orally
- Acute, severe cases: Acetazolamide 15 mg/kg q4h or insulin and glucose infusion, dialysis as last resort

Hypophosphatemia
- $PO_4^{3-} < 2.5$ mg/dL

Mechanisms
- **Decreased Dietary Intake.** Starvation, alcoholism, iatrogenic factors (hyperalimentation without adequate supplementation), malabsorption, vitamin D deficiency, phosphate-binding antacids (eg, AlternaGEL)
- **Redistribution.** Conditions associated with respiratory or metabolic alkalosis (eg, alcohol withdrawal, salicylate poisoning), endocrine abnormalities (eg, insulin, catecholamine), anabolic steroids, hyper- or hypothermia, leukemia and lymphoma, hypercalcemia, hypomagnesemia
- **Renal Losses.** RTA, diuretic phase of ATN, hyperparathyroidism, hyperthyroidism, hypokalemia, diuretics, hypomagnesemia, alcohol abuse, poorly controlled DM
- **Other.** Refeeding in the setting of severe protein-calorie malnutrition, severe burns, management of DKA

Symptoms and Signs: < 1 mg/dL Weakness, muscle pain and tenderness, paresthesia, cardiac and respiratory failure, CNS dysfunction (confusion and seizures), rhabdomyolysis, hemolysis, impaired leukocyte and platelet function

Treatment: IV therapy is reserved for severe, potentially life-threatening hypophosphatemia (< 1.0–1.5 mg/dL) because too rapid correction can lead to severe hypocalcemia. With mild to moderate hypophosphatemia (1.5–2.5 mg/dL), oral replacement is preferred.

- **Severe.** (< 1.0–1.5 mg/dL) Potassium or sodium phosphate. 2 mg/kg given IV over 6 h. (**Caution:** Too rapid replacement can lead to hypocalcemic tetany.)
- **Mild to Moderate.** (> 1.5 mg/dL) Sodium–potassium phosphate (Neutra-Phos) or potassium phosphate (K-Phos): 1–2 tablets (250–500 mg PO_4 per tablet) PO bid or tid. Sodium phosphate (Fleet Phospho-soda) 5 mL PO_4^{3-} bid or tid (128 mg PO_4^{3-})

BLOOD COMPONENT THERAPY

Blood Banking Procedures
Routine Blood Donation
Autologous Blood Donation
Donor-Directed Blood Products
Irradiated Blood Components
Apheresis
Preoperative Blood Set-Up
Emergency Transfusions

Blood Groups
Basic Principles of Blood Component
    Therapy
Blood Bank Products
Transfusion Procedures
Transfusion Reactions
Transfusion-Associated Infectious
    Disease Risk

BLOOD BANKING PROCEDURES

T&S or T&H: The blood bank **types** the patient's blood (ABO and Rh), **screens** for antibodies, and **holds** the blood. If a rare antibody is found, the physician usually is notified. If it is likely that blood will be needed, the T&S order may be changed to a T&C.

T&C: The blood bank does a T&S on the patient's blood and matches specific donor units to the patient. The **cross-match** involves testing the recipient's serum against donor blood cells. A T&C usually takes less than 1 h.

Stat Requests: The bank sets up blood immediately and usually holds it for 12 h. For routine requests, the blood is set up at a date and time that you specify and usually held for 36 h.

ROUTINE BLOOD DONATION

Voluntary blood donation is the mainstay of the blood system in the United States. Donors usually are > 18 y old, are in good health and afebrile, and weigh > 110 lb (50 kg). Donors are usually limited to 1 unit every 8 wk and 6 donations per year. Patients with a history of hepatitis, HBsAg positivity, insulin-dependent DM, IV drug abuse, heart disease, anemia, or homosexual activity are excluded from routine donation. Patients who may have transmissible diseases are counseled about high-risk behaviors that may put the recipient of the blood at risk. Donor blood is tested for ABO, Rh, antibody screen, HBsAg, anti–hepatitis B core antigen, hepatitis C antibody, anti–HIV-1 and -2, and anti–HTLV-1 and -2.

AUTOLOGOUS BLOOD DONATION

Some patients undergoing elective surgery in which blood may be needed use preadmission autologous blood banking (predeposit phlebotomy). General guidelines for autologous banking include good overall health, HCT > 34%, and arm veins that can accommodate a 16-gauge needle. Patients can usually donate up to 1 unit every 3–7 d until 3–7 d before surgery (individual blood banks have

their own specifications), depending on the needs of the planned surgical procedure. Iron supplements (eg, ferrous gluconate 325 mg PO tid) are usually given
before and for several months after the donation. The use of erythropoietin in
this preoperative setting is being investigated. Units of whole blood can be held
for up to 35 d.

DONOR-DIRECTED BLOOD PRODUCTS

A relative or friend can donate blood for a specific patient. This technique cannot be used in the emergency setting because it takes up to 48 h to process the
blood for use.

   This system has some drawbacks: Relatives may be unduly pressured to give
blood; risk factors that would normally exclude the use of the blood (hepatitis or
HIV positivity) become problematic; and the routine donation of blood for
emergency transfusion may be adversely affected. These units are usually stored
as PRBC and released into the general transfusion pool 8 h after surgery unless
otherwise requested.

IRRADIATED BLOOD COMPONENTS

Transfusion-associated graft-versus-host disease (GVHD), a frequently fatal
condition, can be minimized through the use of highly selected irradiated blood
components. Patients who are at risk of GVHD include recipients of donor-
directed units or HLA-matched platelets, fetuses receiving intrauterine transfusions, and selected immunocompromised and bone marrow recipients.

APHERESIS

Apheresis procedures are used to collect single-donor platelets (**plateletpheresis**) or WBC (**leukapheresis**); the remaining components are returned to the
donor. **Therapeutic apheresis** is the separation and removal of a particular
component to achieve a therapeutic effect (eg, **erythrocytapheresis** to treat
polycythemia).

PREOPERATIVE BLOOD SET-UP

Most institutions have established protocols for setting up blood before surgical
procedures. A number of units of PRBC or only a T&S may be needed depending on the procedure. Check with the surgeon.

EMERGENCY TRANSFUSIONS

Non-cross-matched blood is rarely transfused because most blood banks can do
a complete cross-match within 1 h. In cases of massive, exsanguinating hemorrhage, type-specific blood (ABO- and Rh-matched only), usually available in 10
min, can be used. If even this delay is too long, type O, Rh-negative PRBC can
be used as a last resort. When possible, it is generally preferable to support BP
with colloid or crystalloid until properly cross-matched blood is available.

BLOOD GROUPS

Table 10–1, page 197, gives information on the major blood groups and their
relative occurrences. Type O– is the **"universal donor,"** and AB+ is the **"universal recipient."**

TABLE 10–1
Blood Groups and Guidelines for Transfusion

Type (ABO/Rh)	Occurrences	Can Usually Receive[a] Blood From
O+	1 in 3	O (+/−)
O−	1 in 15	O (−)
A+	1 in 3	A (+/−) or O (+/−)
A−	1 in 16	A (−) or O (−)
B+	1 in 12	B (+/−) or O (+/−)
B−	1 in 67	B (−) or O (−)
AB+	1 in 29	AB, A, B, or O (all + or −)
AB−	1 in 167	AB, A, B, or O (all −)

[a]First choice is always the identical blood type; other acceptable combinations are shown. An attempt is also made to match Rh status of donor and recipient; Rh− can usually be given to an Rh+ recipient safely.

BASIC PRINCIPLES OF BLOOD COMPONENT THERAPY

Table 10–2, page 198, shows common indications for and uses of transfusion products. The following are the basic transfusion principles for adults.

10

Red Cell Transfusions

Acute Blood Loss: Healthy persons can usually tolerate up to 30% blood loss without transfusion. Patients may manifest tachycardia and mild hypotension without evidence of hypovolemic shock. Start volume replacement (IV fluids, etc).

- Hgb > 10 g/dL, transfusion rarely indicated.
- Hgb 7–10 g/dL, transfusion based on clinical symptoms, unless patient has severe medical problems (eg, CAD, severe COPD).
- Hgb < 7 g/dL, transfusion usually needed.

"Allowable Blood Loss":   Often used to guide acute transfusion in the operating room. Losses less than allowable are usually managed with IV fluid replacement.

$$\text{Weight in kg} \times 0.08 = \text{Total blood volume}$$

$$\text{Total volume} \times 0.3 = \text{Allowable blood loss (assumes normal Hbg)}$$

Example: A 70-kg adult

$$\text{Estimated allowable blood loss} = 70 \times 0.08 = 5.6\text{L}$$
$$\text{or } (5600 \text{ mL}) \times 0.3 = 1680 \text{ mL}$$

Chronic Anemia: Common in certain chronic conditions, such as renal failure, rarely managed with blood transfusion; typically managed with pharmacologic therapy (eg, erythropoietin). However, transfusion is generally indicated if Hgb < 6 g/dL or in the face of symptoms due to low hemoglobin.

RBC Transfusion Formula: As a guide, 1 unit of PRBC raises the HCT 3% (Hgb, 1 g/dL) in the average adult. To roughly determine the volume of whole blood or PRBC needed to raise the HCT to a known amount, use the following formula:

$$\text{Volume of cells} = \frac{\text{Total blood volume of patient} \times (\text{Desired HCT} - \text{Actual HCT})}{\text{HCT of transfusion product}}$$

(*Text continues on page 202.*)

TABLE 10–2
Blood Bank Products

Product	Description	Common Indications
Whole Blood	No elements removed 1 unit = 450 mL ± 45 mL (HCT ≈ 40%) Contains RBC, WBC, plasma and platelets (WBC & platelets may be nonfunctional) Deficient in factors V & VII	Not for routine use Acute, massive bleeding Open heart surgery Neonatal total exchange
Packed Red Cells (PRBC)	Most plasma, WBC, platelets removed; unit = 250–300 mL. (HCT ≈ 75%) 1 unit should raise HCT 3%	Replacement in chronic and acute blood loss, GI bleeding, trauma
Universal Pedi-Packs	250–300 mL divided into 3 bags Contains red cells, some white cells, some plasma and platelets	Transfusion of infants
Leukocyte-Poor (Leukocyte-Reduced) Red Cells	Most WBC removed by filtration to make it less antigenic $<5 \times 10^6$ WBC, few platelets, minimal plasma 1 unit = 200–250 mL	Potential renal transplant patients Previous febrile transfusion reactions Patients requiring multiple transfusions (leukemia, etc)
Washed RBCs	Like leukocyte-poor red cells, but WBC almost completely removed $<5 \times 10^8$ WBC, no plasma 1 unit = 300 mL	As for leukocyte-poor red cells, but very expensive and much more purified

(continued)

TABLE 10-2
(Continued)

Product	Description	Common Indications
Granulocytes, Pheresis	1 unit = ≈220 mL Some RBC, >1 × 10^{10} PMN/unit, Lymphocytes, platelets	See page 196
Platelets	1 "pack" should raise count by 5000–8000 "6-pack" means a pool of platelets from 6 units of blood 1 pack = about 50 mL >5 × 10^{10} platelets unit, contains RBC, WBC	Decreased production or destruction (aplastic anemia, acute leukemia, postchemo, etc) Counts <5000–10,000 (risk of spontaneous hemorrhage) must transfuse Counts 10,000–30,000 if risk of bleeding (headache, GI losses, contiguous petechiae) or active bleeding Counts <50,000 if life-threatening bleed Prophylactic transfusion >20,000 for minor surgery or >50,000 for major surgery Usually not indicated in ITP or TTP unless life-threatening bleeding or preoperative status
Platelets, Pheresis	>3 × 10^{10} platelets/unit 1 unit = 300 mL	See Platelets, may be HLA matched
Platelets, Leukocyte-Reduced	As above, but <5 × 10^{6} WBC/unit	See Platelets, may decrease febrile reactions and CMV transmission, alloimmunization to HLA antigens

(continued)

10

199

TABLE 10-2
(Continued)

Product	Description	Common Indications
Cryoprecipitated Antihemophilic Factor ("Cryo")	Contains factor VIII, factor XIII, von Willebrand factor, and fibrinogen 1 unit = 10 mL	Hemophilia A (factor VIII deficiency), when safer factor VIII concentrate not available; von Willebrand disease, fibrinogen deficiency, fibrin surgical glue
Fresh-Frozen Plasma (FFP)	Contains factors II, VII, IX, X, XI, XII, XIII, and heat-labile factors V and VII About 1 h to thaw 150–250 mL (400–600 mL if single-donor pheresis)	Emergency reversal of warfarin Massive transfusion (>5 L in adults) Hypoglobulinemia (IV immune globulin preferred) Suspected or documented coagulopathy (congenital or acquired) with active bleeding or before surgery) Clotting factor replacement when concentrate unavailable Not recommended for volume replacement If PT <22 s or PTT <70 s, 1 unit is usually sufficient
Single Donor Plasma	Like FFP, but lacks factors V and VIII About 1 h to thaw; 150–200 mL	No longer routinely used for plasma replacement Stable clotting factor replacement Warfarin reversal, hemophilia B (Christmas disease)
Rho Gam (Rho D immune globulin)	Antibody against Rh factor (volume = 1 mL)	Rh– mother with Rh+ baby, within 72 h of delivery, to prevent hemolytic disease of newborn; autoimmune thrombocytopenia

(continued)

TABLE 10–2
(Continued)

Product	Description	Common Indications
ALL OF THE AFOREMENTIONED ITEMS USUALLY REQUIRE A "CLOT TUBE" TO BE SENT FOR TYPING. THE FOLLOWING PRODUCTS ARE USU-ALLY DISPENSED BY MOST HOSPITAL PHARMACIES AND ARE USUALLY ORDERED AS A MEDICATION.		
Factor VIII (Purified Antihemophilic Factor)	From pooled plasma, pure factor VIII Increased hepatitis risk	Routine for hemophilia A (factor VIII deficiency)
Factor IX Concentrate (Prothrombin Complex)	Increased hepatitis risk Factors II, VII, IX, and X Equivalent to 2 units of plasma	Active bleeding in Christmas disease (hemophilia B or factor IX deficiency)
Immune Serum Globulin	Precipitate from plasma "gamma globulin"	Immune globulin deficiency Disease prophylaxis (hepatitis A, measles, etc)
5% Albumin or 5% Plasma Protein Fraction	Precipitate from plasma (see Drugs, Chapter 22)	Plasma volume expanders in acute blood loss
25% Albumin	Precipitate from plasma	Hypoalbuminemia, volume expander, burns Draws extravascular fluid into circulation

RBC = red blood cells; WBC = white blood cells; HCT = hematocrit; GI = gastrointestinal; ITP = idiopathic thrombocytopenic purpura; TTP = thrombotic thrombocytopenic purpura; HLA = histocompatibility locus antigen; PT = prothrombin time; PTT = partial thromboplastin time.

10

(Text continued from page 197.)

where total blood volume is 70 mL/kg in adults, 80 mL/kg in children. The HCT of PRBC is approximately 70%, and that of whole blood is approximately 40%.

White Cell Transfusions

- The use of white cell transfusions is rarely indicated because genetically engineered myeloid growth factors such as GM-CSF (see Chapter 22) are used instead.
- Indicated for patients being treated for overwhelming sepsis and severe neutropenia (< 500 PMN/µL)

Platelet Transfusions

Indications are in Table 10–2, page 198.

Platelet Transfusion Formula: Platelets are often transfused at a dose of 1 unit/ 10 kg of body weight. After administration of 1 unit of multiple-donor platelets, the count should rise 5000–8000/mm³ within 1 h of transfusion and 4500 mm³ within 24 h. Under normal circumstances, stored platelets that are transfused survive in vivo 6–8 d after infusion. Clinical factors (eg, DIC, alloimmunization) can significantly shorten this time. To standardize the corrected platelet count to an individual patient, use the corrected count increment (CCI). Measure the platelet count immediately before and 1 h after platelet infusion. If the correction is less than expected, do a work-up to determine the possible cause (eg, antibodies, splenomegaly). Many institutions use platelet pheresis units. One platelet pheresis unit has enough platelets to raise the count 6000–8000/mm³. Using a single unit has the advantage of exposing the patient to only one donor versus possibly six to eight donors. This practice limits exposure to different HLA antigens, reducing the risk of antiplatelet antibody production, and also reduces the risk of infection transmission.

$$CCI = \frac{\text{Posttransfusion platelet count} - \text{Pretransfusion count} \times \text{Body surface area (m}^2)}{\text{Platelets given} \times 10^{11}}$$

BLOOD BANK PRODUCTS

Table 10–2, page 198, shows products used in blood component therapy and gives recommendations for use of these products.

TRANSFUSION PROCEDURES

1. Draw a clot tube (red top), and sign the lab slips to verify that the sample came from the correct patient. Identify the patient by referring to the ID bracelet and asking the patient to state, if able, his or her name. Place the patient's name, hospital number, date, and your signature on the tube label. **Prestamped labels are not accepted by most blood banks.**
2. Obtain the patient's informed consent by discussing the reasons for the transfusion and the potential risks and benefits of it. Follow hospital procedure regarding the need for the patient to sign a specific consent form. At most hospitals, chart documentation is usually all that is necessary.
3. When the blood products become available, ensure good venous access for the transfusion (18-gauge needle or larger is preferred for adults).
4. Verify the information on the request slip and blood bag with another person, such as a nurse, and with the patient's ID bracelet. Many hospi-

tals have defined protocols for this procedure; check your institutional guidelines.

5. Mix blood products to be transfused with isotonic (0.9%) NS only. Using hypotonic products such as D_5W can result in hemolysis of the blood in the tubing. Lactated Ringer solution should *not* be used because the calcium can chelate the anticoagulant citrate.

6. Infuse red cells through a special filter. Specific leukocyte reduction filters can be used in highly specific circumstances (history of febrile transfusion reactions, need to reduce potential CMV transmission, need to reduce risk of alloimmunization to WBC antigens).

7. When transfusing large volumes of PRBC (> 10 units), monitor coagulation, Mg^{2+}, Ca^{2+}, and lactate levels. It also usually is necessary to transfuse platelets and FFP. Calcium replacement is sometimes needed because the preservative used in the blood is a calcium binder, and hypocalcemia can occur after large amounts of blood are transfused. For massive transfusions (usually > 50 mL/min in adults and 15 mL/min in children), warm the blood to prevent hypothermia and cardiac arrhythmia.

TRANSFUSION REACTIONS

1. **Acute intravascular hemolysis** (1/240,000–760,000 units transfused) More than 85% of adverse hemolytic reactions involving the transfusion of RBC result from clerical error. Usually caused by ABO-incompatible transfusion. Can result in renal failure.

2. **Nonhemolytic febrile reaction** (~2–3/100 units transfused) Usually mild, fever, chills, rigors, mild dyspnea. Due to a reaction to donor white cells (HLA) and more common in patients who have received multiple transfusions or delivered several children.

3. **Mild allergic reaction** (~1/100 units transfused) Urticaria or pruritus can be caused by sensitization to plasma proteins in transfusion product.

4. **Anaphylactic reaction** (1/150,000 units transfused) Acute hypotension, hives, abdominal pain and respiratory distress; seen mostly in IgA-deficient recipients.

5. **Sepsis** (< 1/500,000 RBC units transfused, 1/12,000 platelet units transfused) Usually caused by transfusion of a bacterially infected transfusion product, with platelet transfusions having the greatest risk. *Escherichia coli, Pseudomonas, Serratia, Salmonella,* and *Yersinia* are the more commonly implicated bacteria.

6. **Acute lung injury** (1/10,000 units transfused) Fever, chills, and life-threatening respiratory failure; probably induced by antibodies from donor against recipient white cells.

7. **Volume overload** (1/100 units transfused) Usually due to excess volume infusion; can exacerbate CHF.

Detection of Transfusion Reaction

1. Spin an HCT to look for a pink plasma layer (indicates hemolysis).

2. Order serum for free Hgb and haptoglobin (haptoglobin decreases with a reaction) and urine for hemosiderin levels. Obtain a stat CBC to determine the presence of schistocytes, suggesting a transfusion reaction.

3. If acute hemolysis is suspected, request a DIC screen (PT, PTT, fibrinogen, and fibrin degradation products).

10

Treatment of Transfusion Reactions

1. Stop the blood product immediately, and notify the blood bank.
2. Keep the IV line open with NS, and monitor the patient's vital signs and urine output carefully.
3. Save the blood bag, and have the lab verify the T&C. Verify that the proper patient received the proper transfusion. Redraw blood samples for the blood bank.
4. **Treat** the patient using the following guidelines and clinical judgment:

   - **Nonhemolytic febrile reaction:** Use antipyretics and continue transfusion monitoring. Use leukocyte-washed transfusion products in the future.
   - **Mild allergic reaction:** After giving diphenhydramine (25–50 mg IM/PO/IV) resume the transfusion only if the patient improves promptly.
   - **Anaphylactic reaction:** Terminate transfusion, monitor closely, give antihistamines (diphenhydramine 25–50 mg IM/PO/IV), corticosteroids (methylprednisolone 125 mg IV, 2 mg/kg pediatric IV), epinephrine (1:1000 0.3–0.5 mL SQ adults, 0.1 mL/kg pediatric), and pressors as needed. Premedicate (antihistamines, steroids) for future transfusions; use only leukocyte-washed red cells.
   - **Acute lung injury:** Provide ventilatory support as needed; use only leukocyte-washed red cells for future transfusions.
   - **Sepsis:** Culture the transfusion product and the patient; treat empirically by monitoring and administering pressors and antibiotics (third- or fourth-generation cephalosporin or piperacillin/tazobactam along with an aminoglycoside) until cultures are returned.
   - **Volume overload:** Use a slow rate of infusion with selective use of diuretics.
   - **Acute intravascular hemolysis:** Prevent acute renal failure. Place a Foley catheter, monitor urine output closely, and maintain brisk diuresis with plain D_5W, mannitol (1–2 g/kg IV), furosemide (20–40 mg IV), and/or dopamine (2–10 mcg/kg/min IV) as needed. Alkalize the urine with bicarbonate and pressure support (fluids, vasopressors). Monitor for DIC. Request renal and hematologic consults.

TRANSFUSION-ASSOCIATED INFECTIOUS DISEASE RISK

For perspective, selected comparative mortality odds ratios are: stroke 1/1,700; pregnancy 1/4,350–1/10,000; MVA 1/6,700; anesthesia 1/7,000–1/339,450; oral contraceptive use 1/50,000; flood 1/455,000; lightning strike 1/10,000,000. (*Transfusion* 2005;45:254–264; http://www.pathology.unc.edu/labs/textfiles/tms_risk.htm [Accessed May 30, 2006])

Hepatitis

One case of posttransfusion hepatitis B occurs for every 205,000–488,000 units transfused; the incidence of hepatitis C is 1/1,8000,000 units transfused. Anicteric hepatitis is more common than hepatitis with jaundice. Donor screening has greatly reduced hepatitis risk. Pooled factor products (concentrates of factor VIII) are associated with the greatest risk; albumin and globulins carry no risk of hepatitis.

HIV

The incidence of transfusion-related HIV infection is 1/2,3000,000 units. Antibody testing is routinely performed on the donor's blood; a positive antibody test means that the donor may have HIV infection; a confirmatory Western blot is necessary. Do a follow-up test on any donor found to be HIV-positive, because false-positives can occur. There is a delay of approximately 22 d between HIV exposure and the development of HIV antibodies. Risk of HIV transmission exists even when HIV-negative donor blood is used. Use of molecular detection decreases the time between infection and detection from 22 d to 11 d.

CMV

The prevalence of CMV infection among donors is very high (approaching 100% in many series). CMV infection represents a major clinical risk mostly for immunocompromised recipients and neonates. Leukocyte filters can reduce the risk of transmission.

HTLV-I, -II

Very rare (1/514,000–2,993,000 units transfused). Use of leukocyte filters can further decrease risk of transmission.

Bacteria, Parasites, and Other Viruses

10

Sepsis caused by bacteria is rare (see page 203). Parasites are very rarely transmitted (< 1/1,000,000 units) for yersiniosis, malaria, babesiosis, and Chagas disease, but careful donor screening is necessary, especially in endemic regions. West Nile virus cases are limited but have been reported.

NUTRITIONAL ASSESSMENT, THERAPEUTIC DIETS, AND INFANT FEEDING

Interplay Between Nutrition and Illness
Nutritional Assessment
Establishing Protein and Energy
    Requirements

Therapeutic Diets
Infant Feeding
Candidates for Nutritional
    Support

INTERPLAY BETWEEN NUTRITION AND ILLNESS

Nutritional factors figure prominently in the pathogenesis of coronary heart disease, cancer, stroke, and type 2 diabetes—diseases that account for more than half of all deaths in the United States. Dietary habits also play an extensive role in other causes of morbidity and mortality, including hypertension, obesity, and osteoporosis. This situation is compounded by the epidemic of obesity in the United States, which is expected to cause sharp increases in the incidence of chronic illness. In recognition of the serious health implications of obesity, current definitions of "malnutrition" include states of overnutrition as well as conditions marked by nutritional deficits.

The link between nutritional status and health risk extends beyond chronic disease to include acute illness. Surveys place the incidence of malnutrition among hospitalized patients between 30% and 55%. Malnutrition increases the risk of adverse clinical outcomes of hospital stays. In short, poor nutrition increases the risk of becoming ill, and when illness does strike, malnutrition complicates treatment and impairs recovery.

Negative Effects of Malnutrition on Clinical Outcome

Greater susceptibility to infectious complications
Reduced immune competence
Poor skin integrity
Delayed wound healing
Higher incidence of surgical complications
Prolonged need for mechanical ventilation
Increased mortality
Extended length of stay, higher health care costs

As the interplay between nutritional status and illness has become better understood, nutritional assessment has taken on greater importance in clinical care. By integrating nutritional assessment into the evaluation of all patients, clinicians not only identify malnutrition but also uncover risk factors for chronic disease and unfavorable clinical outcome, determine nutritional requirements, recognize people likely to benefit from nutritional support, and establish a framework for developing a therapeutic plan.

NUTRITIONAL ASSESSMENT

No single assessment technique has the validity to serve as the sole indicator of nutritional status. Nutritional assessment is a comprehensive process that combines objective data with relevant clinical information. Evaluate body composition, anthropometric measurements, and results of laboratory tests, and use the data in the context of the patient's history, physical examination findings, and clinical condition to make decisions concerning nutritional status.

Body Weight

Body weight is a reliable indicator of nutritional status. Details concerning body weight include deviation of weight from ideal level, change in weight over time, and relation between weight and height. Body weight 20% over or under the ideal level places a patient at nutritional risk. Numerous methods for determining ideal body weight exist, but the Hamwi formula is the most widely used in clinical settings because the calculation is simple and provides a reasonable estimate of ideal body weight:

Formula for Determining Ideal Body Weight

Men: 106 lb for 5 ft of height plus 6 lb for every inch of height over 5 ft
Women: 100 lb for 5 ft of height plus 5 lb for every inch of height over 5 ft
Both: ± 10% based on frame size

11

Changes in body weight from baseline carry important prognostic value. Whether or not usual body weight is over or under the ideal, unintentional weight loss is cause for concern. Both the degree of weight loss and the timeframe in which it occurs are significant variables. In general, involuntary weight loss of 10% of usual weight over a period of 6 mo represents severe nutritional risk that warrants further investigation. Among children, a downward trend in percentile ranking on growth charts is cause for concern even if the child continues to gain weight. Growth charts can also reveal a tendency toward excessive weight gain, allowing early nutritional intervention and management of obesity.

Body Mass Index

Body mass index (BMI), a ratio of weight to height, is a value that eliminates the influence of frame size. BMI is a reliable indicator of adiposity. An elevated BMI is strongly correlated with the risk of development of cardiovascular disease, diabetes, cancer, hypertension, and osteoarthritis. The formula for calculating BMI is:

$$\text{BMI} = \frac{\text{Weight (kg)}}{\text{Height}^2\text{(m)}}$$

Table 11–1 shows the interpretation of BMI values. Each class of obesity represents a higher level of health risk. The BMI formula overestimates body fat in muscular athletes and underestimates fat stores in older persons, limiting the value of the formula in those populations. Online BMI calculators make quick work of the somewhat cumbersome equation.

TABLE 11–1
Body Mass Index

BMI	Interpretation
< 18.5	Underweight
18.5–24.9	Normal
25–29.9	Overweight
30–34.9	Obesity (class 1)
35–39.9	Obesity (class 2)
> 40	Obesity (class 3)

Many BMI calculators are available online; keyword search "BMI"

Anthropometric Measurements

Anthropometric evaluations are body composition assessments derived through direct measurement. A summary of the techniques used to evaluate body composition appears in Table 11–2. In traditional anthropometric evaluations, the circumference of the midarm muscle and the thickness of the triceps skinfold were measured. These techniques have fallen out of favor because the reference tables lack validity and clinical applicability. The preferred method of nutritional assessment includes measuring waist circumference and waist-to-hip ratio to evaluate the distribution of body fat and the health risks associated with abdominal obesity. For men, a waist measurement > 40 in (102 cm) indicates higher risk of cardiovascular disease. Similar risk exists for women with a waist measurement > 35 in (89 cm). For both men and women, a ratio of waist circumference to hip circumference ≥ 1.0 represents increased risk of health problems related to obesity. A favorable waist-to-hip ratio is ≤ 0.90 for men and ≤ 0.80 for women. Abdominal obesity is one feature of **metabolic syndrome,** a cluster of risk factors, such as insulin resistance, dyslipidemia, hypertension, and prothrombotic and proinflammatory states, that increase risk of cardiovascular disease and type 2 diabetes. Table 11–3 details the identification of metabolic syndrome.

Laboratory Tests

In primary care, the lipid profile is perhaps the most frequently ordered laboratory test with nutritional implications. Many other routine laboratory tests, such as CBC, blood glucose, electrolyte levels, creatinine, and BUN, also provide information relevant to nutritional status. Although the lipid profile is important during acute illness, nutritional assessment of hospitalized patients also emphasizes evaluation of serum protein concentration.

Visceral protein markers, such as albumin, transferrin, and prealbumin, are routinely measured in hospitalized patients. Because of its short half-life, prealbumin is the preferred marker in clinical settings. Visceral protein levels are frequently presented as a key part of nutritional assessment. These measurements, however, have limited value as nutritional indicators in acutely ill patients. Studies show a strong link between low visceral protein levels and increased risk of morbidity and mortality, but numerous clinical factors other than nutrition can influence visceral protein levels during acute illness. Visceral protein concentra-

TABLE 11–2
Techniques for Evaluating Body Composition

Method	Description
Body weight	Actual body weight compared with ideal body weight; used to assess changes over time; results are affected by hydration status
BMI	Used to evaluates weight in relation to height; a reliable indicator of adiposity; high levels increase health risks
Anthropometric measurements	Measurement of waist circumference and waist to hip ratio, both values linked to health risks; replaces measurement of triceps skinfold thickness and midarm muscle circumference, which lacks validity
Bioelectrical impedance analysis (BIA)	Assessment of fluid volume and lean body mass by measurement of resistance to electrical current; used in sports medicine; not fully validated for clinical use
Dual-energy x-ray absorptiometry (DEXA)	Measurement of bone density; may help determine fat and lean body compartments; no clear role in predicting clinical outcome
Neutron activation analysis	Use of shielded counters to measure gamma-ray decay of naturally occurring isotopes; estimate of total body potassium, an indicator of body cell mass; safe for pregnant women and children; used primarily in research

tion often reflects hydration status, organ function, or an inflammatory response to injury more than the nutritional state of the patient. In inflammatory states, the liver reprioritizes protein synthesis in favor of acute-phase proteins, causing visceral protein levels to fall. Some investigators have suggested routinely measuring C-reactive protein in conjunction with visceral protein as a way to differentiate low visceral protein levels caused by nutritional factors from those related to the presence of an inflammatory process.

Nutritional assessment does not routinely include assays of specific nutrient levels unless clinical circumstances raise concern about potential imbalances. For instance, order iron studies as part of the assessment of a patient with microcytic anemia, but order vitamin B_{12} and folate levels in the evaluation of macrocytosis.

Health History

The health history obtained in the evaluation of every patient is an indispensable source of information regarding nutritional status. The patient interview not only provides an additional opportunity to detect risk factors related to nutrition but also often reveals the mechanisms underlying nutritional problems. The medical history, for example, indicates the impact of disease or previous surgery on nutrient intake, absorption, and metabolism. A review of the patient's current

TABLE 11–3
Diagnostic Criteria for Metabolic Syndrome

Characteristic	Value
Abdominal obesity	Waist circumference
	Men: > 40 in (102 cm)
	Women: > 35 in (89 cm)
Fasting triglyceride level	> 150 mg/dL
HDL cholesterol	Men: < 40 mg/dL
	Women: < 50 mg/dL
Blood pressure	> 130/85 mm/Hg
Fasting blood glucose	> 110 mg/dL

The presence of three or more of the risk factors identifies the syndrome.

medication profile may reveal drug–nutrient interactions or GI side effects that affect appetite. Symptoms such as nausea, pain, fatigue, dry mouth, and shortness of breath often have negative effects on food intake. Aspects of the patient's social history, such as the presence of substance abuse, financial difficulties, or lack of support systems, also are causes of concern about nutritional status. Whenever possible, request a complete nutritional history by a registered dietitian to obtain complete information about nutritional deficits that may exist.

Physical Examination

Use standard physical assessment procedures to evaluate nutritional status. Physical signs of malnutrition are often nonspecific and require correlation with the patient's history, clinical condition, and results of diagnostic studies. As Table 11–4 shows, muscle wasting, poor skin integrity, and loss of subcutaneous fat are typical findings associated with long-standing deficits in protein and energy intake. Patients rarely exhibit the classic signs of vitamin or mineral deficiency that characterize conditions such as scurvy and beri-beri. Fortification of the food supply in the United States and widespread use of multivitamin supplements have made physical manifestation of nutrient deficiency an uncommon occurrence.

Assessing GI Function

Although not part of nutritional assessment per se, appraisal of GI function often provides insight into the mechanisms underlying nutritional problems and helps to pinpoint specific nutrient deficiencies that may exist. Any alteration in the key GI functions associated with eating—appetite, chewing, swallowing, digestion, absorption, and elimination—can have profound effects on nutritional status. An understanding of GI function is also essential for determining the most appropriate route of nutritional support.

The functional status of the GI tract is a key element in determining when to initiate feeding in postoperative patients. In most cases, patients can safely begin oral intake once they recover consciousness sufficiently to protect their airway. Laparotomy, however, can delay GI motility in the postoperative period. In gen-

TABLE 11-4
Physical Signs of Poor Nutritional Status

Sign	Example	Clinical Implications
Muscle wasting	Loss of muscle mass and tone; concave appearance of the temporal region of the face is evidence of marked muscle wasting, even in the presence of edema	Weakness, reduced stamina and functional status; possible impairment of respiratory effort and ability to cough and clear secretions
Loss of subcutaneous tissue	Loose, elongated skinfolds on the abdomen and in the triceps area; prominent appearance of ribs, scapulae, vertebrae, and pelvic bones	Depletion of fat stores representing marked weight loss and loss of reserves that serve as an energy source during illness
Poor skin integrity	Poor turgor, friability, delayed wound healing; possible edema with severe hypoalbuminemia	Increased risk of pressure ulcers, wound dehiscence, and anastomotic leaks
Obesity	Excess accumulation of body mass and adipose issue	Serious health risks; truncal obesity more serious risk than fat stores on hips and buttocks

11

eral, delayed motility affects the stomach and colon, sparing the small intestine. The stomach regains motility about 24 h postoperatively, and the colon typically recovers 72–96 h after surgery. It is generally believed that by the time a patient reports flatus, oral intake can be resumed.

ESTABLISHING PROTEIN AND ENERGY REQUIREMENTS
Caloric Expenditure

Establishing target ranges for energy and protein intake helps not only to ensure that the patient receives adequate nutrition but also to avoid overfeeding. Numerous studies have shown the deleterious effects of overfeeding, including unwanted weight gain, hyperglycemia, hepatic dysfunction, electrolyte imbalances, azotemia, hyperlipidemia, and elevated respiratory quotient. These effects are especially important in patients fed by vein. Several methods for determining energy expenditure exist, including weight-based calculations, formulas such as the Harris–Benedict equations, and indirect calorimetry techniques. None of these methods is ideal for all situations. Each requires a degree of judgment to account for clinical variables that affect energy needs. The following simple weight-based system is the most practical way to establish goals for caloric intake.

For adults in most clinical settings, a range of 25–30 kcal/kg of body weight is a reasonable estimate of daily energy expenditure. No attempt is made to account for variations in age, sex, body composition, or acuity of illness, hence the need for clinical judgment. Concerns about overfeeding and unfavorable outcome have eliminated the once common practice of providing as much as 35–40 kcal/kg/d to critically ill patients. The weight-based system has a wide margin of error for obese patients. When a patient's BMI falls into an obese category, many clinicians use adjusted body weight (ABW) to determine energy needs. The formula for ABW takes into account that not all of a person's excess weight is adipose tissue but that a portion is metabolically active, lean body mass:

$$\text{ABW} = [(\text{Actual body weight} - \text{Ideal body weight})\ 0.25]$$
$$+ \text{Ideal body weight}$$

Consensus does not exist regarding the optimal level of energy intake for obese patients. Studies in which patients received as little as 50% of estimated energy expenditure or 20 kcal/kg of ABW have shown positive outcomes. Further research is needed, however, for accurate prediction of optimal levels of energy intake for obese patients.

Infants and growing children need much higher energy intake per kilogram of body weight than adults. Infants may need as much as 110 kcal/kg/d. Energy intake remains elevated to support growth through the teenage years, but wide variation occurs. Satisfactory growth is the best indication that a child's energy intake is adequate.

Protein Requirements

Healthy persons with normal renal function need 0.8 g of protein per kilogram of body weight per day, but illness and injury can dramatically increase protein needs. For example, postoperative patients need 1.0–1.5 g/kg/d. Sepsis increases protein needs to 1.2–1.5 g/kg/d. Daily protein intake for patients with multiple trauma should fall within 1.3–1.7 g/kg, and burn victims may need 1.8–2.5 g/kg/d. With the exception of patients with burn injuries, guidelines set the upper limit for protein intake at 2.0 g/kg/d. Research suggests that doses of protein above this level exceed the patient's utilization capacity and can lead to azotemia. As with energy intake, protein intake for obese patients should be based on ABW.

Protein needs for children vary with age. The requirement is greatest in the first year of life and then gradually declines. Healthy infants need 2–3 g/kg/d, and children up to age 10 need 1.0–1.2 g/kg/d. The protein requirement of critically ill children is approximately 1.5 g/kg/d.

Nitrogen Balance

Nitrogen balance studies indicate the adequacy of protein intake by comparing nitrogen intake to nitrogen excretion. Positive nitrogen balance, a state in which nitrogen intake exceeds losses, implies that the amount of protein being administered is sufficient to promote anabolism and prevent erosion of lean body mass. In general, negative nitrogen balance indicates the need to increase protein intake and possibly energy intake as well. Urinary nitrogen losses of 8–12 g/d indicate a mild stress condition; 14–18 g/d, moderate stress; and 20 g/d, severe stress. The extremely high nitrogen losses that characterize critical illness can impede efforts to achieve positive nitrogen balance. In this situation, increasing protein intake to 2.0 g/kg/d may help to achieve nitrogen equilibrium.

Steps to determine nitrogen balance are as follows:

1. **Measure urine urea nitrogen (UUN).** This step requires 24-h urine collection to quantify urinary nitrogen loss. Because this study shows only nitrogen excretion that occurs as urea, a "fudge factor" of 4 g of nitrogen is added to the urinary loss to account for nonurea nitrogen losses through routes such as skin and feces. Therefore 24-h UUN + 4 g = 24-h nitrogen loss.
2. **Determine nitrogen intake.** Calculating nitrogen intake for the 24-h period of the UUN collection is relatively easy for patients who receive a prescribed amount of protein through parenteral or enteral nutrition. For patients who eat orally, a dietitian must work with the patient to maintain accurate records of all food consumed during the study period. To determine 24-h nitrogen intake, divide protein intake (g/24 h) by 6.25.
3. **Formula for calculating nitrogen balance:**

$$N_2 \text{ balance} = \frac{\text{Protein intake (g)}}{6.25} - (\text{Grams UUN } N_2 + 4g)$$

THERAPEUTIC DIETS

The term *therapeutic diet* refers to dietary changes that play a role in the management of a medical condition. The most commonly ordered therapeutic diets and their indications appear in Table 11–5. These dietary modifications, which usually require a physician's order, typically call for a change in the consistency of the food served or an adjustment in the quantity of one or more nutrients in the diet. Most hospitals have diet manuals available for reference, and registered dietitians are usually on staff for consultation in clinical situations that necessitate a therapeutic diet.

TABLE 11-5
Hospital Diets

Diet	Guidelines	Indications
House/regular	Adequate in all essential nutrients All foods are permitted Can be modified according to patient's food preferences	No diet restrictions or modifications
Mechanical soft	Includes soft-textured or ground foods that are easily masticated and swallowed	Decreased ability to chew or swallow Presence of oral mucositis or esophagitis May be appropriate for some patients with dysphagia
Pureed	Includes liquids as well as strained and pureed foods	Inability to chew or swallow solid foods Presence of oral mucositis or esophagitis May be appropriate for some patients with dysphagia
Full liquid	Includes foods that are liquid at body temperature Includes milk/milk products Can provide approximately: 2500–3000 mL fluid 1500–2000 cal 60–80 g high quality protein <10 g dietary fiber 60–80 g fat/d	May be appropriate for patients with severely limited chewing ability Not appropriate for lactase-deficient patients unless commercially available lactase enzyme tablets provided

(continued)

11

TABLE 11-5 (Continued)

Diet	Guidelines	Indications
Clear liquid	Includes foods that are liquid at body temperature Foods are Very low in fiber Lactose-free Virtually fat-free Can provide approximately: 2000 mL fluid 400–600 cal <7 g low-quality protein 1 g dietary fiber <1 g fat/d This diet is inadequate in all nutrients and should not be used >3 d without supplementation	Ordered as initial diet in the transition from NPO to solids Used for bowel preparation before certain medical or surgical procedures For management of acute medical conditions warranting minimized biliary contraction or pancreatic exocrine secretion
Low-fiber	Foods that are low in indigestible carbohydrates Decreases stool volume, transit time, and frequency	Management of acute radiation enteritis and inflammatory bowel disease when narrowing or stenosis of the intestinal lumen is present
Carbohydrate controlled diet (ADA)	Calorie level should be adequate to maintain or achieve desirable body weight (DBW) Total carbohydrates are limited to 50–60% of total calories Ideally fat should be limited to ≈30% of total calories	Diabetes mellitus

(continued)

216

11

TABLE 11-5
(Continued)

Diet	Guidelines		Indications
Acute renal failure	Protein (g/kg DBW)	0.6	For patients in renal failure who are not undergoing dialysis
	Calories	35–50	
	Sodium (g/d)	1–3	
	Potassium (g/d)	Variable	
	Fluid (mL/d)	Urine output + 500	
Renal failure Hemodialysis	Protein (g/kg DBW)	1.0–1.2	For patients in renal failure on hemodialysis
	Calories (per kilogram DBW)	30–35	
	Sodium (g/d)	1–2	
	Potassium (g/d)	1.5–3	
	Fluid (mL/d)	Urine output + 500	
Peritoneal dialysis	Protein (g/kg DBW)	1.2–1.6	For patients in renal failure on peritoneal dialysis
	Calories (per kilogram DBW)	25–35	
	Sodium (g/d)	3–4	
	Potassium (g/d)	3–4	
	Fluid (mL/d)	Urine output + 500	

(continued)

TABLE 11-5
(Continued)

Diet	Guidelines	Indications
Hepatic	In the absence of encephalopathy do not restrict protein In the presence of encephalopathy initially restrict protein to 40–60 g/d then liberalize in increments of 10 g/d as tolerated Specify sodium and fluid restriction according to severity of ascites and edema	Management of chronic liver disorders
Low lactose/lactose-free	Limits or restricts milk products Commercially available lactase enzyme tablets can be used	Lactase deficiency
Low-fat	<50 g total fat per day	Pancreatitis Fat malabsorption
Fat/cholesterol restricted	Total fat >30% total calories Saturated fat limited to 10% of calories <300 mg cholesterol <50% calories from complex carbohydrates	Hypercholesterolemia

(continued)

**TABLE 11–5
(Continued)**

Diet	Guidelines	Indications
Low-sodium	Sodium allowance should be as liberal as possible to maximize nutritional intake yet control symptoms "No added salt" is 4 g/d; no added salt or highly salted food; 2 g/d avoids processed foods (ie, meats) <1 g/d is unpalatable and thus compromises adequate intake	Indicated for patients with hypertension, ascites, and edema associated with the underlying disease

11

Modifying the Consistency of Food

Changing the consistency or texture of the diet is a simple way to make food easier to chew, swallow, and digest. For instance, patients with poor dentition may benefit from a pureed diet. Another use of this type of therapeutic diet is the postoperative diet progression that begins with clear liquids and advances to regular food as tolerated. Although doubt exists concerning the need to step through slow diet advancement postoperatively, the practice remains common after some types of surgery. Patients who have undergone elective colonic resection, for example, can usually receive a regular diet after they tolerate one meal of clear liquids, whereas those who have undergone surgery involving the esophagus, stomach, or small intestine may benefit from a more conservative approach.

Patients with dysphagia frequently need a change in texture or consistency of food to enhance the safety of eating. An evaluation of swallowing function by a speech–language pathologist is essential in determining the appropriate diet for patients with impaired swallowing. Dysphagia occurs most often as a result of neurologic conditions, but many medical and surgical problems can compromise swallowing. A swallowing evaluation is warranted before the start of oral intake in any situation that increases the risk of dysphagia, including cognitive or functional decline, surgery or radiation of structures involved in swallowing, prolonged intubation, and recent tracheostomy.

Modifying Nutrient Content of the Diet

Because illness frequently alters nutrient requirements or nutrient tolerance, diet modification is a common therapeutic intervention in the management of many chronic diseases. In some cases, the therapeutic diet may simply limit a single nutrient, such as sodium. At other times diet prescription may require broad changes in eating habits. The dietary changes recommended for prevention and treatment of cardiovascular disease fall into the latter category. Any diet that restricts one or more nutrients poses nutritional risks. One concern is that in adhering to a dietary restriction, patients may unintentionally omit other essential nutrients. In addition, patients frequently find restrictive diets unpalatable, a problem that leads to poor intake or noncompliance. A patient with a prescription for a therapeutic or modified diet need instruction by a clinical dietitian before discharge or as an outpatient.

Oral Nutritional Supplements

For patients unable to tolerate sufficient food to maintain adequate nutritional status, oral nutritional supplements can halt or reverse nutritional decline and improve clinical outcome. For elderly patients, for example, the use of oral supplements improves nutritional status and reduces mortality. The nutritional products, which are available without a prescription, come in a variety of forms, including high-protein, high-calorie beverages, puddings, snack bars, and soups. Ensure (Ross Laboratories) and Boost (Novartis) are two common examples of liquid oral supplements. These products are flavored for oral consumption, but they are also appropriate for administration through a feeding tube. Depending on the circumstances, patients can consume these products in addition to regular meals or as a meal replacement. Most oral supplements on the market are lactose-free, an important consideration for persons who cannot tolerate milk-based supplements. Unlike most snack foods, commercially prepared oral supplements provide a balanced mix of nutrients, including vitamins and minerals. Encourage patients to try a variety of supplements to avoid taste fatigue, a common problem among patients who consume only one supplement over an extended period. Adding flavoring such as chocolate or coffee syrup to oral supplements can improve palatability. Sustained success with oral supplements frequently requires the creative support of the entire health care team.

INFANT FEEDING

Breast Feeding

Clinical practice guidelines consistently endorse breast feeding as the sole source of infant nutrition for the first 6 mo of life. Breast milk is uniquely suited to the nutritional needs of growing infants, supporting optimal nutritional and reducing the risk of childhood obesity. Research findings suggest that the presence of long-chain polyunsaturated fatty acids in human milk may also enhance neurocognitive development. Breast-fed infants gain protection against infectious disease early in life from immunoglobulins present in the milk and may have fewer infantile allergies than their formula-fed counterparts. In addition to these physiologic advantages, breast feeding offers psychological benefits to both mother and infant and reduces the cost of infant feeding.

Commercial Infant Formulas

Despite compelling evidence of the benefits of breast feeding to both infant and mother, commercial infant formulas continue to play a prominent role as a source of infant nutrition in the United States. Commercial infant formulas serve as an appropriate substitute for breast milk in the presence of medical contraindications to breast feeding, when the mother decides against breast feeding, or if maternal milk production is inadequate. Because manufacturers have refined the nutrient profile of commercial infant formulas to more closely resemble the composition of breast milk, homemade infant formulas are no longer considered an acceptable substitute. Most commercial infant formulas have a cow's milk base, but soy-based formulas are also available. Soy formula does not prevent colic or allergy, as once thought, and has no role as a primary method of infant feeding.

Commonly used formulas are outlined in Table 11–6. Most infant formulas are isoosmolar (eg, Similac 20, Enfamil 20, and SMA 20 with and without iron). These formulas are used most often for healthy infants.

If possible, preterm infants should receive human milk, although breast milk can be fortified to meet the elevated requirements of a rapidly growing infant. Commercial formulas for premature infants contain 24 kcal/oz (eg, Similac 24, Enfamil 24, "preemie" SMA 24). Many other specialty formulas are available for infants with medical conditions such as inborn errors of metabolism, malabsorption syndromes, and milk and protein sensitivity.

Commercial formulas are available with and without iron, but current guidelines call for use of an iron-fortified formula for most infants. Many pediatricians recommend vitamin supplements with some formulas if the infant is taking < 32 oz/d. However, at this point most infants are beginning solid food that serves as an additional source of vitamins and minerals.

Oral Rehydration Solutions

Infants with mild or moderate dehydration, often due to diarrhea or vomiting, may benefit from oral rehydration formulas. These solutions typically include

TABLE 11–6
Commonly Used Infant Formulas

Formula	Indications[a]
Human milk	
Donor	Preterm infant <1200 g
Maternal	All infants
Breast milk fortifiers	
Standard formulas	
Isoosmolar	
Enfamil 20	Full-term infants: as supplement to breast milk
Similac 20	Preterm infants >1800–2000 g
SMA 20[b]	
Higher osmolality	
Enfamil 24	Term infants: for infants on fluid restriction or
Similac 24 & 27	who cannot handle required volumes of
SMA[b] 24 & 27	20-cal formula to grow
Low osmolality	
Similac 13	Preterm and term infants: for conservative initial feeding in infants who have not been fed orally for several days or weeks. Not for long-term use
Soy formulas	
ProSobee (lactose- and sucrose-free)	Term infants: milk sensitivity, galactosemia, carbohydrate intolerance. Do not use in
Isomil (lactose-free)	preterm infants. Phytates can bind calcium
Nursoy (lactose-free)	and cause rickets.
Protein hydrosylate formulas	
Nutramigen	Term infants: Gut sensitivity to proteins, multiple food allergies, persistent diarrhea, galactosemia
Pregestimil	Preterm and term infants: disaccharidase deficiency, diarrhea, GI defects, cystic fibrosis, food allergy, celiac disease, transition from TPN to oral feeding
Alimentum	Term infants: protein sensitivity, pancreatic insufficiency, diarrhea, allergies, colic, carbohydrate and fat malabsorption
Special formulas	
Portagen	Preterm and term infants: pancreatic or bile acid insufficiency, intestinal resection
Similac PM 60/40	Preterm and term infants: problem feeders on standard formula; infants with renal, cardiovascular, digestive diseases that require decreased protein and mineral levels, breastfeeding supplement, initial feeding

(continued)

**TABLE 11–6
(Continued)**

Formula	Indications[a]
Premature formulas	
Low osmolality	
Similac Special Care 20 Enfamil Premature 20 Preemie SMA 20	Premature infants (<1800–2000 g) who are growing rapidly. These formulas promote growth at intrauterine rates. Vitamin and mineral concentrations are higher to meet the needs of growth. Usually started on 20 cal/oz and advanced to 24 cal/oz as tolerated.
Isoosmolar	
Similac Special Care 24 Enfamil Special Care 24 Preemie SMA 24	Same as for low-osmolality premature formulas

[a]Multivitamin supplementation such as Polyvisol (Mead Johnson) 1/2 mL/d may be needed for commercial formulas if baby is taking <2 oz/d.
[b]SMA has decreased sodium content and can be used in patients with congestive heart failure, bronchopulmonary dysplasia, and cardiac disease.
Modified and reproduced with permission from Gomella, TL (ed) *Neonatology*, 5th ed. McGraw-Hill, 2004.

11

glucose, sodium, potassium, and bicarbonate or citrate. Common formulations include **Pedialyte, Lytren, Infalyte, Resol,** and **Hydrolyte.**

Initiating Infant Feeding

Most healthy term infants can begin breast feeding immediately after birth. The initial feeding for bottle-fed infants generally takes place within the first 4 or 5 h of life as long as the infant displays signs of readiness for feeding, such as alertness, active bowel sounds, and rooting and sucking behavior. For preterm and sick infants, conduct a detailed assessment before introducing feeding. In this setting, feedings should begin only if the infant has hemodynamic stability, no excessive oral secretions, no vomiting, no bile-stained gastric aspirate, normal bowel sounds, and a nondistended, soft abdomen and can coordinate breathing, sucking, and swallowing. Because tachypnea increases the risk of aspiration, verify that the infant's respiratory rate is within normal limits before offering a bottle for the first time. Infants who have been weaned from a ventilator should exhibit no evidence of respiratory distress for at least 6 h after extubation before feeding.

Feeding Progression

The initial feeding for bottle-fed infants is usually sterile water or D_5W. Do not use hypertonic solutions such as $D_{10}W$.

Controversy exists regarding the optimal way to introduce commercial infant formula after the initial feeding with water or D_5W. Some clinicians advocate diluting infant formula with sterile water and advancing the concentration as tolerated (eg, start with $1/4$ strength, increase to $1/2$ strength, and then progress to $3/4$ strength before giving full-strength formula). Others believe this gradual progression is unnecessary and start with full-strength formula after the infant tolerates the initial feeding without difficulty. Breast-fed infants typically begin feeding without first receiving a water feeding, and **breast milk is never diluted.**

Considerations for Preterm Infants

Many preterm infants lack the coordination to take oral feedings safely. In this situation, provide nutrients through a feeding tube. Considerable controversy remains concerning the timing of initial enteral feeding of preterm infants. For larger (> 1500 g) premature infants in stable condition, give the first feeding within the first 24 h of life. Early feeding may allow the release of enteric hormones that exert a trophic effect on the intestinal tract. On the other hand, apprehension about necrotizing enterocolitis (mostly in very low birth weight infants) precludes initiation of enteral feeding in the following circumstances: perinatal asphyxia, mechanical ventilation, presence of umbilical vessel catheters, patent ductus arteriosus, indomethacin treatment, sepsis, and frequent episodes of apnea and bradycardia. Consensus does not exist regarding the optimal timing and method of introducing feeding to preterm infants with those conditions. In general, preterm infants begin enteral feeding in the first 3 d of life. The objective is reaching full enteral feeding by 2–3 wk of life. Start parenteral nutrition, including amino acids and lipids, at the same time as enteral feeding to provide adequate caloric intake.

CANDIDATES FOR NUTRITIONAL SUPPORT

When nutritional assessment reveals evidence of poor or declining nutritional status, investigate the causes and develop a plan for intervention. This process includes management of underlying medical problems, management of symptoms that interfere with appetite and eating, and efforts to increase intake with dietary modification and oral supplements. Consider enteral or parenteral nutrition when nutritional deficits persist despite efforts to improve oral intake or when the patient's clinical condition precludes safe or adequate intake by mouth (see Chapter 12).

ENTERAL AND PARENTERAL NUTRITION

Definitions
Enteral Nutrition
Principles of Enteral Tube Feeding
Ordering and Advancing Tube
    Feedings
Complications of Enteral Nutrition
Parenteral Nutrition
Indications
Composition of PN Formulas

Central versus Peripheral
    Administration
Initiating and Managing Parenteral
    Nutrition
Monitoring Response to Therapy
Preventing and Managing
    Complications
Terminating Therapy

DEFINITIONS

Nutritional support is the provision of nutrients with therapeutic intent by either the enteral or the parenteral route. Technically, the term _enteral nutrition_ includes oral supplements as well as tube feeding, but in practice, clinicians use the term to refer strictly to tube feeding. Enteral and parenteral nutrition are important in the management of many medical conditions. Safe and effective nutritional therapy depends on careful selection of patients and a thorough understanding of the complications that can occur.

ENTERAL NUTRITION

If the gut works, use it. This simple adage is the guiding principle of nutritional support. Clinical practice guidelines consistently endorse the use of enteral nutrition for patients who have a functional GI tract but cannot take enough nutrients orally to maintain adequate nutritional status. Enteral nutrition has the following physiologic and practical benefits that make tube feeding superior to parenteral nutrition:

> ### Advantages of Enteral Nutrition
>
> Maintains normal metabolic pathways
> Allows delivery of a full range of nutrients
> Triggers the release of cholecystokinin
> Preserves hepatic lipid metabolism
> Maintains normal intestinal pH and flora
> Supports the GI tract as an organ of the immune system
> Promotes wound healing
> Lowers costs
> Reduces infectious complications

Technological advances in enteral access techniques have increased the numbers of patients who can safely receive tube feeding. The indications for enteral nutrition are as follows:

Indications for Enteral Nutrition

Poor Oral Intake (Won't Eat)
Anorexia
Depression
Disabilities
Eating disorders
Early satiety
Nausea
Painful swallowing

Unsafe Oral Intake (Can't Eat)
Altered level of consciousness
Dysphagia
Endotracheal intubation
Gastroparesis
Impaired sucking and swallowing
Proximal intestinal obstruction

Elevated Needs (Can't Eat Enough)
Burns
Open wounds
Pressure ulcers
Sepsis
Trauma

12 Principles of Enteral Tube Feeding

Timing: The optimal time for initiating enteral nutrition depends on the patient's baseline nutritional status and clinical condition. Well-nourished patients in stable condition can tolerate suboptimal nutritional intake for 7–14 d without harmful effects. On the other hand, a convincing body of evidence has shown that early enteral feeding improves clinical outcome among critically ill patients. Many ICUs have established protocols calling for initiation of tube feeding within 24–36 h of admission to the unit.

Delivery Site: The fundamental decision in planning tube feeding is to determine whether nutrients should be delivered to the stomach or the small intestine. The factors involved in choosing the appropriate location for enteral nutrition include gastric function and risk of aspiration. In general, the gastric route is preferred because feeding into the stomach is better tolerated than intestinal feeding and is technically easier. Although high risk of aspiration is the primary reason for intestinal feeding, other conditions, such as delayed gastric emptying, gastric outlet obstruction, and the presence of a tumor, also limit use of the stomach as a site of tube feeding.

In the past, standard practice was to place feeding tubes just beyond the pylorus, into the first or second portion of the duodenum, to guard against reflux and aspiration. However, there is insufficient evidence that postpyloric feeding protects against aspiration. Reflux of enteral formula and migration of the feeding tube into the stomach can occur, negating any potential benefit of postpyloric feeding. Some evidence suggests that aspiration risk can be reduced by selecting more distal locations for enteral access. As a result, current practice guidelines advocate positioning feeding tubes in the third portion of the duodenum or beyond the ligament of Treitz for patients at risk of aspiration.

Enteral Access Devices: Tubes inserted through the nose or the mouth are most appropriate for short-term use or in situations in which unstable clinical status prevents more invasive placement procedures. In patients with head or facial injuries, insert tubes orally to avoid injury.

The two categories of nasogastric tubes are small-bore and large-bore. Each type has benefits and drawbacks. **Small-bore** feeding tubes are soft and flexible; a guidewire or stylet provides the rigidity needed for insertion. **Large-bore** tubes are usually made of polyvinyl chloride (PVC), a stiff material that allows placement without a stylet. PVC becomes more rigid during use, and this characteristic increases the risk of otitis media, sinusitis, and nasal irritation. Small-bore tubes improve patient comfort and are less likely to cause ear and sinus problems, but small tubes are prone to clogging and become displaced easily. In the past, small-bore feeding tubes were thought to carry a lower risk of aspiration than large-bore tubes, but more recent results suggest that the presence of a tube of any size across the lower esophageal sphincter increases risk of reflux and aspiration.

A key factor in selecting the type of feeding tube is the ability to measure gastric residual volume (GRV) to evaluate gastric emptying. Small-bore tubes do not always allow measurement of GRV. Thus **a larger tube is often used initially and replaced with a small-bore tube** once feeding tolerance is established. Types of feeding tubes and placement procedures are discussed in Chapter 13, page 278.

When enteral feeding is expected to last > 30 d, a **feeding enterostomy** is superior to nasally placed tubes. The most common sites for placement are the stomach and the jejunum, although a feeding enterostomy can be placed in the pharynx or esophagus. A percutaneous endoscopic gastrostomy (PEG) tube is one of the most widely used feeding enterostomies. Other placement options include radiologic, laparoscopic, and open surgical techniques. Less invasive placement methods are preferred, but not all patients are candidates for these procedures. Morbidly obese patients and those with tumors, GI obstruction, adhesions, or abnormal anatomy may need open surgical placement. Techniques for placing percutaneous jejunostomy tubes have replaced older methods that involved threading a small-bore feeding tube through an existing gastrostomy or using a needle–catheter device to achieve access to the jejunum.

Dual-lumen, or combination, feeding tubes are safe and effective conduits for enteral nutrition. With combination tubes, one lumen terminates in the stomach and the second extends into the small intestine, allowing simultaneous gastric decompression and intestinal feeding. These tubes, which are inserted through the nose or through an enterostomy, are especially beneficial for postoperative patients and others with impaired gastric emptying.

Enteral Formulas: A vast number of enteral formulas are available, and many formulas are quite similar in composition. Most hospitals maintain an enteral formulary that contains representative examples of each formula category. With the exception of infant formulas and blenderized adult formulas, enteral formulas are gluten-free and contain no lactose. Characteristics to consider in selecting an appropriate enteral formula include nutrient composition, caloric density, free water content, osmolality, and the presence of fiber. Table 12–1 lists types of enteral formulas and their composition.

The clinical importance of osmolality enteral formulas is debated. At one time, tube feeding was routinely started with half-strength formula to avoid problems

(*Text continues on page 230.*)

TABLE 12-1
Enteral Formulas

Category	Description	Clinical Considerations	Examples (Brand Names)
Standard low residue or fiber enriched: 1.0–1.2 kcal/mL, 270–490 mOsm/L	Contains intact protein, fat, and carbohydrate; free water ~ 84%	For routine tube feeding; not for use in hypermetabolic illness; unflavored products not for oral use	Ensure, FiberSource, Isocal, Isosource, Jevity, Nutren 1.0 Osmolite, Ultracal
Concentrated low residue: 1.5–2.0 kcal/mL, 430–525 mOsm/L	Nutrients similar to standard low residue formulas; contain less free water and more fat; free water ~ 74%	Used to restrict fluid, relieve symptoms from high volume feeding, and to meet elevated nutrient needs. Closely monitor of hydration status.	Comply, Ensure Plus, Deliver 2.0, TwoCal HN, Isosource 1.5, Nutren 1.5, 2.0
Elemental/semielemental: 1.0–1.5 kcal/mL, 270–650 mOsm/L	Nutrients in easily digested form; many contain MCT oil or little long-chain fat, no fiber	For patients with impaired digestion and absorption; appropriate for patients with fat intolerance	Alitraq, Criticare, Isotein, Intensical, Peptamin, Subdue, Vital, Vivonex
Renal failure: 2.0 kcal/mL, 600 mOsm/L	Low protein with emphasis on essential amino acids; may not provide vitamins or electrolytes; free water ~ 70%	Intended to improve nitrogen retention with minimal effect on uremia	Renalcal, Suplena
Renal failure with dialysis: 2.0 kcal/mL, 570–665 mOsm/L	Provides moderate protein; vitamin and mineral content modified for renal failure; free water ~70%	Provides moderate protein for patients with losses from dialysis; vitamin and electrolyte profile adjusted for altered renal metabolism	Magnacal Renal, Nepro

(continued)

228

TABLE 12–1
(Continued)

Category	Description	Clinical Considerations	Examples (Brand Names)
Respiratory failure: 1.5 kcal/mL, 330–650 mOsm/L	Contains low levels of carbohydrate, high fat; no fiber; free water ~ 78%	Developed to reduce CO_2 produced by carbohydrate metabolism; some contain omega three fatty acids and antioxidants	Novasource Pulmonary, Nutrivent, Pulmocare, Respelor, Oxepa
Wound healing: 1.0–1.5 kcal/mL, 340–560 mOsm/L	Very high protein content; some have enhanced vitamin profile; free water ~ 78–83%	Designed to support healing of surgical wounds and pressure ulcers	Isosource VHN, Promote, Protain XL, Resource, Replete, Traumacal
Immune modulation: 1.0–1.5 kcal/mL, 375–630 mOsm/L	Designed for patients with hypermetabolic illness; usually high in protein; many are enriched with specific nutrients arginine, glutamine, and omega-3 fatty acids; some contain fiber	Designed for use during hypermetabolic illness; theoretical benefits for immune function. Use with caution in critically ill, septic patients.	Alitraq, Crucial, Impact, Immunaid
Diabetes: 1.0–1.06 kcal/mL, 300–380 mOsm/L	Low carbohydrate and high ratio of monosaturated fatty acids; contains fiber	Used for patients with abnormal glucose tolerance; nutrient profile meets American Diabetes Association guidelines; many can be consumed orally	Diabetisource, Choice DM, Glytrol, Glucerna

12

(Text continued from page 227.)

related to osmolality. Subsequent research did not show that osmolality contributes significantly to feeding intolerance, especially when rapid infusion rates are avoided.

Feeding intolerance due to osmolality can occur with jejunostomy feeding, but using an enteral pump to control the rate of delivery of formula into the small intestine usually circumvents this problem.

Ordering and Advancing Tube Feedings

Depending on institutional policies and professional licensure laws, responsibility for ordering tube feeding falls to physicians, dietitians, clinical nurse specialists, or pharmacists. As with medication prescriptions, orders for enteral nutrition must specify the name of the enteral formula and the route of delivery. The order must also include the target rate for tube feeding as well as a schedule for advancing the feedings to the goal. Start tube feedings slowly and increase them as the patient's tolerance allows. In hospitalized patients, tube feedings are frequently administered continuously with the aid of an infusion pump. In particular, patients with a jejunal tube usually need a pump control to avoid feeding intolerance. Rapid infusion of enteral formula into the jejunum can produce dumping syndrome, which has symptoms similar to the effects of surgical procedures such as Billroth II gastrectomy. Pump-controlled feedings typically begin at 10–40 mL/h and increase in increments of 10–25 mL/h q4–6h as tolerated. For patients who are eating but are not meeting their needs, an enteral feeding pump can be used to administer nutrients during the night to supplement oral intake.

Under certain circumstances, tube feeding can be administered without a pump. This method, called bolus feeding, is most appropriate for patients with a gastrostomy tube as the sole source of nutrition. With bolus feeding, patients receive 200–400 mL 4–6 times/d. The entire food bolus flows into the stomach through the barrel of a 50- or 60-mL syringe attached to the feeding tube. Bolus feeding is widely used in subacute and home care settings.

Complications of Enteral Nutrition

Aspiration: Aspiration pneumonia is a common and life-threatening complication of enteral nutrition. The following are risk factors for aspiration:

Risk Factors for Aspiration

- Advanced age
- Impaired consciousness
- Neuromuscular disease
- Impaired gag and cough reflex
- Endotracheal intubation
- Mechanical ventilation
- Tracheostomy
- Gastroesophageal reflux (presence of tube)
- Delayed gastric emptying, elevated gastric residual volume

Jejunal feeding can reduce but not eliminate aspiration risk. As for other aspiration precautions, the single most effective measure for preventing aspiration is to elevate the head of the bed during feeding. Enteral feeding protocols also call for measuring GRV approximately every 4–5 h until feeding tolerance is established. Although it is a routine part of the management of tube feedings, measurement of GRV has been the focus of considerable debate. Methods vary considerably, and studies have not identified a GRV value that allows accurate prediction of aspiration risk. The most widely used threshold for intervention is 150–200 mL. For patients receiving continuous feeding, a GRV greater than twice the hourly infusion rate raises concern about the adequacy of gastric emptying. Some protocols stipulate that tube feeding be stopped for an hour or more in response to a single elevated GRV measurement. Others call for monitoring the patient closely and stopping feedings only after two consecutive measurements are elevated. Prokinetic agents may improve gastric emptying and allow feeding to proceed safely. The key point is that clinicians must not rely on GRV as the sole indicator of aspiration risk but evaluate the patient in the context of the entire clinical situation.

Diarrhea: Occurs in 10–60% of patients receiving enteral feedings. Many factors contribute to the incidence of diarrhea among tube-fed patients, including underlying illness, the presence of bacteria, medications, and feeding intolerance. Each of these causes must be systematically ruled out as a cause of the problem. As a starting point, to rule out *Clostridium difficile* colitis, order a stool culture for patients with diarrhea who have received antibiotics. If this test result is negative, administer antidiarrheal agents to control symptoms. Administering a probiotic such as lactobacillus acidophilus (Lactinex) can help restore normal flora and decrease diarrhea. Medications frequently cause diarrhea in patients receiving tube feeding, especially those with a jejunal tube in place. Electrolytes, particularly magnesium, phosphorus, and potassium, are notorious offenders, as are drugs that contain sorbitol. Changing the enteral formula or adjusting the feeding regimen may provide relief.

Constipation: Although less common than diarrhea, constipation can occur in patients receiving enteral nutrition, especially those in long-term care facilities. Switching to a fiber-enriched enteral formula may alleviate the problem. Adequate hydration is important in promoting regular bowel movements. Provide additional free water as periodic water boluses or as a separate enteral infusion.

Dehydration: One of the most common metabolic disorders among tube-fed patients. Numerous factors contribute to the problem, including the use of concentrated, high-protein formulas, poor oral intake of liquids, hyperglycemia, fever, diarrhea, and failure to administer the prescribed volume of formula. Weight loss and elevations in sodium, chloride, and BUN are characteristic of dehydration related to enteral nutrition. Keep in mind that the percentage of free water in enteral formulas ranges from 70% to 84% of the volume administered. On average, patients should receive 30 mL/kg/d of free water. Patients in whom dehydration develops may need a less concentrated enteral formula or additional free water.

PARENTERAL NUTRITION

Indications

In circumstances in which lack of function of the GI tract prevents oral or enteral nutrition, parenteral nutrition (PN) is used. PN is expensive, however, and carries a high risk of complications. IV nutrition therefore is reserved for sit-

TABLE 12–2
Indications for Parenteral Nutrition

Category	Example
Conditions that impair absorption of nutrients	Short-bowel syndrome Enterocutaneous fistula Infectious colitis Radiation or chemotherapy effects Small-bowel obstruction
Need for bowel rest	Inflammatory bowel disease Ischemic bowel Severe pancreatitis Chylous fistula Preoperative status
Motility disorders	Prolonged ileus, scleroderma, pseudoobstruction, visceral organ myopathy
Inability to achieve or maintain enteral access	Unstable clinical condition Hyperemesis gravidarum Eating disorders

uations in which no there are no other options for providing nutritional support. Examples of situations in which PN is indicated appear in Table 12–2. Although well-nourished patients with GI dysfunction can receive conventional IV fluids for 7–10 d without harmful effects, patients with existing nutritional deficits or metabolic stress and those not expected to resume oral intake for 5–10 d need PN within 3–5 d. The decision to initiate PN is not an emergency. Adverse effects of PN are less likely to occur in patients who have good glycemic control, stable hemodynamic status, and electrolyte levels within normal limits. Issues such as prognosis, possibility of benefit, and the patient's views regarding artificial feeding also are factors in the decision to begin PN.

Composition of PN Formulas

PN formulas are highly complex IV fluids containing the nutrients essential for metabolism and growth: protein, carbohydrates, lipids, electrolytes, vitamins, trace elements, and water. The composition of PN formulas can be tailored to meet the demands of hypermetabolic illness and to accommodate limitations in organ function.

Depending on hospital policy, PN formulas can be compounded in two ways. All of the ingredients can be mixed in a single container, a method called **total nutrient admixture** (TNA), or the lipid emulsion can be excluded from the primary solution and administered separately. (Lipid emulsions are isotonic and can be given safely by peripheral vein.) Although TNA offers many advantages over conventional dextrose/amino acid formulas, numerous factors affect the stability of the formula. The integrity of the PN formula is a critical consideration that demands the expertise of a pharmacist familiar with stability and compatibility data.

Protein: Supplied as crystalline amino acids in a mix of essential and nonessential amino acids. Standard amino acid solutions are available in concentrations ranging from 3% to 15%, the upper range being used most frequently in adults. In general, 1 g of amino acids is equivalent to 1 g of protein. As with dietary protein, IV amino acids yield 4 kcal/g.

Manufacturers offer modified amino acids to meet disease- and age-specific requirements. For example, specialty formulas for renal failure contain increased amounts of essential amino acids or provide only essential amino acids. Hepatic failure amino acid mixtures contain higher amounts of branched-chain amino acids and decreased aromatic amino acids. Higher costs and conflicting scientific evidence on effectiveness limit the routine use of specialty amino acid mixtures.

Carbohydrate: Dextrose monohydrate is the principal energy substrate in PN formulas. This form of carbohydrate provides 3.4 kcal in concentrations ranging from 3% to 70%. Studies have shown that dextrose dosages between 4–7 mg/kg/min provide optimal protein sparing, although hyperglycemia occurs less often when the dextrose infusion is limited to 4 mg/kg/min.

Fat: IV fat emulsions contain soybean oil or a mixture of safflower and soybean oils with egg phospholipid added as an emulsifier. Patients allergic to eggs or soybeans may have reactions to lipid emulsions, including hives, back pain, shortness of breath, and anaphylactic shock. Lipid emulsions are available in concentrations of 10%, 20%, and 30% providing 1.1, 2.0, and 3.0 kcal/mL, respectively. More efficient lipid clearance occurs with 20% fat emulsions than with 10% products, making the 20% form preferable, especially for pediatric patients. Provision of 1–4% of the patient's daily energy requirements as lipid emulsion prevents essential fatty acid deficiency, a condition that causes dry skin, hair loss, poor wound healing, and diarrhea after weeks to months of fat-free parenteral feedings. However, in current practice patients typically receive up to 50% of parenteral calories as fat. Current guidelines for adults set the daily limit for lipid dose at 2.5 g/kg, but a growing body of evidence suggests that 1 g/kg may be a safer limit. The ability to furnish a more balanced fuel mix decreases the adverse effects associated with infusing large amounts of dextrose. However, patients with a triglyceride level ≥ 400 mg/dL should not receive lipid emulsions. Monitor triglyceride level to determine whether lipid emulsion can safely be introduced at a later time. On the other hand, a history of type IV hypertriglyceridemia is an absolute contraindication to use of IV fat emulsions.

Electrolytes: PN formulas must contain sufficient electrolytes for critical metabolic activities. The usual electrolyte profile of PN formulas is sodium, potassium, calcium, magnesium, chloride, acetate, and phosphorus. Unlike conventional IV fluids, electrolyte PN formulas contain the acetate or chloride salt of the electrolyte to help maintain acid–base balance. Sodium bicarbonate is used in PN but may precipitate additives, particularly calcium and magnesium. In most cases, hospital pharmacies offer a standard electrolyte product that provides typical maintenance doses of electrolytes. Table 12–3 lists daily electrolyte requirements for adult patients in stable condition. Patients with diarrhea, fistula output, and gastric losses often have altered electrolyte homeostasis and need higher levels of certain electrolytes. On the other hand, the electrolyte content of the PN formula may have to be restricted if a patient has impaired renal function.

Vitamins: All PN formulas must contain the vitamins needed to support normal metabolism. Life-threatening vitamin deficiencies can develop within 2–3 wk in patients who receive PN without vitamins. Table 12–4 lists the composition of a

TABLE 12–3
Electrolytes for Parenteral Nutrition

Electrolyte	Form	Recommended Daily Requirement
Sodium	Sodium chloride Sodium acetate Sodium phosphate	1–2 mEq/kg
Potassium	Potassium chloride Potassium acetate Potassium phosphate	1–2 mEq/kg
Chloride	Sodium chloride Potassium chloride	As needed for acid–base balance
Acetate	Sodium acetate Potassium acetate	As needed for acid–base balance
Phosphate	Sodium phosphate Potassium phosphate	20–40 mmol
Magnesium	Magnesium sulfate	8–20 mEq
Calcium	Calcium gluconate	10–15 mEq

typical parenteral vitamin product for adults. Individual vitamin products, such as A, C, and folic acid, are used to supplement the standard multivitamin combination when a disease-specific or treatment-related deficiency exists.

Trace Minerals: Trace minerals are essential for efficient substrate utilization and other supportive functions. Typical PN solutions contain zinc, chromium, copper,

TABLE 12–4
Parenteral Vitamin Formulas

Vitamin	Dose/10 mL
A (retinol)	1 mg (3300 IU)
B_1 (thiamin)	6 mg
B_2 (riboflavin)	3.6 mg
B_3 (niacin)	40 mg
B_6 (pyridoxine)	6 mg
B_{12} (cobalamin)	5 mcg
Biotin	60 mcg
C (ascorbic acid)	200 mg
D (ergocalciferol)	5 mcg (200 IU)
E (tocopherol)	10 IU
Folic acid	600 mcg
K	150 mcg

TABLE 12–5
Trace Element Requirements for Parenteral Nutrition

Element	Recommended Daily Dose
Zinc	2.5–5.0 mg[a]
Copper	0.3–0.5 mg
Selenium	20–60 mcg
Chromium	10–15 mcg
Manganese	60–100 mcg

[a]Requirements may be as high as 15 mg/d in stress states or in patients with high-output fistulas.

and manganese according to established guidelines. Table 12–5 shows dosing recommendations for trace minerals. Patients receiving long-term PN also need selenium to prevent potentially fatal cardiomyopathy. Commercial trace mineral products do not contain iron. In the past, iron was frequently added to PN formulas in the form of iron dextran, but this practice has fallen out of favor because of concerns about the potential for adverse reactions to IV iron. Current guidelines call for administering iron as a separate infusion as needed. Clinical conditions that impair trace mineral excretion may necessitate restricting certain trace minerals in PN formulas. For example, in patients with biliary disease copper and manganese must be restricted from PN formulas to avoid toxicity.

Central versus Peripheral Administration

PN formulas that rely on glucose as a primary energy source frequently have an osmolarity that approaches 1800 mOsm/L, more than twice the limit for administration through peripheral veins. Safe infusion of such hypertonic fluids requires placement of an IV line in the central venous circulation, as described in Chapter 13. However, the osmolarity of PN formulas that contain lipid emulsion and low concentrations of dextrose may fall below 900 mOsm/L, making these formulas suitable for peripheral administration. Peripheral parenteral nutrition (PPN) is appropriate for patients with adequate peripheral venous access who need PN for a brief time, usually less than 2 wk. Because peripheral PN formulas contain relatively low concentrations of nutrients, this form of nutritional support is more helpful in preventing malnutrition than in correcting existing deficits. For similar reasons, patients with elevated requirements due to hypermetabolism or those who need fluid restriction are not candidates for PPN.

Initiating and Managing Parenteral Nutrition

Beginning Parenteral Nutrition: Because PN can induce metabolic disturbances or worsen existing problems, do not start PN until a patient has a stable fluid and electrolyte profile. It is usually unwise to begin PN in a patient who needs large amounts of fluid, may need resuscitation after trauma, or who is in a septic state. Recommended baseline laboratory tests are serum electrolytes (including ionized calcium, magnesium, and phosphorus), glucose, prealbumin, triglycerides, creatinine, BUN, and liver function tests. These measurements help identify whether the patient is at risk of metabolic complications and help guide the design of the initial PN formula.

Begin PN at a reduced level and advance to goal according to the patient's response. Because carbohydrate is the substrate most likely to induce metabolic disturbances, initial formulas frequently have a limited dextrose load, usually 200–250 g for the first day. Many institutional protocols allow patients to receive the target level of protein and lipid emulsion initially and increase dextrose to goal over 2 d. Some situations call for a more cautious introduction of PN. A patient with a baseline serum glucose level of 120–150 mg/dL, for example, should receive only 100–150 g of dextrose in an initial PN formula. Increase the dextrose in the PN formula over several days while closely observing serum glucose level and insulin requirements.

Refeeding Syndrome: Beginning PN at a reduced level is prudent for patients at risk of refeeding syndrome, a life-threatening metabolic complication that occurs in the setting of severe weight loss or long-standing malnutrition. Risk factors for this problem include anorexia nervosa, chronic alcoholism, cancer cachexia, and other wasting syndromes. In refeeding syndrome, severe fluid and electrolyte disturbances occur in the first few days of therapy. The hallmark of refeeding syndrome is hypophosphatemia, which can be fatal if not recognized and corrected promptly. To avoid refeeding syndrome for patients at risk, current guidelines call for correcting phosphate levels ≤ 2.0 mEq/dL before beginning PN. In this setting, the initial PN formula should limit dextrose to 150 g and begin with only 50% of the patient's caloric requirements. Vigilant electrolyte replacement is essential and may take several days to achieve full repletion. Calorie and protein intake should progress to goal only when fluid and electrolyte status stabilizes.

Ordering PN: Writing orders for PN is a step-by-step process that takes into account energy needs, nutrient requirements, and electrolyte status. The first step is to set goals for energy intake and to distribute the calories among the protein, carbohydrate, and fat in the PN formula. The following example illustrates these steps for a 70-kg man. The formula produced in this process is a reasonable estimated goal. This PN can then be adjusted to account for clinical circumstances that affect nutrient needs, such as severity of illness and organ function.

1. **Establish goals for energy and protein intake.**
   a. Provide 25–30 kcal/kg. For a 70-kg man, the range is 1750–2100 kcal/d. (See Chapter 11 regarding use of adjusted body weight.) Start at the low end of the range to avoid overfeeding.
   b. Give protein 1.0–1.5 g/kg, a range of 70–105 g/d for a 70-kg man. Round the goal to 100 g to meet the patient's needs and to simplify compounding.
2. **Determine nonprotein calories.** Subtract protein calories from total calories (100×4 kcal/g = 400 protein calories). **Example:** $1750 - 400 = 1350$ nonprotein calories.
3. **Determine carbohydrate dose.** The standard lipid dose for most adult patients is 50 g or 500 kcal. Subtract lipid calories from nonprotein calories to determine the amount of dextrose needed to meet the patient's energy needs. **Example:** $1350 - 500 = 850$ carbohydrate calories. Divide the calorie goal for carbohydrate by 3.4 cal/g. Example: $850 \div 3.4 = 250$ g.
4. **Order the PN formula.** Total energy, 1750 kcal; protein, 100 g; carbohydrate, 250 g; fat, 50 g. Safety guidelines for PN call for ordering substrates in grams to avoid confusion. (Some hospitals require that these values be converted to percent solutions in the PN order.) Consult with a pharmacist. As Table 12–6 shows, the identical PN formula can be adjusted to meet the patient's hydration requirements by use of different concentrations of amino acids, dextrose, and fat.

TABLE 12–6
Adjusting the Volume of Parenteral Nutrition Formulas[a]

Example Formula	Standard PN	Fluid Restriction	High Volume
Goal: 1750 kcal			
Protein: 100 g	10% AA 1000 mL	15% AA 500 mL	10% AA 1000 mL
Dextrose: 250 g	$D_{50}W$ 500 mL	$D_{70}W$ 357 mL	$D_{25}W$ 1000 mL
Lipid: 50 g	20% fat 250 mL	30% fat 204 mL	10% fat 500 mL
Volume	1750 mL	1265 mL	2500 mL

[a]Highly concentrated or dilute formulas may affect stability of total nutrient admixture. AA = amino acids.

5. **Make appropriate additions to PN formula.** Individualize the electrolyte content of the PN formula according to the patient's laboratory tests and organ function. Sodium and potassium are available as both chloride and acetate salts. Using higher or lower amounts of these salts can help maintain acid–base balance. Stability and compatibility limits exist for calcium, phosphorus, and magnesium. Many hospitals use standard formulations for vitamins and trace minerals to avoid the need to order each entity individually.

Monitoring Response to Therapy

Carefully monitor patients receiving PN to identify problems and to assess progress toward the therapeutic goal. Measure electrolytes, including calcium, magnesium, and phosphorus, daily until the levels are stable, and order weekly liver function tests and prealbumin and triglyceride levels. Measure blood glucose level by fingerstick every 6 h until the level is stable. Patients receiving insulin or tapering doses of steroids and those with changing clinical status may need closer blood glucose monitoring. Typical PN protocols call for weighing the patient daily and keeping accurate and intake and output records.

No single criterion is a reliable indicator of the effectiveness of PN. Because indicators of protein status are affected by illness, albumin and prealbumin levels are not reliable markers of response to therapy. Nitrogen balance studies do shed light on the adequacy of protein intake, particularly when serial studies are performed. Finally, clinical status is evidence that the a nutritional regimen is appropriate. Adequate wound healing, increased stamina, and improved functional status all suggest the nutritional regimen is meeting the patient's needs.

Preventing and Managing Complications

Hyperglycemia: The most common metabolic complication of PN. Severe hyperglycemia causes osmotic diuresis that depletes electrolytes, especially potassium, sodium, and phosphorus. If left uncorrected, severe hyperglycemia can progress to hyperglycemic hyperosmolar nonketotic (HHNK) syndrome, a rare but potentially fatal condition. Advances in monitoring and delivery techniques have made HHNK an uncommon occurrence. Evidence that tight glucose control during PN greatly improves clinical outcome has made glycemic control a priority during PN therapy.

The goal is to maintain blood glucose level no higher than 120 mg/dL for critically ill patients and no higher than 150 mg/dL for patients in stable condition receiving PN. Keeping dextrose infusion rates ≤ 4 mg/kg/min decreases the incidence of hyperglycemia. Patients with diabetes mellitus and those who are critically ill often need insulin to control blood glucose level during PN. Insulin is stable and is compatible with PN formulas, although a portion of the dose adheres to the administration bags and tubing. Guidelines typically call for 0.05–0.1 units of regular insulin for each gram of dextrose in the PN formula. For example, for an initial dextrose dose of 200 g, 10–20 units of insulin would be added to the PN formula. Closely monitor blood glucose level, and provide additional subcutaneous insulin coverage as needed. The insulin in the PN formula should be increased in increments of 0.05 units per gram of dextrose or by adding 2/3 of the subcutaneous insulin coverage for the previous 24 h to the next PN formula until blood glucose level stays within target range. In cases of extreme hyperglycemia or insulin resistance, a separate continuous insulin drip allows greater flexibility in controlling glucose levels. After glycemic control is achieved, increase the dextrose dose 50 g/d, to maintain the same insulin to dextrose ratio.

Hypoglycemia can develop in patients receiving PN formulas containing insulin. If the blood glucose level stays consistently < 80–100 mg/dL, reassess the insulin dose. This step is particularly necessary for patients with renal insufficiency, which delays insulin clearance, and for patients who are receiving tapering steroid doses. The following are guidelines for maintaining tight glucose control in patients receiving PN:

12

Blood Glucose Management with PN

Goal: Aim for glucose level of 80–120 mg/dL in critically ill patients. Goal for blood glucose for stable patients ranges from 100 to 150 mg/dL.

1. **Order fingerstick blood glucose measurement q6h,** with sliding scale insulin coverage.
2. **Use regular insulin.** Do not use NPH or long-acting insulin to avoid fluctuation in blood glucose levels due to variation in drug action.
3. **For patients with a history of diabetes or baseline blood glucose 120–150 mg/dL,** limit initial dextrose dose to 150 g in PN.
4. **For patients with baseline blood glucose 150–200 mg/dL,** limit initial dextrose dose to 150 g and add insulin 0.1 units/g dextrose (15 units).
5. **Review 24-h insulin coverage.** Add two thirds of the insulin coverage to the next PN *or* increase insulin in PN by 0.05 units/g dextrose to a goal of 0.2 units/g dextrose.
6. **Consider using an insulin drip** for blood glucose levels persistently > 200 mg/dL.
7. **Maintain the insulin/dextrose ratio** when increasing or decreasing dextrose in PN.
8. **Reassess insulin needs daily.** Reduce insulin in PN 30–50% for blood glucose levels that drop below desired level.

Fluid and Electrolyte Disturbances: Candidates for PN often have preexisting nutritional deficits and nutrient losses due to GI disorders, which make fluid and electrolyte shifts especially common in this population. The principles of fluid and electrolyte management for patients receiving PN are similar to those for any patient. In cases in which fluid restriction is called for, PN formulas can contain the most concentrated form of the nutrients to reduce the volume of the solution.

Hepatobiliary Complications: Abnormalities of hepatic function occur frequently in patients receiving PN. Early in therapy adults may have mild, transient elevations in liver enzymes that resolve when PN stops. However, neonates and patients receiving long-term PN may experience progressive, irreversible hepatic failure. Research findings show a strong association between excessive carbohydrate administration and liver dysfunction during PN. A number of additional risk factors have emerged, suggesting a multifactorial cause of PN-related hepatic dysfunction. PN also places recipients at risk of cholelithiasis, particularly patients who cannot tolerate any oral or enteral nutrition.

Strategies for preventing and managing hepatic complications of PN include avoiding overfeeding, limiting dextrose dose to 30–50% of calories, providing 10–30% of calories as lipid, infusing PN over 12–16 h thus giving "time off" to mimic a postabsorptive state, and avoiding complete bowel rest if possible. Treatment with ursodeoxycholic acid may help patients with cholestasis.

Pulmonary Complications: The CO_2 produced by carbohydrate metabolism can place added stress on patients with CO_2 retention and those who are being weaned from mechanical ventilation. To avoid problems related to CO_2 production, the formula must meet, not exceed, the patient's requirements. In addition to avoiding overfeeding, reducing the carbohydrate dose and increasing the proportion of calories provided as fat can help prevent adverse pulmonary effects of PN.

Catheter-Related Bloodstream Infection: PN increases the risk of catheter-related bloodstream infection (CR-BSI). Meticulous protocols for the insertion and maintenance of central venous catheters can greatly reduce the risk of this serious complication. CR-BSI may necessitate removal of the vascular access device or treatment with antibiotics, depending on the type of catheter, clinical status of the patient, and type of organism isolated from the patient's blood. Unexplained fever or elevated WBC count in a patient receiving PN should raise suspicion concerning CR-BSI.

Terminating Therapy

When oral or enteral intake resumes, patients should gradually receive fewer nutrients parenterally. Some clinicians infuse PN only at night in an effort to minimize the risk of rebound hypoglycemia, but no results of controlled trials exist to support this practice. There is rarely a need for a formal schedule of weaning from PN. If concerns about rebound hypoglycemia exist, a 5% dextrose solution can be infused after PN is discontinued.

BEDSIDE PROCEDURES

Procedure Basics
Amniotic Fluid Fern Test
Arterial Line Placement
Arterial Puncture
Arthrocentesis (Diagnostic and
     Therapeutic)
Bone Marrow Aspiration and Biopsy
Central Venous Catheterization
Chest Tube Placement (Closed
     Thoracostomy, Tube
     Thoracostomy)
Cricothyroidotomy (Needle and Surgical)
Culdocentesis
Doppler Pressures
Electrocardiogram
Endotracheal Intubation
Fever Work-Up
Gastrointestinal Intubation
Heelstick and Fingerstick (Capillary
     Blood Sampling)

Internal Fetal Scalp Monitoring
Injection Techniques
Intrauterine Pressure Monitoring
IV Techniques
Lumbar Puncture
Orthostatic Blood Pressure
     Measurement
Pelvic Examination
Pericardiocentesis
Peripheral Insertion of Central
     Catheter (PICC)
Peritoneal Lavage
Peritoneal (Abdominal) Paracentesis
Pulmonary Artery Catheterization
Pulsus Paradoxus Measurement
Skin Biopsy
Skin Testing
Thoracentesis
Urinary Tract Procedures
Venipuncture

PROCEDURE BASICS

Universal Precautions

Universal precautions should be used whenever an invasive procedure exposes
the operator to potentially infectious body fluids. Not all patients infected with
transmissible pathogens can be reliably identified. Because pathogens transmitted by blood and body fluids pose a hazard to personnel caring for such patients,
particularly during invasive procedures, *precautions are required for routine
care of all patients* whether or not they have been placed on isolation precautions of any type. The CDC calls these universal precautions.

1. Wash hands before and after **all** patient contact.
2. Wash hands before and after **all** invasive procedures.
3. Wear gloves in **every** instance in which contact with blood or body fluid is
    certain or likely. For example, wear gloves for all venipunctures, for all IV
    starts, for IV manipulation, and for wound care.
4. Wear gloves once and discard. Do not wear the same pair to perform tasks
    on two different patients or to perform two different tasks at different sites
    on the same patient.
5. Wear gloves in **every** instance in which contact with **any** body fluid is
    likely, including urine, feces, wound secretions, and fluid encountered in
    respiratory tract care, thoracentesis, paracentesis.
6. Wear gown when splatter of blood or body fluids on clothing seems likely.
7. Use additional barrier precautions for invasive procedures in which con-
    siderable splatter or aerosol generation is likely. Such splatter does not
    occur during most routine patient care activities but can occur in the OR,

ER, and ICU, during invasive bedside procedures, and during CPR. Always wear a mask when goggles are called for, and always wear goggles when a mask is called for.

Accidental Needlesticks

The FDA has recommended safer needle devices, including devices that place a barrier between hands and needle after use. Needlestick injury is an occupational injury among health care workers in the United States. OSHA estimates that 600,000–800,000 needlestick injuries occur on the job each year. Health care workers are at risk of transmission of more than 20 blood-borne pathogens (eg, HIV, hepatitis B and C viruses). Although it is not possible to completely eliminate the risk of needlestick injury, it has been estimated that 62–88% of sharps injuries can be reduced through the use of devices and procedures designed to protect health care workers from exposed needles. A variety of self-shielding needle devices are on the market (see Heelstick and Fingerstick [Capillary Blood Sampling], IV Techniques, and Venipuncture for examples).

Informed Consent

Before any procedure, counsel the patient about the reasons for the procedure, alternatives, and the risks and benefits. Explaining the various steps is likely to help gain the patient's cooperation and make the procedure easier on both parties. In general, procedures such as bladder catheterization, NG intubation, and venipuncture do not require written informed consent beyond normal hospital sign-in protocols. More invasive procedures, such as thoracentesis or lumbar puncture, require written consent, which must be obtained by a licensed physician.

Preprocedure Patient Assessment

Conduct a complete pre-procedure assessment with every patient undergoing an invasive procedure that may require sedation or conscious sedation should undergo. Assess the patient's airway (ie, how difficult it would be to intubate the patient in an emergency), past medical history including previous complications with anesthetics, history of bleeding problems, and a complete history of allergies to medications or latex. Be aware of the patient's current medications with emphasis on blood thinners (eg, heparin, warfarin [Coumadin]) and be aware of the most recent coagulation parameters. Review any relevant, recent studies directly associated with the anticipated procedure.

Time Out

Most institutions are following JCAHO regulations that require a time out before surgical intervention. During this time the members of the team (nurses, anesthesiologists, surgeons, and others) review the procedure to be performed, make sure that informed consent has been obtained, and check that the procedure will be performed on the correct patient and on the correct part of the body (eg, right or left side of the chest). Although not mandated for bedside procedures, time out appears to be a reasonable safety measure.

Latex Allergy

People with certain medical conditions or in occupations that are heavily exposed to products containing natural rubber latex (NRL) may became sensitized and develop allergic reactions to NRL. It is estimated that 7% of health care workers have allergic reactions; persons with spina bifida have an 18–40% incidence. Any group of patients frequently and intensely exposed to latex, such as those undergoing repeated surgical procedures and treatments such as intermittent catheterization, are at increased risk. Local and systemic allergic reactions can often be dramatic and occasionally are life-threatening. The treatment is the same as for any allergic reaction (remove exposure, administer epinephrine and steroids; see Chapter 21).

If a patient has a latex allergy, it should be noted on prominently displayed signs and on the patient's chart, and the patient should wear an alert bracelet. Latex is found in medical equipment in addition to gloves (eg, anesthesia masks, catheters, ETs, hemodialysis components, NG tubes, drains, and syringes) and in consumer products (eg, balloons, rubber bands, scuba diving equipment, underwear). Most hospitals have an inventory of latex-free products and ORs have latex allergy procedures in place. Nitrile gloves are becoming common in hospitals because of this growing problem.

Basic Equipment

Table 13–1 lists useful collections of instruments and supplies, often packaged together, that aid in completion of the procedures described in this chapter. Local anesthesia is discussed in Chapter 17.

The size of various catheters, tubes, and needles is often designated by **French unit** (1 Fr = $^1/3$ mm in diameter) or by **needle gauge.** Reference listings for these designations are in Figure 13–1A, page 244. Designations of surgical scalpels used in the performance of many basic bedside procedures and in the OR are shown in Figure 13–1B, page 245.

TABLE 13–1
Instruments and Supplies Used in the Completion of Common Bedside Procedures

13

MINOR PROCEDURE TRAY
Sterile gloves
Sterile towels/drapes
4×4 gauze sponges
Povidone iodine (Betadine) prep solution
Syringes: 5-, 10-, 20-mL
Needles: 18-, 20-, 22-, 25-gauge
1% Lidocaine (with or without epinephrine)
Adhesive tape

INSTRUMENT TRAY
Scissors
Needle holder
Hemostat
Scalpel and blade (no. 10 for adult, no. 15 for children or delicate work)
Suture of choice (2-0 or 3-0 silk or nylon on cutting needle; cutting needle best for suturing to skin)

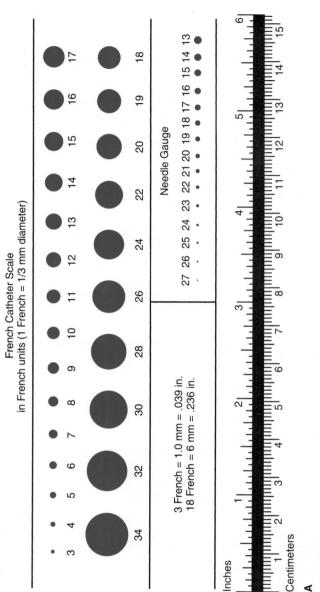

FIGURE 13-1. A. French catheter guide and needle gauge reference. (Courtesy Cook Urological.)

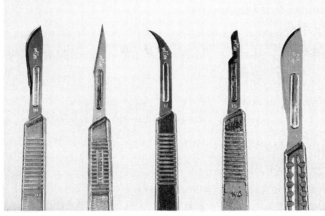

FIGURE 13-1. B. Commonly used scalpel blades. Left to right: no. 10, 11, 12, 15, and 20. No. 10 is the standard surgical blade; no. 11 is useful for incisions into abscesses or to open the skin for placement of large IV devices; no. 12 is designed to open tubular structures; no. 15 is widely used for bedside procedures and for more delicate work; no. 20 is used to make large incisions.

AMNIOTIC FLUID FERN TEST

Indication

- Assessment for rupture of membranes

Materials

- Sterile speculum and swab
- Glass slide and microscope
- Phenaphthazine (Nitrazine) paper (optional)

Procedure

1. Using a sterile speculum, swab a sample of fluid "pooled" in the vaginal vault onto a glass slide and let it air dry.
2. Amniotic fluid yields an arborization, or "fern," pattern seen under 10× magnification. False-positive: cervical mucus collection; however, the ferning pattern of mucus is coarser. Test is unaffected by meconium, vaginal pH, and blood–to–amniotic fluid ratios > 1:10. Samples heavily contaminated with blood may not fern.
3. Another test for ruptured membranes is performed with Nitrazine paper, which has a pH turning point of 6.0. Normal vaginal pH in pregnancy is 4.5–6.0; amniotic fluid pH is 7.0–7.5. Positive Nitrazine test: color change in the paper from yellow to blue. False-positive: more common with the Nitrazine test; blood, meconium, semen, alkalotic urine, cervical mucus, and vaginal infections can raise the pH.

Complication

- Infection

ARTERIAL LINE PLACEMENT

Indications

- Continuous BP readings (eg, critically ill patient)
- Facilitation of frequent ABG measurements (eg, patients who need ventilatory support)

Contraindications

- Arterial insufficiency with poor collateral circulation (see Allen test, page 248)
- Thrombolytic therapy or coagulopathy (relative)
- Planned cardiac surgery if the radial artery has to be preserved for harvest for CABG (relative)

Materials

- Minor procedure and instrument tray
- Heparin flush solution (1:1000 dilution)
- Arterial line set-up according to local ICU routine (transducer, tubing, and pressure bag with preheparinized saline, monitor)
- Arterial line catheter kit *or* 20-gauge catheter over needle, $1^1/2$–2 in (4–5 cm). (Insyte Autoguard shielded IV catheter, Angiocath Autoguard Shielded IV catheter) with 0.025-in (0.6 mm) guidewire (optional)

Procedure (Figure 13–2)

1. The radial artery is most frequently used and is described here. Other sites, in decreasing preference: ulnar, dorsalis pedis, femoral, brachial, and axillary arteries. **Never puncture the radial and ulnar arteries in the same hand;** doing so can compromise the blood supply to the hand and fingers.

2. Using the Allen test or Doppler ultrasonography, verify collateral circulation between the radial and ulnar arteries. Prepare the flush bag, tubing, and transducer, paying particular attention to removing air bubbles.

3. Place the forearm on an armboard with a roll of gauze behind the wrist to hyperextend the joint. Prep with povidone–iodine, and drape with sterile towels. Wear gloves and mask.

4. Palpate the artery, and choose the puncture site where the artery appears most superficial. Using a 25-gauge needle and 1% lidocaine, raise a very small skin wheal at the puncture site. Draw back on the syringe before injecting lidocaine so as not to inadvertently inject into the artery.

5. **a. Standard technique:** (See Figure 13–2). While palpating the path of the artery with your nondominant hand, advance the 20-gauge (preferably $1^1/2$ in [4 cm] long) catheter-over-needle assembly into the artery at a low (< 30-degree) angle. Once "flash" of blood is seen in the hub, advance the entire unit 1–2 mm, so that the needle and catheter are in the artery. If blood flow in the hub stops, carefully pull the entire unit back until flow is reestablished. When flow is established, position the hub of the catheter downward (decreasing the angle between catheter and skin), allowing catheter advancement in a more straight-line direction. Hold the needle

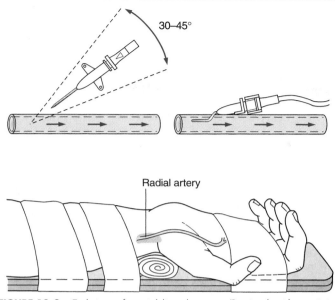

30–45°

Radial artery

FIGURE 13–2. Technique of arterial line placement. (Reprinted, with permission, from: Gomella TL [ed] *Neonatology: Basic Management, On-Call Problems, Diseases, Drugs,* 5th ed. McGraw-Hill, 2004.)

steady, and advance the catheter over the needle into the artery. The catheter should slide smoothly into the artery. Activate the safety button on the catheter to automatically shield the needle. Withdraw the shielded needle completely and check for arterial blood flow from the catheter. A catheter that does not spurt blood is not in position. Briefly occlude the artery with manual pressure while the pressure tubing is being connected. *Note:* The pressure tubing system must be preflushed to clear all air bubbles before connection.

b. **Prepackaged kit technique:** Kits, sometimes called "quick catheters," with a needle and guidewire can be used for the **Seldinger technique** (described in step 8). Place the entry needle at a 30-degree angle to the skin site, and insert until a flash of blood rises in the catheter. The catheter does not have to be advanced, but advance both the guidewire portion (orange handle in some kits) and the catheter into the vessel. Remove the wire and connect it to the pressure tubing.

6. If placement is not successful, apply pressure to the site for 5 min and reattempt one or two more times. If still not successful, move to another site, because the artery may undergo spasm, making cannulation more difficult.

7. Suture the catheter in place with 3-0 silk, and apply a sterile dressing. Splint the dorsum of the wrist to limit mobility and stabilize the catheter.

8. If a larger vessel such as the femoral artery is used, consider the **Seldinger technique** of cannulation: Locate the vessel lumen with a small-gauge, thin-walled needle; pass a 0.035 floppy-tipped J ("J" describes the configuration of the end of the floppy wire) guidewire into the lumen; and use the guidewire to

13

pass a larger catheter into the vessel. Use a 16-gauge catheter assembly at least 6 in (15 cm) long for the femoral artery. *Note:* If a dilator is used with the kit, take care to dilate only skin and subcutaneous tissue; inadvertent dilation of an artery causes excessive bleeding.

9. Any amount of heparin can make coagulation studies (PTT) inaccurate. If an arterial line sample is obtained and unexpectedly high results are seen, repeat the test and consider conventional venipuncture. Even with use of a 5- to 10-mL discard sample from the line, some heparin can contaminate the line.

10. Always compare the arterial line pressure with a standard cuff pressure. An occasional difference of 10–20 mm Hg is normal and should be considered when monitoring the BP.

Complications

Thrombosis, hematoma, arterial embolism, arterial spasm, arterial insufficiency with tissue loss, infection, hemorrhage, and pseudoaneurysm formation.

ARTERIAL PUNCTURE
Indications

- Blood gas determinations and acquisition of arterial blood for chemistry determinations (eg, ammonia levels)

Materials

- Cup of ice
- Blood gas sampling kit

or

- 3- to 5-mL syringe
- 23- to 25-gauge needle (radial artery); 20- to 22-gauge (femoral artery)
- Heparin (1000 U/mL), 1 mL
- Alcohol or povidone–iodine swabs

Procedure

1. Use heparinized syringe for blood gas and nonheparinized syringe for chemistry determinations. If a blood gas kit is not available, heparinize a 3- to 5-mL syringe by drawing up 1 mL of 1:1000 solution of heparin through a small-gauge needle (23–25 gauge) into the syringe, pulling the plunger all the way back. The heparin is then expelled, leaving only a small coating.

2. In order of preference, use the radial, femoral, or brachial artery. For the radial artery, perform an **Allen test** to verify patency of the ulnar artery. You do not want to damage the radial artery if there is no flow in the ulnar artery. To perform the Allen test, have the patient make a tight fist. Occlude both the radial and ulnar arteries at the wrist and have the patient open the hand. While maintaining pressure on the radial artery, release the ulnar artery. If the ulnar artery is patent, the hand flushes red within 6 s, and radial puncture can be safely performed. If flushing is delayed or part of the hand remains pale, do **not** perform the radial puncture because collateral flow is inadequate. Choose an alternative site. Doppler ultrasonography can also be used to determine patency of the ulnar artery.

3. For the femoral artery, use the mnemonic **NAVEL** to locate groin structures. Palpate the femoral artery just below the inguinal ligament. From lateral to medial the structures are **N**erve, **A**rtery, **V**ein, **E**mpty space, **L**ymphatic.

4. Prep the area with either chlorhexidine solution or alcohol swab.

5. With sterile gloves, palpate the chosen artery carefully; lidocaine SQ can be used (small needle such as a 25–27 gauge), but this often turns a one-stick procedure into a two-stick procedure. Palpate the artery proximally and distally with two fingers, or trap the artery between two fingers placed on either side of the vessel. Hyperextension of the joint brings the radial and brachial arteries closer to the surface.

6. Hold the syringe like a pencil with the needle bevel up, and enter the skin at a 60- to 90-degree angle. Often you can feel the arterial pulsations as you approach the artery.

7. Maintaining a slight negative pressure on the syringe, obtain blood on the downstroke or on slow withdrawal (after both sides of the artery have been punctured). Aspirate very slowly. A good arterial sample requires only minimal back pressure. If a glass syringe or special blood gas syringe is used, the barrel usually fills spontaneously, and it is not necessary to pull on the plunger.

8. If the vessel is not encountered, withdraw the needle without coming out of the skin, and redirect.

9. After obtaining the sample, withdraw the needle quickly and apply **firm pressure** at the site for **at least 5 min** (longer if the patient is receiving anticoagulants. To prevent compartment syndrome from extravasated blood, apply pressure even if a sample was not obtained. Activate the needle reshielding mechanism.

10. If the sample is for a blood gas determination, expel any air from the syringe, mix the contents thoroughly by twirling the syringe between your fingers, remove and dispose of the needle assembly, and make the syringe airtight with a cap. Place the syringe in an ice bath if more than a few minutes will elapse before the sample is processed. Note the inspired oxygen concentration and time of day on the lab slip.

13

ARTHROCENTESIS (DIAGNOSTIC AND THERAPEUTIC)
Indications
- **Diagnostic.** Evaluation of new-onset arthritis; ruling out infection in acute or chronic, unremitting joint effusion
- **Therapeutic.** Instillation of steroids, drainage of septic arthritis; relief of tense hemarthrosis or effusion

Contraindications
Cellulitis at injection site. Relative contraindication: bleeding disorder; caution if coagulopathy or thrombocytopenia is present or if the patient is receiving anticoagulants.

Materials
- Minor procedure tray; 18- or 20-gauge needle (smaller for finger or toe)

- Ethyl chloride spray can be substituted for lidocaine.
- Two heparinized tubes for cell count and crystal examination
- Microbiology lab's preferred supplies for transporting fluid for bacterial, fungal, AFB culture, and Gram stain; Thayer–Martin plate for *Neisseria gonorrhoeae* (GC)
- Syringe containing a long-acting corticosteroid such as methylprednisolone (Depo-Medrol) or triamcinolone (see Chapter 22) optional for therapeutic arthrocentesis

General Procedures

1. Obtain consent after describing the procedure and complications.
2. Determine the optimal site for aspiration—knee, wrist, or ankle (see below); identify landmarks and mark site with indentation or sterile marking pen. Avoid injecting into tendons.
3. If aspiration is followed by corticosteroid injection, maintain a sterile field with sterile implements to minimize risk of infection.
4. Clean the area with chlorhexidine. Let the area dry, and wipe the aspiration site with alcohol, because chlorhexidine can render cultures negative. Let the alcohol dry before beginning the procedure.
5. Using a 25-gauge needle, anesthetize the puncture site with lidocaine; **do not inject into the joint space,** because lidocaine is bactericidal. Avoid lidocaine preparations with epinephrine, especially in a digit. Alternatively, spray the area with ethyl chloride ("freeze spray") just before needle aspiration.
6. Insert the aspirating needle (18- or 20-gauge, smaller for finger or toe), applying a small amount of vacuum to the syringe. When the capsule is entered, fluid usually flows easily. Remove as much fluid as possible, repositioning the syringe if necessary.
7. If corticosteroid is to be injected, remove the aspirating syringe from the needle (using a hemostat to hold the needle in place may aid when exchanging syringes), which is still in the joint space. (*Note:* Ensure that the syringe can easily be removed from the needle before step 6). Attach the syringe containing corticosteroid, pull back on the plunger to ensure the needle is not in a vein, and inject contents. Never inject steroids when there is any possibility that the joint is infected. Remove the needle, and apply pressure to the area (leakage of SQ steroids can cause localized atrophy of the skin). In general, the equivalent of 40 mg of methylprednisolone is injected into large joints such as the knee and 20 mg into medium-size joints such as the ankle and wrist. Warn the patient that a postinjection "flare" (pain several hours later) is treated with ice and NSAIDs.
8. Note volume aspirated from the joint. The knee typically contains 3.5 mL of synovial fluid; in inflammatory, septic, or hemorrhagic arthritis, volumes can be higher. A bedside test for viscosity is to allow a drop of fluid to fall from the tip of the needle. Normal synovial fluid is highly viscous and forms a several-inch-long string; viscosity is decreased in infection. A **mucin clot test** (clot normally forms in < 1 min; delayed result suggests inflammation) once a standard test for RA, is no longer routinely performed.
9. Joint fluid is usually sent for:
    - Cell count and diff (purple or green top tube)

13

- Microscopic crystal exam with polarized light microscopy (purple or green top tube); **normally** no debris, crystals, or bacteria; urate crystals present with gout; calcium pyrophosphate in pseudogout.
- Glucose (red top tube) (Table 13–2, page 252)
- Gram stain and cultures for bacteria, fungi, and AFB as indicated (check with your lab or deliver immediately in a sterile tube with no additives)
- Cytology if malignant effusion is suspected

Arthrocentesis of the Knee

1. Fully extend the knee with the patient supine. Wait until the patient has a relaxed quadriceps muscle, because its contraction approximates the patella against the femur, making aspiration painful.
2. Insert the needle posterior to the *lateral* portion of the patella into the patellar–femoral groove. Direct the advancing needle slightly posteriorly and inferiorly (Figure 13–3, page 253).
3. To inject the knee joint, have the patient sitting down with the leg flexed and enter the knee anteriorly over the medial joint line.

Arthrocentesis of the Wrist

1. The easiest site for aspiration is between the navicular bone and radius on the dorsal wrist. Locate the distal radius between the tendons of the extensor pollicis longus and the extensor carpi radialis longus to the second finger. This site is just ulnar to the anatomic snuff box. Direct the needle perpendicular to the mark (Figure 13–4, page 254). The wrist space also can be approached from the ulnar side by placement of the needle just distal to the ulnar bone.

Arthrocentesis of the Ankle

1. The most accessible site is between the tibia and the talus. Position the angle of foot to leg at 90 degrees. Make a mark lateral and anterior to the medial malleolus and medial and posterior to the tibialis anterior tendon. Direct the advancing needle posteriorly toward the heel (Figure 13–5, page 254).
2. The **subtalar ankle joint** does not communicate with the ankle joint and is difficult to aspirate even for an expert. Be aware that "ankle pain" can originate in the subtalar joint rather than in the ankle.

Synovial Fluid Interpretation

Normal synovial fluid values and values in disease states are in Table 13–2, page 252.

Noninflammatory Arthritis: Osteoarthritis, traumatic, aseptic necrosis, osteochondritis desiccans

Inflammatory Arthritis: Gout (usually associated with elevated serum uric acid), pseudogout, RA, rheumatic fever, collagen–vascular disease

Septic Arthritis: Pyogenic bacterial (*Staphylococcus aureus,* GC, and *Staphylococcus epidermidis* most common), TB

Hemorrhagic: Hemophilia or other bleeding diathesis, trauma with or without fracture

TABLE 13–2
Synovial Fluid Analysis and Categories for Differential Diagnosis[a]

Parameter	Normal	Noninflammatory	Inflammatory	Septic	Hemorrhagic
Viscosity	High	High	Decreased	Decreased	Variable
Clarity	Transparent	Transparent	Translucent-opaque	Opaque	Cloudy
Color	Clear	Yellow	Yellow to opalescent	Yellow to green[b]	Pink to red
WBC (per mL)	<200	<3000	3000–50,000	>50,000[b]	Usually <2000
Polymorphonuclear leukocytes (%)	<25%	<25%	50% or more	75% or more	30%
Culture	Negative	Negative	Negative	Usually positive	Negative
Glucose (mg/dL)	Approx. serum	Approx. serum	>25, but <serum	<25, <serum	>25

[a]See page 251 for additional information.
[b]May be lower if antibiotics initiated.
WBC = white blood cells.

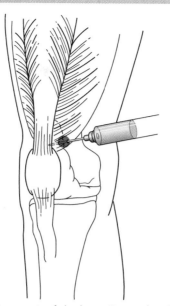

FIGURE 13–3. Arthrocentesis of the knee. (Reprinted, with permission, from: *Internal Medicine on Call,* 4th ed. Haist SA, Robbins JB [eds]. McGraw-Hill, New York, 2005.)

Complications

Infection, bleeding, pain. Postinjection flare of joint pain and swelling can occur after steroid injection and persist for as long as 24 h. This complication is believed to be crystal-induced synovitis caused by the crystalline suspension used in long-acting steroids.

BONE MARROW ASPIRATION AND BIOPSY
Indications

- Evaluation of unexplained anemia, thrombocytopenia, leukopenia
- Evaluation of unexplained leukocytosis, thrombocytosis; search for malignancy primary to the marrow (leukemia, myeloma) or metastatic to the marrow (small-cell lung cancer, breast cancer)
- Evaluation of iron stores; evaluation of possible disseminated infection (tuberculosis, fungal disease)
- Bone marrow donor harvesting (aspiration)

Contraindications

- Infection, osteomyelitis near the puncture site
- Relative contraindications include severe coagulopathy and thrombocytopenia (may be corrected by platelet transfusion); previous radiation to the region

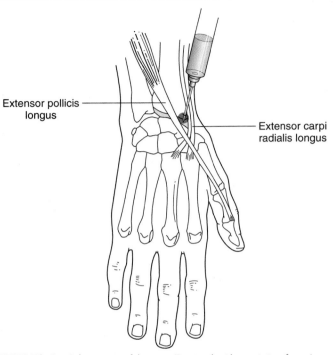

Extensor pollicis longus

Extensor carpi radialis longus

FIGURE 13–4. Arthrocentesis of the wrist. (Reprinted, with permission, from: *Internal Medicine on Call,* 4th ed. Haist SA, Robbins JB [eds]. McGraw-Hill, New York, 2005.)

13

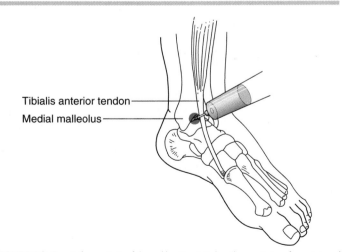

Tibialis anterior tendon
Medial malleolus

FIGURE 13–5. Arthrocentesis of the ankle. (Reprinted, with permission, from: *Internal Medicine on Call,* 4th ed. Haist SA, Robbins JB [eds]. McGraw-Hill, New York, 2005.)

Materials

- Kits contain all the materials necessary. A technician from the hematology lab or BMT facility must be present to ensure delivery and processing of specimens.

Procedure

1. Explain the procedure to the patient and/or the legally responsible surrogate in detail and obtain informed consent.
2. Local anesthesia usually is all that is needed; if a patient is extremely anxious, premedication with an anxiolytic or sedative such as diazepam (Valium) or midazolam (Versed) or an analgesic is reasonable.
3. Bone marrow can be obtained from numerous sites, such as the sternum and anterior or posterior iliac crest. The posterior iliac crest is the safest and the site of choice (described here). Position the patient on either the abdomen or on the side opposite the side from which the biopsy specimen is to be taken.
4. Identify the posterior iliac crest by palpation and mark the desired biopsy site with indelible ink.
5. Use sterile gloves, mask, and gown, and follow strict aseptic technique.
6. Prep the site with povidone–iodine solution and allow it to dry. Use alcohol to wipe the site free of povidone–iodine. Drape the surrounding areas.
7. Administer 1% lidocaine intradermally to raise a skin wheal with a 25- or 26-gauge needle; then use a 22-gauge needle to infiltrate the deeper tissues until the periosteum is reached. Advance the needle just through the periosteum and infiltrate lidocaine subperiosteally. Infiltrate an area approximately 2 cm in diameter, using repeated periosteal punctures.
8. Use a no. 11 scalpel blade to make a 2- to 3-mm skin incision over the biopsy site.
9. Insert the bone marrow biopsy needle through the skin incision and advance it with a rotating motion and gentle pressure until the periosteum is reached. Once the needle is firmly seated on the periosteum, advance it through the outer table of bone into the marrow cavity with the same rotating motion and gentle pressure. In general, a slight change in resistance to needle advancement signals entry into the marrow cavity. At this point, advance the needle 2–3 mm.
10. Remove the stylet from the biopsy needle, and attach a 10-mL syringe to the hub of the biopsy needle. Withdraw the plunger on the syringe briskly, and aspirate 1–2 mL of marrow into the syringe. This step can cause severe, instantaneous pain, but slow withdrawal of the plunger or collection of more than 1–2 mL of marrow with each aspiration results in excessive contamination of the specimen with peripheral blood.
11. Use the specimen to prepare coverslips for viewing under the microscope or send it for special studies (cytogenetics, cell markers, culture). Repeated aspiration may be needed to obtain enough marrow for all studies. Certain studies may require heparin or EDTA for collection. Contact the lab before the procedure to confirm specimen collection procedures.
12. For biopsy, replace the stylet and withdraw the needle. Reinsert the needle at a slightly different angle and location (within the area of periosteum anesthetized). Once the marrow cavity has been reentered, remove the stylet and advance 5–10 mm, using the same rotating motion with gentle pressure. With-

13

draw the needle several millimeters (but not outside the marrow cavity), and redirect it at a slightly different angle and advance again. Repeating several times results in 2–3 cm of core material entering the needle. Rotate the needle rapidly on its long axis in a clockwise and then a counterclockwise manner to sever the specimen from the marrow cavity. Withdraw the needle completely without replacing the stylet. Some physicians prefer to hold a thumb over the open end of the needle to create negative pressure in the needle as it is withdrawn; this step may help prevent loss of the biopsy specimen.

13. Remove the sample by inserting a probe (provided with the biopsy needle) into the distal end of the needle and gently push the specimen the full length of the needle and **out the hub end.** Attempting to push the specimen out the distal end may damage the specimen. Most biopsy needles are tapered at the distal end, presumably allowing the specimen to expand once in the needle and preventing it from being lost when the needle is withdrawn from the patient.

14. The core biopsy specimen is usually placed in formalin. (Confirm with lab before procedure.)

15. Observe for excess bleeding and apply local pressure for several minutes. Clean the area with alcohol and apply an adhesive bandage or gauze patch. Recommend (not required unless coagulopathic) that the patient assume a supine position and place a pressure pack between the bed or examining table and the biopsy site and apply pressure for 10–15 min. A patient who is stable at this point may resume normal activities.

Complications

Local bleeding and hematoma, retroperitoneal hematoma, pain, bone fracture, infection

13

CENTRAL VENOUS CATHETERIZATION

Indications

- Administration of fluids and medications (peripheral access preferred)
- Administration of hyperalimentation solutions or other hypertonic fluids (eg, amphotericin B) that damage peripheral veins
- Measurement of CVP (see Chapter 20, page 410)
- Acute dialysis or plasmapheresis (Shiley or Quinton catheter)
- Insertion of pulmonary artery catheter or transvenous pacemaker

Contraindications

- Coagulopathy dictates the use of the femoral or median basilic vein approach to minimize complications.

Background

A central venous catheter (or **"deep line"**) is a catheter introduced into the superior or inferior vena cava or one of the main branches of these vessels. One technique (**Seldinger technique**) involves puncturing the vein with a small needle through which a thin guidewire is placed. The needle is withdrawn, and the intravascular appliance or a sheath through which a smaller catheter will be placed is introduced into the vein over the guidewire. Another technique involves puncturing the vein with a larger bore needle through which the intravascular catheter will fit. This section focuses on the more common Seldinger technique and placement of either a triple-lumen catheter or a sheath through which a smaller catheter (eg, a pulmonary artery catheter) can be placed. The internal jugular and subclavian approaches are commonly used; the femoral approach, although infrequently used, offers several advantages (see Femoral Vein Approach). The PICC line is designed for more long-term outpatient administration of medications and is described on page 301. Before inserting these catheters, obtain a thorough history, asking about any bleeding diathesis, anticoagulant use, previous catheter placement, history of DVT, and presence of transvenous pacemaker. Note any abnormal laboratory values, especially elevated PT/PTT or low platelets. Correction of any such abnormalities with platelet transfusions, fresh frozen plasma transfusions, vitamin K, or discontinuation of anticoagulation may be required before placement of nonurgent central venous catheters.

Materials

Prepackaged trays contain all the necessary needles, wires, sheaths, dilators, suture materials, and anesthetics needed. If needles, guidewires, and sheaths are collected from different places, make sure that the needle will accept the guidewire, that the sheath and dilator will pass over the guidewire, and that the appliance to be passed through the sheath will fit the inside lumen of the sheath, because sizes are not standard. Supplies should include the following:

- Minor procedure and instrument tray (page 243); 1% lidocaine (mixed 1:1 with sodium bicarbonate 1 mEq/L removes the sting)
- Guidewire (usually 0.035 floppy-tipped J wire)
- Vessel dilator
- Intravascular appliance (triple-lumen catheter or a sheath through which a pulmonary artery catheter can be placed)
- Heparinized flush solution 1 mL of 1:100 units heparin in 10 mL of NS (to fill lumens before placement to prevent clotting during placement)
- Mask, sterile gown, gloves

Subclavian Approach (Left or Right)

The left subclavian approach affords a gentle, sweeping curve to the apex of the right ventricle (preferred site for temporary transvenous pacemaker without fluoroscopy). Hemodynamic measurements are easier from the left subclavian approach; catheters do not have to negotiate an acute angle, as is the case at the junction of the right subclavian vein with the right brachiocephalic vein en route to the superior vena cava. This site is a common one for kinking of the line but is also has the lowest risk of infection. *Caution:* The thoracic duct is on the left side, and the dome of the pleura rises higher on the left.

Procedure

1. Use sterile technique (chlorhexidine prep, gloves, mask, gown, and a sterile field).
2. Place the patient flat or with head slightly down (Trendelenburg position) in the center or turned to the opposite side. (*Note:* The "ideal" position is controversial and based on operator preference.) Placing a towel roll along the patient's spine may help.

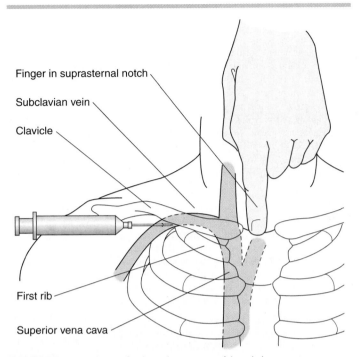

Finger in suprasternal notch

Subclavian vein

Clavicle

First rib

Superior vena cava

FIGURE 13–6. Technique for the catheterization of the subclavian vein.

13

3. Administer 1% lidocaine and use a 25-gauge needle to make a small skin wheal 1 in (2 cm) below the midclavicle. Then use a larger needle (eg, 22-gauge) to anesthetize the deeper tissues and locate the vein.
4. Attach a large-bore, deep-line needle (a 14-gauge needle with a 16-gauge catheter at least 8–12 in [20–30 cm] long) to a 10–20 mL syringe, and introduce it into the site of the skin wheal.
5. Advance the needle under the clavicle, aiming for a location halfway between the suprasternal notch and the base of the thyroid cartilage. Place your index or middle finger in the sternal notch, and aim for just above your finger (Figure 13–6). The vein is encountered under the clavicle, just medial to the lateral border of the clavicular head of the sternocleidomastoid muscle. In most patients the site is roughly two finger breadths lateral to the sternal notch. Apply gentle pressure on the needle at the skin entrance site to assist in lowering the needle under the clavicle, aiming the tip of the needle toward the sternal notch. Do not aim the needle toward the floor; that is how the pleura can be hit, resulting in pneumothorax.
6. Apply back pressure while advancing the needle deep to the clavicle, but above the first rib, and watch for a "flash" of blood.
7. Free return of blood indicates entry into the subclavian vein. Remember that occasionally the vein is punctured through *both* walls, and a flash of blood may not appear as the needle is advanced. Therefore, if free return of blood does not occur on needle advancement, withdraw the

needle slowly with intermittent pressure. Free return of blood heralds entry of the end of the needle into the lumen. Bright red blood that forcibly enters the syringe indicates that the subclavian artery has been entered. If arterial entry occurs, remove the needle. In most patients, the surrounding tissue will tamponade any bleeding from the arterial puncture. *Note:* The artery is under the clavicle; holding pressure has little effect on bleeding.

8. **a.** If you are using an Intracath device, remove the syringe, place a finger over the needle hub, and advance the catheter an appropriate distance through the needle. Withdraw the needle to just outside the skin and snap the protective cap over the tip of the needle.

   b. For the Seldinger wire technique, advance the wire through the needle and withdraw the needle. Pulse or ECG should be monitored during wire passage because the wire can induce ventricular arrhythmias. Arrhythmias usually resolve when the wire is pulled out several centimeters. Nick the skin with a no. 11 blade, and advance the dilator approximately 2 in (5 cm); remove the dilator and advance the catheter in over the guidewire (use the brown port on the triple-lumen catheter). While advancing either the dilator or the catheter over the wire, periodically ensure that the wire moves freely in and out. When placing a Cordis (multiport catheter sheath) system, advance the catheter and dilator over the guidewire as one unit (see Chapter 20, Pulmonary Artery Catheters, page 412). If the wire does not move freely, it usually is kinked; remove the catheter or dilator and reposition it. Maintain a grip on the guidewire at all times. Remove the wire and attach the IV tubing. *Note:* The wire used to insert a single-lumen catheter is shorter than the wire supplied with the triple-lumen catheter. Knowledge of this difference is critical when a triple-lumen is exchanged for a single-lumen catheter; use the longer triple-lumen wire and insert the wire into the brown port. Use the Seldinger wire technique to place Shiley (hemodialysis) catheters.

9. Aspirate blood, remove all the air from each of the ports, and flush with saline solution. Attach the catheter to the appropriate IV solution.

10. Securely suture the assembly in place with 2-0 or 3-0 silk. Apply an occlusive dressing with povidone–iodine ointment.

11. Obtain a CXR immediately to verify the location of the catheter tip and to rule out pneumothorax. Ideally, the catheter tip lies in the superior vena cava at its junction with the right atrium (about T5). Malpositioned catheters into the neck veins can be used only for saline infusion and not for monitoring or TPN infusion.

12. Catheters that cannot be manipulated into the chest at the bedside can usually be positioned properly during an interventional radiology procedure with fluoroscopy.

Right Internal Jugular Vein Approach

There are three sites of access to the right internal jugular vein: anterior (medial to the sternocleidomastoid muscle belly), middle (between the two heads of the sternocleidomastoid muscle belly), and posterior (lateral to the sternocleidomastoid muscle belly). The middle approach is most common and is made with well-defined landmarks. The major disadvantage of the internal jugular site is patient discomfort (difficult to dress, uncomfortable when turning the head).

13

Most larger hospitals are equipped with portable ultrasound scanners and needle guides (Site-Rite Ultrasound by Bard) to facilitate accurate internal jugular cannulation, minimizing the incidence of inadvertent carotid artery puncture.

Procedure

1. Sterilize the site with chlorhexidine, and drape the area with sterile towels. Administer local anesthesia with lidocaine in the area to be explored, as noted in the previous section.
2. Place the patient in the **Trendelenburg** (head down) position.
3. If using a portable ultrasound scanner, pass the head of the scanner through the sterile sheath, and after applying ultrasound gel locate the internal jugular vein (it is larger and more compressible than the carotid artery). Advance the large bore, deep-line needle through the needle guide and watch it enter the vein on the ultrasound monitor. If not using ultrasonography, use a small-bore (21-gauge) needle with syringe to locate the internal jugular vein. It may help to have a small amount of anesthetic in the syringe to inject during exploration if the patient feels discomfort. Some clinicians prefer to leave this needle and syringe in the vein and place the large-bore needle directly over the smaller needle, into the vein. This method is commonly called the "seeker needle" technique.
4. Make sure the internal diameter of the needle used to locate the internal jugular vein is large enough to accommodate the passage of the guidewire (typically 22-gauge or larger).
5. Make the percutaneous entry at the apex of the triangle formed by the two heads of the sternocleidomastoid muscle and the clavicle (Figure 13–7).

13

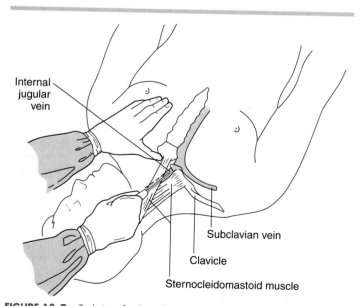

Internal jugular vein

Subclavian vein

Clavicle

Sternocleidomastoid muscle

FIGURE 13–7. Technique for the catheterization of the right internal jugular vein.

6. Direct the needle slightly lateral toward the ipsilateral nipple and enter at a 45-degree angle to the skin.

7. A notch can sometimes be palpated on the posterior surface of the clavicle; this step can help locate the vein in the mediolateral plane because the vein lies deep to this shallow notch.

8. Vein puncture often is accomplished at an unnerving depth of needle insertion and is heralded by sudden aspiration of nonpulsatile venous blood. Bedside Doppler ultrasonography is available in most ORs or ICUs and can aid in localization of the internal jugular vein if the standard techniques fail.

9. Inadvertent carotid artery puncture is common if the needle is inserted medial to where it should be on the middle approach and is common with the anterior approach. With arterial puncture, the syringe fills without negative pressure because of arterial pressure, and bright red blood pulsates from the needle after the syringe is removed. In this case remove the needle and apply manual pressure for 10–15 min.

10. Follow steps 8–12 as for subclavian line (page 259) to confirm position and end procedure.

Complications

Overall, a safe procedure when the small-bore needle is used to identify the vein.

- Pneumothorax may be detected when a sudden gush of air is aspirated instead of blood. Always obtain a postprocedure CXR to rule out pneumothorax and check line placement. Pneumothorax necessitates chest tube placement in almost all cases, especially when the patient is receiving mechanical ventilation or is a trauma patient. The left-sided approach is associated with higher pneumothorax risk (higher dome of the left pleura).
- Perforation of ET cuffs
- Hemothorax (vascular injury) or hydrothorax (administration of IV fluids into the pleural space)
- **Deep venous thrombosis:** Greatest risk factor for upper extremity DVT is a history of or the presence of a subclavian or an internal jugular deep line.
- **Catheter tip embolus: Never** withdraw the catheter through the needle (can shear off the tip).
- **Air embolus: Always** keep the open end of a deep line covered with a finger. As little as 50–100 mL of air in a vein can be fatal. For suspected **air embolization, place the patient's head down, and turn the patient to his or her left side to keep the air in the right atrium.** A stat portable CXR will show whether air is present in the heart.

Left Internal Jugular Vein Approach

The left internal jugular vein approach is not commonly used for central lines. Try one of the better options before using this approach. The procedure is similar to the right internal jugular vein approach. In addition to the usual complications, left internal jugular vein approach has unique complications, including inadvertent left brachiocephalic vein and superior vena caval puncture with intravascular wires, catheters, and sheaths and laceration of the thoracic duct with chylothorax.

13

External Jugular Vein Approach

The external jugular vein is a safe approach to central venous catheterization, but the method is technically demanding owing to difficulty threading the catheter into the central venous system. This site is uncomfortable for the patient because the dressing and IV tubing are on the neck. If the central venous system cannot be entered, the external jugular vein is also a site of last resort for placing a standard IV catheter ("peripheral") for administration of routine nonsclerosing IV fluids. The external jugular vein is usually visible with the patient in a 30-degree Trendelenburg position. The vein, located in the SQ tissues, crosses the sternocleidomastoid muscle arising from just behind the angle of the jaw inferiorly where it drains into the subclavian vein just lateral to the inferior aspect of the sternocleidomastoid muscle.

Procedure

1. Place the patient in the Trendelenburg position with the head turned away from the side of insertion. Prep and drape the neck from the ear to the subclavicular area.
2. Have the patient perform the Valsalva maneuver or gently occlude the vein near its insertion into the subclavian vein to help engorge the vein.
3. At the midpoint of the vein, make a skin wheal with a 25-gauge needle and lidocaine solution. Use a 21-gauge needle to anesthetize the deeper SQ tissue and to locate the vein.
4. Remove the syringe from the needle and insert a floppy-tipped J wire into the needle. Use the guidewire with gentle pressure to negotiate the turns into the intrathoracic portion of the venous system. With difficult wire passage, have the patient turn his or her head slightly to help direct the wire. **Never forcibly push the wire.** As a last resort, use fluoroscopy to direct the wire into the superior vena cava.
5. Once a sufficient length of guidewire is passed, remove the needle.
6. Nick the skin with a no. 11 blade to accommodate the catheter; advance the catheter over the guidewire, and remove the guidewire. Aspirate blood from the end of the catheter to confirm venous placement.
7. Follow steps 8–12 as for placement through the subclavian vein (page 259).

Complications

See Right Internal Jugular Vein Approach, page 261.

Femoral Vein Approach

The femoral vein approach is safe (arterial and venous sites are easily compressible), and pneumothorax is not possible. Placement can be accomplished without interrupting CPR. This site can be used to place a variety of intravascular appliances, including temporary pacemakers, pulmonary artery catheters (expertise with fluoroscopy may be needed), and triple-lumen catheters. The main disadvantages are high risk of sepsis, the immobilization it causes, and the need for fluoroscopy to ensure proper placement of pulmonary artery catheters and transvenous pacemakers.

Procedure

1. Place the patient in the supine position.

2. Use sterile preparation and appropriate draping. Administer local anesthesia in the area to be explored.
3. Palpate the femoral artery. Use the NAVEL technique to locate the vein (see page 249). If the arterial pulse is difficult to palpate, Doppler ultrasonography may aid in locating the artery.
4. Guard the artery with the fingers of one hand.
5. Explore for the vein just medial to your fingers with a needle and syringe as described previously.
6. It may be helpful to have a small amount of anesthetic in the syringe to inject with exploration.
7. Direct the needle cephalad at about a 30-degree angle and insert it below the femoral crease.
8. Puncture is heralded by the return of venous, nonpulsatile blood on application of negative pressure to the syringe.
9. Advance the guidewire through the needle.
10. The guidewire should pass with ease into the vein to a depth at which the distal tip of the guidewire is always under your control, even when the sheath–dilator or catheter is placed over the guidewire.
11. Remove the needle once the guidewire has advanced into the femoral vein.
12. For catheter size > 6 Fr, make a skin incision with a no. 11 scalpel blade and use a vessel dilator. Advance the catheter along with the guidewire into the femoral vein. Maintain control on the distal end of the guidewire.
13. Follow steps 8–12 as for the subclavian line.

Complications

The femoral site has the highest risk of contamination and sepsis. If an occlusive dressing can remain in place and free from contamination, this option is safe.

DVT has occurred after femoral vein catheterization. The risk of DVT increases if the catheter remains in place for a prolonged period.

Uncontrolled retroperitoneal bleeding can occur if the iliac or common femoral artery is inadvertently punctured above the inguinal ligament.

Removal of a Central Venous Catheter (Any Site)

1. Turn off the IV flow.
2. Place the patient lying down in slight Trendelenburg position. Cut the retention sutures, and gently withdraw the catheter. Visually inspect the catheter to ensure it is intact.
3. Apply pressure for at least 2–3 min, and apply a sterile dressing. Undo the Trendelenburg positioning, and place the patient in reverse Trendelenburg to decrease venous engorgement.

Removal of Tunneled Catheters

Permacath (or Hickman or Broviac) catheters are tunneled catheters placed in the OR or interventional radiology suite. These catheters pass through from the internal jugular or the subclavian vein, and are then tunneled subcutaneously and emerge from the chest wall. They also have an antibiotic-impregnated cuff near the skin exit site to prevent infection and promote tissue growth.

1. Wearing sterile gloves, gown, and mask, prep the patient as if placing a central line. Be sure to prep the catheter outside of the skin as well.

2. Cut skin sutures holding catheter in place.
3. Infiltrate field with 1% lidocaine using 25-gauge needle. Use caution to not inject directly into catheter (infiltrate only surrounding tissue). Palpate the antibiotic cuff through the skin. It should be a few centimeters from skin exit site, although this distance varies by catheter type and length of catheter outside the skin.
4. If it has been placed within the past 2–4 wk, the catheter may slide out with gentle traction, much like other central lines. More commonly, however, the antibiotic disk causes an inflammatory response that creates a tissue cuff around the cuff and catheter track. Begin by using a hemostat or scissors placed through the exit site to bluntly separate the surrounding connective tissue from the cuff. You may have to use a scissors to sharply cut some of this soft tissue. Take great care not to cut the catheter itself.
5. Once the cuff is free, gently attempt to pull out the catheter. If it does not release with gentle traction, do not pull harder because the catheter can snap, part of it being drawn into right atrium.
6. If the catheter is still not free, continue to cut tissue immediately surrounding it down to the catheter itself. Once you see the white color of the catheter, gently pull again and slide it out.
7. Once the catheter is removed, hold pressure for at least 5 min both at the site of entry into the vein (the internal jugular or subclavian) and at the exit site from the skin. Undo the Trendelenburg positioning.
8. If the cuff is very far from the skin exit site of the catheter, make a counterincision through the skin higher on the chest wall to aid in freeing the cuff from surrounding tissue at that location.

CHEST TUBE PLACEMENT (CLOSED THORACOSTOMY, TUBE THORACOSTOMY)

13

Indications

- Pneumothorax (simple or tension)
- Hemothorax, hydrothorax, chylothorax, or empyema evacuation
- Pleurodesis for chronic recurring pneumothorax or effusion refractory to standard management (eg, malignant effusion)

Materials

- Chest tube (Adult, 16–24 Fr for pneumothorax, 28–36 Fr for hemothorax or pleural effusion; newborn, 12–18 Fr; 1–2 y, 14–24 Fr; 5 y, 20–32; > 5 y, as for adult)
- Water-seal drainage system (eg, Pleur-Evac) with connecting tubing to wall suction
- Minor procedure tray and instrument tray (see page 243)
- Silk or nylon suture (0 to 2-0)
- Petrolatum gauze (Vaseline) (optional)
- 4 × 4 gauze dressing and cloth tape
- Pulse oximeter monitoring (recommended)

Background

A chest tube is usually placed to manage an ongoing intrathoracic process that cannot be managed with simple thoracentesis (page 310). The traditional methods of chest tube placement are described. Use of percutaneous tube thoracostomy kits for the Seldinger technique (used for small pneumothoraces when there is no risk of ongoing air leak) is contraindicated in severe conditions (eg, empyema, major pneumothorax > 20%, tension pneumothorax, chronic effusion). This procedure can be painful and may require conscious sedation.

Procedure

1. Before placing the tube, review the CXR unless an emergency does not allow time. For pneumothorax, choose a high anterior site (2nd or 3rd ICS, midclavicular line, or subaxillary position). Subaxillary placement leaves the best appearance. Place a low lateral chest tube in the 5th or 6th ICS in the midaxillary line and direct it posteriorly for fluid removal (usually corresponds to the inframammary crease.) In traumatic pneumothorax, use a low lateral site because it is usually associated with bleeding. In rare instances loculated apical pneumothorax or effusion may necessitate placement of an anterior tube in the 2nd ICS at the midclavicular line. When a tube is placed on the right side, the right hemidiaphragm may be slightly elevated because of the anatomic position of the liver. Insert the tube above the diaphragm in the pleural space.

2. Choose the appropriate chest tube. Use a 16- to 24-Fr tube for pneumothorax and 28–36 Fr for fluid removal. A **"thoracic catheter"** has multiple holes and works best for nearly all purposes.

3. Position the patient in an appropriate manner. If the patient is supine, have him or her raise the ipsilateral arm over the head to expose the rib space. If the patient is in the lateral decubitus position, have him or her place the ipsilateral arm on a bedside tray table.

4. Wear mask, hat, gown, and sterile gloves. Prep the area with chlorhexidine solution and drape it with sterile towels. Use lidocaine (with or without epinephrine) to anesthetize the skin, intercostal muscle, and periosteum of the rib; start at the center of the rib and gently work over the top. Remember, the neurovascular bundle runs under the rib (Figure 13–8). The needle then can be gently "popped" through the pleura, and the aspiration of air or fluid confirms the correct location for the chest tube. Back out the needle slowly until no fluid or air is aspirated just outside the parietal pleura, and inject lidocaine. There is no benefit in injecting lidocaine inside the pleural space. If the procedure is elective, the patient is extremely anxious, and the patient's respiratory status is not compromised, sedation **occasionally** is helpful. When the procedure is performed under conscious sedation with anxiolytics and IV narcotics, place the patient in a monitored setting.

5. Make a 2- to 3-cm transverse incision over the center of the rib with a no. 15 or no. 11 scalpel blade. Use a blunt-tipped clamp to dissect over the top of the rib and make a SQ tunnel (see Figure 13–8).

6. Puncture the parietal pleura with the hemostat, and spread the opening. **Be careful not to injure the lung parenchyma with the hemostat tips.** If the tube is inserted for a pneumothorax, a rush of air usually is heard on entry into the pleural cavity. If the tube is placed for effusion, fluid under pressure may be released at this time. Insert a gloved finger into the pleural cavity to gently clear any clots or adhesions and to make certain the lung is not accidentally punctured by the tube.

7. Carefully insert the tube into the desired position with a hemostat or gloved finger as a guide. Make sure all the holes in the tube are in the chest cavity. Attach the end of the tube to a water-seal or Pleur-Evac suction system. One indication of proper placement in the pleural place is fogging on the inner tubing of the

13

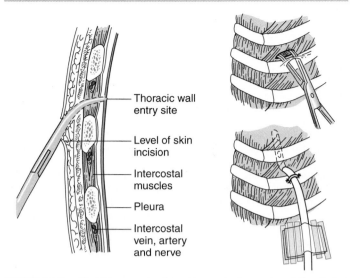

Thoracic wall
entry site

Level of skin
incision

Intercostal
muscles

Pleura

Intercostal
vein, artery
and nerve

FIGURE 13–8.   Chest tube procedure for making a subcutaneous tunnel. The skin incision is lower than the thoracic wall entry site. If a patient has signs of tension pneumothorax (acute shortness of breath, hypotension, distended neck veins, tachypnea, tracheal deviation) before a chest tube is placed, urgent treatment is needed. Insert a 14-gauge needle into the chest in the 2nd ICS in the midclavicular line to rapidly decompress the tension pneumothorax and proceed with chest tube insertion. Do not wait for chest x-ray confirmation before inserting a needle into the chest if the diagnosis of tension pneumothorax is suspected. (Reprinted, with permission, from: Gomella TL [ed] *Neonatology: Basic Management, On-Call Problems, Diseases, Drugs*, 5th ed. McGraw-Hill, 2004.)

13

chest tube that varies with respiration. To guarantee intrapleural position, make sure you observe respiratory variation within the tube or suction system to guarantee intrapleural position. Some chest tubes have sharp trocars that are used to pierce the chest wall and place the chest tube simultaneously with minimal amounts of dissection. These instruments are extremely dangerous and are usually placed in the anterior high position (ie, 2nd, 3rd, or 4th ICS).

8. Suture the tube in place. Place a heavy silk or polypropylene (0 or 2-0) suture through the incision next to the tube. Tie the incision together, then tie the ends around the chest tube. Make sure to wrap the suture around the tube several times. Tie the suture around the tube tightly enough that the tubing dimples slightly but not so tightly as to occlude the lumen. This step prevents the tube from slipping through the suture. As an alternative, place a purse-string suture (or "U stitch") around the insertion site. Make sure all of the suction holes are in the chest cavity before the tube is secured.

9. Cover the insertion site with plain gauze. Make the dressing as airtight as possible with tape, and secure all connections in the tubing to prevent accidental loss of the water seal. Some physicians wrap the insertion site with petrolatum (Vaseline or Xeroform) gauze, but these materials can be troublesome (ie, they are not water soluble and act as a foreign body), inhibit wound healing, and may not actually seal the site.

10. Start suction (usually −20 cm water in adults, −16 cm in children) and obtain a portable CXR immediately to check placement of the tube and to evaluate for residual pneumothorax or fluid.

Chest Tube Placement Using Seldinger Technique

Kits for chest tube insertion by the Seldinger technique are good for nonemergency chest tube placement, make the tube easier to insert, and cause less patient discomfort than other equipment.

1. After sterile prepping and draping, anesthetize the skin over the desired ICS (see details above). Insert the needle over the rib space to avoid injury to the intercostal bundle.

2. Once air (from pneumothorax) or fluid (from effusion) is aspirated, introduce a wire, serial dilators, and finally the desired chest tube. Secure the chest tube to the skin and connect it to the Pleur-Evac system as described earlier.

Chest Tube Removal

1. Verify that the pneumothorax or hemothorax is cleared. Check for air leak by having the patient cough; observe the water-seal system for bubbling that indicates either a system (tubing) leak or persistent pleural air leak.

2. Take the tube off suction **but not off water seal,** and cut the retention suture. Have the patient inspire deeply and perform the Valsalva maneuver while you apply pressure with petrolatum gauze or with a sufficient amount of antibiotic ointment on 4 × 4 gauze with additional 4 × 4 gauze squares. Pull the tube rapidly while the patient performs the Valsalva maneuver, and make an airtight seal with tape. Check an "upright" exhalation CXR for pneumothorax.

13

Pleurodesis

1. Used for recurrent pneumothorax or in recurrent malignant effusion with the goal to obliterate pleural space. It is an uncomfortable procedure, and sedation with a short-acting narcotic is recommended. Sclerosing agents used include doxycycline (500–1000 mg in 100 mL NS), talc (2 g/100 mL NS), and bleomycin (60 units/100 mL NS).

2. After the chest tube is in place, inject 20–40 mL 1% lidocaine into the tube and allow to enter the pleural space. Clamp the tube, and move the patient through various positions (Trendelenburg, reverse Trendelenburg, right and left lateral decubitus) to allow the lidocaine to disperse.

3. Connect the syringe containing the sclerosing agent to the chest tube and release the clamp. Inject the agent and clamp the tube for 4 h. It is important to use sterile technique when injecting into the tube because the pleural cavity is a sterile one. If at any time during clamping the patient experiences severe dyspnea or hypoxia, unclamp the tube because the lung may have collapsed and needs to be re-expanded.

4. Unclamp the tube and connect it to the Pleur-Evac suction device for 24–48 additional hours. Remove the tube after drainage is minimal and a CXR shows no pneumothorax.

5. To prevent tension pneumothorax or subcutaneous emphysema if sclerosing is performed for a persistent air leak, do not clamp the chest tube.

Place the chest tubing system on water-seal mode over an IV pole to prevent drainage of sclerosing agent but to allow air to escape if pressure develops within the chest. After 4 h, take down the tubing system from the IV pole, and place the chest tube back on suction for 24–48 h.

Complications

Infection, bleeding, lung damage, SQ emphysema, persistent pneumothorax or hemothorax, poor tube placement, cardiac arrhythmia

CRICOTHYROIDOTOMY (NEEDLE AND SURGICAL)

Indications

- Immediate mechanical ventilation when an endotracheal or orotracheal tube cannot be placed (eg, severe maxillofacial trauma, excessive oropharyngeal hemorrhage)

Contraindications

- Child < 12 y; use needle approach instead

Basic Materials

- Oxygen connecting tubing, high-flow oxygen source (tank or wall)
- Bag ventilator

Needle Cricothyroidotomy

- 12- to 14-gauge catheter-over-needle assembly (Angiocath or other)
- 6–12-mL syringe
- 3-mm pediatric ET adapter

13

Surgical Cricothyroidotomy (Minimum Requirements)

- Minor procedure and instrument tray (page 243) plus tracheal spreader if available
- No. 5–7 tracheostomy tube (6- to 8-Fr ET can be substituted)
- Tracheostomy tube adapter to connect to bag–mask ventilator

Procedure

Needle Cricothyroidotomy
1. With the patient supine, place a roll behind the shoulders to gently hyperextend the neck.
2. Palpate the cricothyroid membrane, which resembles a notch between the caudal end of the thyroid cartilage and the cricoid cartilage. Prep the area with povidone–iodine solution. Local anesthesia can be used if the patient is awake.
3. Mount the syringe on the 12- or 14-gauge catheter-over-needle assembly, and advance the syringe through the cricothyroid membrane at a 45-degree angle, applying back pressure on the syringe until air is aspirated.
4. Advance the catheter, and remove the needle. Attach the hub to a 3-mm ET adapter that is connected to the oxygen tubing. Use a Y-connector or a hole in the side of the tubing to turn the flow on and off, allowing oxygen to flow at 15 L/min for 1–2 s on, then 4 s off.

5. The needle technique is only useful for about 45 min because the exhalation of CO_2 is suboptimal.

Surgical Cricothyroidotomy

1. Follow steps 1 and 2 as for needle cricothyroidotomy.
2. Make a 3- to 4-cm vertical skin incision through the cervical fascia and strap muscles in the midline over the cricothyroid membrane. Expose the cricothyroid membrane, and make a horizontal incision. Insert the knife handle and rotate it 90 degrees to open the hole in the membrane. As an alternative, use a hemostat or tracheal spreader to dilate the opening.
3. Insert a small (5–7 mm) tracheostomy tube, inflate the balloon (if present), and secure it in position with the attached cotton tapes. Because the procedure is performed in an emergency, if a tracheostomy tube is not immediately available, use a smaller diameter ET (6–7 Fr).
4. Attach to oxygen source and ventilate. Listen to the chest for symmetrical breath sounds.
5. Replace a surgical cricothyroidotomy with a formal tracheostomy after the patient's condition has stabilized, generally within 24–36 h.

Complications

Bleeding, esophageal perforation, SQ emphysema, pneumomediastinum and pneumothorax, CO_2 retention (especially with the needle procedure)

CULDOCENTESIS
Indications

- Diagnostic technique for problems of acute abdominal pain in women
- Evaluation of female patient with signs of hypovolemia and possible intraabdominal bleeding
- Evaluation of ascites, especially in possible cases of gynecologic malignant disease

13

Materials

- Speculum
- Antiseptic swabs
- Chlorhexidine
- 1% lidocaine
- 18- to 21-gauge spinal needle
- 2 (10 mL) syringes and tenaculum

Procedure

1. Perform a careful pelvic exam to document uterine position and rule out pelvic mass at risk of perforation by the culdocentesis.
2. Obtain informed consent, and prep the vagina with antiseptic (eg, chlorhexidine).
3. Using the long needle, inject 1% lidocaine submucosally in the posterior cervical fornix before applying the tenaculum.
4. Improve traction by applying the tenaculum to the posterior cervical lip.
5. Connect an 18- to 21-gauge spinal needle to a 10-mL syringe filled with 1 mL of air.

6. Moving the needle forward through the posterior cervical fornix, apply light pressure to the syringe until the air passes. Maintain traction on the tenaculum while advancing the spinal needle to maximize the surface area of the cul-de-sac for needle entry.

7. After the abdomen has been entered, ask the patient to elevate herself on her elbows to allow gravity drainage into the area of needle entry. Apply negative pressure to the syringe. Slowly rotating the needle and slowly removing it may aid in detection and aspiration of a pocket of fluid.

8. If the first culdocentesis attempt is not successful, repeat the procedure with a different angle of approach.

9. Although perforation of a viscus is a possibility, the complication rate of culdocentesis is low. Fresh blood that clots rapidly is probably the result of traumatic tap, and the procedure can be repeated.

10. If blood is aspirated, spin it for HCT, and place it in an empty glass test tube to determine the presence or absence of a clot. Failure of blood to clot suggests old hemorrhage.

11. If pus is aspirated, send specimens for GC, aerobic, anaerobic, *Chlamydia, Mycoplasma,* and *Ureaplasma* cultures.

12. If a malignant tumor is suspected, send fluid for cytologic evaluation.

Complications

Infection, hemorrhage, air embolus, perforated viscus

DOPPLER PRESSURES
Indications

- Evaluation of peripheral vascular disease (ankle/brachial [A/B] or ankle/ arm [A/I] index)
- Routine BP measurement in infants or critically ill adults

Materials

- Doppler flow monitor
- Conductive gel (lubricant jelly can also be used)
- BP cuff

Procedure (A/B or A/A Index)

1. Determine the BP in each arm.

2. Measure the pressures in the popliteal arteries by placing a BP cuff on the thigh. The pressures in the dorsalis pedis arteries (on the top of the foot) and the posterior tibial arteries (behind the medial malleolus) are determined with a BP cuff on the calf.

3. Apply conductive jelly and place the Doppler transducer over the artery. Inflate the BP cuff until the pulsatile flow is no longer heard. Deflate the cuff until the flow returns. This is the systolic, or Doppler, pressure. *Note:* The Doppler examination does not give the diastolic pressure, and a palpable pulse need not be present for Doppler studies.

4. The **A/B** or **A/A index** is often computed from Doppler pressure. It is equal to the best systolic pressure in the ankle (usually from the posterior tibial artery) divided by the systolic pressure in the arm. An A/B index > 0.9 is usually normal, and an index < 0.5 is usually associated with sig-

nificant peripheral vascular disease. In patients with long-standing diabetes, the foot arteries can be severely calcified, and thus ankle systolic pressures may be falsely elevated because of the pressure needed to compress the calcified arteries.

ELECTROCARDIOGRAM

Basic ECG interpretation is described in Chapter 19.

Indications

- Evaluation of chest pain and other cardiac conditions

Materials

- ECG machine with paper and lead electrodes
- Adhesive electrode pads

Procedure

Most hospitals have fully automated ECG machines. Become acquainted with the machine at your hospital before using it. The following is a general outline.

1. Start with the patient in a comfortable, recumbent position. Explain the steps of the procedure to the patient. Instruct the patient to lie as still as possible to cut down on artifacts in the tracing.
2. Plug in the ECG machine and turn it on.
3. Attach the electrodes as follows:
    a. **Patient Cables.** A standard ECG machine has five lead wires, one for each limb and one for the chest leads. Newer machines have six precordial electrodes, all of which are placed in the proper positions before the procedure. The leads may be color-coded in the following manner:

    - RA: White—right arm
    - LA: Black—left arm
    - RL: Green—right leg
    - LL: Red—left leg
    - C: Brown—chest

    b. **Limb Electrodes.** Newer machines have self-adhering electrode pads. Older machines have flat, rectangular plates held in place by straps that encircle the limb. Place each electrode on the limb indicated, wrist or ankle, usually on the ventral surface. In case of amputation or presence of a cast, placing the lead on the shoulder or groin has minimal effect on the tracing.
    c. **Chest (Precordial) Electrodes.** With newer machines all leads can be placed before the ECG is run with all pads applied at the same time. This makes locating the proper positions quick and easy (Figure 13–9, page 272). Older units have a suction cup chest electrode that is brown and designated by the letter "C." It is attached in sequence to each of the positions on the precordium. Precordial leads are placed as follows:

    - V_1 = 4th ICS just to the **right** of the sternal border
    - V_2 = 4th ICS just to the **left** of the sternal border

13

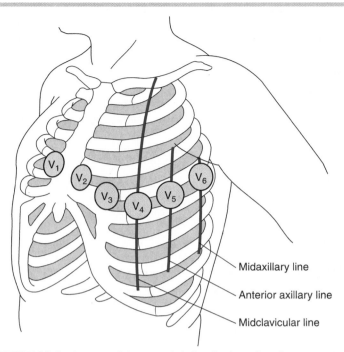

FIGURE 13–9. Location of the precordial chest leads used in obtaining a routine ECG.

13

- V_3 = midway between leads V_2 and V_4
- V_4 = midclavicular line in the 5th ICS
- V_5 = anterior axillary line at the same level as V_4
- V_6 = midaxillary line at the same level as leads V_4 and V_5

4. When everything is ready, follow the directions for your particular machine to obtain the ECG tracing. It should include 12 leads: I, II, III, AVR, AVL, and V_1–V_6. Standard paper speed is 25 mm/s.
5. Label the tracing with the patient's name, date, time, and any other useful information, such as medications, and your name. A routine 12-lead ECG should take 4–8 min.

Helpful Hints

1. The second rib inserts at the sternal angle, and therefore the second ICS is directly inferior to the sternal angle. Feel down two more ICSs and you have the fourth ICS to position V_1 and V_2.
2. Learn the color scheme for the leads; doing so can be very useful in an emergency. Some memory aids include
   a. Red and green go to the legs: "Christmas on the bottom" or "When driving your car you use your left leg to brake (red light) and your right leg to go (green light)."

b. Black (left) and white (right) go to the arms: "Remember white is right and black is left."
c. Brown is for the chest.

ENDOTRACHEAL INTUBATION
Indications

- Airway management during CPR
- Any indication for using mechanical ventilation (eg, respiratory failure, coma, general anesthesia)

Contraindications

- Massive maxillofacial trauma (relative)
- Fractured larynx
- Suspected cervical spinal cord injury (relative)

Materials

- Endotracheal tube of appropriate size (Table 13–3)
- Laryngoscope handle and blade (straight [Miller] or curved [MAC]; size no. 3 for adults, no. 1–1.5 for small children)
- 10-mL syringe, adhesive tape, benzoin
- Suction equipment (Yankauer suction)
- Malleable stylet (optional)
- Oropharyngeal airway

Procedure

1. Orotracheal intubation is most commonly used and is described here. In suspected cervical spine injury, nasotracheal intubation is preferred.
2. Before attempting endotracheal intubation (bag–mask or mouth to mask), ventilate any patient who is hypoxic or apneic. Avoid prolonged periods of no ventilation if the intubation is difficult. A rule of thumb is to hold your

13

TABLE 13–3
Recommended Endotracheal Tube Sizes

Patient	Internal Diameter (mm)	
Premature infant	2.5–3.0	(uncuffed)
Newborn infant	3.5	(uncuffed)
3–12 mo	4.0	(uncuffed)
1–8 y	4.0–6.0	(uncuffed)a
8–16 y	6.0–7.0	(cuffed)
Adult	7.0–9.0	(cuffed)

aRough estimate is to measure the little finger.

breath while attempting intubation. When you need to take a breath, so must the patient. Resume ventilation, and reattempt intubation in a minute or so.

3. Extend the laryngoscope blade to 90 degrees to verify the light is working, and check the balloon on the tube (if present) for leaks.

4. Place the patient's head in the "sniffing position" (neck extended anteriorly and the head extended posteriorly). Use suction to clear the upper airway if needed.

5. Hold the laryngoscope in your left hand, hold the mouth open with your right hand, and use the blade to push the tongue to patient's left while keeping it anterior to the blade. Advance the blade carefully toward the midline until the epiglottis is visualized. Use suction if needed.

6. If a **straight laryngoscope blade** is used, pass it under the epiglottis and **lift** upward to visualize the vocal cords (Figure 13–10, below). If the **curved blade** is used, place it anterior to the epiglottis (into the vallecula) and gently lift anteriorly. In either case, **do not use the handle to pry the epiglottis open,** but rather gently lift to expose the vocal cords (ie, minimize torquing action).

7. While maintaining visualization of the cords, grasp the tube in your dominant hand and pass it through the cords. With more difficult intubations, use the malleable stylet to direct the tube.

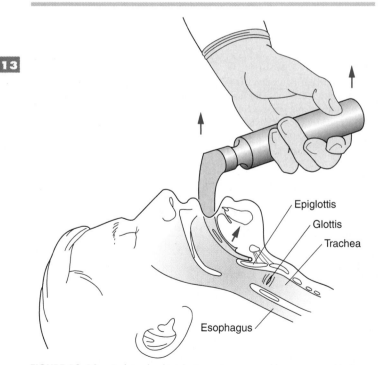

FIGURE 13–10. Endotracheal intubation using a curved laryngoscope blade.

8. If the patient may have eaten recently, have an assistant place gentle pressure over the cricoid cartilage to occlude the esophagus and prevent aspiration during intubation. "Cricoid pressure" can also facilitate visualization of the vocal cords in patients whose larynx is situated more anteriorly than usual.

9. When using a cuffed tube (adults and older children), gently inflate with air using a 10-mL syringe until the seal is adequate (about 5 mL). Ventilate the patient while auscultating and visualizing both sides of the chest to verify positioning. Failure of the left side to ventilate may signify that the tube has been advanced down the right mainstem bronchus. Withdraw the tube 1–2 cm, and recheck the breath sounds. Also auscultate over the stomach to ensure the tube is not mistakenly placed in the esophagus. Confirm positioning with a CXR. The tip of the ET should be a few centimeters above the carina. If a CO_2 colorimetric device is available, confirm placement of the tube by connecting the device to the ET between the adapter and the ventilating device.

10. Tape the tube in position, and insert an oropharyngeal airway to prevent the patient from biting the tube. Consider an orogastric tube to prevent regurgitation.

Complications

Bleeding, oral or pharyngeal trauma, improper tube positioning (esophageal intubation, right mainstem bronchus), aspiration, tube obstruction or kinking

FEVER WORK-UP

Although not a standard "bedside procedure," fever work-up involves judicious use of invasive procedures. The true definition of a *fever* can vary from service to service. General guidelines to follow are that a fever is an oral temperature > 100.4°F (38°) on a medical or surgical service and a rectal temperature of ≥ 101°F (38.3°C) or oral temperature ≥ 100°F (37.7°C) in an infant or immunocompromised patient. When evaluating a patient for a fever, consider whether the temperature is oral, rectal, tympanic, or axillary (rectal and tympanic temperatures are about 1°F higher and axillary temperatures are about 1°F lower than oral); whether the patient has drunk hot or cold liquids or smoked around the time of the determination; and whether the patient is taking antipyretics. Also, remember body temperature is highest at about 8 PM (+ 0.5°F from 98.6°F) and lowest at about 4 AM (−1 to 1.5°F). Differential diagnosis of fever and fever of unknown origin are discussed in Chapter 3.

General Fever Work-Up

1. Quickly review the chart and medication record if the patient is not familiar to you.
2. Question and examine the patient to locate any obvious sources of fever.
   a. **Ears, nose, sinuses and throat:** Especially in children
   b. **Neck:** Pain with flexion
   c. **Nodes:** Adenopathy
   d. **Lungs:** Rales (crackles), rhonchi (wheezes), decreased breath sounds, or dullness to percussion. Can the patient generate an effective cough?
   e. **Heart:** A new or changing heart murmur, which may suggest endocarditis

    f.   **Abdomen:** Presence or absence of bowel sounds, guarding, rigidity, tenderness, bladder fullness, or costovertebral angle tenderness

    g.   **Genitourinary:** If a Foley catheter is in place, note appearance of the urine, grossly and microscopically

    h.   **Rectal Exam:** Tenderness or fluctuance that suggests an abscess or acute prostatitis

    i.   **Pelvic Exam:** Especially in the postpartum patient or sexually active woman with multiple partners

    j.   **Wounds:** Erythema, tenderness, swelling, or drainage from surgical sites

    k.   **Extremities:** Signs of inflammation at IV sites. Look for thigh or calf tenderness and swelling.

    l.   **Miscellaneous:** Consider the possibility of a drug fever (eosinophil count on the CBC may be elevated) or NG tube fever. Look at every IV site looking for cellulitis or IV infiltrates and also remember central lines, Infus-a-port devices, and PICC lines as potential sources of fever. Do all of the above before beginning to investigate the less common or less obvious causes of a fever.

3.   **Laboratory Studies**

    a.   **Basic:** CBC with diff, UA, cultures and Gram stains: urine, blood, sputum, wound, spinal fluid (**especially** in children < 4–6 mo old)

    b.   **Other:** Order based on clinical findings:

        (i)   **Radiographic:** Chest or abdominal films, CT or ultrasound exam

        (ii)   **Invasive:** LP, thoracentesis, paracentesis are more aggressive procedures that may be indicated.

Miscellaneous Fever Facts

1.   **Causes of Fever in the Postop Patient:** Think of the "Six Ws":

    a.   **Wind:** Atelectasis secondary to intubation and anesthesia is the most common cause of immediate postop fever. To treat, have the patient sitting up and ambulating, using incentive spirometry, P&PD, etc.

    b.   **Water:** UTI; may be secondary to presence of a bladder catheter

    c.   **Wound:** Infection; a very high fever in the immediately postoperative period can be indicative of a clostridial or group A streptococcal soft-tissue necrotizing infection. Examine the wound for signs of necrosis, including crepitus deep to the epidermis. If necrosis is present, debride the wound to clean edges immediately, and order antibiotics.

    d.   **Walking:** Phlebitis, DVT

    e.   **Wonder Drugs:** Drug fever (common causes are listed on page 39).

    f.   **Woman:** Endometritis, mastitis (common only in postpartum period)

2.   **Elevated WBC Count:** Commonly elevated secondary to catecholamine discharge after stress such as surgery or childbirth. However, very low white counts can also be a sign of overwhelming sepsis or immunocompromise.

3.   **Temperatures of 103–105°F** (39.4–40.5°C) In adults, think of lung or kidney infections, or bacteremia.

4.   **Lethargy, Combativeness, Inappropriate Behavior:** Strongly consider doing an LP to rule out meningitis.

5.   **Elderly Patients:** Can be extremely ill without many of the typical manifestations; they may be hypothermic or may deny any tenderness that

13

could point toward an obvious source. On laboratory examination, elderly patients may not mount the same WBC response to an infection that an otherwise young, healthy individual might. Be aggressive in identifying the cause.

6. **Infants and Children:** Have normally elevated baseline temperatures (up to 3 mo, 99.4°F [37.4°C]; 1 y, 99.7°F [37.6°C]; 3 y, 99.0°F [37.2°C]).

7. **Immunosuppressed patients** after solid organ transplantation or patients being treated with high doses of steroids may not be able to mount a fever in response to stress or infection. In this patient population, normal temperatures do not exclude infection.

GASTROINTESTINAL INTUBATION

Indications

- GI decompression: ileus, obstruction, pancreatitis associated with emesis, postoperative period
- Lavage of the stomach with GI bleeding or drug overdose
- Prevention of aspiration in an obtunded patient
- Feeding a patient who is unable to swallow

Materials

- GI tube of choice (see following list)
- Lubricant jelly
- Catheter tip syringe
- Glass of water with a straw, stethoscope

Types of GI Tubes

13

1. **Nasogastric Tubes**
   a. **Levin:** A tube with a single lumen, a perforated tip, and side holes for the aspiration of gastric contents. Connect the tube to an intermittent suction device to prevent the stomach lining from obstructing the lumen. Sometimes it is necessary to cut off the tip to allow aspiration of larger pills and tablets. The size varies from 10 to 18 Fr (1 Fr unit = 1/3 mm in diameter, see page 244).
   b. **Salem Sump:** A double-lumen tube; the smaller tube is an air intake vent so that continuous suction can be applied. The best tube for irrigation and lavage because it will not collapse on itself. If a Salem sump tube stops working even after it is repositioned, often a "shot" of air from a catheter-tipped syringe in the air vent will clear the tube. Both the Salem sump and Levin tubes have radiopaque markings. In general, for suspected obstruction place an 18-Fr tube; smaller diameter tubes are less effective at suctioning and become clogged more easily than wider tubes.

2. **Intestinal Decompression Tubes** ("long intestinal tubes"). These tubes have largely fallen out of favor because of a lack of data supporting their use in intestinal obstruction.
   a. **Cantor Tube:** A long single-lumen tube with a rubber balloon at the tip. The balloon is partially filled with mercury (5–7 mL through a tangentially directed 21-gauge needle, then the air is aspirated), which

allows it to gravitate into the small bowel with the aid of peristalsis. Used for decompression of distal bowel obstruction.

b. **Miller–Abbott Tube:** A long double-lumen tube with a rubber balloon at the tip. One lumen is used for aspiration; the other connects to the balloon. After the tube is in the stomach, inflate the balloon with 5–10 mL of air, inject 2–3 mL of mercury into the balloon, and then aspirate the air. Functioning and indications are essentially the same as for the Cantor tube. **Do not** tape these intestinal tubes to the patient's nose, or the tube will not descend. The progress of the tube can be followed on radiographs.

3. **Feeding Tubes.** Although any NG tube can be used as a feeding tube, it is preferable to place a specially designed nasoduodenal feeding tube. These tubes are of smaller diameter (usually 8 Fr) and are more pliable and comfortable for the patient. Weighted tips tend to travel into the duodenum, which may help prevent regurgitation and aspiration. Most feeding tubes are supplied with stylets that facilitate positioning, especially if fluoroscopic guidance is needed. Always verify the position of the feeding tube with a radiograph before starting tube feeding. Commonly used tubes include mercury-weighted varieties **(Keogh tube, Duo-Tube, Dobbhoff),** tungsten-weighted **(Vivonex tube),** and unweighted pediatric feeding tubes. Take great care with these tubes because complications such as tracheobronchial intubation can easily occur.

4. **Miscellaneous Gastrointestinal Tubes**

a. **Sengstaken–Blakemore Tube:** A triple-lumen tube used exclusively for the control of bleeding esophageal varices by tamponade. One lumen is for gastric aspiration, one is for the gastric balloon, and the third is for the esophageal balloon. Other types include the **Linton** and **Minnesota** tubes. These tubes are no longer routinely used; quick access to endoscopy allows for more efficient treatment under direct visualization.

b. **Ewald Tube:** An orogastric tube used almost exclusively for gastric evacuation of blood or drug overdose. The tube is usually double lumen and large diameter (18–36 Fr).

c. **Dennis, Baker, Leonard Tubes:** Used for intraoperative decompression of the bowel and are manually passed into the bowel at the time of laparotomy.

Procedure (for Nasogastric and Feeding Tubes)

1. Inform the patient of the nature of the procedure and encourage cooperation if the patient is able. Choose the nasal passage that appears most open. The patient should sit up if able. Before beginning the procedure, ask the patient about recent facial or skull base fractures or trauma and recent transphenoidal and other neurosurgical or otolaryngologic procedures.

2. Lubricate the distal 3–4 in (8–10 cm) of the tube with a water-soluble jelly (K-Y Jelly or viscous lidocaine), and insert the tube gently along the floor of the nasal passageway. Maintain gentle pressure that will allow the tube to pass into the nasopharynx. Have the patient flex the neck slightly from neutral. Inform the patient that it may be slightly uncomfortable and to avoid gasping, which can cause inadvertent tracheal intubation.

3. When the patient can feel the tube in the back of the throat, ask him or her to swallow small amounts of water through a straw as you advance the tube 2–3 in (5–8 cm) at a time.

4. To be sure that the tube is in the stomach, aspirate gastric contents or blow air into the tube with a catheter-tipped syringe and listen over the stomach with a stethoscope for a "pop" or "gurgle." To prevent accidental bronchial instillation of tube feedings, **verify** the position of feeding tubes with radiography before starting feedings. Most Salem sump tubes have four black markers at the end of the tube. Proper placement in most adults is achieved when two of the markers are inside the patient and two are outside.

5. NG tubes are attached either to low continuous wall suction (Salem sump tubes with a vent) or to intermittent suction (Levin tubes); the latter allows the tube to fall away from the gastric wall between suction cycles.

6. Feeding and pediatric feeding tubes in adults are more difficult to insert because they are more flexible. Many are provided with stylets that make passage easier. Feeding tubes are best placed into the duodenum or jejunum to decrease the risk of aspiration. Administer 10 mg of metoclopramide (Reglan) IV 10 min before insertion to aid in placing the tube into the duodenum. Once the feeding tube is in the stomach, place the bell of the stethoscope on the right side of the middle portion of the patient's abdomen. While advancing the tube, inject air to confirm progression of the tube to the right, toward the duodenum. If the sound of the air becomes fainter, the tube is probably curling in the stomach. Pass the tube until a slight resistance is felt, heralding the presence of the tip of the tube at the pylorus. Holding constant pressure and slowly injecting water through the tube is often rewarded with a "give," which signifies passage through the pylorus. The tube often can be advanced far into the duodenum with this method. The duodenum usually provides constant resistance that will give with slow injection of water. Placing the patient in the right lateral decubitus position may help the tube enter the duodenum. Always confirm the location of the tube with an abdominal radiograph.

7. Tape the tube securely in place, but do not allow it to apply pressure to the ala of the nose. (*Note:* Intestinal decompression tubes should not be taped because they are allowed to pass through the intestine.) Patients have been disfigured because of ischemic necrosis of the nose caused by a poorly positioned NG tube.

8. Be extremely careful with sedated and intubated patients because it is possible to introduce these small feeding tubes past the ET into the trachea and furthermore into the distal bronchial tree, causing pneumothorax. If you meet any resistance, stop immediately and obtain a CXR to assess placement.

13

Complications

- Inadvertent passage into the trachea can provoke coughing or gagging in the patient.
- Aspiration
- If the patient is unable to cooperate, the tube often becomes coiled in the oral cavity.
- The tube is irritating and may cause a small amount of bleeding in the mucosa of the nose, pharynx, or stomach. The drying and irritation can be lessened with throat lozenges or antiseptic spray.

- Intracranial passage in a patient with a basilar skull fracture
- Esophageal perforation
- Esophageal reflux caused by tube-induced incompetence of the distal esophageal sphincter
- Sinusitis from edema of the nasal passages that blocks drainage from the nasal sinuses

HEELSTICK AND FINGERSTICK (CAPILLARY BLOOD SAMPLING)

Indication

- Collection of blood samples from infants
- Fingerstick also can be used for small samples in older children and adults

Materials

- Alcohol swabs
- Lancet (BD QuikHeel lancet, BD Genie Lancet for fingersticks that require high volume of blood. BD Genie needle lancet for glucose determinations)
- Collection container: capillary tube, BD Microtainer tube (with Micro-Guard closure) or Caraway tubes
- Clay or other capillary tube sealer

Heelstick Technique

To avoid the risk of repeated venous punctures, especially in infants, assays have been developed that rely on small volumes of blood. Although called "heelstick" and "fingerstick," any highly vascularized capillary bed can be used (finger pad, earlobe, and great toe).

13

1. The heel can be warmed for 5–10 min by wrapping it in a warm washcloth. Wipe the area with an alcohol swab. Use Figure 13–11A to choose the site for the puncture; use of these sites helps decrease risk of osteomyelitis.
2. Use a lancet, and make a quick, deep puncture so that blood flows freely (see Figure 13–11A). An automated safety lancet (BD QuikHeel Lancet in neonatal and infant sizes) for heelstick is held over the site at a 90-degree angle to the foot (Figure 13–11B). A button activates the blade, after which the blade retracts into its casing.
3. Wipe off the first drop of blood. Gently squeeze the heel and touch a collection tube to the drop of blood. The tube should fill by capillary action and is sealed.
4. Labs can make determinations on small samples from pediatric patients. A **Caraway tube** can hold 0.3 mL of blood. One to three Caraway tubes can be used for most routine tests. For a capillary blood gas, the blood is usually transferred to a 1-mL heparinized syringe and placed on ice. BD Microtainer tubes with Microgard closure are available in color-coded styles for specific blood determinations similar to those of larger Vacutainer tubes (See Table 13–8, page 318).
5. Samples should flow freely enough that the specimen can be collected in less than 2 min. Longer time periods may be affected by microclotting of the sample.
6. Wrap the site with 4 × 4 gauze squares, or apply an adhesive bandage.

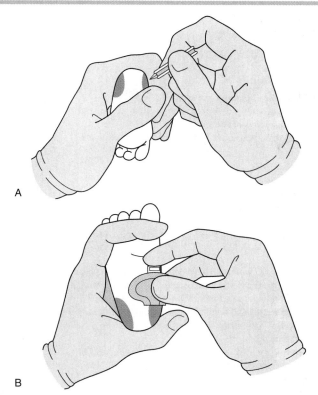

A

B

13

FIGURE 13-11. **A.** Preferred sites and technique of heelstick in an infant. (Reprinted, with permission, from: Gomella TL [ed] *Neonatology: Basic Management, On-Call Problems, Diseases, Drugs,* 5th ed. McGraw-Hill, 2004.) **B.** Use of an automated lancet (BD QuikHeel Lancet [BD Biosciences]) for heelstick in an infant. The device is held 90 degrees to the axis of the foot and activated.

Fingerstick Technique

1. Clean the puncture site with alcohol, and allow to air dry.
2. Remove the protective cap from the safety lancet (BD Genie lancet) and position the lancet over pad of finger.
3. Press the white activation button with your thumb. Discard device.
4. Gently massage from base of finger to puncture site to collect sample. Holding the patient's hand below level of elbow will enhance blood flow. For glucose determinations with a device such as the Genie needle lancet, only a drop of blood is needed to apply to the reagent strip for glucose determination. A lancet style device is not necessary because of the small amount of blood needed.
5. Follow steps 3–6 as for heelstick.

Complications

Cellulitis at site, osteomyelitis for heelstick in infants

INTERNAL FETAL SCALP MONITORING

Indication

- Accurate assessment of fetal heart rate (FHR) patterns during labor to screen for possible fetal distress

Contraindications

- Presence of placenta previa
- Lack of ability to identify the portion of the fetal body where device application is being considered
- Active herpes, active hepatitis, or HIV in the mother

Materials

- Fetal scalp monitoring electrode
- Sterile vaginal lubricant or povidone–iodine spray
- Spiral electrode
- Leg plate, fetal monitor

Procedure

1. Position the woman in the dorsal lithotomy position (knees flexed and abducted), and perform an aseptic perineal prep with sterile vaginal lubricant or povidone–iodine spray.
2. Perform a manual vaginal exam, and clearly identify the fetal presenting part. The membranes **must** be ruptured before attachment of the spiral electrode.
3. Remove the spiral electrode from the sterile package and place the guide tube firmly against the fetal presenting part. Electrode should not be applied to fetal face, fontanels, or genitalia.
4. Advance the drive tube and electrode until the electrode contacts the presenting part. Maintaining pressure on the guide tube and drive tube, rotate the drive tube clockwise until mild resistance is met (usually one turn).
5. Press together the arms on the drive tube grip, which releases the locking device. Carefully slide the drive and guide tubes off the electrode wires while holding the locking device open.
6. Attach the spiral electrode wires to the color-coded leg plate, which is then connected to the electronic fetal monitor.
7. Clean the area of electrode placement on the baby's scalp after delivery.

Complications

- Fetal or maternal hemorrhage, fetal infection (usually scalp abscess at the site of insertion)
- Malpositioning of the monitor on the maternal cervix making it impossible to obtain FHR. Test placement by gently pulling on the catheter; if the woman feels discomfort, the electrode may be inappropriately placed.

Interpretation

Normal FHR is 120–160 beats/min.

Accelerations: Increases in FHR can be associated with fetal distress (usually in association with late decelerations) but are almost always a sign of fetal well-being.

Decelerations: Transient decreases in FHR are related to a uterine contraction and are of three types:

1. **Early Deceleration:** In normal labor, slowing of FHR associated with the onset of a contraction. FHR promptly returns to normal after the contraction is over. Usually due to head compression, occasionally by cord compression.

2. **Late Deceleration:** Slowing of the FHR that occurs after the uterine contraction starts and the rate does not return to normal until well after the contraction is over. This pattern is often associated with uteroplacental insufficiency (fetal acidosis or hypoxia).

3. **Variable Deceleration:** Irregular pattern of deceleration unassociated with contractions; caused by cord compression.

Other Patterns

1. **Beat-to-Beat Variability:** Small fluctuations in FHR 5–15 beats/min over the baseline FHR usually associated with fetal well-being

2. **Bradycardia:** Associated with maternal and fetal hypoxia, fetal heart lesions including heart block. If bradycardia persists, evaluate with scalp pH.

3. **Tachycardia:** Often an early sign of fetal distress, seen with febrile illnesses, hypoxia, fetal thyrotoxicosis

4. **Sinusoidal Pattern:** Can be drug-induced and is seen occasionally with severe fetal anemia

INJECTION TECHNIQUES

Indications

- **Intradermal:** Most commonly used for skin testing (eg, PPD)
- **Subcutaneous:** Useful for low-volume medications such as insulin, heparin, and some vaccines
- **Intramuscular:** Administration of parenteral medications that cannot be absorbed from the SQ layer or of high volume (≤ 10 mL)

13

Contraindications

- Allergy to any components of the injectate
- Active infection or dermatitis at the injection site
- Coagulopathy (IM injections)

Procedure

Intradermal: (See Skin Testing, page 308.)

Subcutaneous

1. Deposit the drug within the fat but above the muscle. With careful placement of the injection, nerve injury is rarely a danger.

2. Choose a site free of scarring and active infection. Injection sites include the outer surface of the upper arm, anterior surface of the thigh, and lower abdominal wall. For repeated injections (eg, for diabetic patients), rotate the sites.

3. 25–27 gauge 3/4–1 in (2–2.5 cm) needles are most commonly used; volume of medication must not exceed 5 mL. Draw up the medication, making certain to expel any air bubbles.

4. Clean the site with an alcohol swab. Bunch up the skin with your thumb and forefinger so that the SQ tissue is off the underlying muscle.

5. Warn the patient that there will be "pinch" or "sting," and insert the needle firmly and rapidly at a 45-degree angle until a sudden release signifies penetration of the dermis.

6. Release the skin, aspirate to make certain a blood vessel has not been entered, and inject slowly.

7. Withdraw the needle and apply gentle pressure. Activate the automatic needle shield (eg, BD SafetyGlide shielding hypodermic needle) and discard the needle. A dressing is not usually necessary. Apply pressure longer if there is bleeding from the site.

Intramuscular

1. Common sites include the deltoid, gluteus, and vastus lateralis.
   - **Deltoid Muscle:** The safe zone includes only the main body of the deltoid muscle lying lateral and a few centimeters beneath the acromion. There is low risk of radial nerve injury unless the needle strays into the middle or lower third of the arm.
   - **Gluteus Muscles:** This muscle is the preferred site for children > 2 y and adults. Draw an imaginary line from the femoral head to the posterior superior iliac spine. This site (upper outer quadrant of the buttocks) is safe for injections because it is away from the sciatic nerve and superior gluteal artery.
   - **Vastus Lateralis Muscle** (anterior thigh): A very safe site for all patients and the site of choice for infants. The only disadvantage of this site is that the firm fascia lata overlying the muscle can make needle insertion somewhat more painful.

2. A 22-gauge, 1 1/2 in (4 cm) needle is acceptable for most IM injections. Remove air bubbles from the syringe and needle. Wipe the skin with alcohol.

3. Gently stretch the skin to one side and warn the patient of a sting. Penetrate the skin at a 90-degree angle, and advance the needle approximately 1 in (2.5 cm) into the muscle. (Obese patients may require deeper penetration with a longer needle.)

4. Aspirate to make sure a blood vessel has not been entered. Administer the medication. Gently massage the site with an alcohol swab or gauze to promote absorption.

Complications

- Nerve and arterial injury
- Abscesses (sterile or septic). Use good technique and rotate injection sites.
- Bleeding can usually be controlled with pressure.

INTRAUTERINE PRESSURE MONITORING

Indication

- Accurate assessment of uterine contraction during labor

Contraindication

- Placenta previa

Materials

- Pressure catheter and introducer
- Transducer connected to fetal monitor

- Sterile gloves, vaginal lubricant, povidone–iodine spray
- 10-mL syringe, 30 mL sterile water

Procedure

1. Prime the transducer with sterile water.
2. Position the patient in the dorsal lithotomy position (knees flexed and abducted), and perform an aseptic perineal prep with sterile vaginal lubricant or povidone–iodine spray.
3. Perform a manual vaginal exam, and clearly identify the fetal presenting part. The patient must be in labor with a cervix dilated at least 1–2 cm, and the membranes **must** be ruptured before insertion of the catheter.
4. Remove the catheter from the sterile package, and place the guide tube through your fingers around the presenting part into the uterine cavity.
5. Prime the catheter with sterile water and thread through the guide tube.
6. Attach the distal catheter to the transducer and zero to air.

Complications

Infection, placental perforation if the placenta is low lying

IV TECHNIQUES

Indication

- IV access for administration of fluids, blood, or medications (other techniques include Central Venous Catheterization, page 256, and Peripheral Insertion of Central Catheter (PICC), page 301.)

Materials

- IV fluid
- Connecting tubing
- Tourniquet
- Alcohol swab
- IV cannulas (a catheter over a needle [eg, BD Insyte Autoguard shielded IV catheter, BD Angiocath Autoguard shielded IV catheter] or a butterfly-style needle)
- Antiseptic ointment, dressing, and tape

Procedure

1. It helps to rip the tape into strips, attach the IV tubing to the solution, and flush the air out of the tubing before you begin.
2. The upper, nondominant extremity is the site of choice for an IV, unless the patient is being considered for placement of permanent hemodialysis access. In this instance, the upper nondominant extremity should be "saved" as the access site for hemodialysis. If the patient has previously undergone axillary lymph node dissection (eg, some breast cancer operations), start the IV on the side opposite the surgical site. Choose a distal vein (dorsum of the hand) so that if the vein is lost, you can reposition the IV more proximally. Figure 13–12 shows common upper extremity veins; avoid veins that cross a joint space. Also avoid the leg because of the increased risk of thrombophlebitis.

13

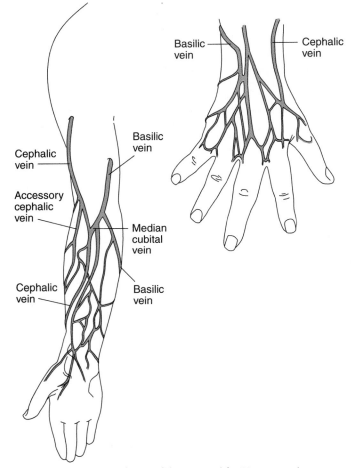

FIGURE 13–12. Principal veins of the arm used for IV access and in venipuncture. The pattern can be highly variable. (Reprinted, with permission, from: Stillman RM [ed] *Surgery, Diagnosis, and Therapy,* Appleton & Lange, Norwalk, CT, 1989.)

3. Apply a tourniquet above the proposed IV site. Use the techniques described in Venipuncture (page 316) to help expose the vein. Carefully clean the site with an alcohol or povidone–iodine swab. If a large-bore IV needle is to be used (16- or 14-gauge), local anesthesia (lidocaine injected with a 25-gauge needle) is helpful.

4. Stabilize the vein distally with the thumb of your free hand. Using the catheter-over-needle assembly, either enter the vein directly or enter the skin alongside the vein first and then stick the vein along the side at about a 20-degree angle. Direct-entry and side-entry IV techniques are illustrated in Figures 13–13 and 13–14. Once the vein is punctured, blood should

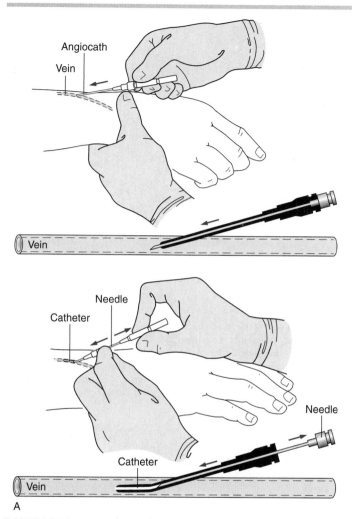

FIGURE 13–13. A. Technique for insertion of a standard catheter-over-needle device for IV access. Stabilize the vein with gentle traction. Enter the vein; when a flash of blood is observed in the chamber, advance the entire assembly slightly to ensure that the catheter tip is in the lumen of the vein. Advance the catheter off the end of the needle, and remove the needle.

appear in the "flash chamber." Lower the needle assembly. The next steps vary if you are using a standard catheter-over-needle device or a self-shielding device:

a. **Standard Catheter-over-Needle** (Figure 13–13A). Advance a few more millimeters to be sure that **both** the needle **and** the tip of the catheter have entered the vein. Thread the catheter into the vein while

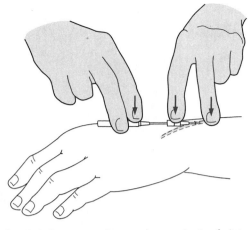

B

FIGURE 13–13. **B.** When using a device such as an Angiocath Autoguard (BD Biosciences), before pressing the autoshield button, apply digital pressure as shown to stabilize the catheter and to prevent blood from escaping after the needle is removed. Activate the self-shielding needle by pushing the white button on the needle device.

maintaining traction on the skin. Remove the tourniquet, compress the vein, and stabilize the catheter hub. Connect the IV fluid.

b. **Self Shielding Device.** After seeing the flashback, lower the catheter assembly to almost parallel to the skin. Advance the entire unit before attempting to thread the catheter. Thread the catheter into the vein while maintaining traction. Release the tourniquet and apply pressure

13

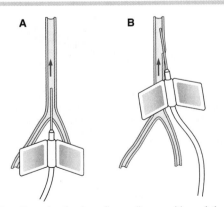

A   **B**

FIGURE 13–14. Example of a butterfly needle assembly and the two different techniques of entering a vein for IV access. **A.** Direct puncture. **B.** Side entry. (Reprinted, with permission, from: Gomella TL [ed] *Neonatology: Basic Management, On-Call Problems, Diseases, Drugs,* 5th ed. McGraw-Hill, 2004.)

beyond the catheter tip, making sure to maintain digital pressure beyond the catheter tip (Figure 13–13B). Press the white button, and the needle retracts into a shield. Connect the IV line to the catheter.

5. With the IV fluid running, observe the site for signs of induration and swelling, which indicate improper placement or damage to the vein. (See Chapter 9 for choosing IV fluids and how to determine infusion rates.)

6. Tape the IV securely in place; apply a drop of povidone–iodine or antibiotic ointment and apply a sterile dressing. Ideally, the dressing should be changed every 24–48 h to help reduce the likelihood of infection. Arm boards are also useful to help maintain an IV site.

7. **Never reinsert the needle into the catheter.** Doing so can cause shearing in the catheter.

8. **A butterfly,** or **scalp vein** needle can sometimes be used (see Figure 13–14). This small metal needle has plastic "wings" on the side. It is very useful in infants (who often have poor peripheral veins but prominent scalp veins), children, and in adults who have small, fragile veins.

9. **Troubleshooting difficult IV placement**

   • If the veins are deep and difficult to locate, a 3- to 5-mL syringe can be mounted on the catheter assembly. Determine proper positioning inside the vein by aspirating blood. If blood specimens are needed for a patient who also needs an IV, use this technique to start the IV and collect samples at the same time.

   • A **Whaid maneuver** can be attempted (*J Emerg Nurs* 1993;19: 186). Spend about 1 min using both hands to "milk" blood from the arm toward the forearm. While holding the arm compressed with both hands, place a tourniquet above the elbow. Milk the blood from the fingers to the forearm for 3–5 min. When a vein becomes prominent, wrap your hand around the patient's wrist and place the IV.

   • If no extremity vein can be found, try the external jugular vein. Placing the patient in the head-down position (deep Trendelenburg) can help distend the vein.

   • If all these maneuvers fail, insert a central venous line insertion (page 256).

13

LUMBAR PUNCTURE

Indications

   • **Diagnosis:** Analysis of CSF for conditions such as meningitis, encephalitis, Guillain–Barré syndrome, and staging work-up for lymphoma
   • **Measurement of CSF pressure** or its changes with various maneuvers (eg, Valsalva)
   • **Injection of agents** eg, contrast media for myelography, antitumor drugs, analgesics, antibiotics

Contraindications

   • Increased intracranial pressure (papilledema, mass lesion)
   • Infection near the puncture site
   • Planned myelography or pneumoencephalography
   • Coagulation disorders

Materials

- Sterile, disposable LP kit

or

- Minor procedure tray (see page 243)
- Spinal needles (21-gauge for adults, 22-gauge for children)

Background

The objective of LP is to obtain a sample of CSF from the subarachnoid space. Specifically, during LP the fluid is obtained from the **lumbar cistern,** the CSF located between the termination of the spinal cord (conus medullaris) and the termination of the dura mater at the coccygeal ligament. The cistern is surrounded by the subarachnoid membrane and the overlying dura. Located within the cistern are the filum terminale and the nerve roots of the cauda equina. When LP is done, the main body of the spinal cord is avoided, and the nerve roots of the cauda are simply pushed out of the way by the needle. The termination of the spinal cord in adults is usually between L1 and L2, and in pediatric patients between L2 and L3. The safest site for LP is the interspace between L4 and L5. An imaginary line drawn between the iliac crests (the supracristal plane) intersects the spine at either the L4 spinous process or the L4–L5 interspace. A spinal needle introduced between the spinous processes of L4 and L5 penetrates the layers in the following order: skin, supraspinous ligament, interspinous ligament, ligamentum flavum, epidural space (contains loose areolar tissue, fat, and blood vessels), dura, "potential space," subarachnoid membrane, and subarachnoid space (lumbar cistern) (Figure 13–15, page 291).

Procedure

1. Examine the fundus for evidence of papilledema, and review the CT or MRI of the head if available. Discuss the relative safety and lack of discomfort to the patient to dispel any myths. Some clinicians prefer to call the procedure "subarachnoid analysis" rather than a spinal tap. As long as the procedure and the risks are outlined, most patients agree to the procedure. Have the patient sign an informed consent form.

2. Place the patient in the lateral decubitus position close to the edge of the bed or table. The patient (held by an assistant, if possible) should be positioned with knees pulled up toward stomach and head flexed onto chest (Figure 13–16, page 292). This position enhances flexion of the vertebral spine and widens the interspaces between the spinous processes. Place a pillow beneath the patient's side to prevent sagging and ensure alignment of the spinal column. If the patient is obese or has arthritis or scoliosis, the sitting position, leaning forward, may be preferred.

3. Palpate the supracristal plane (see Background) and carefully determine the location of the L4–L5 interspace.

4. Open the kit, put on sterile gloves, and prep the area with povidone–iodine solution in a circular manner and covering several interspaces. Drape the patient.

5. With a 25-gauge needle and lidocaine, raise a skin wheal over the L4–L5 interspace. Anesthetize the deeper structures using a 22-gauge needle.

6. Examine the spinal needle (20- or 22-gauge) with stylet for defects and then insert it into the skin wheal and into the spinous ligament. Hold the

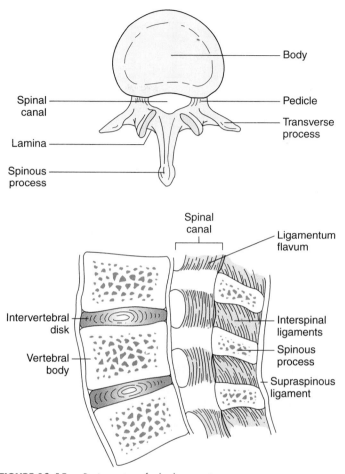

FIGURE 13–15. Basic anatomy for lumbar puncture.

needle between your index and middle fingers with your thumb holding the stylet in place. Direct the needle cephalad at a 30- to 45-degree angle in the midline and parallel to the bed (see Figure 13–16).

7. Advance the needle through the major structures and pop into the subarachnoid space through the dura. An experienced operator can feel these layers, but an inexperienced one may need to periodically remove the stylet to look for return of fluid. It is important to always replace the stylet before advancing the spinal needle. The needle may be withdrawn, however, with the stylet removed. This technique may be useful if the needle has passed through the back wall of the canal. Direct the bevel of the needle parallel to the long axis of the body so that the dural fibers are separated rather than sheared. This method helps cut down on "spinal headaches."

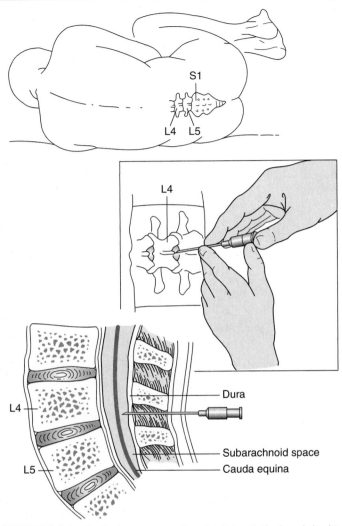

FIGURE 13–16. For lumbar puncture, place the patient in the lateral decubitus position, and locate the L4–L5 interspace. Control the spinal needle with two hands, and enter the subarachnoid space.

8. If no fluid returns, it is sometimes helpful to rotate the needle slightly. If still no fluid appears, and you believe the needle is within the subarachnoid space, inject 1 mL of air; it is not uncommon for a piece of tissue to clog the needle. **Never** inject saline solution or distilled water. If no air returns and if spinal fluid cannot be aspirated, the bevel of the needle is probably in the epidural space; advance it with the stylet in place.

9. When fluid returns, attach a manometer and stopcock and measure the pressure. Normal opening pressure is 70–180 mm water in the lateral position. Increased pressure may be due to a tense patient, CHF, ascites, subarachnoid hemorrhage, infection, or a space-occupying lesion. Decreased pressure may be due to CSF leak, needle position, or obstructed flow (you may need to leave the needle in for a myelogram because if it is moved, the subarachnoid space may be lost).

10. Collect 0.5- to 2.0-mL samples in serial, labeled containers. Send them to the lab in this order:

- **First tube for bacteriology:** Gram stain, routine C&S, AFB, and fungal cultures and stains.
- **Second tube for glucose and protein:** In addition, if MS is suspected, order electrophoresis to detect oligoclonal banding and assay for myelin basic protein.
- **Third tube for cell count:** CBC with diff
- **Fourth tube for special studies as clinically indicated:** VDRL (neurosyphilis), CIEP (counter-immunoelectrophoresis) for bacterial antigens such as *Haemophilus influenzae, Streptococcus pneumoniae, Neisseria meningitidis*, PCR assay for tuberculous meningitis and herpes simplex encephalitis (allows rapid diagnosis). If *Cryptococcus neoformans* is suspected (most common cause of meningitis in AIDS patients), India ink preparation and cryptococcal antigen (latex agglutination test).
- *Note:* Some clinicians prefer to send the first and last tubes for CBC because this procedure allows better differentiation between **subarachnoid hemorrhage and a traumatic tap.** In a traumatic tap, the number of RBCs in the first tube should be much higher than in the last tube. In subarachnoid hemorrhage, the cell counts should be equal, and **xanthochromia** of the fluid should be present, indicating the presence of old blood.

11. Withdraw the needle, and place a dry, sterile dressing over the site.

12. Instruct the patient to remain lying down for 6–12 h, and encourage increased fluid intake to help prevent "spinal headaches."

Interpret the results using Table 13–4, page 294.

Complications

- **Spinal headache:** The most common complication (about 20%), appears within the first 24 h after LP. It is relieved when the patient lies down and is aggravated when the patient sits up. Spinal headache is characterized by severe throbbing pain in the occipital region and can last a week. It is thought to be caused by intracranial traction caused by acute volume depletion of CSF and by persistent leakage from the puncture site. To help prevent spinal headache, keep the patient recumbent for 6–12 h, encourage intake of fluids (especially caffeinated drinks such as coffee, tea, and soft drinks), use the smallest needle possible, and keep the bevel of the needle parallel to the long axis of the body to help prevent persistent CSF leak. If the headache persists, a blood patch (peripheral blood injected into the epidural space, usually performed by anesthesia service) may be needed to seal the leak.
- **Trauma to nerve roots or to the conus medullaris:** Much less frequent (some anatomic variation does exist, but it is very rare for the cord to end

TABLE 13-4
Differential Diagnosis of Cerebrospinal Fluid

Condition	Color	Opening Pressure (mm H$_2$O)	Protein (mL/100 mL)	Glucose (mg/100 mL)	Cells (#/mm^3)
NORMAL					
Adult	Clear	70–180	15–45	45–80	0–5 lymphocytes
Newborn	Clear	70–180	20–120	2/3 serum	40–60 lymphocytes
INFECTIOUS					
Viral infection ("aseptic meningitis")	Clear or opalescent	Normal or slightly increased	Normal or slightly increased	Normal	10–500 lymphocytes PMN early
Bacterial infection	Opalescent yellow, may clot	Increased	50–10,000	Decreased, usually <20	25–10,000 PMN
Granulomatous infection (TB, fungal)	Clear or opalescent	Often increased	Increased, but usually <500	Decreased, usually <20–40	10–500 lymphocytes

(continued)

294

13

TABLE 13-4
(Continued)

Condition	Color	Opening Pressure (mm H$_2$O)	Protein (mL/100 mL)	Glucose (mg/100 mL)	Cells (#/mm^3)
NEUROLOGIC					
Guillain–Barré syndrome	Clear or cloudy	Normal	Markedly increased	Normal	Normal or increased lymphocytes
Multiple sclerosis	Clear	Normal	Normal or increased	Normal	0–20 lymphocytes
Pseudotumor cerebri	Clear	Increased	Normal	Normal	Normal
MISCELLANEOUS					
Neoplasm	Clear or xanthochromic	Increased	Normal or increased	Normal or decreased	Normal or increased lymphocytes
Traumatic tap	Bloody, no xanthochromia	Normal	Normal	Increased	RBC = peripheral blood; fewer RBC in tube 4 than in tube 1
Subarachnoid hemorrhage	Bloody or xanthochromic after 2–8 h	Usually increased	Increased	Normal	WBC/RBC ratio same as blood, RBC in tube 1 = tube 4

WBC = white blood cells; RBC = red blood cells; PMN = polymorphonuclear neutrophils.

13

295

below L3). If the patient suddenly complains of paresthesia (numbness or shooting pain in the legs), stop the procedure.

- **Herniation of either the cerebellum or the medulla:** Occurs rarely during or after spinal tap, usually in a patient with increased intracranial pressure. This complication can often be reversed medically if it is recognized early.
- **Meningitis**
- **Bleeding** in the subarachnoid or subdural space can occur with resulting paralysis, especially if the patient is receiving anticoagulants or has severe liver disease with coagulopathy.

ORTHOSTATIC BLOOD PRESSURE MEASUREMENT
Indication
- Assessment of volume depletion

Materials
- BP cuff and stethoscope

Procedure
1. Changes in BP and pulse when a patient moves from supine to the upright position are very sensitive guides for detecting early volume depletion. Even before a person becomes overtly tachycardic or hypotensive because of volume loss, the demonstration of orthostatic hypotension aids in the diagnosis.
2. Have the patient assume a supine position for 5–10 min. Determine the BP and pulse.
3. Have the patient stand up. If the patient is unable to stand, have the patient sit at the bedside with legs dangling.
4. After about 1 min, measure BP and pulse again.
5. A drop in systolic BP greater than 10 mm Hg or an increase in pulse rate greater than 20 beats/min (16 beats/min in the elderly) suggests **volume depletion.** A change in heart rate is more sensitive and occurs with a lesser degree of volume depletion. Other causes of a drop in BP with body position change (usually without an increase in heart rate) include peripheral neuropathy, surgical sympathectomy, diabetes, and medications (prazosin, hydralazine, or reserpine).

PELVIC EXAMINATION
Indications
- Physical examination of female patients
- Diagnosis of diseases and conditions of the female genital tract

Materials
- Sterile gloves
- Vaginal speculum and lubricant
- Slides, fixative (eg, Pap smear aerosol spray), cotton swabs, endocervical brush and cervical spatula prepared for a Pap smear

Materials for Other Diagnostic Tests

- Culture media to test for gonorrhea, *Chlamydia,* herpes
- Sterile cotton swabs
- Plain glass slides
- KOH
- NS solutions, as needed

Procedure

1. Perform the pelvic exam in conditions that are as comfortable as possible for both patient and physician. Either the physician or the assistant must be a woman. Drape the patient appropriately and help her place her feet in the stirrups on the examining table. Prepare a low stool, a good light source, and all needed supplies before starting the exam. In unusual situations examinations are conducted on a gurney or bed; raise the patient's buttocks on one or two pillows to elevate the perineum off the mattress.

2. Inform the patient of each movement in advance. Glove hands before proceeding.

3. **General inspection**
   a. Observe the skin of the perineum for swelling, ulcers, condylomata (venereal warts), and color changes.
   b. Separate the labia to examine the clitoris and vestibule. Multiple clear vesicles on an erythematous base on the labia suggest herpes.
   c. Observe the urethral meatus for developmental abnormalities, discharge, neoplasm, and abscess of Bartholin glands at the 4 and 8 o'clock positions.
   d. Inspect the vaginal orifice for discharge and protrusion of the walls (cystocele, rectocele, urethral prolapse).
   e. Note the condition of the hymen.

4. **Speculum examination**
   a. Use a speculum moistened with warm water *not* with lubricant (lubricant interferes with Pap tests and slide studies). Touch the speculum to the patient's leg to see whether the temperature is comfortable.
   b. Because the anterior wall of the vagina is close to the urethra and bladder, do not exert pressure in this area. Place pressure on the posterior surface of the vagina. With the speculum directed at a 45-degree angle to the floor, spread the labia and insert the speculum fully, pressing posteriorly. The cervix should pop into view with some manipulation as the speculum is opened.
   c. Inspect the cervix and vagina for color, lacerations, growths, nabothian cysts, and evidence of atrophy.
   d. Inspect the cervical os for size, shape, color, and discharge.
   e. Inspect the vagina for secretions and obtain specimens for Pap smear, other smear, or culture (see tests for vaginal infections and Pap smear in step 7).
   f. Inspect the vaginal wall; rotate the speculum as you draw it out to see the entire canal. Use caution when removing the speculum (especially it if is metal) because it can close quickly if not held open while being withdrawn and can trap vaginal mucosa.

13

5. **Bimanual examination**
   a. Stand up for this part of the exam. Use whichever hand is comfortable to do the internal vaginal exam. Remove the glove from the hand used to examine the abdomen.
   b. Place lubricant on the first and second gloved fingers, and keeping pressure on the posterior fornix, introduce the fingers into the vagina.
   c. Palpate the tissue at the 5 and 7 o'clock positions between the first and second fingers and the thumb to rule out any abnormality of the Bartholin glands. Likewise, palpate the urethra and paraurethral (Skene) glands.
   d. Place the examining fingers on the posterior wall of the vagina to further open the introitus. Ask the patient to bear down. Look for evidence of prolapse, rectocele, and cystocele.
   e. Palpate the cervix. Note the size, shape, consistency, and motility and test for tenderness (**"chandelier" sign**) and cervical motion tenderness, which is suggestive of PID or ruptured ectopic pregnancy.
   f. With your fingers in the vagina posterior to the cervix and your hand on the abdomen placed just above the symphysis, force the corpus of the uterus between the two examining hands. Note size, shape, consistency, position, and motility.
   g. Move the fingers in the vagina to one or the other fornix, and place the hand on the abdomen in a more lateral position to bring the adnexal areas under examination. Palpate the ovaries, if possible, for masses, consistency, and motility. Unless they are diseased, the fallopian tubes usually are not palpable.

6. **Rectovaginal examination**
   a. Insert your index finger into the vagina, and place the well-lubricated middle finger in the rectum.
   b. Palpate the posterior surface of the uterus and the broad ligament for nodularity, tenderness, and masses. Examine the uterosacral and rectovaginal septum. Nodularity may represent endometriosis.
   c. It may also be helpful to do a test for occult blood if a stool specimen is available.

7. **Papanicolaou (Pap) smear**
   The Pap smear is helpful in early detection of cervical intraepithelial neoplasia and carcinoma. Endometrial carcinoma is occasionally identified on routine Pap smears. It is recommended that once they reach age 18 or are sexually active, low-risk patients undergo routine Pap smears done every 2–3 y, but only after three annual Pap smears are negative. High-risk patients such as those exposed in utero to DES; patients with HPV infection or history of HIV infection; history of cervical dysplasia or cervical intraepithelial neoplasia; more than two sexual partners in their lifetime; and intercourse before age 20 should undergo an annual Pap smear.
   a. With an unlubricated speculum in place, use a wooden cervical spatula to obtain a scraping from the squamocolumnar junction. Rotate the spatula 360 degrees around the external os. Smear on a frosted slide that has the patient's name written on it in pencil. Fix the slide either in a bottle of fixative or with spray fixative. Fix the slide within 10 s, or a drying artifact may occur.
   b. Obtain a specimen from the endocervical canal using a cotton swab or endocervical brush and prepare the slide as described in part **a**.

    c. Using a wooden spatula, obtain an additional specimen from the posterolateral vaginal pool of fluid and smear it on a slide.

    d. Complete the appropriate lab slips. Forewarn the patient that she may experience spotty vaginal bleeding after the Pap smear.

8. Tests for cervical and vaginal infections

    a. GC and *Chlamydia* culture: Use a sterile cotton swab to obtain a specimen from the endocervical canal and plate it out on **Thayer–Martin** medium for GC. *Chlamydia* testing varies but can include DNA probe, EIA, or direct fluorescent antibody (DFA) testing.

    b. Vaginal saline (wet) prep: Helpful in the diagnosis of *Trichomonas vaginalis* and bacterial vaginosis. Mix a drop of discharge with a drop of NS on a glass slide and cover it with a coverslip. Observe the slide while it is still warm to see the flagellated, motile trichomonads. Bacterial vaginosis is most often caused by *Gardnerella vaginalis* and can be diagnosed by the presence of "clue cells," which represent PMNs dotted with the *G. vaginalis* bacteria; vaginal pH > 4.5; and a fishy amine odor with addition of KOH to the secretions. It is also possible to see these cells by using a hanging drop of saline and a concave slide. *Lactobacillus* organisms are normally the predominant bacteria in the vagina in the absence of specific infection, and the normal pH is usually < 4.5.

    c. Potassium hydroxide prep: If a thick, white, curdy discharge is present, the patient may have *Candida albicans* (monilial) yeast infection. Prepare a slide with one drop of discharge and one drop of aqueous 10% KOH solution. The KOH dissolves the epithelial cells and debris and facilitates viewing of the hyphae and mycelia of the fungus that causes the infection.

    d. Gram stain: Material can easily be stained in the usual manner (Chapter 7, page 121). Gram-negative intracellular diplococci (so-called GNIDs) are pathognomonic of *N. gonorrhoeae* infection. The bacteria most commonly found in Gram stains are large gram-positive rods (lactobacilli), which are normal vaginal flora.

    e. Herpes cultures: A routine Pap smear of the cervix or a Pap smear of the herpetic lesion (multiple, clear vesicles on a painful, erythematous base) may show herpes inclusion bodies. Swab the suspicious lesion or the endocervix to obtain a specimen for herpes viral culture.

13

PERICARDIOCENTESIS

Indications

- Emergency treatment of cardiac tamponade
- Diagnosis of cause of pericardial effusion

Contraindications

- Minimal pericardial effusion (< 200 mL)
- Aftermath of CABG because of risk of injury to grafts
- Uncorrected coagulopathy

Materials

- ECG machine

- Prepackaged pericardiocentesis kit or procedure and instrument tray (page 243) with pericardiocentesis needle or 16- to 18-gauge needle 10 cm long

Background

Cardiac tamponade results in decreased cardiac output, increased right atrial filling pressure, and pronounced pulsus paradoxus.

Procedure

1. If time permits, use sterile prep and draping with gown, mask, and gloves.
2. Use a left paraxiphoid or left parasternal approach through the 4th ICS. The paraxiphoid approach is safer, more commonly used, and described here (Figure 13–17, see below).
3. Anesthetize the insertion site with lidocaine. Connect the needle with an alligator clip to the chest lead (brown) on the ECG machine. Attach the limb leads, and monitor the machine.
4. Insert the pericardiocentesis needle just to the left of the xiphoid process and directed upward 45 degrees toward the left shoulder.
5. Aspirate while advancing the needle until the pericardium is punctured and the effusion is tapped. If you feel the ventricular wall, withdraw the needle

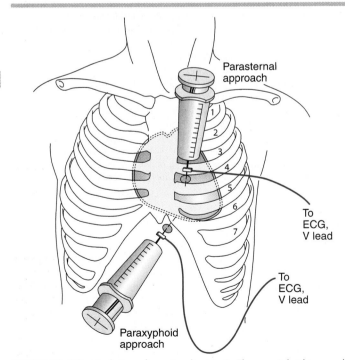

FIGURE 13–17.   Techniques for pericardiocentesis. The paraxiphoid approach is the most frequently used.

slightly. If the needle contacts the myocardium, pronounced ST segment elevation will be recorded on the ECG.

6. If pericardiocentesis is performed for cardiac tamponade, removal of as little as 50 mL of fluid dramatically improves BP and decreases right atrial pressure.

7. Blood from a bloody pericardial effusion is usually defibrinated and does not clot, whereas blood from the ventricle does clot.

8. Send fluid for HCT, cell count, or cytology if indicated.
    - **Serous fluid:** Consistent with CHF, bacterial infection, TB, hypoalbuminemia, or viral pericarditis
    - **Bloody fluid (HCT > 10%):** May result from trauma; be iatrogenic; or be due to MI, uremia, coagulopathy, or malignant disease (lymphoma, leukemia, breast, lung most common)

9. If continuous drainage is necessary, use a guidewire to place a 16-gauge IV catheter and connect to a closed drainage system.

Complications

Arrhythmia, ventricular puncture, lung injury

PERIPHERAL INSERTION OF CENTRAL CATHETER (PICC)
Indications

- Home infusion of hypertonic or irritating solutions and drugs
- Long-term infusion of medications (antibiotics, chemotherapeutics)
- TPN
- Repeated venous blood sampling

Contraindications

- Infection over placement site
- Inability to identify veins in an arm with a tourniquet in place

13

Materials

- PICC catheter kit (contains most items necessary, including the Silastic long arm line, eg, Introsyte Autoguard system)
- Tourniquet, sterile gloves, mask, sterile gown, heparin flush, 10-mL syringes

Background

Installation of a PICC allows for central venous access through a peripheral vein. Typically, a long arm catheter is placed into the basilic or cephalic vein, usually with bedside portable ultrasound guidance (see Figure 13–12, page 286) and is threaded into the subclavian vein and superior vena cava. PICCs are useful for long-term home infusion therapy. The design of PICC catheters can vary, and the operator should be familiar with the features of the device (attached hub or detachable hub designs). Usually these catheters are placed by specialized PICC nurses at the bedside or by interventional radiologists under fluoroscopic guidance, but it is prudent to be aware of the technique because any trained medical personnel can be called on to place these catheters.

Procedure

1. Explain the procedure to the patient and obtain informed consent. Have the patient sit or lie down with the elbow extended and the arm in a dependent position. The arm should be externally rotated.

2. Using a measuring tape, determine the length of the catheter required. Measure from the extremity vein insertion site to the subclavian vein.

3. Wear mask, gown, protective eyewear, and sterile gloves. Prep and drape the skin in the standard manner. Set up an adjacent sterile working area.

4. Anesthetize the skin at the proposed area of insertion. Apply a tourniquet above the proposed IV site.

5. Trim the catheter to the appropriate length. Most PICC lines have an attached hub, and the distal end of the catheter is cut to the proper length. Flush with heparinized saline.

6. Insert the catheter and introducer needle (usually 14-gauge) into the chosen arm vein as detailed in IV Techniques (page 285). Once the catheter is in the vein, push the white button on the Introsyte device to shield the needle. Discard the needle assembly.

7. Place the PICC line in the catheter and advance it (using a forceps if provided by the manufacturer of the kit). Remove the tourniquet and gradually advance the catheter the requisite length. Remove the inner stiffening wire slowly once the catheter has been adequately advanced.

8. Peel away the introducer catheter. Attach the Luer-Lock, and flush the catheter again with heparin solution. Attempt to aspirate blood to verify patency.

9. Attach the provided securing wings, and suture them in place. Apply a sterile dressing over the insertion site.

10. Confirm placement in the central circulation with a CXR. Always document the type of PICC, the length inserted, and the site of its radiologically confirmed placement.

11. If vein cannulation is difficult, a surgical cutdown may be necessary to cannulate the vein. If the catheter will not advance, fluoroscopy may be helpful.

12. Instruct the patient on the maintenance of the PICC. The PICC should be flushed with heparinized saline solution after each use. Dressing changes should be performed at least every 7 d under sterile conditions. Instruct the patient to evaluate the PICC site for signs and symptoms of infection. Also instruct the patient to come to the ER for evaluation if a fever develops.

13. For venous samples, withdraw a specimen of at least the catheter volume (1–3 mL) and discard it. The PICC must always be flushed with heparinized saline solution after each blood draw.

PICC Removal

1. Position the patient's arm at a 90-degree angle to the body. Remove the dressing and gently pull the PICC out.

2. Apply pressure to site for 2–3 min. Always measure the length of the catheter and check previous documentation to ensure that the PICC line has been removed in its entirety. If a piece of a catheter is left behind, an emergency interventional radiology consult is in order.

Complications

Site bleeding, clotted catheter, subclavian thrombosis, infection, broken catheter (leakage or embolization), arrhythmia (catheter inserted too far)

PERITONEAL LAVAGE

Indications

- **Diagnostic peritoneal lavage (DPL)** is used in the evaluation of intraabdominal trauma (bleeding, perforation) (*Note:* Spiral CT of the abdomen has largely replaced DPL as an initial screening tool for intraabdominal trauma in the emergency setting.)
- Acute peritoneal dialysis and management of severe pancreatitis.

Contraindications

- No absolute complications. Relative contraindications: multiple abdominal procedures, pregnancy, known retroperitoneal injury (high false-positive rate), cirrhosis, morbid obesity, coagulopathy

Materials

- Prepackaged DPL or peritoneal dialysis tray

Procedure

1. A Foley catheter and an NG or orogastric tube **must** be in place to decompress the bladder and viscera. Prep the abdomen from above the umbilicus to the pubis.
2. The site of choice is in the midline 1–2 cm below the umbilicus. Avoid the sites of old surgical scars (danger of adherent bowel). If a subumbilical scar or pelvic fracture is present, use a supraumbilical approach.
3. Infiltrate the skin with lidocaine with epinephrine. Incise the skin in the midline vertically, and expose the fascia.
4. Either pick up the fascia and incise it or puncture it with the trocar and peritoneal catheter. Exercise caution to avoid puncturing any organs. Use one hand to hold the catheter near the skin and to control the insertion while using the other hand to apply pressure to the end of the catheter. After the peritoneal cavity is entered, remove the trocar and direct the catheter inferiorly into the pelvis.
5. During a diagnostic lavage, gross blood indicates a positive tap. If no blood is encountered, instill 10 mL/kg (about 1 L in adults) of RL or NS into the abdominal cavity.
6. Gently agitate the abdomen to distribute the fluid; after 5 min drain off as much fluid as possible into a bag on the floor. (Minimum fluid for a valid analysis is 200 mL in an adult.) If the drainage is slow, try instilling additional fluid, carefully repositioning the catheter.
7. Send the fluid for analysis (amylase, bile, bacteria, hematocrit, cell count). Interpret the findings using Table 13–5.
8. Remove the catheter and suture the skin. If the catheter is inserted because of pancreatitis or for peritoneal dialysis, suture the catheter in place.
9. Negative DPL does not exclude retroperitoneal trauma. False-positive DPL can be caused by a pelvic fracture or bleeding induced by the procedure (eg, laceration of an omental vessel).

Complications

Infection, peritonitis, superficial wound infection, bleeding, perforated viscus (bladder, bowel)

TABLE 13–5
Criteria for Evaluation of Peritoneal Lavage Fluid

Positive	>20 mL gross blood on free aspiration (10 mL in children)
	≥100,000 RBC/mL
	≥500 WBC/mL (if obtained >3 h after the injury)
	≥175 units amylase/dL
	Bacteria on Gram stain
	Bile (by inspection or chemical determination of bilirubin content)
	Food particles (microscopic analysis of strained or spun specimen)
Intermediate	Pink fluid on free aspiration
	50,000–100,000 RBC/mL in blunt trauma
	100–500 WBC/mL
	75–175 units amylase/dL
Negative	Clear aspirate
	≤ 100 WBC/μL
	≤ 75 units amylase/dL

Source: Reprinted, with permission, from: Way, L., Doherty GM (eds): *Current Surgical Diagnosis and Treatment*, 11th ed. McGraw-Hill, 2003.
RBC = red blood cells; WBC = white blood cells.

PERITONEAL (ABDOMINAL) PARACENTESIS

Indications

- Determining the cause of ascites
- Determining whether intraabdominal bleeding is present or whether a viscus has ruptured (DPL is considered a more accurate test. See preceding procedure.)
- Therapeutic removal of fluid when distention is pronounced or respiratory distress is associated with it (acute treatment only)

Contraindications

- Abnormal coagulation factors
- Bowel obstruction, pregnancy
- Uncertainty whether distention is caused by peritoneal fluid or due to a cystic structure (usually can be differentiated with ultrasonography)

Materials

- Minor procedure tray (see page 243)
- Catheter-over-needle assembly (Angiocath Autoguard, Insyte Autoguard 18- to 20-gauge with 1 1/2-in [4 cm] needle)
- 20–60-mL syringe
- Sterile specimen containers

Procedure

Peritoneal paracentesis is surgical puncture of the peritoneal cavity for aspiration of fluid. Ascites is indicated by abdominal distention, shifting dullness, and a palpable fluid wave; generally ultrasonography is used to confirm ascites.

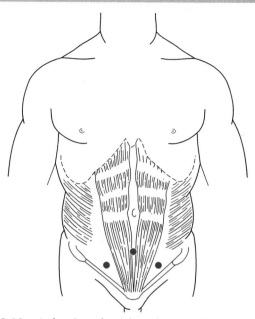

FIGURE 13–18. Preferred sites for abdominal (peritoneal) paracentesis. Be sure to avoid old surgical scars.

13

1. Explain the procedure and have the patient sign an informed consent form. Have the patient empty the bladder, or place a Foley catheter if voiding is impossible or if marked changes in mental status are present.
2. The entry site is usually the midline 1–1 1/2 in (3–4 cm) below the umbilicus. Avoid old surgical scars because the bowel may be adherent to the abdominal wall. An alternative entry site is the left or right lower quadrant midway between the umbilicus and the anterior superior iliac spine or the patient's flank, depending on the percussion of the fluid wave (Figure 13–18). Avoid the rectus abdominus because of bleeding potential.
3. Prep and drape the area and raise a skin wheal with the lidocaine over the entry site.
4. A Z track technique helps limit persistent leakage of peritoneal fluid after the tap. Manually retract the skin caudally and release traction on the skin when the peritoneum is entered. With the catheter mounted on the syringe, go through the anesthetized area while aspirating. There is resistance as the fascia is entered. When there is free return of fluid, leave the catheter in place, and remove the needle or activate the self-shielding mechanism. Begin to aspirate; reposition the catheter as needed because of abutting bowel.
5. Aspirate the amount of fluid needed for tests (20–30 mL). If the tap is therapeutic, 10–15 L can be safely removed. The removal of a large volume can be facilitated by the use of vacuum container bottles (500 mL–1 L) supplied at most hospitals. Tubing is first connected to the catheter and then to the vacuum container bottles.

TABLE 13–6
Differential Diagnosis of Ascitic Fluid

Albumin Gradient:
Serum Alb – Ascites Alb = X
    if X > 1.1 g/dL, then portal hypertension
    if X < 1.1 g/dL, then not from portal hypertension

Total Protein: < 1.0 g/dL, high risk of spontaneous bacterial peritonitis

Cell Count: Absolute neutrophil count > 250/μL, presume infected

Bacterial Culture: Blood culture bottles 85% sensitivity
Routine cultures 50% sensitivity

Bacterial Peritonitis: Spontaneous versus secondary
Secondary: (1) polymicrobial; (2) total protein > 1.0 g/dL; (3) LDH > normal serum value; (4) glucose < 50 mg/dL

Food Fibers: Found in most cases of perforated viscus

Cytology: Bizarre cells with large nuclei may represent reactive mesothelial cells and not malignancy. Malignant cells suggest a tumor.

Source: Reprinted with permission. From: Haist SA, Robbins JB (eds.) *Internal Medicine on Call*, 4th ed. McGraw-Hill, 2005.

6. Apply a sterile 4 × 4 gauze square, and apply pressure with tape. In patients with chronic ascites, a purse-string suture may be placed at the puncture site to minimize ongoing leakage of ascitic fluid from the tap.
7. Depending on the patient's clinical condition, send samples for cell count including differential, total protein, albumin, amylase, LDH, glucose, cytology, and C&S.

Complications

Peritonitis, perforated viscus (bowel, bladder), hemorrhage, precipitation of hepatic coma if patient has severe liver disease, oliguria, hypotension

Diagnosis of Ascitic Fluid

A differential diagnosis is in Chapter 3, page 35. The older classification of ascitic fluid as either transudative or exudative is no longer used. The cause of ascites is more likely to be found by determining the serum-to-ascites albumin gradient. See Table 13–6, above, to interpret the results of ascitic fluid analysis.

PULMONARY ARTERY CATHETERIZATION

(See Chapter 20)

PULSUS PARADOXUS MEASUREMENT (PARADOXICAL PULSE)

(See also Chapter 20)

Indication

- Used in the evaluation of cardiac tamponade and other diseases (eg, severity of asthma)

Materials

- BP cuff and stethoscope

Background

Pulsus paradoxus is an exaggeration of the normal inspiratory drop in arterial pressure. Inspiration decreases intrathoracic pressure. The result is increased right atrial and right ventricular filling with an increase in right ventricular output. Because the pulmonary vascular bed also distends, these changes lead to a delay in left ventricular filling and subsequently decreased left ventricular output. This drop in systolic BP is usually < 10 mm Hg. In the case of cardiac compression (eg, acute asthma or pericardial tamponade), the right side of the heart fills more with inspiration and decreases the left ventricular volume to an even greater degree as a result of compression of the pericardial sac. This exaggerated decrease in left ventricular output decreases systolic pressure > 10 mm Hg. See Figure 20–1 (page 408) for a graphic representation of a paradoxical pulse.

Procedure

1. For a simple, **qualitative method** palpate the radial pulse, which "disappears" on normal inspiration.
2. For a more precise **quantitative method** measure systolic BP at end-exhalation during tidal breathing.
   a. Determine systolic BP at end-inspiration during tidal breathing.
   b. The difference in systolic pressure between end-exhalation and end-inspiration should be < 10 mm Hg. If not, a so-called paradox exists.
3. Differential diagnosis includes pericardial effusion, cardiac tamponade, pericarditis, COPD, bronchial asthma, restrictive cardiomyopathy, hemorrhagic shock, massive PE, tricuspid stenosis, and mitral stenosis.

SKIN BIOPSY

Indications

- Any skin lesion or eruption for which the diagnosis is unclear
- Any refractory skin condition

Contraindications

- Any skin lesion suspected of being malignant (eg, melanoma) should be referred to a plastic surgeon or dermatologist for excisional biopsy rather than punch biopsy; full-thickness biopsy is critical for diagnosis and accurate staging.

Materials

- 2-, 3-, 4-, or 5-mm skin punch
- Minor procedure tray (see page 243)
- Curved iris scissors and fine-toothed forceps (ordinary forceps may distort a small biopsy specimen and should not be used)

13

- Specimen bottle containing 10% formalin
- Suture material (3-0 or 4-0 nylon)

Procedure

1. If more than one lesion is present, choose one that is well developed and representative of the dermatosis. For patients with vesiculobullous disease, choose an early edematous lesion rather than a vesicle. Avoid lesions that are excoriated or infected.
2. Mark the biopsy area with a skin-marking pen. Inject lidocaine to form a skin wheal over the site of the biopsy.
3. After putting on sterile gloves and preparing a sterile field, obtain the punch biopsy specimen. Immobilize the skin with the fingers of one hand, applying pressure perpendicular to the skin wrinkle lines with the skin punch. Core out a cylinder of skin by twirling the punch between the fingers of the other hand. As the punch enters into the SQ fat, resistance lessens. At this point, remove the punch. The core of tissue usually pops up slightly and can be cut at the level of the SQ fat with a curved iris scissors without forceps. If a tissue core does not pop up, elevate it using a hypodermic needle or fine-toothed forceps. Be sure to include a portion of the SQ fat in the specimen.
4. Place the specimen in the specimen container.
5. Apply pressure with the gauze pad to achieve hemostasis.
6. Defects from 1.5- and 2-mm punches usually do not require suturing and heal with minimal scarring. Punch defects measuring 2–4 mm can generally be closed with a single suture.
7. Apply a dry dressing and remove it the following day.
8. Sutures can be removed as early as 3 d from the face and 7–10 d from other areas.

13

Complications

Infection (unusual); hemorrhage (usually controlled by simple application of pressure); keloid formation, especially in a patient with a history of keloid formation

SKIN TESTING
Indications

- Screening for current or past infection (eg, TB, coccidioidomycosis)
- Screening for immune competency (so-called anergy screen) in debilitated patients

Materials

- Appropriate antigen (usually 0.1 mL) (eg, 5 TU PPD)
- A small, short needle (25-, 26-, or 27-gauge)
- 1-mL syringe
- Alcohol swab

Procedure

1. Skin tests for **delayed type hypersensitivity (type IV, tuberculin)** are the most commonly administered and interpreted. Delayed hypersensitivity

(so called because a lag time of 24–48 h is required for a reaction) is caused by the activation of sensitized lymphocytes after contact with an antigen (cell-mediated arm of the immune system). The inflammatory reaction results from direct cytotoxicity and the release of lymphokines. Allergy tests (immediate wheal and flare) are rarely performed by students or house officers.

2. The most commonly used site is the flexor surface of the forearm, approximately 4 in (10 cm) below the elbow crease.

3. Prep the area with alcohol. With the bevel of the 27-gauge needle up, introduce the needle into the upper layers of skin, but **not** into the subcutis. Inject 0.1 mL of antigen, such as PPD. The goal is to inject the antigen intradermally. If the injection has been done properly, a discrete white bleb approximately 10 mm in diameter (known as the **Mantoux test**) rises. The bleb should disappear soon, and no dressing is needed. If a bleb is not raised, move to another area and repeat the injection. Do not inject too superficially (in the epidermis); doing so causes epidermal–dermal separation resulting in blister formation and an inaccurate test result.

4. Mark the test site with a pen; if multiple tests are being administered, identify each one. Document the site or sites in the patient's chart.

5. To interpret the skin test, examine the site 48–72 h after injection. If nonreactive, check again at 72 h. **Measure the area of induration (the firm raised area), not the erythematous area.** Use a ballpoint pen held at approximately a 30-degree angle and bring it lightly toward the raised area. Where the pen touches is the area of induration. Measure two diameters and take the average.

6. It is important to check the PPD and other tests at intervals. If the patient develops a severe reaction to the skin test, apply hydrocortisone cream to prevent skin sloughing.

13

Specific Skin Tests

TST (Tuberculin Skin Testing):   Routine TST on persons at low risk is not recommended. Persons at high risk should undergo periodic TST: those with CXR findings suspicious for TB or recent contact with known or suspected TB cases (includes health care workers); immigrants from high-risk areas (Asia, Africa, Middle East, Latin America), the medically underserved (IV drug abusers, persons with alcoholism, homeless persons); persons undergoing long-term institutionalization; and persons with HIV infection and others who are immunosuppressed.

The **Mantoux test** is the standard technique for TST and relies on the intradermal injection of **PPD**. The **tine test** for TB is no longer recommended by the CDC. The PPD comes in three tuberculin unit strengths: 1 TU (first), 5 TU (intermediate), and 250 TU (second). One TU is used if the patient is expected to be hypersensitive (history of a positive skin test); 5 TU is the standard initial screening test. A patient who has a negative response to a 5-TU test dose may react to the 250-TU solution. A patient who does not respond to 250-TU is considered nonreactive to PPD. A patient may not react if he or she has not been exposed to the antigen or is anergic and unable to respond to any antigen challenge. A positive TST indicates the presence of *Mycobacterium tuberculosis* infection, either active or past (dormant), and intact cell-mediated immunity.

Interpretation of a positive PPD test is based on the clinical scenario. **Patients who have been previously immunized with percutaneous BCG may give a false-positive PPD, usually 10 mm or less.**

- 0–5 mm induration: Negative response
- ≥ 5 mm: Considered positive in contacts of known TB cases, CXR findings consistent with TB infection or HIV infection or in patients who are immunosuppressed, occasionally in non-TB mycobacterial infection due to cross reactivity
- ≥ 10 mm induration: Considered positive in patients with chronic disease (diabetes, alcoholism, IV drug abuse, other chronic diseases), homeless persons, immigrants from known TB regions, and children < 4 y
- > 15 mm induration: Positive in persons who are healthy and otherwise do not meet the preceding risk categories

Anergy Screen (Anergy Battery): An anergy screen is based on the assumption that a patient has been exposed in the past to certain common antigens and that a healthy person is able to mount a reaction to them. In the screen, an antigen such as mumps or *Candida* is applied, and the results are read as in a PPD test (a reaction of > 5 mm induration is considered a positive test and indicates intact cellular immunity). Anergy screens are sometimes used to evaluate a patient's immunologic status. Test is not commonly used today.

THORACENTESIS
Indications

- Determining the cause of a pleural effusion
- Therapeutic removal of pleural fluid in the event of respiratory distress
- Aspirating small pneumothoraces when the risk of recurrence is small (eg, postoperative without lung injury)
- Instilling sclerosing compounds (eg, tetracycline) to obliterate the pleural space

13

Contraindications

- No absolute contraindications. Relative: pneumothorax, hemothorax, any major respiratory impairment on the contralateral side; coagulopathy

Materials

- Prepackaged thoracentesis kit with either needle or catheter (preferred)

or

- Minor procedure tray (page 243)
- 20- to 60-mL syringe, 20- or 22-gauge needle 1^1/2-in (4 cm) needle, three-way stopcock
- Specimen containers

Background

Thoracentesis is a surgical puncture on the chest wall for aspiration of fluid or air from the pleural cavity. The area of pleural effusion is dull to percussion with decreased breath sounds. Pleural fluid causes blunting of the costophrenic angles on CXR. Blunting usually indicates that at least 300 mL of fluid is present. If you suspect that less than 300 mL of fluid is present or that the fluid is loculated (trapped and not free-flowing), obtain a lateral decubitus film. Loculated effusions do not layer out. Thoracentesis can be done safely on fluid visualized on a lateral decubitus film if at least 10 mm of fluid is measurable on the decubitus x-ray. Ultrasonography may also be used to localize a small or loculated effusion.

Procedure

1. Explain the procedure, and have the patient sign an informed consent form. Have the patient sit up comfortably, preferably leaning forward slightly on a bedside tray table. Ask the patient to practice increasing intrathoracic pressure using the Valsalva maneuver or by humming.
2. The usual site for thoracentesis is the posterior lateral aspect of the back superior to the diaphragm but inferior to the top of the fluid level. Confirm the site by counting the ribs on the basis of the CXR and percussing out the fluid level. Avoid going below the 8th ICS because of the risk of peritoneal perforation. A good frame of reference is the inferior angle of the scapula, which is located horizontally at the 7th rib or 7th intercostal space.
3. Use sterile technique, including gloves, chlorhexidine, and drapes. Thoracentesis kits come with an adherent drape with a hole in it.
4. Make a skin wheal over the proposed site with a 25-gauge needle and lidocaine. Change to a 22-gauge, 1 1/2-in (4 cm) needle and infiltrate up and over the rib (Figure 13–19); try to anesthetize the deeper structures and the pleura. During this time, aspirate back for pleural fluid. Once fluid returns, note the depth of the needle and mark it with a hemostat. This maneuver gives you an approximate depth. Remove the needle.
5. Use a hemostat to measure the 14- to 18-gauge thoracentesis needle to the same depth as the first needle. Penetrate through the anesthetized area with the thoracentesis needle. **Make sure that you "march" over the top of**

13

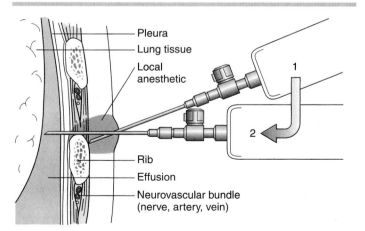

FIGURE 13–19. In thoracentesis, the needle is passed over the top of the rib to avoid the neurovascular bundle.

the rib to avoid the neurovascular bundle that runs below the rib (see Figure 13–19). With the three-way stopcock attached, advance the thoracentesis catheter through the needle, withdraw the needle from the chest, and place the protective needle cover over the end of the needle to prevent injury to the catheter. Next, aspirate the amount of pleural fluid needed. Turn the stopcock, and evacuate the fluid through the tubing. **Never remove more than 1000–1500 mL per tap in patients with chronic effusions (eg, malignant effusions).** Doing so can cause hypotension or development of pulmonary edema due to reexpansion of compressed alveoli. In acute effusions (eg, traumatic hemothorax or postoperative pleural effusions after cardiac surgery) > 1000 mL can be removed at one time without major side effects. In the event of reexpansion pulmonary edema, treat the patient with aggressive diuresis, supplemental oxygenation, potential endotracheal intubation, and continuous hemodynamic and saturation monitoring.

6. Have the patient hum or do the Valsalva maneuver as you withdraw the catheter. This maneuver increases intrathoracic pressure and decreases the risk of pneumothorax. Place a sterile dressing over the site.

7. Obtain a CXR to evaluate the fluid level and to rule out pneumothorax. An expiratory film is preferred because it is superior in identification of a small pneumothorax.

8. Distribute specimens in containers, label slips, and send them to the lab. Always order pH (collect in an ABG syringe), specific gravity, protein, LDH, cell count and differential, glucose, Gram stain and cultures, acid-fast cultures and smears, and fungal cultures and smears. Optional lab studies are cytology if malignancy is suspected, amylase if effusion secondary to pancreatitis (usually on the left) or esophageal perforation is suspected, and Sudan stain and triglycerides (> 110 mg/dL) if chylothorax is suspected.

13

Complications

Pneumothorax, hemothorax, infection, pulmonary laceration, hypotension, hypoxia due to $\dot{V}/\dot{Q}$ mismatch in the newly aerated lung segment

Differential Diagnosis of Pleural Fluid

(See Chapter 3) **Transudate** suggests nephrosis, CHF, cirrhosis; **exudate,** infection (pneumonia, TB), malignancy, empyema, peritoneal dialysis, pancreatitis, or chylothorax. Table 13–7 shows the differential diagnosis.

URINARY TRACT PROCEDURES
Bladder Catheterization
Indications

- Relief of urinary retention
- Collection of an uncontaminated urine specimen for diagnostic purposes
- Monitoring of urinary output in critically ill patients
- Bladder tests (cystogram, cystometrogram)

Contraindications

- Urethral disruption, often associated with pelvic fracture

TABLE 13–7
Differential Diagnosis of Pleural Fluid

Lab Value	Transudate	Exudate
Appearance	Clear yellow	Clear or turbid
Specific gravity	<1.016	>1.016
Absolute protein	<3 g/100 mL	>3 g/100 mL
Protein (pleural to serum ratio)	<0.5	>0.5
LDH (pleural to serum ratio)	<0.6	>0.6
Absolute LDH	<200 IU	>200 IU
Glucose (serum to pleural ratio)	<1	>1
Fibrinogen (clot)	No	Yes
WBC (pleural)	Very low	>2500/mm^3
Differential (pleural)		PMN early, monocytes later

OTHER SELECTED TESTS

Cytology: Bizarre cells with large nuclei may represent reactive mesothelial cells and not malignancy. Malignant cells suggest a tumor.

pH: Generally > 7.3. If between 7.2 and 7.3, suspect TB or malignancy or both. If < 7.2, suspect empyema.

Glucose: Normal pleural fluid glucose is 2/3 serum glucose. Pleural fluid glucose is much lower than serum glucose in effusions due to rheumatoid arthritis (0–16 mg/100 mL); low ,< 40 mg/100 mL in empyema.

Triglycerides and positive Sudan stain: Chylothorax

LDH = lactate dehydrogenase; WBC = white blood cells; RBC = red blood cells; PMN = polymorphonuclear neutrophils; TB = tuberculosis.

13

- Acute prostatitis (relative contraindication)

Materials

- Prepackaged bladder catheter tray (may or may not include a Foley catheter)
- Catheter (Figure 13–20, page 314):

Foley: Balloon at the tip to keep it in the bladder. Use a 16- to 18 Fr for adults (the higher the number, the larger the diameter). Irrigation catheters (three-way Foley) should be larger (20–22 Fr).

Coudé (pronounced "coo-DAY"): An elbow-tipped catheter useful in men with prostatic hypertrophy (the catheter is passed with the tip pointing to the 12 o'clock position).

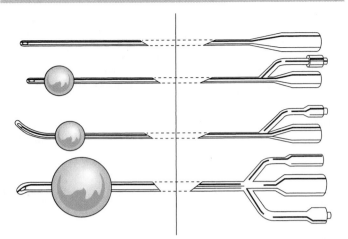

FIGURE 13–20. Bladder catheters, top to bottom: straight Robinson or red rubber catheter, Foley catheter with standard 5-mL balloon, Coudé catheter, and three-way irrigating catheter with 30-mL balloon. Catheters have been shortened for illustrative purposes.

Red rubber catheter (Robinson): Plain rubber or latex catheter without a balloon, usually used for in-and-out catheterization, in which urine is removed but the catheter is not left indwelling.

13 Procedure

1. Use strict aseptic technique.
2. Have the patient lie supine in a well-lighted area; female patients with knees flexed wide and heels together to get adequate exposure of the meatus.
3. Get all the materials ready before attempting to insert the catheter. Open the kit, and put on the gloves. Open the prep solution, and soak the cotton balls. Apply the sterile drapes.
4. Inflate and deflate the balloon of the Foley catheter to ensure its proper function. Coat the end of the catheter with lubricant jelly.
5. In **female patients,** use one gloved hand to prep the urethral meatus in a pubis-toward-anus direction; hold the labia apart with the other gloved hand. For uncircumcised male patients, retract the foreskin to prep the glans; use a gloved hand to hold the penis still.
6. Do not let the hand used to hold the penis or labia touch the catheter to insert it; use the disposable forceps in the kit insert the catheter. Or, use the forceps to prep, and then use the gloved hand to insert the catheter.
7. For **male patients,** stretch the penis upward perpendicular to the body to eliminate any internal folds in the urethra that might lead to a false passage. Use **steady, gentle** pressure to advance the catheter. The bulbous urethra is the most likely part to tear. Any significant resistance encountered may represent a stricture and requires urologic consultation. In men with BPH, a Coudé tip catheter may facilitate passage. Tricks used to get a

catheter to pass in a male patient are to make sure that the penis is well stretched and to instill 3050 mL of sterile water-based surgical lubricant (K-Y jelly) into the urethra with a catheter-tipped syringe before passing the catheter. Viscous lidocaine jelly for urologic use can help lubricate and relieve the discomfort of difficult catheter placement. Allow at least 5 min after instillation of the lidocaine jelly for the anesthetic effect to take place.

8. For both male and female patients, insert the catheter to the hilt of the drainage end. In male patients, compress the penis toward the pubis. These maneuvers ensure that the balloon inflates in the bladder and not in the urethra. Inflate the balloon with 5–10 mL of sterile water or, occasionally, air. After inflation, pull the catheter back so that the balloon comes to rest on the bladder neck. There should be good urine return when the catheter is in place. If a large amount of lubricant jelly was placed into the urethra, you may have to flush the catheter with sterile saline to clear the excess lubricant. A catheter that will not irrigate is probably **in the urethra, not the bladder.**

9. In uncircumcised male patients, reposition the foreskin to prevent massive edema of the glans after the catheter is inserted.

10. Catheters in female patients can be taped to the leg. In male patients, the catheter should be taped to the abdominal wall to decrease stress on the posterior urethra and help prevent stricture formation. The catheter is usually attached to a gravity drainage bag or a device for measuring the amount of urine. Many new kits come with the catheter already secured to the drainage bag. These systems are considered closed; do not open them if at all possible.

"In-and-Out" Catheterized Urine

1. If urine is needed for analysis or for C&S, especially for a female patient, a so-called in-and-out catheterization can be done. This procedure is also useful for measuring residual urine in male or female patients. The incidence of inducing infection with this procedure is about 3%.

2. The procedure is identical to that described for bladder catheterization. The main difference is that a red rubber catheter (no balloon) is often used and is removed immediately after the specimen is collected.

Clean-Catch Urine Specimen

1. A clean-catch urine is useful for routine urinalysis, is usually good for culturing urine from male patients, but is only fair for culturing urine from female patients because of the potential for contamination.

2. For male patients:
   a. Expose the glans, clean with a povidone–iodine solution and dry the area with a sterile pad.
   b. Collect midstream urine in a sterile container after the initial flow has escaped.

3. For female patients:
   a. Separate the labia widely to expose the urethral meatus; keep the labia spread throughout the procedure.
   b. Cleanse the urethral meatus with povidone–iodine solution from front to back, and rinse with sterile water.
   c. Catch the midstream portion of the urine in a sterile container.

Percutaneous Suprapubic Bladder Aspiration

Indications

Used most frequently in young children.

- Inability to obtain urine with a less invasive method
- Urethral abnormalities
- Refractory UTI

Contraindications

- Voiding within the last hour (children)
- Inability to percuss the bladder

Procedure

1. This procedure is almost exclusively limited to infants younger than 6 mo.
2. Immobilize the child. Do not attempt this procedure if the child has voided within the last hour.
3. Palpate the bladder above the pubic symphysis (the bladder sticks out high above the pubis in a young child when it is full). Some clinicians suggest occluding the urethra in boys by holding the penis and in girls by inserting a finger in the rectum to exert pressure. Percuss out the limits of the bladder.
4. Obtain a 20-mL syringe with a 23- or 25-gauge, $1^{1}/2$-in (4 cm) needle. Prep with povidone–iodine and alcohol $^{1}/2$–$1^{1}/2$ in (1.5–4 cm) above the pubis. Anesthesia is not routinely used.
5. Insert the needle perpendicular to the skin in the midline; maintain negative pressure on the downstroke and on withdrawal until urine is obtained (Figure 13–21).
6. If no urine is obtained, wait at least 1 h before reattempting the procedure.

VENIPUNCTURE

Indications

- Venipuncture **(phlebotomy)** is the puncture of a vein to obtain a sample of venous blood for analysis.

Materials

- Tourniquet ($1^{1}/2$-in [4 cm] Penrose drain or BP cuff is acceptable replacement)
- Alcohol prep pad, gauze pad, and adhesive bandage
- Proper specimen tubes for desired studies (red top, purple top, etc) (Table 13–8, page 318)
- Appropriate-sized syringe for volume of blood needed (5 mL, 10 mL, etc), or Vacutainer tube and appropriate needle and Vacutainer holder. The BD Eclipse blood collection system includes a manually activated needle shield.
- A 20- to 22-gauge needle (Larger needles are uncomfortable, and smaller ones can cause hemolysis or clotting; the higher the gauge number, the smaller the needle, see Figure 13–1A.)

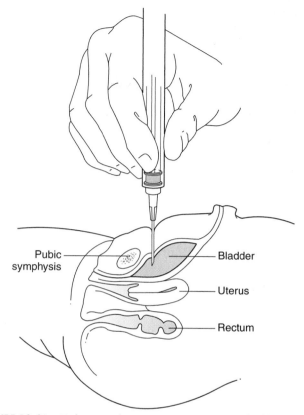

FIGURE 13–21.   Technique and anatomic structures in suprapubic bladder aspiration. (Reprinted, with permission, from: Gomella TL [ed] *Neonatology: Basic Management, On-Call Problems, Diseases, Drugs,* 5th ed. McGraw-Hill, 2004.)

Procedure

Blood cultures, IV techniques, and arterial punctures are discussed in other sections of the chapter.

1. Collect the necessary materials before you begin, including extras in case there is a problem.
2. The common sites for routine venipuncture are the veins of the antecubital fossa (see Figure 13–12, page 286). Alternative sites include the dorsum of the hand, the forearm, the saphenous vein near the medial malleolus, and the external jugular vein. If peripheral sites are unacceptable, use the femoral vein. **Never draw a blood sample proximal to an IV site** because of the high concentration of IV fluid in the veins.
3. Apply the tourniquet at least 2–3 in (5–8 cm) above the venipuncture site. Have the patient make a fist to help engorge the vein. If veins are difficult to locate, try gently slapping or flicking the vein to cause reflex dilation,

TABLE 13-8
Tube Guide for Venipuncture Using the Vacutainer System (from BD Biosciences)

Vacutainer Tube	Vacutainer Hemogard Closure	Additive	Number or Inversions at Blood Collection (Invert gently, do not shake)	Laboratory Use
Black/red marbled ("tiger top")	Gold	Clot activator and gel for serum separation	5	SST brand tube for serum demonstrations in chemistry. Tube inversions ensure mixing of clot activator with blood and clotting within 30 min
Green/red marbled	Light green	Lithium heparin and gel for plasma separation	8	PST brand tube for plasma determinations in chemistry. Tube inversions prevent clotting
Red	Red	None	0	For serum determinations in chemistry, serology, and blood banking
Yellow/black marbled	Orange	Thrombin	8	For stat serum determinations in chemistry. Tube inversions prevent clotting, usually in less than 5 min
Royal blue	Royal blue	Sodium heparin Na EDTA None	8 8 0	For trace element, toxicology, and nutrient determinations. Special stopper formulation offers the lowest verified levels of trace elements available (see package insert)

(continued)

318

13

TABLE 13-8
(Continued)

Vacutainer Tube	Vacutainer Hemogard Closure	Additive	Number or Inversions at Blood Collection (Invert gently, do not shake)	Laboratory Use
Green	Green	Sodium heparin	8	For plasma determinations in chemistry. Tube inversions prevent clotting
		Lithium heparin	8	
		Ammonium heparin	8	
Gray	Gray	Potassium oxalate/ Sodium fluoride	8	For glucose determinations. Tube inversions ensure proper mixing of additive and blood. Oxalate and heparin, anticoagulants, will give samples that are serum
		Sodium fluoride	8	
		Lithium iodoacetate	8	
Brown	Brown	Sodium heparin	8	For lead determinations. This tube is certified to contain less than .01 mcg/mL (ppm) lead. Tube inversions prevent clotting
Yellow	Yellow	Sodium polyanethole-sulfonate (SPS)	8	For blood culture specimen collections in microbiology. Tube inversions prevent clotting

(continued)

13

TABLE 13–8
(Continued)

Vacutainer Tube	Vacutainer Hemogard Closure	Additive	Number or Inversions at Blood Collection (Invert gently, do not shake)	Laboratory Use
Lavender	Lavender	Liquid EDTA Freeze-dried Na EDTA	8 8	For whole blood hematology determinations. Tube inversions prevent clotting
Light blue	Light blue	0.105 M sodium citrate (3.2%) 0.129 M sodium citrate (3.8%)	8 8	For coagulation determinations on plasma specimens. Tube inversions prevent clotting. Note: Certain tests require chilled specimens. Follow recommended procedures for collection and transport of specimen

hanging the extremity in a dependent position, wrapping the extremity in a warm wet towel, substituting a BP cuff for the standard tourniquet, or applying nitroglycerin paste below and over the area to help dilate the veins.

4. Swab the site with the alcohol prep pad, and allow the alcohol to evaporate.

5. The **Vacutainer system** has become the standard means of collecting blood for analysis. Screw a 20- to 22-gauge Vacutainer needle on the Vacutainer cup, and rotate the safety shield back. In the Eclipse needle system (BD Biosciences) a shield covering the end of the needle is manually activated after the sample is collected. Remove the protective needle cap.

6. Keep the needle bevel up, and puncture the skin alongside the vein. After the needle is through the skin, use the thumb of your free hand to stabilize the vein and prevent it from rolling. Enter the vein on the side at about a 30-degree angle. An alternative technique is to enter both the skin and vein in one stick. This maneuver requires practice because the vein is often punctured through and through.

7. Advance the appropriate collection tube (see Table 13–8, page 318) onto the needle inside the Vacutainer cup. The vacuum inside the tube automatically collects the sample. If you hold the Vacutainer steady, several tubes can be collected in this manner.

8. After the blood is collected, remove the tourniquet, withdraw the needle, and apply firm pressure with the alcohol swab or sterile gauze for 2–3 min. The BD Eclipse needle allows rapid one-handed reshielding of the needle tip. Elevation of the extremity is helpful for limiting hematoma. Bending the arm actually increases the size of the venipuncture site and should be discouraged.

9. If no peripheral veins can be located, attempt to puncture the **femoral vein.** Locate the femoral artery using the **NAVEL** system (see page 249). The femoral vein should be just medial to the femoral artery. After prepping the skin, insert the needle perpendicular to the skin, and gently aspirate. The vein should be about 1–1 1/2 in (2.5–4 cm) below the skin. Apply firm pressure after collecting the sample; hematomas are frequent complications of femoral venipuncture. If the the femoral artery is accidentally entered, it is acceptable to collect the sample. Apply pressure for a longer period (5 min) if the artery is entered.

10. In children and elderly persons with fragile veins, a butterfly (21–25 gauge) can be used to obtain a sample (see Figure 13–14, page 288). Attach a syringe, or use a needleless Vacutainer system.

PAIN MANAGEMENT

Defining Pain and Educating the Patient   Assessing Pain
Classification of Pain   Pain Management (Acute vs Chronic)
Adverse Physiologic Effects of Pain   Patient-Controlled Analgesia

DEFINING PAIN AND EDUCATING THE PATIENT

The International Association for the Study of Pain defines pain as an "unpleasant sensory and emotional experience associated with actual or potential tissue damage." Pain is the most common symptom that brings patients to see a physician, and it is frequently the first alert of an ongoing pathologic process. Whenever possible, inform the patient beforehand about the nature and the degree of pain to be expected during a hospital stay. Make the pain control options clear during and after hospitalization so that the patient will have realistic expectations.

CLASSIFICATION OF PAIN

Somatic Pain

A well-localized constant, achy area in skin and subcutaneous tissues and less well-localized in bone, connective tissues, blood vessels, and muscles. Examples are incisional pain, bone fractures, bony metastasis, osteoarthritis and rheumatoid arthritis, and peripheral vascular disease.

Visceral Pain

Poorly localized, crampy, diffuse, and deep sensation originating from an internal organ or a cavity lining. Examples are bladder distention and spasms, intestinal distention, inflammatory bowel disease, hiatal hernia, organ metastasis, and pericarditis.

Neuropathic Pain

A poorly localized, electric-shock-like, lancinating, shooting sensation originating from injury to a peripheral nerve, the spinal cord, or the brain. Examples are diabetic neuropathy, radiculopathy, postherpetic neuralgia, phantom limb pain, and tumor-related nerve compression.

ADVERSE PHYSIOLOGIC EFFECTS OF PAIN

Table 14–1, page 324, shows adverse effects of pain as they relate to specific organ systems.

ASSESSING PAIN

Pain assessment has physiologic, emotional, and psychological aspects. Ask the patient about discomfort. Conduct a detailed history interview to gather information about the patient's pain.

TABLE 14–1
Adverse Effects of Pain as They Relate to
Specific Organ Systems

Organ System	Adverse Effect
RESPIRATORY	
Increased skeletal muscle tension	Hypoxia, hypercapnia
Decreased total lung compliance	Ventilation–perfusion abnormality, atelectasis, pneumonitis
ENDOCRINE	
Increased adrenocorticotropic hormone	Protein catabolism, lipolysis, hyperglycemia
Decreased insulin, decreased testosterone	Decreased protein anabolism, decreased sex drive
Increased aldosterone, increased antidiuretic hormone	Salt and water retention, congestive heart failure, edema
Increased catecholamines	Vasoconstriction, hypertension
Increased angiotensin II	Increased myocardial contractility
CARDIOVASCULAR	
Increased myocardial work	Dysrhythmias, angina, ischemia
IMMUNOLOGIC	
Lymphopenia, depression of reticuloendothelial system leukocytosis	Decreased immune function, increased susceptibility to infection
Reduced killer T-cell cytotoxicity	
COAGULATION EFFECTS	
Increased platelet adhesiveness, diminished fibrinolysis	Increased incidence of thromboembolic phenomena
Activation of coagulation cascade	
GASTROINTESTINAL	
Increased sphincter tone	Ileus
Decreased smooth muscle tone	
GENITOURINARY	
Increased sphincter tone	Urinary retention
Decreased smooth muscle tone	

14

Information about what relieves the pain and what makes it worse is as important as how long the pain lasts. Is the pain constant or intermittent? Does it have any precipitating factors? Does the pain radiate to a specific extremity, or is it referred from an internal source? An example of a pain radiating to a limb is lower back pain with associated right or left leg radiation. An example of referred pain is a ureteral calculus referring pain to the ipsilateral testicle. Are there any accompanying symptoms, such as nausea, vomiting, or headache?

In addition to a thorough physical exam, consider using a pain assessment instrument or rating scale to further stratify the level of pain.

Visual Analog Scales

Often called the "fifth vital sign." Ask the patient to indicate on a visual scale the intensity of pain. These scales are particularly useful for assessing pain management interventions. Examples of commonly used visual scales are shown in Figure 14–1.

McGill Pain Questionnaire: The MPQ (Malzack RR: The McGill Pain Questionnaire: Major properties and scoring methods. *Pain* 1975;1:227–299) is a checklist of words describing symptoms. Analyze scores in various sensory and affective dimensions to identify the quality of pain. Consider using this tool in the detailed management of pain syndromes.

Psychological Evaluation: A psychological evaluation is indicated if medical evaluation does not reveal an apparent cause of pain. Two tools frequently used for evaluating chronic pain and depression are the Minnesota Multiple Personality Inventory (Hathway SR and McKinley JC: *MMPI.* University of Minneapolis Press, Minneapolis, 1989) and Beck Depression Inventory (Beck AT, Steer RA: Internal consistencies of the original and revised Beck Depression Inventory. *J Clin Psychol* 1984;40:1365–1367). Use these questionnaires to determine the patient's psychological status and to his or her behavior and response to pain and its management.

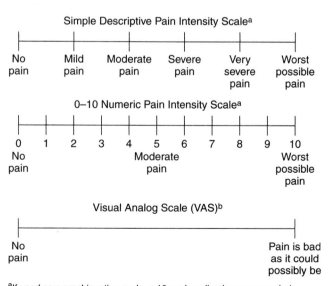

FIGURE 14–1. Scales used to determine pain intensity. The patient is asked to indicate where on the scale their pain would fall. (From Clinical Practice Guidelines Number 9: Management of Cancer Pain, Rockville, MD, US Department of Health and Human Services, ACHPR publication 94-0592).

Electromyography and Nerve Conduction Testing: Used to differentiate neurogenic from myogenic causes of pain and to confirm a diagnosis of nerve entrapment, neural trauma, or polyneuropathy.

Thermography: Under normally circumstances, heat from body surfaces is emitted in the form of infrared energy; this emission is symmetrical in homologous areas. Neurogenic pathophysiologic changes result in asymmetry. This infrared energy can be measured and displayed: Hyperemission indicates an acute stage and hypoemission a chronic stage.

Diagnostic and Therapeutic Neural Blockade: Neural blockade with local anesthetics used in the diagnosis and management of both acute and chronic pain.

PAIN MANAGEMENT (ACUTE VS CHRONIC)

The goal of pain management is to provide the patient adequate relief with minimum side effects (eg, drowsiness). Always begin therapy with the lowest dose of any medicine that provides significant relief.

Pain management can be generally divided into:

- Pharmacologic
- Nonpharmacologic
- Combinations according to patient response and compliance

Pharmacologic

The World Health Organization has made specific recommendations concerning pain management. These principles apply primarily to cancer pain but can be used in any clinical setting. Start at step 1 and advance to the next level on the basis of the patient's response.

Step 1: Nonopioid agents (eg, NSAIDs, acetaminophen, aspirin, COX-2 inhibitors)
Step 2: Weak opioids (codeine, oxycodone) or opioid-like agents

- Use concurrently with step 1 agents (eg, oxycodone, hydrocodone combinations)
- Weak opioids as single agents (immediate-release codeine, propoxyphene)
- Opioid agonists and antagonists (pentazocine, butorphanol)
- Other agents such as ketorolac or tramadol

Step 3: Strong opioids. Controlled-release oxycodone, morphine, or fentanyl
Step 4: Multimodal approach (eg, neurolysis)

Specific pharmacologic agents are reviewed in the following section and in Table 14–2 with additional information in Chapter 22. Supplemental agents can enhance the effects of analgesics and allow dose reduction of some agents.

Nonopioid Analgesics: A multimodal approach may involve pharmacologic and nonpharmacologic methods. Aspirin, acetaminophen, and NSAIDs are the principal nonopioid analgesics used to manage mild and moderate pain. NSAIDs are primarily cyclooxygenase inhibitors that prevent prostaglandin-mediated amplification of chemical and mechanical irritants of the sensory pathways. Short-term (maximum 5 d of use) perioperative use of ketorolac (Toradol) can reduce pain medication requirements. **Side effects:** Possible hepatotoxicity (large dose of acetaminophen); stomach upset, nausea, dyspepsia, ulceration of gastric mucosa; dizziness; platelet dysfunction; exacerbation of bronchospasm; acute renal insufficiency (aspirin and NSAIDs).

(*Text continues on page 337.*)

TABLE 14-2
List of Commonly Used Analgesic Agents

Generic and (Brand) Names	Dose Range/ Interval (Adults)	Dose Range/ Interval (Children)	Indications	Contraindications	Comments
Acetaminophen (Tylenol)	650–1000 mg q4–6h and PRN; daily max 4000 mg	10–15 mg/kg q4h	Mild to moderate pain. Use in aspirin-sensitive patients.	Use with caution in liver disease or history of alcohol abuse	No peripheral antiinflammatory effects, unlike NSAIDs
Tramadol	50–100 mg q4–6h; daily max 400 mg	Not recommended under age 16	Moderate to moderately severe pain	Caution if used with hypnotics, centrally acting analgesics, opioids, or psychotropic drugs or acute intoxication with alcohol	Risk of nausea, dizziness, seizure in patients with SSRIs, tricyclics, MAO inhibitors, neuroleptics and history of seizures
SALICYLATES–ACETYLATES					
Aspirin	650–975 mg q4h; daily max 4000 mg	10–15 mg/kg q4h	Mild to moderate pain	Do not use in children <12 w/ viral illness because of risk of Reye syndrome	Risk of GI bleeding, ulcers, perforation, platelet dysfunction. Must be discontinued for 7–10 d if patient is to undergo surgery

(*continued*)

14

TABLE 14-2
(Continued)

Generic and (Brand) Names	Dose Range/ Interval (Adults)	Dose Range/ Interval (Children)	Indications	Contraindications	Comments
SALICYLATES—NONACETYLATED					
Choline magnesium trisalicylate (Trilisate)	1000–1500 mg bid; daily max 2000–3000 mg	25 mg/kg bid	Long-term management of OA, RA; acute pain of shoulder or knee	Sensitivity to nonacetylated salicylates	Useful in patients with bony metastasis and those who are allergic to ASA. The drug has minimal antiplatelet activity.
Diflunisal (Dolobid)	1000 mg initial, followed by 500 mg q12h; daily 1500 mg	Not recommended < age 12	Acute and long-term mild to moderate pain; OA, RA	Hypersensitivity to aspirin or other NSAIDs	Potential for life-threatening (NSAID) hypersensitivity syndrome; disrupts platelet function with high doses; Reye syndrome
Salsalate (Disalcid)	500 mg q4h; daily max varies	Not indicated	Pain related to OA, RA, other rheumatic disorders	Hypersensitivity or allergy to salsalate	Minimal antiplatelet activity; useful in patients with bony metastasis and those who are allergic to ASA
NONSELECTIVE NSAIDS					
Ibuprofen (Advil, Motrin, Nuprin, Mediprin, Rufen)	400 mg q4–6h; 800 mg q8h; daily max 2400 mg	5–10 mg/kg q6–8h; daily max 40 mg/kg	Mild to moderate pain, fever in children, RA, OA, other pain	Hypersensitivity to aspirin or other NSAIDs; severe kidney disease	Increases risk of GI bleeding, ulcers, perforation, platelet dysfunction

(continued)

TABLE 14–2
(Continued)

Generic and (Brand) Names	Dose Range/ Interval (Adults)	Dose Range/ Interval (Children)	Indications	Contraindications	Comments
Indomethacin (Indocin)	25 mg q8–12h; daily max 100 mg	6 mo, 0.5 mg/kg IM/ IV q6h, max 30 mg/ dose	Mild to severe acute pain, OA, RA, other rheumatic disorders	Hypersensitivity to aspirin or other NSAIDs	Usually a second-line drug because of high incidence of GI and CNS sensory adverse effects
Ketorolac (Toradol)	30–60 mg IM or 30 mg IV initial, 15 or 30 mg IV or IM q6h, also available PO	Not indicated for pediatric use	Short-term management of moderate to severe acute pain, eg, postoperative	Hypersensitivity to aspirin or other NSAIDs; GI disease; bleeding disorders; renal disorders; labor and delivery; nursing	Increases risk of renal failure in dehydrated patients; may cause fluid retention, CHF. **Treatment should be limited to 5 d max.**
Nabumetone (Relafen)	1000–2000 mg/d q12–24h; daily max 2000 mg	Not indicated for pediatric use	Signs or symptoms of OA, RA, ankylosing spondylitis	Hypersensitivity to aspirin or other NSAIDs	Has increased risk of GI bleeding, ulcers, and perforation like any other NSAID

(continued)

14

TABLE 14–2
(Continued)

Generic and (Brand) Names	Dose Range/ Interval (Adults)	Dose Range/ Interval (Children)	Indications	Contraindications	Comments
Naproxen (Aleve, Anaprox, Naprosyn)	550 mg initial, 250 subsequent q6–8h; daily max 1250–1375 mg (depends on formulation)	5 mg/kg q12h	Acute and chronic pain of OA, RA, other rheumatic disorders	Hypersensitivity to aspirin or other NSAIDs	Risk of GI bleeding, ulcers, perforation
Oxaprozin (Daypro)	600–1200 mg q24h; daily max 1800 mg	For juvenile RA > age 6 10–20 mg/kg q24h; daily max 1200 mg	Acute and long-term management of OA, RA	Hypersensitivity to aspirin or other NSAIDs	Increased NSAID-related, risk of GI bleeding, ulcers, perforation
Piroxicam (Feldene)	20 mg/d, q12–24h; daily max 20 mg	Not indicated for pediatric use	Acute and long-term management of OA, RA	Hypersensitivity to aspirin or other NSAIDs	Increases risk of GI bleeding, ulcers, perforation; steady-state blood levels are reached in 7–12 d

(continued)

14

TABLE 14–2
(Continued)

Generic and (Brand) Names	Dose Range/ Interval (Adults)	Dose Range/ Interval (Children)	Indications	Contraindications	Comments
MUSCLE RELAXANTS					
Carisoprodol (Soma)	350 mg q8h and at bedtime	Not indicated	Acute, painful musculo-skeletal conditions; does not directly relax tense skeletal muscles	Acute intermittent porphyria; sensitivity to related compounds	Use with caution in patients with altered kidney/liver function; it has potential for abuse
Cyclobenzaprine HCl (Flexeril)	20–40 mg/d q6–8h; daily max 60 mg	Not indicated	Muscle spasm associated with acute painful musculoskeletal conditions	Use of MAO inhibitors; acute MI; heart disorders; hyperthyroidism	Enhances the effects of alcohol, barbiturates, and other CNS depressants
OPIOID ANALGESICS					
Codeine	15–60 mg q4–6h; daily max varies	> 1 y old; 0.5–1 mg/kg q4–6h	Mild to moderate pain	Hypersensitivity to codeine	Drug effects may be exaggerated in head injury, may obscure its clinical course; caution with liver/kidney disease. May cause significant respiratory depression; patients should be monitored judiciously with pulse oximetry or respiratory checks or both

(continued)

14

**TABLE 14-2
(Continued)**

Generic and (Brand) Names	Dose Range/ Interval (Adults)	Dose Range/ Interval (Children)	Indications	Contraindications	Comments
Hydromorphone (Dilaudid)	Start tabs 2–4 mg q3–4h; liq-uid 2.5–10 mL q3–6h; daily max varies	> 6 mo: 0.03–0.08 q4–6h	Moderate to severe pain	Impaired respiration	Caution in head injury, abdominal conditions; decrease dose for older patients. Significant respiratory depression may occur; monitor respiration carefully.
Meperidine (Demerol, Mepergan)	Tabs/syrup: 50–150 mg q3–4h; daily max 600 mg	Tabs/syrup: 0.5–1 mg/lb q3–4h or 1–1.75 mg/kg q3–4h	Moderate to severe pain	Do not use concomitantly with MAO inhibitors. Avoid its use in elderly patients and in renal disease.	Caution in head injury, abdominal conditions, sickle cell disease, impaired respiration; may cause sei-zures, psychosis, anxiety, delirium; toxic metabolites; normeperidine can accumulate, especially in patients with renal insufficiency and the elderly
Methadone (Dolophine)	Tabs/soln 2.5–10 mg q4h	Not indicated	Severe acute and chronic pain; heroin withdrawal	Hypersensitivity to methadone	Use with caution in head injury, abdominal conditions, or concomi-tant use of other CNS depressants

(continued)

TABLE 14-2
(Continued)

Generic and (Brand) Names	Dose Range/Interval (Adults)	Dose Range/Interval (Children)	Indications	Contraindications	Comments
Morphine immediate release (MSIR, Roxanol)	Oral form given q4h to establish daily opioid requirement	Some forms may be used in children; most are not indicated	Moderate to severe pain; used most often in terminal illness	Respiratory depression, severe asthma, paralytic ileus	Use with caution in head injury, abdominal conditions, renal disease, use of other CNS depressants, and older patients. Respiratory depression precautions.
Morphine sustained release (Kadian, MS Contin, Oramorph SR, Avinza)	Given only after establishing daily opioid requirement; 1/2 daily requirement given q12h	Some forms may be used in children; most are not indicated	Moderate to severe pain; used most often in terminal illness	Respiratory depression severe asthma, paralytic ileus	Use with caution in head injury, abdominal conditions, renal disease, use of other CNS depressants, and older patients. Respiratory depression precautions.
Oxycodone immediate release (OxyIR, Roxicodone)	Regimen can be individualized according to opioid/non-opioid requirements	Dosage forms should be adjusted for weight	Moderate to severe pain	Respiratory depression, severe asthma, paralytic ileus	Use with caution in head injury, abdominal conditions, renal disease, use of other CNS depressants

14

(continued)

333

**TABLE 14-2
(Continued)**

Generic and (Brand) Names	Dose Range/ Interval (Adults)	Dose Range/ Interval (Children)	Indications	Contraindications	Comments
Oxycodone sustained release (OxyContin)	Regimen can be individualized according to opioid/non-opioid requirements	Not indicated < age 18	Moderate to severe pain	Respiratory depression, severe asthma, paralytic ileus	Use with caution in head injury, abdominal conditions, renal disease, use of other CNS depressants
Propoxyphene (Darvon, Darvon-N)	Darvon: 65 mg q4h; Darvon-N: 100 mg q4h	Not indicated	Mild to moderate pain w/wo fever	Suicidal or addiction-prone patients; do not use with alcohol; hypersensitivity to propoxyphene	Propoxyphene metabolites may accumulate. Overdose may cause seizures. Drug carries risk of renal toxicity.
COMBINATION ANALGESICS					
Codeine/acetaminophen (Tylenol w/ codeine)	15–60 mg/300–100 mg on varying schedule; daily max 360/4000 mg; elixir form is available	> age 3 y 0.5–1 mg/kg q4h based on codeine	Tabs for mild to moderately severe pain; elixir for mild to moderate pain	Hypersensitivity to any component	Use with caution in head injury, abdominal conditions and in older patients

(continued)

14

TABLE 14–2
(Continued)

Generic and (Brand) Names	Dose Range/ Interval (Adults)	Dose Range/ Interval (Children)	Indications	Contraindications	Comments
Hydrocodone/ acetamino-phen (Hydrocet, Lorcet, Lortab, Vicodin)	1–2 (2.5–10 mg/500 mg) caps q4–6h; daily max 8 caps	Not indicated	Moderate to moderately severe pain	Hypersensitivity to hydrocodone or acetaminophen	Use with caution in head injury, abdominal conditions; respiratory depression may ensue; monitor respiratory function closely
Oxycodone/acet-aminophen (Percocet, Roxicet, Tylox)	1–2 (2.5–10 mg/325 mg) tab q4–6h; daily max varies	Not indicated	Moderate to moderately severe pain	Hypersensitivity to oxycodone or acetaminophen	Use with caution in head injury, abdominal conditions, and elderly population
Propoxyphene/ acetamino-phen (Darvocet)	100 mg/650 mg q4h; propoxyphene daily max 600 mg	Not indicated	Mild to moderate pain w/wo fever	Hypersensitivity to propoxyphene or acetaminophen	Caution in head injury, abdominal conditions and impaired hepatic or renal functions

(continued)

14

TABLE 14-2
(Continued)

Generic and (Brand) Names	Dose Range/ Interval (Adults)	Dose Range/ Interval (Children)	Indications	Contraindications	Comments
Pentazocine/aspirin (Talwin)	2 (12.5 mg/325 mg) caplets q6–8h; daily max varies	Not recommended < age 12 30 mg IM/IV q3–4h; IM max 60 mg; IV max 30 mg	Moderate pain	Hypersensitivity to pentazocine or acetaminophen	High potential for abuse. Caution in head injury, abdominal conditions; may cause respiratory depression, renal/hepatic disorders, and risk or Reye syndrome. Subcutaneous injections may cause severe tissue damage.
Hydrocodone/ibuprofen (Vicoprofen)	1 (7.5 mg/200 mg) tablet q4–6h; max 5 tabs daily	Not recommended < age 16	Best for short-term (< 10 d) of moderate to severe acute pain treatment	Hypersensitivity to hydrocodone, ibuprofen, aspirin, or other NSAIDs	Increases risk of anaphylactic reaction; possible GI ulceration, bleeding, perforation. Use with caution in head injury, abdominal conditions. Can cause respiratory depression.

ASA = aspirin; CHF = congestive heart failure; CNS = central nervous system; GI = gastrointestinal; MAO = monoamine oxidase; MI = myocardial infarction; NSAID = nonsteroidal antiinflammatories; OA = osteoarthritis; RA = rheumatoid arthritis; SSRI = selective serotonin reuptake inhibitors.

14

336

(Text continued from page 326.)

Opioids: Attach to opioid receptors, which are responsible for their analgesic effect. **Side effects:** In acute pain, nausea and vomiting are the most common side effects and usually resolve with time or antiemetics. In chronic pain, constipation is the most common side effect and persists until treatment cessation. Other side effects include sedation, miosis, and dizziness with smaller doses. Larger doses can precipitate respiratory depression, apnea, circulatory arrest, comma, and death. These more serious side effects may necessitate supplemental oxygen therapy, pulse oximetry monitoring, and close patient supervision. Opioids can be taken orally or parenterally or by the neuroaxillary route (intrathecal/epidural). Opioids are available in short- (q4h) and long-duration forms (eg, q12h, q24h). Opioids can also be given IV as a patient-controlled analgesia (PCA) (see page 338). Comparison of opioids can be found in Table 14–2, page 327.

Antidepressants: Work well as adjuncts and are an appropriate consideration mostly for chronic pain associated with diabetic neuropathy, postherpetic neuralgia, and chemotherapy. **Side effects:** Antimuscarinic effects (dry mouth, impaired visual accommodation, urinary retention), antihistaminic (sedation), and alpha-adrenergic blockage (orthostatic hypotension).

Neuroleptics: Used to treat patients with agitation and psychological symptoms. **Side effects:** Extrapyramidal and neuroleptic drug symptoms; mask-like facies, festinating gait, cogwheel rigidity (bradykinesia) managed with benztropine or diphenhydramine.

Anticonvulsants: Suppress spontaneous neural discharge. **Side effects:** Bone marrow depression, hepatotoxicity, possible ataxia, dizziness, confusion, and sedation (at higher doses).

Corticosteroids: Antiinflammatory agents. **Side effects:** Hyperglycemia, increased risk of infections, peptic ulcer, osteoporosis, HTN, myopathy, Cushing syndrome.

Local Anesthetics: Bind to sodium channels, exerting effect on the cellular level. Effect usually localized to the area where the drug is injected. **Side effects:** Relatively few side effects. Allergic reactions usually due to PABA-like preservatives in the solution and not the agents themselves. Toxicity (usually due to overdose) includes tonic–clonic seizures, respiratory arrest, and subsequent cardiovascular collapse.

Benzodiazepines: Used to manage anxiety and muscle spasms associated with acute pain. **Side effects:** No analgesic effects and must be used with caution because of abuse potential.

Nerve Blocks or Neurolysis: Destruction of nerves. **Side effects:** Permanent nerve damage

Nonpharmacologic

Physical Therapy: Heat and cold can provide pain relief by alleviating muscle spasm. Heat decreases joint stiffness and increases blood flow; cold vasoconstricts and reduces tissue edema.

Osteopathic or Chiropractic Treatment: Physical manipulation can relax soft tissues, increase range of motion, and alleviate pain. Biweekly or monthly treat-

14

ments are recommended and are best for chronic pain. Acute treatment minimizes musculoskeletal pain.

Radiation: Beneficial in management of cancer pain (eg, bony metastasis).

Psychological Intervention: Cognitive therapy, behavioral therapy, or biofeedback relaxation technique and hypnosis. Pain is often associated with depression, especially when it becomes chronic.

Acupuncture: Needles are inserted into discrete anatomically defined points or meridians and stimulated by mild electric current. This method is believed to release endogenous opioids.

Electrical Stimulation of Nervous System: Analgesia is achieved using various methods of treatment. The three methods are:

1. Transcutaneous electrical stimulation (TENS) with electrodes applied to skin.
2. Spinal cord stimulators: Electrodes connected to an external generator into the epidural space. Patient is under general anesthesia and is awakened half-way through the procedure in the lateral recumbent position. The patient is asked specific questions, and the programming is adjusted accordingly. The patient is put back under anesthesia, and the surgeon can close the skin.
3. Intracerebral stimulation with electrodes implanted in the periaqueductal or periventricular area.

PATIENT-CONTROLLED ANALGESIA (PCA)

Most commonly used after surgery. Allows the patient to self-administer doses of narcotics with an IV pump. The patient manages the pain as soon as he or she feels it coming on, thus avoiding the peak and trough of a narcotic dosing regimen that can lead to extremes of pain or risk of oversedation. The pain management team can titrate the dose of the drug as required with a computerized system that controls the total dose and the interval between doses with or without a continuous basal infusion. PCA duration varies according to procedure and patient response (eg, gynecologic procedures, 1–2 d; bowel operations, 2–5 d; thoracotomy, 4–6 d). Reduce dose in elderly ($1/3$–$2/3$), and consider discontinuation of PCA when patients are able to take analgesics PO.

PCA Ordering Parameters

Table 14–3, page 339, shows examples of PCA orders.

- **Dose:** Number of milliliters (typically morphine concentration or its equivalent) given on activation of button by patient
- **Lockout:** Minimum interval of time in minutes between PCA doses
- **Hourly Max:** Maximum volume (milliliters) that machine will administer in an hour
- **Basal Rate:** Continuous infusion rate may be programmed in addition to the bolus dosing; not recommended unless a qualified member of the anesthesiology department pain team has evaluated the patient. Basal infusions increase risk of significant respiratory depression and should be monitored more closely with hourly respiratory checks.
- **Nursing PRN Bolus:** Number of milliliters nurses can administer at their discretion in addition to PCA dose for breakthrough pain.

PCA Opioid Concentration at Equipotent Levels

Drug	Dose
Morphine	1.0 mg/mL
Meperidine[a]	10 mg/mL
Hydromorphone	0.2 mg/mL
Fentanyl	10–15 mcg/mL

[a]Use only if a patient has allergies to other medications greater side effects profile, ie, seizure from metabolites.

PCA in Renal Failure (nonencephalopathic patient):

Use fentanyl or hydromorphone only, avoiding morphine and meperidine because of their renal excretion.

1. Load with fentanyl 25 mcg or hydromorphone 0.5 mcg IV in postanesthetic care unit and repeat every 5–10 min until patient is comfortable.
2. Maintenance: PCA dose 1 mL; lockout 6 min; hourly max 3–5 mL

TABLE 14–3
Illustrative PCA Orders

Typical Procedure	Dose (mL)	Lockout (min)	Hourly Max (mL)	Basal
Somewhat painful (lower abdominal, incisions, minor orthopedic, gynecologic, or plastic surgical procedures)	1	6	10	None
Fairly painful (upper abdominal incisions)	1–1.5	6	10–15	None Nursing PRN bolus 2–3 mL q1–2h PRN
Very painful (thoracotomy, total knee replacement, shoulder joint repairs)	1–2.0	6	10–20	None Nursing PRN bolus 2–4 mL q1–2h PRN

14

IMAGING STUDIES

X-Ray Preparations
Common Studies: Noncontrast
Common X-Ray Studies: Contrast
Ultrasonography
Computed Tomography (CT)

Spiral (Helical) CT
Magnetic Resonance Imaging (MRI)
Nuclear Scans
Positron Emission Tomography (PET)
How to Read a Chest X-Ray

X-RAY PREPARATIONS

In general, follow this principle: Obtain plain films before obtaining films that require contrast. Each hospital has its own guidelines for patient preps. Consult the radiology department before ordering any x-ray that requires a prep. Examinations that require no specific bowel preparation are routine CXR, flat and upright abdominal films, cystograms, C-spines, skull series, extremity films, CT scans of the head and chest, and many others.

Studies that usually require preps such as enemas, laxatives, or oral contrast agents or those that require that the patient be NPO before the examination include upper GI series, small-bowel follow-through (SBFT), barium enema, IVP, and others. IV contrast studies are discussed below.

COMMON X-RAY STUDIES: NONCONTRAST

Chest

Chest X-Ray (Routine): Includes posteroanterior (PA) and lateral chest films. (PA means the film is placed in front of the patient with the beam coming from the back.) Evaluation of pulmonary, cardiac, and mediastinal diseases and traumatic injury. See How to Read a Chest X-Ray on page 353 and Figures 15–1, page 342, and 15–2, page 343.

Expiratory Chest: Visualization of small pneumothorax

Lateral Decubitus Chest: Allows small amounts of pleural effusion or subpulmonic effusion to layer out; as little as 175 mL of pleural fluid can be detected

Lordotic Chest: Evaluation of apices and lesions of the right and left upper lobes, TB

Portable Chest and AP Films: Imaging of critically ill patients who cannot stand for a routine PA CXR; diagnosis of pneumothorax, pneumonia, and edema; verification of vascular line or tube placement. Not accurate in evaluation of heart or mediastinal size because the standard x-ray is PA (beam from behind), and the AP technique magnifies these structures

Rib Details: Delineation of rib abnormalities when plain CXR or bone scan findings suggest fracture or other metastatic lesions

Abdominal

Abdominal Decubitus: Obtain instead of upright abdominal film for imaging of debilitated patients. Patient's left side is down to show free air outlining the liver and right lateral gutter.

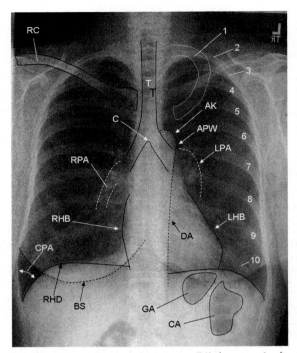

FIGURE 15–1. Structures seen on a posteroanterior (PA) chest x-ray. 1 = first rib; 2–10 = posterior aspect of ribs 2–10; AK = aortic knob; APW = aortopulmonary window, BS = breast shadow (labeled only on right); C = carina; CA = colonic air; CPA = costophrenic angle, DA = descending aorta; GA = gastric air; LHB = left heart border (*Note:* Most of the left heart border represents the left ventricle; the superior aspect of the left heart border represents the left atrial appendage.); LPA = left pulmonary artery; RC = right clavicle (left clavicle not labeled); RHB = right heart border (*Note:* The right heart border represents the right atrium.); RHD = right hemidiaphragm (left hemidiaphragm not labeled); RPA = right pulmonary artery; T = tracheal air column.

15

Acute Abdominal Series ("Obstruction Series"):   Includes flat and upright abdominal films (KUB) and CXR. Initial evaluation of acute abdomen (See KUB.)

Cross-Table Lateral Abdominal: Identification of free air in debilitated patients.

KUB, Supine and Erect: Short for "kidneys, ureter, and bladder"; also known as **flat and upright abdominal, scout film,** and **flat plate.** Useful when the patient complains of abdominal pain or distention, and for initial evaluation of the urinary tract (80% of kidney stones and 20% of gallstones are visualized on KUBs). Look for calcifications, foreign bodies, the gas pattern, psoas shadows, renal and liver shadows, flank stripes, the vertebral bodies, and the pelvic bones. On the upright, look for air–fluid levels of adynamic ileus and mechanical obstruction and for free air under the diaphragm, which suggests a perforated viscus or recent surgery; however, an upright CXR (especially the lateral view) is often best for spotting pneumoperitoneum.

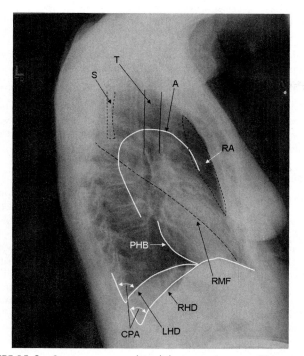

FIGURE 15–2. Structures seen on a lateral chest x-ray. A = aorta; CPA = posterior costophrenic angle; LHD = left hemidiaphragm; PHB = posterior heart border (*Note:* The posterior heart border represents the left atrium superiorly and left ventricle inferiorly; the anterior heart border is not clearly defined on this film but represents the right ventricle.); RA = retrosternal airspace; RHD = right hemidiaphragm; RMF = right major fissure (left major fissure and minor fissures not well visualized on these films but can occasionally be seen); S = scapula; T = tracheal air column.

15

Other Noncontrast X-Rays

C-Spine: Usually includes PA, lateral, and oblique films. Evaluation of trauma, neck pain, and neurologic evaluation of the upper extremities. All seven cervical vertebrae must be seen for this study to be acceptable. Add an "open mouth" view to identify odontoid fractures in trauma.

DEXA Scan (Dual Energy X-Ray Absorptiometry, Bone Densitometry):   Quantification of osteoporosis by measurement of bone mineral density (BMD). Assessment of fracture risk and effect of drugs such as bisphosphonates in osteoporosis. Central DEXA measures BMD in the spine or hip. Results are reported as a T and a Z score. T score shows the amount of bone compared with that of a young adult of the same sex with peak bone mass. A score above –1 is normal, –1 to –2.5 indicates osteopenia, and below –2.5 indicates osteoporosis. Z score reflects the amount of bone compared with an age-matched group.

Mammography: Detection of tumors > 5 mm. Two forms are equal in diagnostic quality:

- **Screen film.** Produces standard black and white x-ray with a specially designed mammographic machine; 3–5 % smaller radiation dose
- **Digital mammography.** Digital images may improve the resolution over film techniques

Sinus Films (Paranasal Sinus Radiographs): Evaluation of sinus trauma, sinusitis, neoplasms, and congenital disorders

Skull Films: Detection of fractures and identification of pituitary tumors and congenital anomalies; not generally as useful as other imaging studies

Thoracic, Lumbar, Sacral Vertebral Radiography: Evaluation of fractures, dislocations, subluxations, disk disease, and the effects of arthritic and metabolic disorders of the spine

COMMON X-RAY STUDIES: CONTRAST

A visualizing agent is used (such as barium, Gastrografin, or an IV contrast agent). If a GI tract fistula or perforation is suspected, inform the radiologist because the presence of such a lesion can affect the choice of contrast agent (eg, using a water-soluble agent such as Gastrografin rather than barium to prevent "barium peritonitis"). Standard IV contrast media are ionic, potentially nephrotoxic, and may be associated with rare adverse reactions when administered systemically (see following section). The use of nonionic contrast media can limit these side effects. In general, for use of an IV contrast agent, the creatinine must be < 1.8–2.0 mg/dL. Patients with elevated creatinine should be well hydrated to minimize nephrotoxicity.

    Contrast reactions to IV agents can occur. The overall incidence is 5%. Severe reactions occur in 1/1000 cases, and death due to anaphylaxis occurs in 1/40,000 cases. Reactions can be mild (nausea, vomiting, sneezing, diaphoresis, headache), intermediate (urticaria, angioneurotic edema, wheezing), or severe (cardiovascular collapse, pulmonary edema, shock, laryngeal edema, respiratory arrest). Vagal reactions (hypotension and bradycardia) are another adverse effect. A history of asthma is a risk factor, and a previous reaction to a contrast agent does not necessarily preclude use of IV contrast material (allergy to seafood or iodine is no longer considered an important risk factor). Premedication with two doses of PO methylprednisolone, one 12 h before and the other 2 h before IV contrast injection, as well as oral antihistamines **may limit** symptoms. For patients with a known history of allergic reaction, a nonionic agent or an alternative imaging technique is recommended.

Angiography: A rapid series of films obtained after a bolus contrast injection through a percutaneous catheter. Imaging of aorta, major arteries and branches, tumors, and venous drainage with late "run-off" films. Helical CT scans also generate angiographic images.

- **Digital subtraction angiography (DSA).** Allows reverse negative views and requires less contrast load
- **Cardiac angiography.** Definitive for diagnosis and assessment of severity of CAD. Significant (> 70% occlusion) stenotic lesions can be seen: 30% involve single vessels, 30% involve two, and 40% involve three vessels.
- **Cerebral angiography.** Evaluation of intra- and extracranial vascular disease, atherosclerosis, aneurysms, and A–V malformations. Not used for detection of cerebral structural lesions (use MRI or CT instead)

- **Pulmonary angiography.** Visualization of emboli, intrinsic or extrinsic vascular abnormalities, A–V malformations, and bleeding due to tumors. Most accurate diagnostic procedure for PE but only used if findings on helical CT or lung $\dot{V}/\dot{Q}$ scan are not diagnostic
- **Bronchial angiography.** Visualization of bleeding vessels from the systemic circuit. Evaluation of hemoptysis in cases of known bronchiectasis

Barium Enema (BE):   Examination of colon and rectum. Indications include diarrhea, crampy abdominal pain, heme-positive stools, change in bowel habits, and unexplained weight loss

- **Air-contrast BE.** Done with the double-contrast technique (air and barium) to better delineate the mucosa. More likely to show polyps than standard BE
- **Gastrografin enema.** Similar to barium enema, but water-soluble contrast agent is used (clears colon more quickly than barium). If Gastrografin leaks from the GI tract, it is less irritating to the peritoneum (does not cause barium peritonitis). Therapeutic in evaluation of obstipation and colonic volvulus; depicts postop anastomotic leak

Barium Swallow (Esophagogram):   Evaluation of swallowing mechanism, esophageal lesions, and abnormal peristalsis

Cystogram: Bladder is filled and emptied with a catheter in place; used to evaluate bladder filling defects (tumors, diverticula) and bladder perforation. Can also be done with CT (CT cystogram is more sensitive for perforation with trauma) (see also Voiding Cystourethrography)

Enteroclysis: Intubation of the proximal jejunum and rapid infusion of contrast material. Better than an SBFT in evaluation of polyps and obstruction (eg, adhesions, internal hernia); used to evaluate small-bowel sources of chronic bleeding after negative upper and lower endoscopy

Endoscopic Retrograde Cholangiopancreatography (ERCP):   Contrast material is endoscopically injected into the ampulla of Vater to visualize the common bile and pancreatic ducts for obstruction, stones, and ductal pattern

Intravenous Pyelography (IVP):   Contrast study of the kidneys and ureters; limited usefulness for evaluating bladder. Indications include flank pain, kidney stones, hematuria, UTI, trauma, and malignancy. Bowel prep helpful but not essential. Creatinine must be < 1.8 mg/dL. Largely replaced by CT urography. **Nephrotomograms** are images of kidney sections for further definition of the three-dimensional location or nature of renal lesions and stones.

Fistulography (Sinogram):   Injection of water-soluble contrast medium into any wound or body opening to determine the connection with other structures

Hysterosalpinogography (HSG):   Evaluation of uterine abnormalities (congenital anomalies, fibroids, adhesions) or tubal abnormalities (occlusion or adhesion), often as part of infertility evaluation. Contraindicated during menses, undiagnosed vaginal bleeding, and acute PID and if pregnancy is suspected. Place the patient in pelvic exam position, insert a speculum, cannulate the uterine os, and inject contrast material.

Lymphangiography: Iodinated oil is injected to opacify lymphatics of the leg and the inguinal, pelvic, and retroperitoneal areas. Test of the integrity of the

15

lymphatic system, evaluation for metastatic tumors (eg, testicular) and lymphoma

Myelography: Evaluation of subarachnoid space for tumors, herniated disks, and other cause of nerve root injury. Use LP technique to inject contrast material into the subarachnoid space.

Oral Cholecystography (OCG): Oral agent is used to visualize gallbladder; generally replaced by ultrasonography

Percutaneous Nephrostography: Management of renal obstruction; percutaneous catheter placement through the renal parenchyma and into the collecting system to relieve and evaluate level and cause of obstruction

Percutaneous Transhepatic Cholangiography (PTHC): Visualization of biliary tree in patients unable to concentrate contrast medium (bilirubin > 3 mg/dL). Needle inserted percutaneously into dilated biliary duct; contrast material injected.

Retrograde Pyelography (RPG): Contrast material injected into the ureters through a cystoscope. Imaging of patients allergic to IV contrast medium or with elevated creatinine, if kidney or ureter cannot be visualized with other imaging techniques, and in the presence of renal mass, ureteral obstruction, or filling defects in the collecting system

Retrograde Urethrography (RUG): Visualization of traumatic disruption of the urethra and urethral strictures

Small Bowel Follow-Through (SBFT): Usually done after a UGI series. Delayed films show jejunum and ileum. Evaluation of diarrhea, abdominal cramps, malabsorption, and UGI bleeding

T-Tube Cholangiography: Contrast injection into T-tube placed in the common bile duct after gallbladder or bile duct surgery. Evaluation of degree of swelling, find residual stones, and evaluate patency of bile duct drainage

Upper GI (UGI) Series: Includes esophagography and imaging of stomach and duodenum. Visualization of ulcers, masses, hiatal hernia and to evaluate heme-positive stools and upper abdominal pain

Venography, Peripheral: Contrast material is injected into a small foot or ankle vein for evaluation of patency of deep veins of leg and calf and detection of filling defect or outline of a thrombus. Noninvasive exams for DVT, such as Doppler ultrasonography and compression ultrasonography; highly sensitive (> 90%) for proximal thrombi. Has largely replaced contrast venography.

Voiding Cystourethrography (VCUG): Bladder is filled with contrast material through a catheter, then catheter is removed, and the patient voids. Diagnosis of vesicoureteral reflux, examination of urethral valves, and evaluation of UTI

ULTRASONOGRAPHY

Abdominal: Gallbladder (95% sensitivity in diagnosis of stones), cholecystitis, biliary tree obstruction, pancreas (pseudocyst, tumor, pancreatitis), aorta (aneurysm), kidneys (obstruction, tumor, cyst), abscesses, ascites

Echocardiography
- **M-mode.** Valve mobility, chamber size, pericardial effusions, septal size

- **Two-dimensional.** Valvular vegetations, septal defects, wall motion, chamber size, pericardial effusion, valve motion, wall thickness
- **Doppler.** Cross-valvular pressure gradients, blood flow patterns, and valve orifice areas in work-up of cardiac valvular disease

Endovaginal: Diagnosis of abnormalities of uterus and ovaries

Pelvic: (*Note:* A full bladder is desirable)

- **Pregnancy.** Fetal dating (biparietal diameters); diagnosis of multiple gestations; determination of intrauterine growth retardation, hydrocephalus, and hydronephrosis; localization of placenta
- **Gynecologic.** Ovarian and uterine masses (eg, tumors, cysts, fibroids), ectopic pregnancy, abscesses

Thyroid: Thyroid nodules (cyst versus solid) and direct biopsy. Ultrasonographic findings alone cannot be used to differentiate benign from malignant lesions.

Transrectal: Rectal wall and prostate abnormalities, prostate needle biopsy in diagnosis of prostate cancer, drainage of pelvic and prostatic abscesses

Other: Testicular and scrotal masses (eg, hydrocele versus tumor), intraoperative determination of bladder emptying

COMPUTED TOMOGRAPHY (CT)

Performed with or without contrast agent. Administration of a dilute oral contrast agent (eg, Tomocat) before abdominal or pelvic scans helps delineate the bowel. IV contrast is used to obtain vascular and tissue enhancement for some CT scans; check the creatinine level to determine the suitability of IV contrast administration. Any body part can be scanned depending on the indications, but CT is most helpful in evaluating the brain, lung, mediastinum, retroperitoneum (pancreas, kidney, nodes, aorta), and liver and to a lesser extent pelvis, colon, and bone.

In CT density, measurements called **Hounsfield units** are used to differentiate cysts, lipomas, hemochromatosis, vascular (enhancing) and avascular (nonenhancing) lesions. In Hounsfield units, bone is +1000, water is 0, fat is –1000, and other tissues fall within this scale, depending on the machine settings. Metal and barium can cause distortion of the image.

Abdominal CT: Imaging of all intraabdominal and retroperitoneal organs and define disease processes. Accurate for abscesses, but ultrasonography may show smaller collections adjacent to the liver, spleen, or bladder. Surgical clips or undiluted barium in the gut can cause artifacts. An IV contrast usually is given, so check creatinine level. Oral contrast helps identify the bowel; give the oral contrast agent at least 45 minutes before imaging.

Chest CT: Depicts 40% more nodules than whole-lung tomograms, which show 20% more nodules than plain CXR. Although calcifications suggest benign disease (eg, granuloma), no definite density value can reliably separate malignant from benign lesions. Useful in differentiating hilar adenopathy from vascular structures seen on plain CXR, especially when contrast-enhanced images are obtained. High-resolution images are useful for characterizing interstitial lung disease. PE-protocol scans are obtained with contrast enhancement on spiral scanners (see below); this protocol frequently includes CT venography of the lower pelvis and legs.

Head CT: Evaluation of tumors, subdural and epidural hematomas, A–V malformations, hydrocephalus, and sinus and temporal bone abnormalities. Initial test of choice for trauma; may be superior to MRI in detection of hemorrhage within first 24–48 h

Mediastinal CT: Masses, nodes, ectopic parathyroid tissue

Neck CT: Work-up of neck masses, abscesses, and other diseases of the throat and trachea

Pelvic CT: Staging and diagnosis of bladder, prostate, rectal, and gynecologic carcinoma; diagnosis of appendicitis, diverticulitis, and complications of pregnancy

Retroperitoneal CT: Evaluation of pancreatitis; pancreatic masses; nodal metastasis from colon, prostate, renal, and testicular tumors; adrenal masses (> 3 cm suggests carcinoma); psoas mass; aortic aneurysm, retroperitoneal hemorrhage

Spinal CT: MRI generally preferred over CT. However, rare conditions, contraindication to MRI, and artifact from metal may make the CT the preferred test.

SPIRAL (HELICAL) CT

Spiral technique can be used for any type of CT. It minimizes motion artifact and allows capture of a bolus of contrast material at peak levels in the region being scanned. Conventional CT is too slow to capture this peak flow. From a practical standpoint, almost all newer CT scanners have multidetector rows for acquisition of multiple (4, 8, 16) spiral scans at one time. These scanners provide higher-resolution images than do older units. Contrast-enhanced spiral CT scans allow detailed 3D reconstruction and angiographic evaluation (aortic, renal, peripheral, carotid, CNS, cardiac). Bony structures can also be visualized without contrast administration. The term *spiral* or *helical* is derived from the fact that the tube spins around the patient while the table moves. Spiral CT can compensate for "streak" artifact due to implanted metallic devices. Diagnosis of PE, pretransplantation angiography, evaluation of flank pain, detection of kidney stones (largely replacing emergency IVP), and rapid evaluation of trauma.

Coronary CT angiography is used to evaluate common causes of acute chest pain and other cardiac indications. It requires a 64-slice scanner that acquires up to 192 images of the heart per second. Calcium scoring is an emerging technology for evaluation of coronary artery disease.

MAGNETIC RESONANCE IMAGING (MRI)

How MRI Works

Measurements of the magnetic movements of atomic nuclei are used to delineate tissues. When placed in a strong magnetic field, nuclei, such as hydrogen, resonate and emit radio signals when pulsed with radio waves. A defined sequence of magnetic pulses and interval pauses produces measured changes in the magnetic vectors of the tissue, which results in an MR image. T1, or longitudinal relaxation time, is the measurement of magnetic vector changes in the z-axis during the relaxation pause. T2, or transverse relaxation time, is the magnetic vector changes in the x-axis and the y-axis.

Each tissue, normal or pathologic, has unique T1 and T2 for a given MRI field strength. In general T1 > T2. T1 = 0.1–2 s and T2 = 0.03–0.6 s. The inherent tissue differences between various T1 and T2 values give the visual contrast seen between tissues on the MR image. An image is **T1-weighted** if it depends on the differences in T1 measurements for visual contrast and **T2-weighted** if it depends on T2 measurements.

The oldest, most common pulse sequence is called spin echo (SE). Partial saturation (PS) and inversion recovery (IR) are variations of the traditional SE sequence. A gradient echo technique now is used to obtain tissue contrast similar to that obtained with older SE methods. MR images are obtained in the transverse, sagittal, oblique, and coronal views.

MRI Contrast: Gadolinium (gadopentetic dimeglumine) is an ionic contrast agent that acts as a paramagnetic agent and enhances vessels and lesions of abnormal vascularity.

How to Read MR Images

SE T1-Weighted Images: Provide good anatomic planes because of the wide variance in T1 values among normal tissues.

- Brightest (high signal intensity): Fat
- Dark or black: Pathologic tissues, tumor or inflammation, fluid collections
- Black (low signal intensity): Respiratory tract, GI tract, calcified bone and tissues, blood vessels, heart chambers, and pericardial effusions

SE T2-Weighted Images: Pathologic lesions prolong T2 measurements, and normal tissues have a very small range of T2 values. T2-weighted images depict pathologic lesions best and normal tissue anatomy not as well. Tumor surrounded by fat may be lost on T2-weighted images.

- Brightest: Fat and fluid collections
- Bright: Pheochromocytoma

When to Use MRI

MRI provides better soft-tissue contrast than CT. MRI also is better than CT for imaging of the brain, spinal cord, musculoskeletal soft tissues, and areas of high CT bony artifact. However, spiral CT may overcome some of these disadvantages.

Advantages

- No ionizing radiation
- Display of vascular anatomy without contrast
- Visualization of linear structures: spine and spinal cord, aorta, vena cava
- Visualization of posterior fossa and other difficult-to-see CT areas
- High-contrast soft-tissue images

Disadvantages

- Claustrophobia because of confining magnet; **open MRI** systems may help, but some may have more motion artifact
- Longer scanning time, resulting in motion artifacts
- Inability to image critically ill patients who need life support equipment
- Metallic foreign bodies (eg, pacemakers, shrapnel, CNS vascular clips, metallic eye fragments, and cochlear implants) are contraindications

Uses of MRI

MRI is sensitive to motion artifact; anxious or agitated patients may have to be sedated for acquisition of optimal images. Intramuscular glucagon can be used to suppress intestinal peristalsis on abdominal studies. If the presence of metallic eye fragments is likely, obtain screening CT scans of the orbits before MRI. MRI is generally contraindicated in patients with intracranial aneurysm clips, intraocular metallic fragments, and pacemakers. Dental fillings and dental prostheses have not been a problem.

Abdomen: Detection of adrenal lesions, tumor staging (renal, GI, pelvic), evaluation of abdominal masses, examination of almost all intraabdominal organs and retroperitoneal structures, and differentiation of benign adenoma from metastasis

Chest: Evaluation of mediastinal masses, differentiation of nodes from vessels, detection of cardiac disease, tumor staging, detection of aortic dissection or aneurysm

Head: Analysis of all intracranial lesions, identification of demyelinating diseases; some conditions, including acute trauma, are better evaluated with CT (see previous section). Magnetic resonance spectroscopy **MRS** may increase the sensitivity of diagnosis of many neurologic diseases by providing a biochemical "fingerprint" of tissues in the brain. Performed in conjunction with MRI equipped with MRS capability. Differentiation of causes of dementia, tumors, MS, and many other conditions.

Musculoskeletal System: Detection of bone tumors and bone and soft-tissue infection, evaluation of joint spaces (unless a prosthesis is in place), marrow disorders, aseptic necrosis of femoral head

Pelvis: Evaluation of all pelvic organs in male and female patients, differentiation of endometrium from myoma and adenomyosis, diagnosis of congenital uterine anomalies (eg, bicornuate, septate). Endorectal surface coil allows enhanced imaging of structures such as the prostate.

Spine: Diagnosis of diseases of the spinal column (eg, herniated disk, tumors)

15

NUCLEAR SCANS

The following are the more commonly used nuclear scans and their purposes. Most are contraindicated in pregnancy; check with your nuclear medicine department.

Adrenal Scan: Localization of pheochromocytoma when MRI or CT findings are equivocal. Performed with labeled **MIBG;** patient must return for imaging several days after MIBG administration.

Bleeding Scan: Detection of source of GI tract bleeding.

- **Technetium-99m** (^{99m}Tc) Sulfur Colloid Scan. Detection of bleeding of 0.05–0.1 mL/min.
- **Technetium-99m** (^{99m}Tc)-Labeled Red Cell Scan. Same as sulfur colloid scan, but may be superior for localizing intermittent bleeding

Bone Scan: Metastatic work-ups (cancers most likely to go to bone: prostate, breast, kidney, thyroid, lung); evaluation of delayed union of fractures, osteomyelitis, avascular necrosis of femoral head; evaluation for hip prosthesis; differentiation of pathologic and traumatic fractures

Brain Scan: Metastatic work-up, determination of blood flow (in brain death or atherosclerotic disease), evaluation of space-occupying lesions (tumor, hematoma, abscess, AV malformation), encephalitis

Cardiac Scans: Diagnosis of MI, stress testing, measurement of ejection fractions and cardiac output, diagnosis of ventricular aneurysms

- **Thallium-201** (^{201}Tl). Measurement of myocardial perfusion by uptake of ^{201}Tl by normal myocardium. Normal myocardium appears hot, and ischemic or infarcted areas cold. AMI (< 12 h) seen as a hotspot, old MI (scar) seen as cold on both resting and exercise scans. Ischemia is cold on exercise scan and returns to normal after rest.
- **Technetium-99m** (^{99m}Tc) Pyrophosphate. Recently damaged myocardium concentrates ^{99m}Tc pyrophosphate, producing a myocardial hotspot. Most sensitive 24–72 h after AMI
- **Technetium-99m** (^{99m}Tc) Ventriculogram. ^{99m}Tc-labeled serum albumin or RBCs are used. Shows abnormal wall motion, cardiac shunt, size and function of heart chambers, cardiac output, and ejection fraction. Another form of this study is a **MUGA scan,** in which data collected are synchronized to an ECG and used to produce a "moving picture" of cardiac function. Performed with patient at rest or during exercise stress test.

Gallium Scan: Location of abscesses (5–10 d old) and chronic inflammatory lesions, lymphoma staging and follow-up for disease detection, diagnosis of lung cancer, melanoma, other neoplasms

Hepatobiliary Scan (HIDA-Scan, BIDA-Scan):   Differential diagnosis of biliary obstruction (when bilirubin > 1.5 mg/dL and < 7 mg/dL), acute cholecystitis, biliary atresia; not good for stones unless cystic duct is completely occluded and acute cholecystitis is present

Indium-111 (^{111}In) Octreotide (OctreoScan):   Imaging of tumors with somatostatin receptors (pheochromocytoma, gastrinomas, insulinomas, small-cell lung cancer)

Iodine-125 (^{125}I) Fibrinogen Scanning: Detection of venous thrombosis in the lower extremities. Patient is scanned several hours and several days after injection of tracer. Identification of clots at or below knees. False-positives with varicosities, cellulitis, incisions, arthritis, hematomas, and recent venography. Tracer availability is a problem.

Liver–Spleen Scan: Estimating organ size; evaluation of parenchymal disease (eg, hepatitis), abscess, cysts, primary and secondary tumors

Lung Scan (V̇/Q̇ Scan):   With CXR, evaluation of PE. Normal scan excludes PE; indeterminate scan necessitates further study with pulmonary angiography; clear perfusion deficit coupled with a normal ventilation is highly suggestive of PE. Shows evidence of pulmonary disease, COPD, and emphysema

Renal Scans: Agents are generally classified as functional tracers or morphologic tracers.

- **Iodine-131** (^{131}I) Hippuran. Evaluation of function in renal insufficiency; visualization is poor, and radiation dose can be high

- **Technetium-99m (99mTc) Glucoheptonate.** Combination renal cortical imaging and renal function; evaluation of overall function but can be used to determine vascular flow and visualize renal parenchyma and collecting system
- **Technetium-99m** (^{99m}Tc) DMSA (dimercaptosuccinic acid). Renal cortical imaging only
- **Technetium-99m** (^{99m}Tc) DTPA (diethylenetriamine pentaacetic acid). Renal function; renal blood flow studies, estimation of GFR, evaluation of collecting system
- **Technetium-99m** (^{99m}Tc) Mercaptoacetyltriglycine (MAG3). Renal function; imaging of the parenchyma within minutes of injection and with low radiation dose. May eventually replace all other renal agents.

Single-Photon Emission CT (SPECT):   Multiple nuclear images are sequentially displayed as in CT; can be applied to many nuclear scans.

Strontium-89 (^{89}Sr)(Metastron):   Palliative therapy for multiple painful bony metastasis (eg, prostate or breast cancer). Because agent is a pure beta emitter, radioactivity remains in the body, so no special precautions (other than blood and urine) are needed.

Thyroid Scan: Most often technetium-99m pertechnetate. Evaluation of nodules (solitary cold nodules require a tissue diagnosis because 25% are cancerous). Scan patterns in correlation with lab tests may help diagnose hyperfunctioning adenoma, Plummer and Graves diseases, multinodular goiter; localization of ectopic thyroid tissues (especially after thyroidectomy for cancer); identification of superior mediastinal thyroid masses

POSITRON EMISSION TOMOGRAPHY (PET)

PET involves injection of a positron-emitting tracer that is attached to a metabolically active molecule and accumulates in areas of increased metabolic activity. Tomographic images localize the tracer within the body. PET is often performed with CT or MRI, and the functional information obtained with PET scan is correlated with the precise anatomic detail obtained from CT or MRI. The most commonly used PET tracer is 18-fluoro-deoxyglucose (18-FDG). Fluorine-18 decays by positron emission.

The positron emitters used in PET generally have a short half-life. The half-life of ^{18}F is 110 min. This short half-life results in a low dose to the patient but means that a cyclotron must be available to produce the agent a short time before it is to be used. Clinical applications of PET are:

- **Cancer:** Because malignant tissue has a higher metabolic rate than benign tissue, PET tracers of glucose metabolism are selectively concentrated in living tumor. PET depicts small foci of cancer that may be missed with conventional CT or MRI. PET can also be used to differentiate live tumors from treated dead tissue and fibrosis. Any metabolically active tissue will "light up," however. Areas of inflammation can cause false-positive results. The tumors most commonly imaged with PET include colorectal cancer, lung cancer, brain cancer, breast cancer, lymphoma, and melanoma. PET can be used in both diagnosis and staging of these cancers.
- **Neurologic Imaging:** Localization of specific functions and definition of functional neuroanatomy. Localization of epileptogenic foci in patients

with seizures; diagnosis of various brain disorders, including dementia, depression, and schizophrenia.

- **Cardiac Imaging:** Definition of myocardial viability; findings complementary to anatomic information obtained with cardiac angiography, may be used in treatment planning.

HOW TO READ A CHEST X-RAY

A CXR is a basic part of the evaluation of an ill patient. Understanding the basic principles of CXR interpretation is considered a key learning step for all physicians.

Determine the Adequacy of the Film

- **Inspiration:** Diaphragm below ribs 8–10 posteriorly and 5–6 anteriorly
- **Rotation:** Clavicles are equidistant from the spinous processes
- **Penetration:** Disk spaces are seen, but bony details of spine cannot be seen

PA Film

The film is in front of the patient, and the x-ray beam passes from back (posterior) to front (anterior). The following structures are shown in Figure 15–1, page 342.

Soft Tissues: Check for symmetry, swelling, loss of tissue planes, and subcutaneous air.

Skeletal Structures: Examine the clavicles, scapulas, vertebrae, sternum, and ribs. Look for symmetry. In a good x-ray, the clavicles are symmetrical. Check for osteolytic or osteoblastic lesions, fractures, and arthritic changes. Look for rib-notching.

Diaphragm: Sides should be equal and slightly rounded, although the left is usually slightly lower by one rib interspace. Costophrenic angles should be clear and sharp. Blunting suggests scarring or fluid. It takes about 100–200 mL of pleural fluid to cause blunting. Check below the diaphragm for the gas pattern and free air. A unilateral high diaphragm suggests paralysis (from nerve damage, trauma, or an abscess), eventration, or loss of lung volume on that side because of atelectasis or pneumothorax. A low, flat diaphragm suggests COPD.

Mediastinum and Heart: The aortic knob should be visible and distinct. Widening of the mediastinum is seen with traumatic disruption of the thoracic aorta. In children, do not mistake the normally prominent thymus for widening. Mediastinal masses can be associated with Hodgkin disease and other lymphomas. The trachea should be in a straight line with a sharp carina. Tracheal deviation suggests a mass (tumor), goiter, unilateral loss of lung volume (collapse), or tension pneumothorax. The heart should be less than one-half the width of the chest wall on a PA film. If greater than one half, consider the presence of CHF or pericardial fluid.

Hilum: The left hilum should be up to 2–3 cm higher than the right. Vessels are seen. Look for any masses, nodes, or calcifications.

Lung Fields: Note the presence of any shadows from CVP lines, NG tubes, pulmonary artery catheters, etc. The fields should be clear with normal lung markings all the way to the periphery. The vessels should taper to become almost invisible at the periphery.

15

Vessels in the lower lung should be larger than those in the upper lung. A reversal of this difference (called cephalization) suggests pulmonary venous hypertension and heart failure. **Kerley B lines,** small linear densities found usually at the lateral base of the lung, are associated with CHF. Check the margins carefully; look for pleural thickening or calcification, masses, and pneumothorax. If the lungs appear hyperlucent with a relatively small heart and flattening of the diaphragms, COPD is likely. Thin, plate-like linear densities are associated with atelectasis. To locate a lesion, do not forget to check a lateral film and remember the "silhouette sign." Obliteration of all or part of a heart border means the lesion is anterior in the chest and lies in the right middle lobe, lingula, or anterior segment of the upper lobe. A radiopacity that overlaps the heart but does not obliterate the heart border is posterior and lies in the lower lobes.

Examine carefully for the following:

1. Coin lesions: Caused by granulomas (50% of cases and usually calcified and caused by histoplasmosis, 25%; TB, 20%, or coccidioidomycosis, 20%; varies with locale); primary carcinoma (25%), hamartoma (< 10%), and metastatic disease (< 5%)
2. Cavitary lesions: Caused by abscess, cancer, TB, coccidioidomycosis, Wegener granulomatosus
3. **Infiltrates:** Two major types
   a. **Interstitial Pattern.** "Reticular." Caused by granulomatous infections, miliary TB, coccidioidomycosis, pneumoconiosis, sarcoidosis, CHF. "Honeycombing" represents end-stage fibrosis caused by sarcoid, RA, and pneumoconiosis.
   b. **Alveolar Pattern.** Diffuse, quick progression and regression. "Butterfly" pattern or air bronchograms. Caused by PE, pneumonia, hemorrhage, or PE associated with CHF.

Lateral Film

Examine the structures shown in Figure 15–2, page 343. Check for 3D location of lesions. Pay close attention to retrosternal clear space, costophrenic angles, and the path of aorta.

INTRODUCTION TO THE OPERATING ROOM

Sterile Technique
Entering the OR
Surgical Hand Scrub
Preparing the Patient
Gowning and Gloving

Draping the Patient
Finding Your Place
Universal Precautions
Latex Allergy

Prepare before you get to the OR by knowing the patient thoroughly and having a basic understanding of what is planned. Avoid stereotyping the nurses as "cranky," the surgeons as "egotistical," and the medical students as "clueless" by learning the OR routine. Be alert, attentive, and, above all, patient. Don't be afraid to admit to the scrub nurse and the circulating nurse that you're new in the OR. They are usually happy to help you follow correct procedures.

STERILE TECHNIQUE

The members of the OR team include the surgeons, anesthesia staff, and the nursing staff. Members of the surgical team are the surgeon, surgical assistants, students, and scrub nurse or technician responsible for the instruments, gowning the surgical team, and maintaining a sterile field. The circulating nurse acts as a go-between between the sterile and nonsterile areas.

Sterile areas include the front of the gown to the waist, gloved hands and arms to the shoulder, draped part of the patient down to the tabletop, covered part of the Mayo stand (the small table where the most commonly used instruments are kept), and the top of the back table where additional instruments are kept. The sides of the back table are not considered sterile, and anything that falls below the level of the patient table is considered contaminated.

ENTERING THE OR

In the OR everything is geared toward maintaining a sterile field. Use of sterile technique begins in the locker room. Change into scrub clothing. Remove your T-shirt, tuck the scrub shirt into the pants, and tuck the ties of the scrub pants inside the pants. In some hospitals scrub clothes are allowed on the wards, provided they are covered by a coat or other form of gown; check your hospital's requirements. If you wear scrub clothing out of the OR, be sure that it is not bloodstained.

Pass into the surgical anteroom to get your mask, cap, and shoe covers. The mask should cover your entire nose and mouth. Full hoods are necessary for men with beards. The cap must cover all of your hair. Because of universal precautions, protective eyewear is required while you are at the operative field. If you wear regular glasses, use a mask with adhesive at the bridge of the nose to prevent fogging. Tape the glasses to your forehead if you think they may be loose enough to fall onto the table during the operation. Do not wear nail polish, and remove any loose jewelry, watches, and rings before scrubbing. Make sure that shoelaces are tucked inside the shoe covers.

At most hospitals you do not have to wear the mask in the hallway of the OR suite, but you do have to wear everything else. The mask must be worn in the OR itself, near the scrub sinks, and in the substerile room between ORs.

Find the OR where your patient's procedure is taking place, and assist in transport, if necessary. Introduce yourself to the intern or resident and nurse, and try to get an idea of when to begin scrubbing (usually when the first surgeon starts to scrub). If you have a pager or cell phone, follow local OR procedures, and remove the pager or cell phone if you are going to scrub into the case. If the electronic device is allowed, keep it in the room, identifying it with your name and informing the circulating nurse about its presence.

SURGICAL HAND SCRUB

The purpose of the surgical scrub is to decrease the bacterial flora of the skin by mechanical cleansing of the arms and hands before the operation. Key points to remember: (1) If contamination occurs during the scrub, start over, and (2) In emergency situations exceptions are made to the time allowed for scrubbing (as in obstetrics, when the baby is brought out from the delivery room and the student is still scrubbing!). Properly position your cap and mask before starting the scrub.

Povidone–Iodine (Betadine) Hand Scrub

Scrubbing technique depends somewhat on local policies. Some ORs require a timed scrub in which you determine the duration of scrubbing by watching the clock. Other ORs use an "anatomic" scrub in which the duration of scrubbing is determined by counting strokes. Some ORs use brush-free or waterless scrubs.

Timed Scrub
1. Perform a general prewash with surgical soap and water up to 2 in (5 cm) above the elbows.
2. Aseptically open one brush and place it on the ledge above the sink for the second half of the scrub. Open another brush, and begin the scrub with povidone–iodine. Use the nail cleaner to clean under all fingernails.
3. Scrub both arms during the first 5 min. Start at the fingertips and end 2 in (5 cm) above the elbows; pay close attention to the fingernails and inter-digital spaces. Discard the brush and rinse from fingertips to elbows.
4. Take the second brush and repeat step 3. Always start at the fingertips and work up to the elbows.
5. Always allow water to drip off the elbows by keeping the hands above the level of the elbows.
6. Move into the OR to dry your hands and arms (back into the room to push the door open).
7. Scrubbing times:
   a. Ten minutes at the start of the day or with no previous scrub within the last 12 h and on all orthopedic cases
   b. Five minutes with a previous scrub or between cases if you have not been out of the OR working with other patients

Chlorhexidine (Hibiclens) 6-Min Hand Scrub (Timed)
1. Wet your hands and forearms to the elbows with water.
2. Dispense about 5 mL of chlorhexidine into your cupped hands and spread it over both hands and arms to the elbows.

3. Scrub vigorously for 3 min without adding water. Use a sponge or brush for scrubbing, and pay particular attention to fingernails, cuticles, and interdigital spaces.
4. Rinse thoroughly with running water.
5. Dispense another 5 mL of chlorhexidine into your cupped hands.
6. Wash for an additional 3 min. There is no need to use a brush or sponge at this point. Rinse thoroughly. Move into the OR back first to dry your hands.

Anatomic Scrub

1. Perform a general prewash with surgical soap and water, up to 2 in (5 cm) above the elbows.
2. Use disposable brushes if available. Aseptically open one brush and place it on the ledge above the sink for the second half of the scrub. Open another brush and begin the scrub. Use the nail cleaner to clean under all fingernails.
3. Scrub each surface vigorously 10 times. Start with each finger (each of which has four surfaces), proceeding to the hand, the forearm, and the arm above the elbow. After finishing one extremity, scrub the other from fingers to above the elbow. Be sure to include all parts of your hand, especially the interdigital spaces.
4. Rinse both arms and rescrub each extremity, this time not going above the elbow. The method is the same as that for step 3: 10 times on each surface from fingers to elbow.
5. Rinse thoroughly and proceed into the OR.

Waterless Surgical Scrub (Handrub)

1. Most waterless surgical hand rubs are alcohol based (usually > 60% ethyl alcohol with chlorhexidine). The CDC recommends that surgical staff prewash with nonantimicrobial soap and dry hands and arms completely before using an alcohol-based product, such as Avagard or Triseptin.
2. For the first scrub of the day, make sure your hands are visibly clear of any soiling (the same is true for subsequent scrubs), and clean the nails with the provided cleaner.
3. **Apply the product to clean, dry hands.** Dispense one pump (2 mL) into the palm of one hand. Dip the fingertips of the other hand into the hand prep and work under the fingernails. Spread the remaining hand prep over the hand and up to just above the elbow.
4. Dispense one pump (2 mL) and repeat the procedure with the other hand.
5. Dispense the final pump (2 mL) of hand prep into either hand and reapply it to all aspects of both hands up to the wrists. Allow the prep to air dry; do not use towels. Air dry completely before gowning and gloving.

PREPARING THE PATIENT

Most ORs have instituted a time-out policy whereby all attention is directed at reading the surgical permit aloud and clearly identifying the patient, operation, and site of procedure to reduce medical errors. The patient prep technique can vary but involves mechanically cleansing the patient's skin in the region of the surgical site to reduce bacterial flora. Ask the resident to guide you through the procedure; it is always better to prep a wider area than you think necessary. For example, for midline laparotomy, prep the patient from nipples to pubis and from the flank at table level on one side to the flank at table level on the other side.

Materials

Small prep table containing gloves, towels, povidone–iodine or other scrub soap (optional), povidone–iodine or other paint solution, 4 × 4 gauze squares or sponges, ring forceps (optional)

Technique

1. Prep the patient before putting on the sterile gown. Using sterile technique, put on a pair of gloves, and scrub the area designated with the soap solution. At many centers, wound scrubbing is no longer routine and is used only in specific conditions, such as contaminated wounds.

2. **Cover** the area with a towel, and then gently pat the area dry if the wound was scrubbed. Gently peel off the towel from one side, being careful not to allow the towel to fall back on the prepped area.

3. Use 4 × 4s to paint the exposed area with the povidone–iodine or other solution, using the proposed incision site as the center. Move circumferentially away from the incision site. Never bring the 4 × 4s back to the center after they have painted peripheral areas. Paint in a series of concentric circles.

4. After the prep, remove the gloves using sterile technique and put on your gown.

GOWNING AND GLOVING

1. If you have just completed the hand scrub, back into the room to push the door open; keep your hands above your elbows.

2. Ask the scrub nurse for a towel. Do not be impatient; the scrub nurse is often very busy. Stick out one hand, palm up and well away from the body. The nurse drapes the towel over your hand.

3. Bend at the waist to maintain sterility of the towel. It should never touch your clothing.

4. With one half of the towel, dry one arm, beginning at the fingers; change hands and dry the other arm with the other half of the towel. Never go back to the forearm or hands after drying your elbows.

5. Drop the towel in the hamper. Again, remember to keep your hands above your elbows.

6. Ask for a gown and hold your arms out straight. The scrub nurse places the gown on you, and the circulator ties the back.

7. The nurse holds out a right glove with the palm toward you. Push your hand through the glove. Gloves come in several sizes—small (5 1/2–6 1/2), medium (7–7 1/2), and large (8–8 1/2)—and materials: standard latex gloves, hypoallergenic (powder free), reinforced (orthopedic), and latex free. Ask the resident or scrub nurse for guidance on the type of glove to request. It is good form to ask the circulating nurse to open your gloves before you actually begin to scrub.

8. Repeat the procedure with the left glove. It is easier if you use two fingers of your gloved right hand to help hold the left glove open.

9. Visually inspect the gloves for holes. Double gloving is becoming commonplace because of increased awareness of universal precautions and may be mandatory depending on the procedure being performed.

10. Give the scrub nurse the long string of your front gown-tie. Hold the other string yourself and turn around in place. Tie the strings.

11. The nurse may offer you a damp sponge to clean the powder off the gloves (powder is implicated in some postoperative complications, eg, adhesions); however, most gloves are powder free.

12. Wait patiently; stay out of the way, and keep your hands above your waist. Hold them together to prevent yourself from accidentally dropping them or touching your mask. This is one of the most difficult things to remember. Be attentive. The only sterile area is the front of your body from chest to waist and hands to shoulders. Your back is not sterile, nor is your body below the waist. Do not cross your arms.

DRAPING THE PATIENT

Draping the patient is usually done by the surgeon and assistants. Watch how they do it, and consider helping in a future procedure. It is more difficult to keep sterile than it looks.

FINDING YOUR PLACE

As a student, stand where the senior surgeon indicates. The first thing to remember is that once you are scrubbed, you must not touch anything that is not sterile. Put your hands on the sterile field and do not move about unnecessarily. If you need to move around someone else, pass back to back. When passing by a sterile field, try to face it. When passing a nonsterile field, pass it with your back toward it. If you are observing an operation and are not scrubbed in, do not go between two sterile fields, and stay about 1 ft (30 cm) away from all sterile fields to avoid contamination (and condemnation!). When not scrubbed in, keep your hands behind your back, being careful not to back into the instrument table.

When scrubbed, do not drop your hands below your waist or table level. Do not grab at anything that falls off the side of the table—it is considered contaminated. If something falls, inform the circulating nurse. Do not reach for anything on the scrub nurse's small instrument stand (the Mayo stand); ask for the instrument to be given to you.

If someone tells you that you have contaminated a glove, light handle, or anything else, do not move and do not complain or disagree. Remember that the focus of the OR is maintaining a sterile field, so if anyone says, "You're contaminated," accept the statement, and change gloves, gown, or whatever is needed. If a glove alone is contaminated, hold the hand out away from the sterile field, fingers extended and palms up, and a circulating nurse will pull the glove off. The same is true if a needle sticks you or if a glove tears. Tell the surgeon and scrub nurse and change gloves. For a skin break event such as a needle stick, follow local infectious disease policies.

If you have to change your gown, step away from the table. The circulator will remove first the gown and then the gloves. This procedure prevents the contaminated inside of the gown from passing over the hands. Regown and reglove without scrubbing again.

Always be aware of "sharps" on the field. When passing a potentially injurious instrument, alert the other members of the team aware that you are passing a sharp (eg, "needle back," "knife back"). Learn the names and functions of the common instruments. A knowledgeable student is more likely to actively participate in the operation.

16

At the end of the operation (once the dressing is on the wound), remove the gown and gloves but not the mask, cap, or shoe covers. To protect yourself, remove the gown first, and remove your own gloves last. This system keeps your hands clean of blood or fluids that got onto your gown during the procedure.

In accordance with the OSHA Bloodborne Pathogens Standard, **wash your hands with soap and water after the surgical procedure.** Assist in the transfer of the patient to the recovery room. Write postop orders and a brief operative note immediately (see Chapter 2 on how to write postop notes and orders). It is good form to offer to write the postop note and orders if you are comfortable with the process. Because of regulations that affect attending physicians at teaching hospitals, the attending may be required to write the note personally. At the very least, the attending of record annotates an "attestation" to your note saying that the surgeon was "personally present during the critical portions of the procedure."

UNIVERSAL PRECAUTIONS

All operating room personnel are at risk of infection with blood-borne infectious agents (eg, HIV, hepatitis). To reduce the incidence of such transmission, the CDC has developed a set of guidelines called universal precautions. The underlying principle is that because patients cannot be routinely tested for HIV and are rarely tested preoperatively for transmissible diseases such as hepatitis, the safest policy is to treat all patients as though they have an infection. This approach ensures evenhanded treatment of all patients and the safest work environment for those exposed to the blood of others.

Minimizing the risks to all who are in the OR requires constant vigilance. Movements must be coordinated among surgeon, assistant, and technician. Never use your fingers to pick up needles; pick them up only with another instrument. DO not use your fingers and hands as retractors. Two people should never be holding the same sharp instrument. Placing a sharp instrument down or handing it to another member of the team is always preceded by a verbal warning that notifies the recipient that a sharp object is about to be passed. Protective eyewear must be worn by all members of the operating team.

The practice of double gloving is often reserved for operations in which the patient is known to carry a transmissible agent. This technique reduces the incidence of blood–skin contact, especially in light of the extraordinarily high incidence of unrecognized glove perforations. Until puncture-resistant gloves are developed, double gloving is the best approach.

LATEX ALLERGY

People with medical conditions or occupations heavily exposed to products containing natural rubber latex may became sensitized to it and develop allergic reactions (~7% of health care workers). Some conditions, such as spina bifida and cerebral palsy, predispose patients to an 18–40% incidence of allergy. Reactions vary from mild rash and itching to anaphylaxis and death. Latex products are found in a wide array of products, from gloves and drapes, to IV tubing and syringes. Some patients have documented latex allergy. Hospitals have latex allergy protocols, and hospitals maintain an inventory of latex-free products that should be used in these cases.

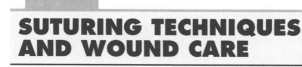

17

SUTURING TECHNIQUES AND WOUND CARE

Wound Healing	Suturing Patterns
Vacuum-Assisted Closure	Surgical Knots
Suture Materials	Suture Removal
Suturing Procedure	Tissue Adhesives

WOUND HEALING

The process of wound healing is generally divided into four stages: inflammation, fibroblast proliferation, contraction, and remodeling. There are three types of wound healing:

- **First intention.** The wound is closed by routine primary suturing, stapling, or gluing. Epithelialization occurs in 24–48 h.
- **Secondary intention.** The wound is not closed by suturing, stapling, or gluing but closes by spontaneous contraction and epithelialization at a rate of 1 mm/d). Most often used for wounds that are infected and packed open.
- **Third intention** (also called delayed primary closure). The wound is left open for a time and then sutured at a later date. Often used with grossly contaminated wounds.

VACUUM-ASSISTED CLOSURE

Used for healing both acute and chronic wounds. Continuous negative pressure is distributed over the wound surface. The system consists of a soft sponge cut to fit and occupy the volume of the wound, a plastic tube imbedded in the center of the sponge and extending out of the wound to a controlled suction pump, and a gas- and fluid-impermeable plastic outer film that adheres to the back of the sponge and the surrounding normal skin. Vacuum-assisted closure allows "active" removal of extracellular debris (exudate). Soft-tissue defects heal faster when subatmospheric pressure is applied. Used for wounds resulting from pressure, trauma, infection, IV extravasation, A–V insufficiency, and skin grafting.

SUTURE MATERIALS (SEE TABLES 17–1 AND 17–2, PAGES 362–363)

Suture materials can be broadly defined as absorbable and nonabsorbable. **Absorbable sutures** can be thought of as temporary and include plain catgut, chromic catgut, and synthetic materials such as polyglactin 910 (Vicryl), polyglycolic acid (Dexon), and polyglecaprone (Monocryl). Left inside the body, these materials are resorbed after a variable period. Polydioxanone (PDS) is a long-lasting absorbable suture. **Nonabsorbable sutures** can be thought of as "permanent" unless they are removed; these materials include silk, stainless steel wire, polypropylene (Prolene), and nylon.

TABLE 17–1
Common Absorbable Suture Materials

Suture (Brand Names)	Description	Tensile Strength[a]	Absorbed	Common Uses
Fast catgut	Twisted/fast absorption	3–5 d	30 d	Facial lacerations in children
Plain catgut	Twisted/rapidly absorbable	7–10 d	70 d	Vessel ligation, subcutaneous tissues
Chromic catgut	Twisted/absorbable	10–14 d	90 d	Mucosa
Polyglycolic acid (Dexon)	Braided/absorbable	14–21 d	60–90 d	GI, subcutaneous tissues
Polyglactin 910 (Vicryl Rapide)	Braided/absorbable	5 d	42 d	Skin repair needing rapid absorption
Polyglactin 910 (Vicryl)	Braided/absorbable	21 d	56–70 d	Bowel, deep tissue
Poliglecaprone 25 (Monocryl)	Monofilament/absorbable	7–14 d	91–119 d	Skin, bowel
Polydioxanone (PDS)	Monofilament/absorbable	28 d	6 mo	Fascia, GI
Polyglyconate (Maxon)	Braided/absorbable	28 d	6 mo	GI, muscle, fascia
Panacryl	Braided/absorbable	>6 mo	>24 mo	Fascia, tendons

[a]When suture loses approximately 50% strength.

17

TABLE 17–2
Common Nonabsorbable Suture Materials

Suture (Brand Names)	Description	Common Uses
Polytetrafluoroethylene (PTFE) (Gore-Tex)	Monofilament	Vascular grafts, hernia, valve repair
Nylon (Dermalon, Ethilon)	Monofilament	Skin, drains
Nylon (Nurolon)	Braided	Tendon repair
Polyester (Ethibond, Tycron)	Braided	Cardiac, tendon
Polypropylene (Prolene)	Monofilament	Vessel, fascia, skin
Silk	Braided	GI, vessel ligation, drains
Stainless steel	Monofilament	Fascia, sternum

The size of a suture is defined by the number of zeros. The more zeros in the number, the smaller is the suture. For example, 5-0 suture (00000) is much smaller than 2-0 (00) suture. Most sutures come prepackaged and mounted on needles ("swaged on"). **Cutting needles** are used for tough tissues such as skin, and **tapered needles** are used for more delicate tissues such as intestine. The most common needle for skin closure is the $3/8$-circle cutting needle.

SUTURING PROCEDURE

The following guidelines cover repair of lacerations in the emergency setting. Similar principles hold true for closure of wounds in the OR. The choice of suture material is based on many factors, including location, extent of the laceration, strength of the tissues, and preference of the physician.

- **Face:** 5-0 or 6-0 nylon or polypropylene when appearance is important
- **Scalp:** 3-0 nylon or polypropylene
- **Trunk and extremities:** 4-0 or 5-0 nylon or polypropylene
- Use 3-0 and 4-0 absorbable sutures such as Dexon or Vicryl to approximate deep tissues. Close skin with interrupted sutures placed with good approximation and minimal tension or with a running subcuticular suture. Use tissue adhesives selectively (see page 373). Suture patterns are discussed in the next section. Suture marks ("tracks") are the result of excessive tension on the tissue or leaving the sutures in too long. In most cases the length of time and the technique used are more important in determining the final result than is the type of suture used.

1. Remove all foreign materials and devitalized tissues by sharp excision (debridement). Clean the wound with plain saline solution (avoid antiseptic solutions for wound cleansing because they can be toxic to viable cells). A useful technique involves irrigation with at least 200 mL of saline through a 35-mL syringe and a 19-gauge needle. Anesthesia may be necessary before any of these steps. If all the debris is not removed, traumatic "tattooing" of the skin can result.

17

TABLE 17-3
Local Anesthetic Comparison Chart for Commonly Used Injectable Agents

Agent	Proprietary Names	Onset	Duration	Maximum Dose	
				mg/kg	Volume in 70-kg Adult[a]
Bupivacaine	Marcaine, Sensorcaine	7–30 min	5–7 h	3	70 mL of 0.25% solution
Lidocaine	Xylocaine, Anestacon	5–30 min	2 h	4	28 mL of 1% solution
Lidocaine with epinephrine (1:200,000)		5–30 min	2–3 h	7	50 mL of 1% solution
Mepivacaine	Carbocaine	5–30 min	2–3 h	7	50 mL of 1% solution
Procaine	Novocain	Rapid	30 min–1 h	10–15	70–105 mL of 1% solution

[a]To calculate the maximum dose if the patient is not a 70kg adult, use the fact that a 1% solution has 10 mg of drug per milliliter.

17

364

2. Obtain a surgical consultation before suturing infected or contaminated wounds, lacerations more than 6–12 h old (24 h on the face), missile wounds, and human or animal bites.

3. Anesthetize the wound by infiltrating it with an agent such as 0.5% or 1% lidocaine (Xylocaine). The maximum safe dose is 4.5 mg/kg (about 28 mL of a 1% solution in an adult). Lidocaine and other local anesthetic agents are available with epinephrine (1:100,000 or 1: 200,000) added to produce local vasoconstriction that prolongs the anesthetic effect and helps decrease systemic side effects and bleeding. Use epinephrine with caution, particularly in treatment of patients with a history of hypertension, and do not used epinephrine on the fingers, toes, or penis. One milliliter of 1:10 NaHCO$_3$ can be mixed with 9 mL of lidocaine to help minimize the discomfort of the injection. Commonly used local anesthetics are compared in Table 17–3, page 364.

4. When using local anesthetics, always aspirate before injecting to prevent intravascular injection of the drug. Anesthetize with a 26- to 30-gauge needle. Symptoms of toxicity from local anesthetics include twitching, restlessness, drowsiness, light-headedness, and seizures.

5. Close the wound using one of the suturing patterns discussed in the next section. To decrease trauma, use a fine-toothed forceps (Adson or Brown–Adson) with gentle pressure to handle the skin edges. A toothed forceps is *less damaging* to the skin than other forceps with flat surfaces that can crush the tissue.

6. Cover the wound and keep it dry for at least 24–48 h. Dry gauze or Steri-Strips are sufficient. On the face, simply cover the wound with antibiotic ointment, especially around the eyes and mouth. After that time, *epithelialization is complete* in healthy patients with uninfected wounds, and the patient may shower and wet the wound without increasing the risk of infection.

7. Address tetanus and antibacterial prophylaxis, particularly for contaminated wounds (Table 17–4).

SUTURING PATTERNS

Opinions vary greatly on the ideal technique for skin closure. The following are the common techniques of skin approximation. Critical to any suturing technique is making certain that the edges of the wound closely approximate without overlapping or inversion and that there is no tension. Remember "approximation without strangulation" or eversion of the skin edges gives the best results (Figure 17–1). Figures 17–2 through 17–6 illustrate the commonly used suturing patterns. These include simple interrupted suture (Figure 17–2), running (locked or unlocked) suture (Figure 17–3), vertical mattress suture (Figure 17–4), horizontal mattress suture (Figure 17–5), and subcuticular suture (Figure 17–6).

SURGICAL KNOTS

There are three basic knot-tying techniques: one-handed and two-handed ties and the instrument tie. The most advanced knot-tying technique is a one-handed tie, not recommended for medical students or junior residents. Although one-handed ties can be more useful in certain situations (eg, deep cavities or need for speed), the two-handed tie is easier to learn. Instrument ties are more useful for

TABLE 17–4
Tetanus Prophylaxis

History of Absorbed Tetanus Toxoid Immunization	Clean, Minor Wounds		All Other Wounds[a]	
	Td[b]	TIG[c]	Td[b]	TIG[c]
Unknown or <3 doses	Yes	No	Yes	Yes
<3 doses[d]	No[e]	No	No[f]	No

[a]Such as, but not limited to, wounds contaminated with dirt, feces, soil, saliva, etc; puncture wounds; avulsions; and wounds resulting from missiles, crushing, burns, and frostbite.
[b]Td = tetanus–diphtheria toxoid (adult type), 0.5 mL IM.
- For children <7 y of age, DPT (DT, if pertussis vaccine is contraindicated) is preferred to tetanus toxoid alone.
- For persons >7 y of age, Td is preferred to tetanus toxoid alone.
- DT = diphtheria-tetanus toxoid (pediatric), used for those who cannot receive pertussis.
[c]TIG = tetanus immune globulin, 250 U IM.
[d]If only three doses of fluid toxoid have been received, then a fourth dose of toxoid, preferably an absorbed toxoid, should be given.
[e]Yes, if >10 y since last dose.
[f]Yes, if >5 y since last dose.
Source: Based on guidelines from the CDC and reported in MMWR.

closing skin and for emergency department laceration repair. Figure 17–7, page 370, shows the technique for tying a two-handed square knot, the standard surgical knot that should be learned first. Figure 17–8, pages 372 and 373, shows the technique for a one-handed tie. Figure 17–9, page 374, shows the technique for an instrument tie.

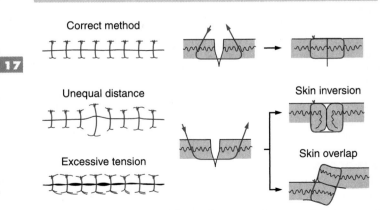

Correct method

Unequal distance

Excessive tension

Skin inversion

Skin overlap

FIGURE 17–1. Proper method for simple interrupted suturing of a skin wound compared with incorrect techniques that result in poor scars from skin overlap, skin inversion, or necrosis of the skin edges due to excessive tension.

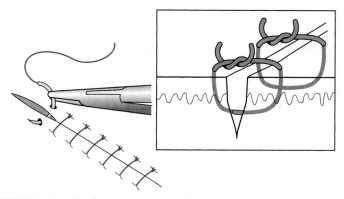

FIGURE 17–2. Simple interrupted sutures. "Bites" are taken through the thickness of the skin, and the width of each stitch should equal the distance between sutures to avoid inverting the skin edges.

SUTURE REMOVAL

The longer a permanent suture material is left in place in the skin, the more scarring it produces. Using a topical antibiotic ointment (eg, Polysporin) on the wound is helpful in decreasing suture tract epithelialization. Epithelialization results from crusting around the suture that increases suture marks and subsequent scarring. Sutures can be safely removed when a wound has developed sufficient tensile strength. Situations vary greatly, but general guidelines for removing sutures from different areas of the body are as follows: face and neck, 3–5 d; scalp and body, 5–7 d; extremities, 7–12 d. Any suture material or skin clips can be removed earlier if they have been reinforced with a deep absorbable suture or with application of Steri-Strips after the suture is removed. Steri-Strips stay in place more securely if tincture of benzoin (spray or solution) is applied to the skin and allowed to dry

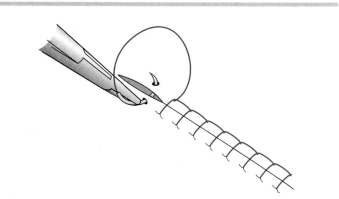

17

FIGURE 17–3. Continuous running suture. Technique allows rapid closure but depends on only two knots for security and may not allow precise approximation of the skin edges. "Locking" each stitch, as shown, may increase scarring.

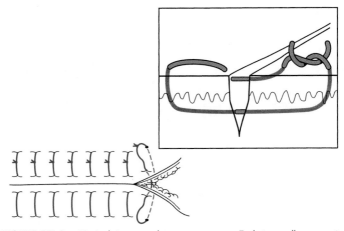

FIGURE 17–4. Vertical interrupted mattress sutures. Technique allows precise approximation of skin edges with little tension but can result in more scarring than simple stitches. Needle is placed in the skin in a "far, far, near, near" sequence.

17

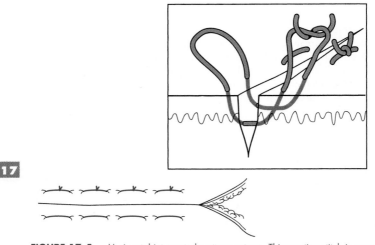

FIGURE 17–5. Horizontal interrupted mattress sutures. This everting stitch is more frequently used in fascia than in skin. It is often used in calloused skin, such as the palms and soles.

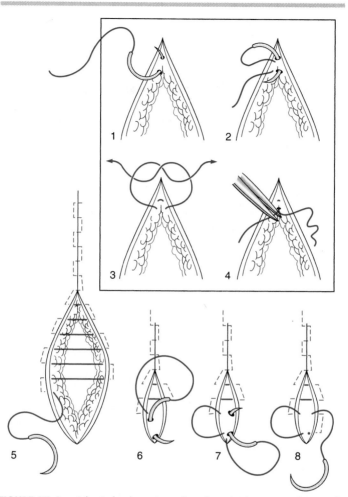

FIGURE 17–6. Subcuticular closure is usually performed with continuous, horizontally applied intradermal sutures. These sutures are ideal for linear cosmetic closure because they eliminate possible cross-hatching deformities. If nonabsorbable suture material (eg, 5-0 or 6-0 Prolene) is used, the knot is placed on the skin and pulled taut. If absorbable (5-0 or 6-0 Dexon or Vicryl) is used, the knot is usually buried as shown. The knot is tied in part 8, the needle passed through the skin, and the suture material cut flush.

before the Steri-Strips are applied. The length of time absorbable sutures remain in tissues is shown in Table 17–1.

Suture Removal Procedure

1. Gently clear away any dried blood with saline solution and gauze. Verify that the wound is sufficiently healed to allow suture removal. Use a forceps to gently elevate the knot off the skin. This step can be uncomfortable for the patient.

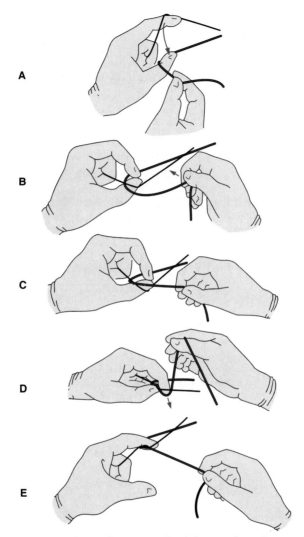

FIGURE 17-7. Technique for tying two-handed square knot. Suture ends are uncrossed as step A begins (continued on next page).

17

2. Cut the suture as close to the skin as possible so that a minimal amount of "dirty suture" is dragged through the wound. When removing continuous sutures, cut and pull out each section individually. **Never** pull a knot through the skin. Often the suture material is pulled tight to the skin, and it is difficult to remove the stitch with thick scissors. A no. 11 scalpel with the blade pointed up is helpful in this situation.

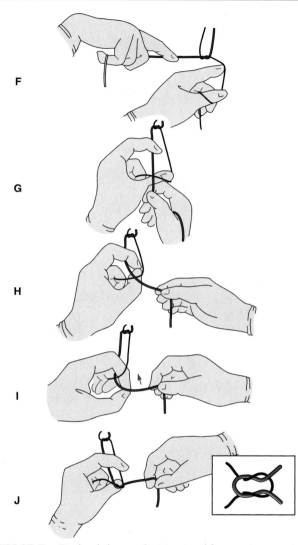

F

G

H

I

J

FIGURE 17-7. Two-handed square knot (continued from previous page). Hands must be crossed at the end of the first loop tie (step F) to give a flat knot; hands are not crossed at the end of the second loop tie (step J).

17

3. Use of skin staples is commonplace in the OR because of the rapidity of closure and the nonreactive nature of the steel staples. Staples are typically removed 3–5 d after surgery (abdominal incisions) as shown in Figure 17–10. Because staples are removed fairly quickly, reinforce the incision with Steri-Strips and benzoin. When removing skin staples, make sure

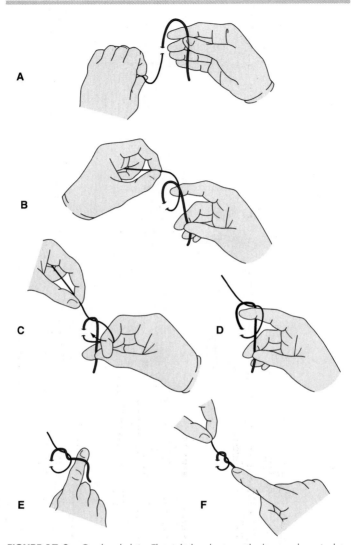

FIGURE 17–8. One-handed tie. The right hand sets up the loop and manipulates the working strand (continued on next page).

that the staple is completely reformed (see Figure 17–10) before pulling it out of the skin to decrease patient discomfort. Before removal, verify that the wound is epithelialized and that there is no sign of infection or wound leakage. If the wound gaps or if a discharge appears as the staples are removed, stop the removal procedure and ask a senior physician to evaluate the wound.

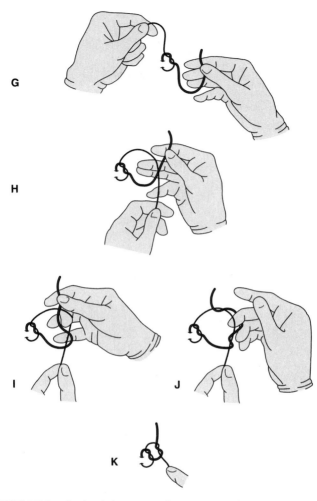

FIGURE 17–8. One-handed tie continued.

17

TISSUE ADHESIVES

Octyl cyanoacrylate (Dermabond) and *n*-butyl-2-cyanoacrylate (Indermil) are topical skin adhesives similar to cyanoacrylate glue that hold wound edges together. These substances are useful in closure of topical skin incisions and lacerations in areas of low skin tension that are simple, thoroughly cleansed, and have easily approximated skin edges. Adhesives can be used in conjunction with, but not in place of, deep dermal stitches. They are particularly useful in treatment of young children, for whom suture removal may be a problem. The wound should be nonmucosal on the face, torso, or extremity. Adhesives are

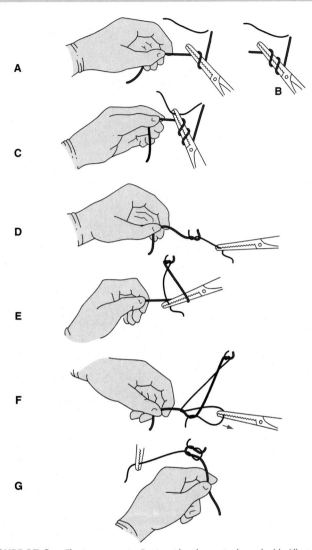

A

B

C

D

E

F

G

FIGURE 17–9. The instrument tie. Begin with either a single or double (illustrated) looping of the lower end of the suture around the needle holder. The first loop is laid flat without crossing the hands. Hands must be crossed after the second loop tie (step G) to produce a flat square knot.

recommended for wounds < 8 cm with minimal tension (skin gap < 0.5 cm) and for stabilizing wounds after early suture removal to minimize suture marks. Do not use tissue adhesives for puncture wounds, bites, or wounds that need debridement or in anatomic regions subjected to frequent movement (eg, joints). The patient may shower for brief periods with this type of closure.

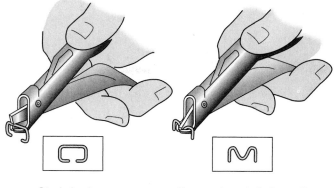

Staple in place   Removed staple "reformed"

FIGURE 17–10.   Removal of skin staples. The staple remover is passed beneath the staple and completely closed. To decrease patient discomfort, be sure that the staple is completely "reformed" before removal. (Courtesy of Ethicon, Inc.)

1. Gently approximate the wound edges with fingers or a forceps and place a small coating of the glue directly on the wound. Dermabond has a direct-contact applicator tip; Indermil has a noncontact applicator tip.
2. Wait 2–3 min for the glue to dry, and apply an additional one or two coats if needed. The glue sheds in 5–10 d.
3. Once the glue is in place and stable, it is not necessary to use topical medication or ointment. If the adhesive remains tacky, too much glue has been applied.

RESPIRATORY CARE

Respiratory Therapy
Pulmonary Function Tests (PFTs)
Differential Diagnosis of PFTs
Oxygen Supplements

Postoperative Pulmonary Care
Bronchopulmonary Hygiene
Topical Medications
Metered-Dose Inhalers

RESPIRATORY THERAPY

Respiratory therapy is a vital component of health care. For any patient initial medical care begins with assessment of the ABCs: **A**irway, **B**reathing, and **C**irculation. Respiratory therapy includes key components of airway and breathing support. The objective is the care of all types of patients with cardiopulmonary diseases. Functions of the respiratory therapist include emergency care, airway management, ventilatory support, oxygen therapy, humidity and aerosol therapies, chest physiotherapy, physiologic monitoring, and pulmonary diagnostics.

PULMONARY FUNCTION TESTS (PFTs)

PFTs are useful in the diagnosis of a variety of pulmonary disorders. Common PFTs include spirometry, lung volume determinations, and diffusion capacity. Important measurements include FVC and FEV_1. Spirometry results indicate the presence of obstructive airway diseases such as asthma and emphysema when the FEV_1/FVC ratio is < 0.70. They indicate the presence of restrictive lung diseases such as sarcoidosis and ankylosing spondylitis when the FVC/FEV_1 ratio > 80%.

Spirometry can be an important part of a preoperative evaluation. Obtain spirograms before and after administration of bronchodilators if they are not contraindicated (ie, history of intolerance). Bronchodilator responsiveness helps in predicting the response to treatment and in identifying asthma. Asthmatic patients typically have at least 15% improvement in FEV_1 after bronchodilator therapy.

Order lung volumes, commonly determined by helium dilution, to definitively diagnose restrictive lung disease. This test is usually indicated when TLC < 80% of predicted normal value. Diffusion capacity is important in the diagnosis of interstitial lung disease and pulmonary vascular disease, in which it is reduced. Diffusion capacity is frequently monitored to determine response to therapy for interstitial diseases.

Obstructive pulmonary diseases include asthma, chronic bronchitis, emphysema, and bronchiectasis. **Restrictive pulmonary diseases** include interstitial pulmonary disease, diseases of the chest wall, and neuromuscular disorders. Interstitial disease can be caused by inflammatory conditions (usual interstitial pneumonitis [UIP]), inhalation of organic dust (hypersensitivity pneumonitis), inhalation of inorganic dust (asbestosis), and systemic disorders with lung involvement (sarcoidosis).

Normal PFT values vary with age, sex, race, and body size. Normal values for a given patient are established from studies of healthy populations and are provided along with the results. ABG should be included in all PFTs. Typical volumes and capacities are illustrated in Figure 18–1, page 378.

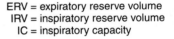

IRV	IC	
TV		VC
ERV	FRC	
RV		RV

VC = vital capacity   ERV = expiratory reserve volume
RV = residual volume   IRV = inspiratory reserve volume
FRC = functional residual capacity   IC = inspiratory capacity
TV = tidal volume

FIGURE 18–1. Lung volumes in interpretation of pulmonary function tests.

- **Tidal Volume (TV).** Volume of air moved during a normal breath on quiet respiration
- **Forced Vital Capacity (FVC).** Maximum volume of air that can be forcibly expired after full inspiration
- **Functional Residual Capacity (FRC).** Volume of air in the lungs after a normal tidal expiration (FRC = reserve volume + expiratory reserve volume)
- **Total Lung Capacity (TLC).** Volume of air in the lungs after maximal inspiration
- **Forced Expired Volume in 1 Second (FEV$_1$).** Measured after maximum inspiration, the volume of air that can be expelled in 1 s
- **Vital Capacity (VC).** Maximum volume of air that can be exhaled from the lungs after a maximal inspiration
- **Residual Volume (RV).** The volume of air remaining in the lungs at the end of a maximal exhalation

18

DIFFERENTIAL DIAGNOSIS OF PFTS

Table 18–1 shows the differential diagnosis of various PFT patterns. When interpreting PFTs, remember that some patients may have combined restrictive and obstructive diseases, such as coexistence of emphysema and asbestosis.

TABLE 18-1
Differential Diagnosis of Pulmonary Function Tests

Test	Restrictive Disease	Obstructive Disease		
FVC	↓	N or ↓		
TLC	↓	↑		
FEV_1/FVC	N or ↑	↓		
FEV_1	↓	↓		

OBSTRUCTIVE AIRWAYS DISEASE (COPD)

Test	Normal	Mild	Moderate	Severe
FEV_1 (% of VC)	>75	60–75	40–60	<40
RV (% of predicted)	80–120	120–150	150–175	>200

RESTRICTIVE LUNG DISEASE

Test	Normal	Mild	Moderate	Severe
FVC (% of predicted)	>80	60–80	50–60	<50
FEV_1 (% of VC)	>75	>75	>75	>75
RV (% of predicted)	80–120	80–120	70–80	70

N = normal; ↑ = increased, ↓ = decreased; FVC = forced vital capacity; TLC = total lung capacity; RV = residual volume; FEV_1 = forced expiratory volume in 1s; VC = vital capacity.

OXYGEN SUPPLEMENTS

Table 18–2, page 380 describes various methods of oxygen supplementation. Use a bubble-diffuser humidifier to bring the percentage of inspired gas up to room humidity (30–40% of relative humidity [RH]) when using the nasal cannula, simple oxygen mask, partial rebreathing mask, or nonrebreathing mask.

POSTOPERATIVE PULMONARY CARE (SEE ALSO CHAPTER 20)

After a surgical procedure with general anesthesia, the patient needs close observation and good respiratory support. This care includes good suctioning and lateral turning of the head to prevent aspiration. The airway must be patent, and adequate oxygenation and ventilation ensured. For high-risk patients, maintain intubation until it has been clearly determined that the patient can maintain spontaneous ventilation and wakefulness. Determine the capability for maintaining spontaneous ventilation by using the following parameters:

- Ability to follow commands
- Vital capacity > 15 mL/kg
- Inspiratory force >~20 cm water
- Expiratory force 25 cm water
- Blood gases with normal $PaCO_2$ (< 44 mm Hg) and pH (> 7.35) during spontaneous breathing
- Adequate PaO_2

18

TABLE 18–2
Various Methods of Oxygen and Humidity Supplementation

Device	O$_2$ Range	L/min	FIO$_2$	Uses
Nasal cannula	Low	1–6	0.24–0.5	COPD, general oxygen needs
Simple face mask	Medium	6–8	0.5–0.6	General oxygen needs
Partial rebreathing face mask	High	8–12	0.6–0.7	High oxygen emergency needs
Nonrebreathing face mask	High	8–12	0.7–0.95	High oxygen emergency needs
Venturi mask	Low–medium	—	0.24–0.50	COPD (can specify exact FIO$_2$)

Note: FIO$_2$ vary with fluctuations in the patient's minute ventilation with use of a nasal cannula. This is not true with use of a Venturi mask because it is a "high-flow oxygen enrichment system" that supplies three times the patient's minute ventilation, thus providing an exact FIO$_2$.
COPD = chronic obstructive pulmonary disease; FIO$_2$ = fraction of inspired oxygen.

Administer a judicious regimen of analgesics to control pain but not inhibit the respiratory center. Avoid dressings that restrict chest wall and abdominal excursion. Administer postoperative incentive spirometry, which has been shown effective in decreasing the incidence of postoperative pulmonary complications after upper abdominal operations. Other options include deep breathing exercises and intermittent positive pressure breathing.

BRONCHOPULMONARY HYGIENE

The following techniques are used by the respiratory care and nursing services of most hospitals. All are designed to help patients with bronchopulmonary hygiene, more commonly called "pulmonary toilet." Bronchopulmonary hygiene is defined as maintenance of clear airways and removal of secretions from the tracheobronchial tree. This therapy is important for routine postoperative surgical patients, medical patients with obstructive pulmonary diseases, and any patient with excessive respiratory secretions.

Aerosol (Nebulizer) Therapy

Aerosolized medications such as bronchodilators and mucolytic agents can be delivered via nebulizer to spontaneously breathing, awake patients or intubated patients.

Indications
- Management of COPD, acute asthma, CF, and bronchiectasis
- Help in inducing sputum for diagnostic tests

Goals
- Relief of bronchospasm
- Help in decreasing the viscosity and in clearing of secretions

To Order: Specify the following:

- Frequency
- Heated or cool mist
- Medications: In sterile water or NS
- FIO_2
- *Example:* Albuterol 2.5 mg in 3 mL of sterile saline, FIO_2 0.28.

Chest Physiotherapy

Percussion and postural drainage (P&PD) along with coughing and deep breathing exercises (TC&DB). Position the patient so that the involved lobes of the lung are in a dependent drainage position. Using a cupped hand or vibrator, percuss the chest wall. Nasotracheal (NT) suctioning is quite uncomfortable for patients but is still useful in the appropriate clinical setting in the absence of severe coagulopathy.

Indications
- Management of pneumonia, atelectasis, and diseases resulting in weak or ineffective coughing

To Order
1.   **P&PD:** Specify the following:

     - Frequency
     - Segments or lobes involved (eg, right upper lung [RUL])
     - Duration
     - Drainage only

2.   **TC&DB:** Order on a timed schedule or as needed

     - *Example:* P&PD qid of RUL and RML 5 min/lobe or TC&DB q4h

Incentive Spirometry

Encourages the patient to make a maximal and sustained inspiratory effort to help reinflate the lungs or prevent atelectasis.

Indications
- Treatment of patients at risk of postoperative pulmonary complications
- Management and prevention of atelectasis, especially in the postoperative setting

Goals: Set for the patient depending on the device used:

- Lighting lights
- Moving "Ping-Pong" balls

To Order: Specify the following:

- Frequency (eg, 10 min q1–2h while patient is awake or 10 repetitions q1h while patient is awake)
- Device (if you have a preference)
- *Example:* Incentive spirometry 10 repetitions every hour while awake

TOPICAL MEDICATIONS

The following agents can be added to aerosol therapy to prevent or manage pulmonary complications caused by bronchospasm, mucosal congestion, and inspissated secretions. Even though these are primarily topical agents, systemic absorption can occur.

Acetylcysteine (Mucomyst):   A mucolytic agent useful for managing retained mucoid secretions, inspissated secretions, and impacted mucoid plugs that develop in diseases such as COPD, CF, and pneumonia. A bronchodilator should be given along with Mucomyst. *Usual Adult Dosage:* 1–3 mL of 20% acetylcysteine in 3 mL albuterol

Albuterol (Ventolin, Proventil):   A short-acting selective bronchodilator with principally beta-2 activity; can cause tachycardia. Onset 15 min after administration. Peak effect at 0.5–1 h, duration 3–5 h. *Usual Adult Dosage:* 2.5 mg in 3 mL NS q4h

Levalbuterol (Xopenex):   L-isomer of short-acting albuterol; more expensive but this form causes less tachycardia. Onset 15 min after administration. Peak effect at 0.5–1 h, duration 3–5 h. *Usual Adult Dosage:* 0.63–1.25 mg in 3 mL NS q6h

Racemic Epinephrine: Contains both D- and L- forms of epinephrine. Alpha effects cause mucosal vasoconstriction to reduce mucosal engorgement, and bronchodilation lessens the risk of hypoxemia. Most useful for laryngotracheobronchitis and immediately after extubation in children. *Usual Adult Dosage:* 0.125–0.5 mL (3–10 mg) in 2.5 mL NS

Ipratropium Bromide (Atrovent):   A parasympatholytic agent that causes bronchodilation and decreases secretions with "drying" of the respiratory mucosa. Minimally absorbed and rarely causes tachycardia. Onset 45 min after administration. Duration 4–6 h. *Usual Adult Dosage:* 0.5 mg in 3 mL NS qid

Atropine: A parasympatholytic agent; causes bronchodilation and decreases secretions with "drying" of the respiratory mucosa. Readily absorbed and therefore has cardiac effects (tachycardia). *Usual Adult Dosage:* 0.025–0.05 mg/kg of 1% solution

METERED-DOSE INHALERS

(See Chapter 22 for additional prescribing information). All bronchodilating agents can be effectively delivered by metered-dose inhaler as long as the patient can cooperate and proper technique is used. For these devices to be successful, inpatients must be well trained or have the assistance of a nurse or respiratory therapist. Albuterol and ipratropium bromide (Atrovent) can be delivered two puffs q4h. A combination bronchodilator (Combivent) containing the equivalent of one puff of each provides synergistic bronchodilation.

18

BASIC ECG READING

Basic Information
Axis Deviation
Heart Rate
Rhythm

Cardiac Hypertrophy
Myocardial Infarction
Electrolyte and Drug Effects
Miscellaneous ECG Changes

The formal procedure for obtaining an ECG is given in Chapter 13, page 271. Every ECG should be approached in a systematic, stepwise way. Many automated ECG machines can give a preliminary interpretation of a tracing; however, all automated interpretations require analysis and sign-off by a physician. Determine each of the following:

- **Standardization.** With the ECG machine set on 1 mV, a 10-mm standardization mark (0.1 mV/mm) is evident (Figure 19–1).
- **Axis.** If the QRS is upright (more positive than negative) in leads I and aVF, the axis is normal. The normal axis range is –30 degrees to +105 degrees.
- **Intervals.** Determine the PR, QRS, and QT intervals (Figure 19–2). Intervals are measured in the limb leads. The PR should be 0.12–0.20 s, and the QRS, < 0.12 s. The QT interval increases with decreasing heart rate, usually < 0.44 s. The QT interval usually does not exceed one half of the RR interval (the distance between two R waves).
- **Rate.** Count the number of QRS cycles on a 6-s strip and multiply that number by 10 to roughly estimate the rate. If the rhythm is regular, you can be more exact in determining the rate by dividing 300 by the number of 0.20-s intervals (usually depicted by darker shading) and then extrapolating for any fraction of a 0.20-s segment.
- **Rhythm.** Determine whether each QRS is preceded by a P wave, look for variation in the PR interval and RR interval (the duration between two QRS cycles), and look for ectopic beats.
- **Hypertrophy.** One way to detect LVH is to calculate the sum of the S wave in V_1 or V_2 plus the R wave in V_5 or V_6. A sum > 35 indicates LVH. Some other criteria for LVH are R > 11 mm in aVL or R in I + S in III > 25 mm.
- **Infarction or Ischemia.** Check for ST-segment elevation or depression, Q waves, inverted T waves, and poor R-wave progression in the precordial leads (see later, Myocardial Infarction).

BASIC INFORMATION

Equipment

Bipolar Leads
- Lead I: Left arm to right arm
- Lead II: Left leg to right arm
- Lead III: Left leg to left arm

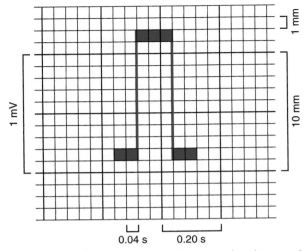

FIGURE 19–1. Examples of 10-mm standardization mark and time marks and standard ECG paper running at 25 mm/s.

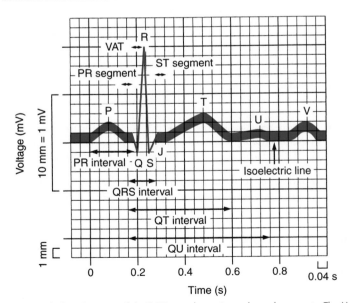

FIGURE 19–2. Diagram of the ECG complexes, intervals, and segments. The U wave is normally not well seen.

19

Precordial Leads: V_1 to V_6 across the chest (see Figure 13–9, page 272).

ECG Paper: With the ECG machine set at 25 mm/s, each small box represents 0.04 s, and each large box 0.2 s (see Figure 19–1). Most ECG machines automatically print a standardization mark.

Normal ECG Complex

Note: A small amplitude in the Q, R, or S wave is represented by a lowercase letter. A large amplitude is represented by an uppercase letter. The pattern shown in Figure 19–2 can also be noted qRs.

- **P Wave.** Caused by depolarization of the atria. With normal sinus rhythm, the P wave is upright in leads I, II, aVF, V_4, V_5, and V_6 and inverted in aVR.
- **QRS Complex.** Represents ventricular depolarization
- **Q Wave.** The first negative deflection of the QRS complex (not always present and, if present, may be pathologic). To be significant, the Q wave should be > 25% of the QRS complex.
- **R Wave.** The first positive deflection that sometimes occurs after the S wave
- **S Wave.** The negative deflection following the R wave
- **T Wave.** Caused by repolarization of the ventricles and follows the QRS complex, normally upright in leads I, II, V_3, V_4, V_5, and V_6 and inverted in aVR

AXIS DEVIATION

Axis represents the sum of the vectors of the electrical depolarization of the ventricles and gives an idea of the electrical orientation of the heart in the body. In a healthy person, the axis is downward and to the left (Figure 19–3). The QRS

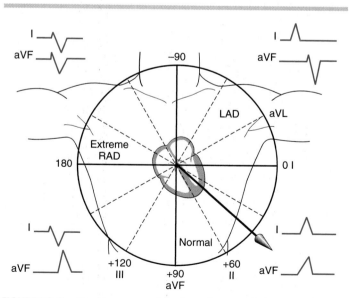

FIGURE 19–3. Graphic representation of axis deviation. ECG representations of each type of axis are shown in each quadrant. Large arrow indicates normal axis.

axis is midway between two leads that have QRS complexes of equal amplitude, or the axis is 90 degrees to the lead in which the QRS is isoelectric (ie, R amplitude wave equals S-wave amplitude).

- **Normal Axis.** QRS positive in I and aVF (0–90 degrees). Normal axis is actually –30 to 105 degrees.
- **Left Axis Deviation (LAD).** QRS positive in I and negative in aVF, –30 to –90 degrees
- **Right Axis Deviation (RAD).** QRS negative in I and positive in aVF, +105 to +180 degrees
- **Extreme RAD.** QRS negative in I and negative in aVF, +180 to +270 or –90 to –180 degrees

Clinical Correlations

- **RAD.** Seen with RVH, RBBB, COPD, and acute PE (a sudden change in axis toward the right) and occasionally in healthy persons
- **LAD.** Seen with LVH, LAHB (–45 to –90 degrees), LBBB, and in some healthy persons

HEART RATE

Bradycardia: Heart rate < 50 beats/min

Tachycardia: Heart rate > 100 beats/min

Rate Determination: Figure 19–4, below

- **Method 1.** Note the 3-s marks along the top or bottom of the ECG paper (15 large squares). The approximate rate equals the number of cycles (ie, QRSs) in a 6-s strip × 10.
- **Method 2** (for regular rhythms). Count the number of large squares (0.2-s boxes) between two successive cycles. The rate equals 300 divided by the number of squares. Extrapolate if the QRS complex does not fall exactly on the 0.2-s marks (eg, if each QRS complex is separated by 2.4 0.20-s segments, the rate is 120 beats/min. The rate between two 0.20-s segments is 150 beats/min, and between three 0.20-s segments is 100 beats/min). Each of the five smaller 0.04-s marks between the second and third 0.20 mark would be 10 beats/min (150 – 100 = 50 ÷ 5). Because the rate is three of the 0.04-s marks from the third 0.20-s segment, the rate is 100 + 30, or 130 beats/min.

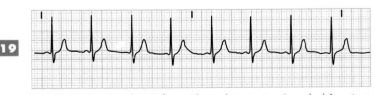

FIGURE 19–4. Sample strip for rapid rate determination. In method 1, estimate the rate by counting the number of beats (eight) in two 3-s intervals. The rate is 8 × 10, or 80 beats/min (method 1). In method 2, each beat is separated from the next by four 0.20-s intervals, so divide 300 by 4, and the rate is 75 beats/min. Because the beats are separated by exactly four beats, extrapolation is not necessary.

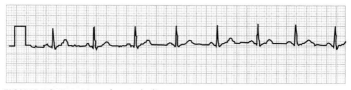

FIGURE 19–5. Normal sinus rhythm.

Remember that the number of beats per minute for each 0.04-s mark varies depending on which two 0.20 marks they are associated with (eg, between the fifth and sixth 0.20-s mark each 0.04 mark is 2 beats/min).

RHYTHM

Sinus Rhythms

Normal: Each QRS preceded by a P wave (which is positive in II and negative in aVR) with a regular PR and RR interval and a rate between 60 and 100 beats/min (Figure 19–5, above)

Sinus Tachycardia: Normal sinus rhythm with a heart rate > 100 beats/min and < 180 beats/min (Figure 19–6, below)

Clinical Correlations. Anxiety, exertion, pain, fever, hypoxia, hypotension, increased sympathetic tone (secondary to drugs with adrenergic effects [eg, epinephrine]), anticholinergic effect (eg, atropine), PE, COPD, AMI, CHF, hyperthyroidism, and others

Sinus Bradycardia: Normal sinus rhythm with heart rate < 50 beats/min (Figure 19–7, page 388)

Clinical Correlations. Well-trained athlete, normal variant, secondary to medications (eg, beta-blockers, digitalis, clonidine, nondihydropyridine calcium channel blockers [verapamil, diltiazem]), hypothyroidism, hypothermia, sick sinus syndrome (tachy–brady syndrome), and others

Treatment

- If asymptomatic (good urine output, adequate BP, and normal sensorium), no treatment.
- If hypotension, support blood pressure (see page 441)

19

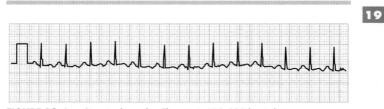

FIGURE 19–6. Sinus tachycardia. The rate is 120–130 beats/min.

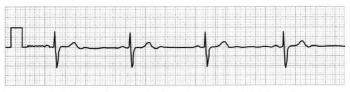

FIGURE 19-7. Sinus bradycardia. Rate is approximately 38 beats/min.

Sinus Arrhythmia: Normal sinus rhythm with irregular heart rate. Inspiration causes a slight increase in rate; expiration decreases rate. Normal variation between inspiration and expiration is 10% or less.

Atrial Arrhythmias

PAC: Ectopic atrial focus firing prematurely followed by a normal QRS (Figure 19–8, below). The compensatory pause following the PAC is partial; the RR interval between beats 4 and 6 is less than between beats 1 and 3 and beats 6 and 8.

Clinical Correlations. Usually no clinical significance; caused by stress, caffeine, and myocardial disease

PAT: A run of three or more consecutive PACs. The rate is usually 140–250 beats/min. The P wave may not be visible, but the RR interval is very regular (Figure 19–9, page 389). Falls under the more general category of **supraventricular tachycardia (SVT)** because it is indistinguishable from **AV nodal reentry tachycardia (AVNRT)** and paroxysmal junctional tachycardia and the treatments are similar.

Clinical Correlations. Some healthy persons; heart disease. Symptoms: palpitations, light-headedness, and syncope

Treatment

- **Increase Vagal Tone.** Valsalva maneuver or carotid massage
- **Medical Treatment.** Can include adenosine, verapamil, digoxin, edrophonium, or beta-blockers (propranolol, metoprolol, esmolol). Use verapamil and beta-blockers cautiously at the same time because asystole can occur.
- **Cardioversion with Synchronized DC Shock.** Particularly in patients in hemodynamically unstable condition (see Chapter 21, page 465)

19

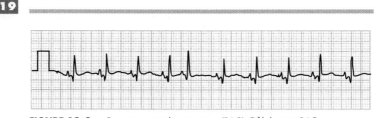

FIGURE 19-8. Premature atrial contraction (PAC). Fifth beat is PAC.

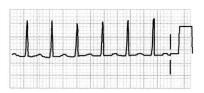

FIGURE 19–9.   Paroxysmal atrial tachycardia.

MAT: Originates from ectopic atrial foci; characterized by varying P-wave morphology and PR interval and irregular (Figure 19–10).

Clinical Correlations. COPD, advanced age, CHF, diabetes, and theophylline use. Antiarrhythmics are often ineffective. Manage the underlying disease.

AFib: Irregularly irregular rhythm, no discernible P waves. Ventricular rate varies 100–180 beats/min (Figure 19–11, page 390). The ventricular response may be < 100 beats/min if the patient is taking digoxin, verapamil, or a beta-blocker or has AV nodal disease.

Clinical Correlations. Some healthy persons; organic heart disease (CAD, hypertensive heart disease, valve disease), thyrotoxicosis, alcohol abuse, pericarditis, PE, and postoperative state

Treatment

- **Pharmacologic Therapy.** IV adenosine, verapamil, diltiazem, digoxin, and beta-blockers (propranolol, metoprolol, esmolol) can be used to slow the ventricular response. Quinidine, procainamide, propafenone, ibutilide, and amiodarone can be used to maintain or convert to sinus rhythm (see individual agents in Chapter 21, Emergencies)
- **DC-Synchronized Cardioversion.** If associated with increased myocardial ischemia, hypotension, or pulmonary edema (see Chapter 21, page 465)

Atrial Flutter: Sawtooth flutter waves with an atrial rate of 250–350 beats/min; rate may be regular or irregular depending on whether the atrial impulses are conducted through the AV node at a regular interval or at a variable interval (Figure 19–12, page 390).

Example: One ventricular contraction (QRS) for every two flutter waves = 2:1 flutter. A flutter wave is buried within each QRS complex so if you see two flutter waves before each QRS complex, that is 3:1 flutter; one flutter wave before each QRS complex is 2:1 flutter (the second flutter is hidden in the QRS complex or the T-wave).

19

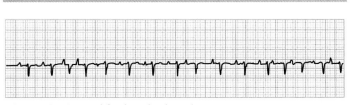

FIGURE 19–10.   Multifocal atrial tachycardia.

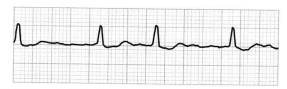

FIGURE 19–11. Atrial fibrillation.

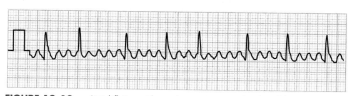

FIGURE 19–12. Atrial flutter with varying atrioventricular (AV) block (3:1 to 5:1 conduction).

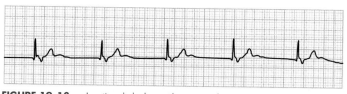

FIGURE 19–13. Junctional rhythm with retrograde P waves (inverted) following QRS complex.

Clinical Correlations. Valvular heart disease, pericarditis, ischemic heart disease; pulmonary disease, including PE; alcohol abuse

Treatment. Do *not* use quinidine or procainamide (atrial conduction may decrease to the point where 1:1 atrial to ventricular conduction can occur, and the ventricular rate increases and causes hemodynamic compromise); otherwise, similar to management of atrial fibrillation. Ibutilide (class III antiarrhythmic) or radiofrequency ablation

19

Nodal Rhythm

AV Junctional or Nodal Rhythm: Rhythm originates in the AV node. Associated with retrograde P waves that precede or follow the QRS. If the P wave is present, it is negative in lead II and positive in aVR (opposite of normal sinus rhythm) (Figure 19–13). Three or more premature junctional beats in a row constitute junctional tachycardia, which has the same clinical significance as PAT.

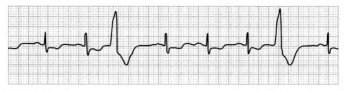

FIGURE 19–14.   Premature ventricular contractions (PVCs). Third and seventh beats are PVCs.

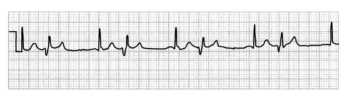

FIGURE 19–15.   Ventricular bigeminy.

1   2   3   4   5   6   7   8   9

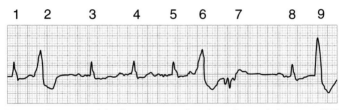

FIGURE 19–16.   Multifocal PVCs. Second, sixth, and seventh beats are PVCs. Second and sixth PVCs have the same morphology.

Ventricular Arrhythmias

PVC: A premature beat arising in the ventricle. P waves may be present but have no relation to the QRS of the PVC. The QRS is usually > 0.12 s with an LBBB pattern. A compensatory pause follows a PVC that is usually longer than after a PAC (Figure 19–14, above). The RR interval between beats 2 and 4 is equal to that between beats 4 and 6. Thus the pause following the PVC (the third beat) is fully compensatory. The following patterns are recognized:

- **Bigeminy.** One normal sinus beat followed by one PVC in an alternating manner (Figure 19–15, above)
- **Trigeminy.** Sequence of two normal beats followed by one PVC
- **Unifocal PVCs.** Arise from one site in the ventricle. Each has the same configuration in a single lead (see Figure 19–14).
- **Multifocal PVCs.** Arise from different sites and therefore have various shapes (Figure 19–16, above)

19

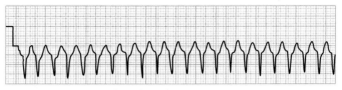

FIGURE 19–17.   Ventricular tachycardia.

Clinical Correlations. Healthy persons; excessive caffeine ingestion, anemia, anxiety; organic heart disease (ischemic, valvular, or hypertensive); medications (epinephrine and isoproterenol; digitalis and theophylline toxicity); predisposing metabolic abnormalities (hypoxia, hypokalemia, acidosis, alkalosis, hypomagnesemia)

Criteria for Treatment.

- No treatment if **asymptomatic.** Studies have shown increased mortality among patients treated for PVCs; however, > 10 PVCs per hour does increase death risk in patients with heart disease.
- If **symptomatic,** beta-blockers. Radiofrequency ablation for **right ventricular outflow tract (RVOT) tachycardia** in structurally normal hearts.

Ventricular Tachycardia: Three or more PVCs in a row (Figure 19–17). A wide QRS usually with an LBBB pattern (vs narrow complex seen with supraventricular tachycardia). May occur as short paroxysm or sustained run (> 30 s) with rate of 120–250 beats/min. Can be life-threatening (hypotension and degeneration into ventricular fibrillation). Management of nonsustained ventricular tachycardia is controversial.

Clinical Correlations. See PVCs. Patients with ventricular aneurysm are more susceptible to arrhythmias, especially in the presence of cardiac disease.

Treatment. See Chapter 21, page 464.

Ventricular Fibrillation: Erratic electrical activity from the ventricles, which fibrillate or twitch asynchronously; no cardiac output (Figure 19–18).

Clinical Correlations. One of two patterns seen with cardiac arrest (the other is asystole/flat line)

Treatment. See Chapter 21, page 464.

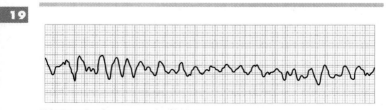

FIGURE 19–18.   Ventricular fibrillation.

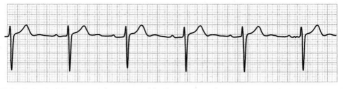

FIGURE 19–19. First-degree AV block. PR interval is 0.26 s.

Heart Block

First-Degree Block: PR interval > 0.2 s (or five small boxes). Usually not clinically significant (Figure 19–19). Caused by drugs (beta-blockers, digitalis, calcium channel blockers)

Second-Degree Block

Mobitz Type I (Wenckebach). Progressive prolongation of PR interval until P wave is blocked and not followed by a QRS complex (Figure 19–20). Can occur as a 2:1, 3:2, or 4:3 block. The ratio of the atrial to ventricular beats can vary. With 4:3 block, every fourth P wave is not followed by a QRS.

Clinical Correlations. Acute myocardial ischemia such as inferior MI, ASD, valvular heart disease, rheumatic fever, and digitalis or propranolol toxicity. Can be transient or rarely progress to life-threatening bradycardia.

Treatment. Usually expectant; if bradycardia occurs: atropine, isoproterenol, or a pacemaker

Mobitz Type II. A series of P waves with conducted QRS complexes followed by a nonconducted P wave. The PR interval for the conducted beats remains constant. Can occur as 2:1, 3:2, or 4:3 block. The ratio of the atrial to ventricular beats can vary. With 4:3 block, every fourth P wave is not followed by a QRS. (*Note:* 2:1 AV block can be either Mobitz type I or Mobitz type II, which can be difficult to differentiate. Mobitz I has a prolonged PR with a narrow QRS; Mobitz II has a normal PR interval with an LBBB pattern [wide QRS]).

Clinical Correlations. Implies severe conduction system disease that can progress to complete heart block; acute anterior MI and cardiomyopathy

Treatment. Temporary cardiac pacemaker, particularly when associated with acute anterior MI

19

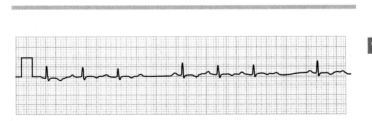

FIGURE 19–20. Second-degree AV block, Mobitz type I (Wenckebach) with 4:3 conduction.

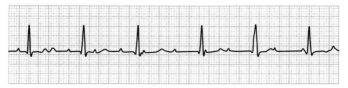

FIGURE 19–21. Third-degree AV block (complete heart block). Atrial rate is 100 beats/min; ventricular rate is 57 beats/min.

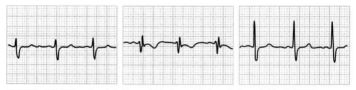

FIGURE 19–22. Leads I, V_1, and V_6 show right bundle branch block (RBBB) pattern.

Third-Degree Block: Complete AV block with independent atrial and ventricular rates. The ventricular rate is usually 20–40 beats/min (Figure 19–21).

Clinical Correlations. Degenerative changes in conduction system in elderly persons, digitalis toxicity, transient finding with an acute inferior MI (ischemia of the AV junction), aftermath of acute anterior MI (higher probability of mortality than after inferior MI); can result in syncope or CHF

Treatment. Placement of a temporary or permanent pacemaker

BBB: Complete BBB is present when the QRS complex is > 0.12 s (or three small boxes on the ECG). Look at leads I, V_1, and V_6. Degenerative changes and ischemic heart disease are the most common causes.

RBBB: The RSR pattern seen in V_1, V_2, or both. Also a wide S in leads I and V_6 (Figure 19–22)

Clinical Correlations. Healthy persons; diseases affecting the right side of the heart (pulmonary hypertension, ASD, ischemia); sudden onset associated with PE and acute exacerbation of COPD

LBBB: RR' in leads I, V_6, or both. QRS complex may be more slurred than double-peaked as in RBBB. A wide S wave is seen in V_1 (Figure 19–23).

19

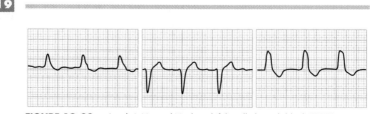

FIGURE 19–23. Leads I, V_1, and V_6 show left bundle branch block (LBBB) pattern.

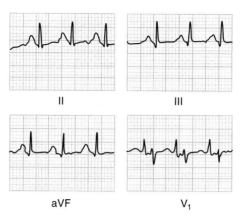

FIGURE 19–24. Right atrial enlargement, leads II, III, aVF, and V_1. Note tall P waves in II, III, and aVF and tall, slender P waves in V_1.

Clinical Correlations. Organic heart disease (hypertensive, valvular, and ischemic), severe aortic stenosis. New LBBB after AMI can be an indication for inserting a temporary cardiac pacemaker. Consider new LBBB MI until proven otherwise.

CARDIAC HYPERTROPHY

Atrial Hypertrophy

P wave > 2.5 mm in height and > 0.12 s wide (three small boxes on the ECG)

RAE: Tall (> 2.5 mm), slender, peaked P waves (P pulmonale pattern) in leads II, III, aVF (Figure 19–24). Tall (> 1.5 mm) P may be present in V_1 and V_2.
Clinical Correlations. Chronic diffuse pulmonary disease, pulmonary hypertension, congenital heart disease (ASD)

LAE: Notched P wave (P mitrale pattern) in leads I and II. Wide (≥ 0.11 s), slurred biphasic P in V_1 with wider terminal than initial component (negative deflection) (Figure 19–25)

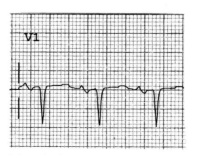

FIGURE 19–25. Left atrial enlargement.

19

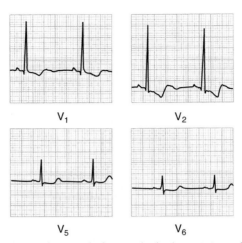

FIGURE 19–26.   Right ventricular hypertrophy, leads V_1, V_2, V_5, and V_6. Note the tall R waves in V_1 and V_2, greater than the R waves in V_5 and V_6. Also note strain pattern in V_1 and V_2 with down-sloping ST-segment depression and T-wave inversion.

Clinical Correlations. Mitral stenosis or mitral regurgitation or secondary to LVH with hypertensive cardiovascular disease

Ventricular Hypertrophy

RVH: Tall R wave in V_1 (R wave > S wave in V_1), persistent S waves in V_5 and V_6, progressively smaller R wave from V_1 to V_6, slightly widened QRS intervals (Figure 19–26), and strain pattern with ST-segment depression and T-wave inversion in V_1 to V_3. Pattern of small R waves with relatively large S waves in V_1 to V_6 may be present. Right axis deviation (> 105 degrees) invariably present.

Clinical Correlations. Mitral stenosis, chronic diffuse pulmonary disease, chronic recurrent PE, congenital heart disease (eg, tetralogy of Fallot), Duchenne muscular dystrophy, biventricular hypertrophy (LVH and RVH, LVH findings often predominating)

LVH: Voltage criteria (> age 35 y): S wave in V_1 or V_2 plus R wave in V_5 or V_6 > 35 mm, or R wave in aVL > 11 mm or R wave in I + S wave in III > 25 mm, or R wave in V_5 or V_6 > 26 mm. QRS complex may be > 0.10 s wide in V_5 or V_6. ST-depression and T-wave inversion in anterolateral leads (I, aVL, V_5 or V_6) suggest LVH with strain (Figure 19–27, page 397)

Clinical Correlations. HTN, aortic stenosis, aortic insufficiency, long-standing CAD, some forms of congenital heart disease

MYOCARDIAL INFARCTION

(See also Chapter 21, page 466.)

Myocardial Ischemia: Inadequate myocardial oxygen supply (coronary artery blockage or spasm). The ECG can show ST-segment depression (subendocardial ischemia) (Figure 19–28, page 397), ST elevation (transmural ischemia) (Figure 19–29, page 397), or symmetrically inverted (flipped) T waves (Figure 19–30,

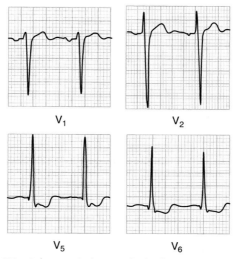

FIGURE 19–27. Left ventricular hypertrophy, leads V_1, V_2, V_5, and V_6. S wave in V_2 + R wave in V_5 is 55 mm. Note ST changes and T-wave inversion in V_5 and V_6, suggesting strain.

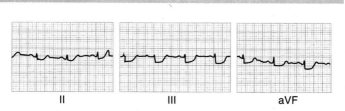

FIGURE 19–28. ST segment depression in leads II, III, and aVF in a patient with acute subendocardial ischemia and infarction.

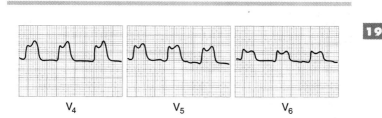

FIGURE 19–29. ST elevation in leads V_4, V_5, and V_6 in a patient with acute anterolateral ischemia.

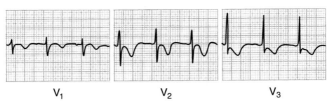

FIGURE 19–30.   Inverted T waves.

above) in the area of ischemia (eg, inferior ischemia in II, III, and F; anterior ischemia in V_1 to V_6; lateral ischemia in I, aVL; anterolateral ischemia in I, aVL, V_5, and V_6; anteroseptal ischemia in V_1, V_2, V_3, and V_4.

MI: Myocardial necrosis caused by severe ischemia. Can be **transmural MI** (ST elevation early, T-wave inversion, Q waves late) or **subendocardial MI** (ST depression, T-wave inversion without evidence of Q waves). Table 19–1, below, outlines the localization of MIs.

- **Acute Injury Phase (transmural).** Hyperacute T waves, then ST-segment elevation. Hyperacute T waves return to normal in minutes to hours. ST elevation usually regresses after hours to days. Persistent ST elevation suggests a left ventricular aneurysm.
- **Evolving Phase (transmural).** Hours to days after MI. Deep T-wave inversion occurs and then replaces ST-segment elevation, and T wave may return to normal.

TABLE 19–1
Localization of Transmural Myocardial Infarction on ECG

Location of MI	Presence of Q Wave or ST-Segment Elevation	Reciprocal ST Depression
Anterior	V_1 to V_6 (or poor R-wave progression in leads V_1 to V_6)[a]	II, III, aVF
Lateral	I, aVL, V5, V6	V_1, V_3
Inferior	II, III, aVF	I, aVL, possibly anterior leads
Posterior	Abnormally tall R and T waves in V_1 to V_3	V_1 to V_3
Subendocardial	No abnormal Q wave. ST-segment depression in the anterior, lateral, or inferior leads	

[a]Normally in V_1 to V_6, the R-wave amplitude gradually increases and the S wave decreases with a "biphasic" QRS (R = S) in V_3 or V_4. With an anterior MI, there will be a loss of R-wave voltage (instead of Q waves) and the biphasic QRS will appear more laterally in V_4 to V_6, hence the term *poor R-wave progression*.

19

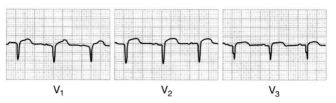

FIGURE 19–31.   Q waves in leads V₁, V₂, and V₃ in a patient with acute anteroseptal MI. Note ST elevation to determine acute nature of infarction.

- Q Waves (transmural). Hours to days after transmural MI, a Q wave is the initial negative deflection of the QRS complex. A significant Q wave is 0.04 s in duration and > 25% the height of the R wave (Figure 19–31). May regress to normal after years.

ELECTROLYTE AND DRUG EFFECTS

Electrolytes

Hyperkalemia: Narrow, symmetrical, diffuse, peaked T waves. In severe hyperkalemia, PR prolongation occurs, the P wave flattens and is lost, and the QRS widens and can progress to ventricular fibrillation (Figure 19–32).

Hypokalemia: ST-segment depression with the appearance of U waves (positive deflection after the T wave) (Figure 19–33)

Hypercalcemia: Short QT interval

Hypocalcemia: Prolonged QT interval

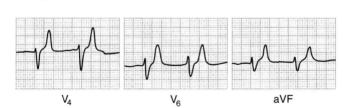

FIGURE 19–32.   Diffuse tall T waves in leads V₄, V₆, and aVF with widened QRS and junctional rhythm (loss of P waves) secondary to hyperkalemia.

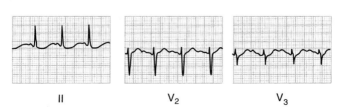

FIGURE 19–33.   Leads II, V₂, and V₃ in a patient with hypokalemia. A U wave is easily seen in V₂ and V₃ but difficult to distinguish from the T wave in II.

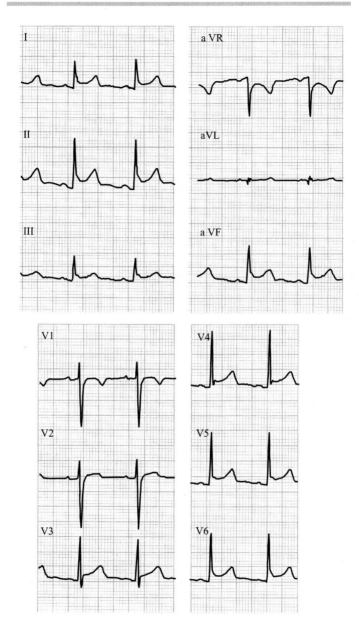

FIGURE 19–34. Acute pericarditis.

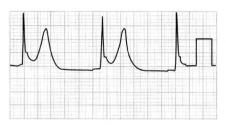

FIGURE 19–35.   Sinus bradycardia, Osborne wave. J-point elevation with ST-segment elevation and prolonged QT interval (0.56 s) in patient with hypothermia.

Drugs

Digitalis Effect: Down-sloping ST segment

Digitalis Toxicity
- **Arrhythmias.** PVCs, bigeminy, trigeminy, ventricular tachycardia, ventricular fibrillation, PAT, nodal rhythms, accelerated junctional tachycardia and sinus bradycardia
- **Conduction Abnormalities.** First-degree, second-degree, and third-degree heart blocks

Quinidine and Procainamide: With toxic levels, prolonged QT, flattened T wave, and QRS widening

MISCELLANEOUS ECG CHANGES

Pericarditis: Diffuse ST elevation concave upward, diffuse PR depression, diffuse T-wave inversion, or a combination of these findings (Figure 19–34, page 400)

   Clinical Correlations. Idiopathic conditions; viral, bacterial, and fungal infections, such as TB; AMI, postpericardiotomy syndrome, Dressler syndrome; collagen–vascular diseases; uremia; cancer

Hypothermia: Sinus bradycardia, AV junctional rhythm, ventricular fibrillation. Classically, **J point** (the end of the QRS complex and the beginning of the ST segment) elevation, intraventricular conduction delay, and prolonged QT interval possible (Figure 19–35). Known as an **Osborne wave.**

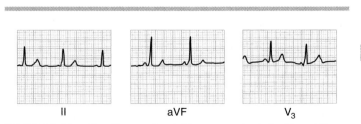

| II | aVF | V$_3$ |

19

FIGURE 19–36.   Short PR interval and delta waves in leads II, aVF, and V$_3$ in a patient with Wolff–Parkinson–White syndrome.

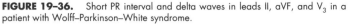

WPW Pattern and Syndrome: The WPW (Wolff–Parkinson–White) pattern is a short PR interval along with a delta wave (a delay in initial deflection of the QRS complex) on the ECG (Figure 19–36). WPW syndrome is the WPW pattern on ECG *and* documented tachyarrhythmias, usually SVT or Afib. Tachyarrhythmia (preexcitation syndrome) due to conduction from the SA node to the ventricle through an accessory pathway that bypasses the AV node (bundle of Kent).

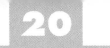

CRITICAL CARE

Care of the Critically Ill Patient
ICU Progress Note
Routine Monitoring
Transporting Critically Ill Patients
Central Nervous System
Cardiovascular System
Cardiovascular Physiology
Central Venous Pressure
Pulmonary Artery Catheters
Clinical Pulmonary Physiology

Indications for Intubation
Securing the Airway
Mechanical Ventilation Modes
Ventilator Management
Nutrition in the ICU
Complications in Critical Care
Quick Reference to Critical Care
    Formulas
Guidelines for Adult Critical Care
    Drug Infusions

CARE OF THE CRITICALLY ILL PATIENT

Patients admitted to the ICU often have multisystem disease, have traumatic injuries, or are under intensive treatment regimens to avoid or manage end-organ dysfunction. The interactions between dysfunctional organ systems are complicated and can be overwhelming to students and new house officers. This chapter describes an organ-system approach to evaluating and treating critically ill patients as well as commonly encountered critical care complications. The field of critical care medicine is rapidly advancing, and evidence-based protocols and pathways are becoming an important part of clinical practice. Become familiar with unit protocols in the following major areas:

1. Sedation and analgesia
2. Delirium and substance withdrawal
3. Nutrition
4. Intensive insulin therapy
5. Transfusion of blood products
6. DVT and stress ulcer prophylaxis
7. Weaning from mechanical ventilation
8. Antibiotics
9. Management of sepsis including:
    a. Goal-directed therapy
    b. Activated protein C (drotrecogin alfa)
    c. Adrenal insufficiency and use of steroids
    d. Vasopressors
    e. ARDS

ICU PROGRESS NOTE

The ICU progress note is a concise summary of the events of the past 24 h, medications, physical exam, laboratory data, and the assessment and treatment plan. Although the information can be found elsewhere in the chart, the physician's interpretation of the data communicates the medical decision-making process. The daily progress note includes:

1. Problem list and injury summary
    a. Active problems and major inactive problems

     b. Allergies

     c. Past medical or surgical history relevant to the present illness

     d. Notation of hospital day, post trauma day, postoperative day, etc

2. Events and procedures over the past 24 h

3. Current medications

4. System-specific physical exam and pertinent flow sheet data

     a. **CNS:** CNS functioning or other neurologic assessment and sedation level (eg, Modified Ramsay Sedation scale, Richmond Agitation–Sedation Scale [RASS], Confusion Assessment Method [CAM-ICU])

     b. **CV:** Cardiovascular function, including indicators of systemic perfusion, blood pressure, heart rate, and pulmonary artery (PA) catheter data

     c. **Pulm:** Pulmonary function, including ventilator settings and ABG values

     d. **GI/Nut:** GI function and nutritional status

     e. **F/E/R:** Fluids, electrolytes, and renal function

     f. **Heme/ID:** Hematologic function, including CBC, coagulation values; infectious disease status (recent culture data, antibiotic regimen, treatment duration)

     g. **Prophylaxis:** DVT, ethanol withdrawal, stress gastritis, etc

5. Other relevant laboratory and radiographic data

6. Assessment and plan

ROUTINE MONITORING

1. **Continuous ECG:** Computerized arrhythmia detection systems facilitate rapid detection of rhythm abnormalities and increase the likelihood of successful resuscitation.

2. **Blood Pressure:** Intermittent (sphygmomanometer) or continuous (intravascular) assessment of BP (systolic, diastolic, mean arterial, and central venous pressures). Assessment of response to treatment and titration of vasoactive drugs. Continuous intravascular methods are warranted in patients with marked hemodynamic instability.

3. **Pulse Oximetry:** Continuous, quantitative arterial O_2 saturation (SaO_2); ensures adequate oxygenation of systemic arterial blood for tissue delivery.

4. **Temperature:** Critically ill patients are at high risk of thermoregulatory disorders due to their pathophysiologic condition (eg, fluid resuscitation, burns, sepsis); continuous measurements in the esophagus (esophageal probe) and central venous blood compartment (PA catheter) are accurate methods for monitoring core body temperature. ATLS definitions of hypothermia are mild, 35°C; moderate 32°C; and severe 28°C.

5. **Capnography:** Continuous measurement of expired CO_2. Changes imply alteration in clinical status (eg, hypoventilation, overfeeding, fever, sepsis).

TRANSPORTING CRITICALLY ILL PATIENTS

20

"Whatever can go wrong, will go wrong" is especially true during the transport of critically ill patients. Adherence to common sense guidelines helps to minimize the risk of adverse events:

1. Maintain the patient's **airway;** if the airway is tenuous, intubate the patient *before* transport.

2. Transport only stable patients (unless the role of transport is to provide a life-saving intervention).

3. Pay attention to IV catheters and pumps and their connections.
4. Bring sufficient oxygen, IV fluids, medications, etc.
5. Adequate assistance must be available to safely transport the patient and associated equipment; the destination should be prepared to accept the patient.
6. Expect the unexpected; have personnel, equipment, and supplies available that can make the difference in a crisis (eg, drugs and equipment for reintubation, bag valve mask).

CENTRAL NERVOUS SYSTEM

Severe acute illness often results in altered mental status (AMS). AMS manifests a spectrum of disability from simple, mild delirium to complex, life-threatening coma.

Critically ill patients are often intubated, and medications must be administered for sedation and analgesia. Inadequate sedation and pain control have adverse effects such as increased catabolism, tachycardia and higher myocardial O_2 consumption, immunosuppression, hypercoagulability, and severe anxiety, so great care must be taken in finding the proper balance of medications.

When acute agitation occurs, first rule out *life-threatening pathology* (ie, inadequate blood flow and nutrient availability to the brain). Evaluate vital signs, oxygenation and ventilation status, and serum glucose and electrolytes before administering CNS-altering medications.

Sedation

Benzodiazepines are potent inducers of sedation, amnesia, muscle relaxation, and anxiolysis. These properties make this class of drug ideal for short- to intermediate-term use. Take great care to choose a drug that will not accumulate in the patient's system if end-organ dysfunction is present:

- **Lorazepam:** Good intermediate-duration benzodiazepine; metabolized by the liver with inactive metabolite excreted in the urine; very potent but has a long time to peak effect (ideal agent for longer-term sedation)
- **Midazolam:** Shorter-onset, shorter-acting benzodiazepine; metabolism altered by calcium channel blockers, erythromycin, and triazole antifungals

Titrate either agent to achieve a sedation level according to published scales (eg, RASS). The reliability and validity of the RASS for titration of sedation has been validated in numerous studies (eg, *Am J Respir Crit Care Med* 2002;166: 1338–1344 and *JAMA* 2003;289:2983–2991).

The **RASS** (*Am J Respir Crit Care Med* 2000;161:A506 and *JAMA* 2001; 286:2703–2710) is scored as follows:

+4 Combative—Combative, violent, immediate danger to staff
+3 Very agitated—Pulls or removes tubes and catheters; aggressive
+2 Agitated—Frequent nonpurposeful movement; fights ventilator
+1 Restless—Anxious, apprehensive but no aggressive movement
 0 Alert and calm
−1 Drowsy—Sustained (> 10 s) awakening to voice
−2 Light sedation—Briefly (< 10 s) awakens to stimulation
−3 Moderate sedation—Movement or eye opening to voice
−4 Deep sedation—Response to physical stimulation but not voice
−5 Unarousable—No response to voice or physical stimulation

20

If overmedication occurs (eg, inadvertent overadministration, accumulation of metabolites), stop the medication, prepare to institute cardiopulmonary support, and use flumazenil (a benzodiazepine antagonist) to reverse the overly sedated state. Carefully review the contraindications to flumazenil use before administering the drug.

- **Propofol:** Nonbenzodiazepine, lipid-based sedative–hypnotic; little analgesic properties; extremely short onset and half-life make accumulation unlikely (ultra-short-term drug); expensive; longer-term use has adverse financial and infectious consequences. One approach is to initiate at 10 mcg/kg/min and adjust by increments of 10–20 mcg/kg/min q5–15 min to achieve desired level of sedation (reconsider dosing > 50 mcg/kg/min). To discontinue, decrease infusion 25% q10–15 min, then halt the infusion when the patient is conscious.
- **Haloperidol:** Short-term management of agitation, especially with components of delirium. Relevant considerations in the ICU setting are as follows:

1. Prolongation of the QT interval; discontinue if QT interval increases > 50% of baseline or exceeds 450 ms.
2. Lowering of the seizure threshold; be cautious with use in the presence of alcohol withdrawal, traumatic brain injury, etc
3. Potential CNS effects, such as extrapyramidal symptoms, tardive dyskinesia, and the uncommon but potentially devastating neuroleptic malignant syndrome

Analgesia (See Also Chapter 14)

Critically ill patients may have acute pain due to recent operations or prehospital trauma. Opioid narcotic agents are best for acute pain control.

- **Morphine:** IV opioid narcotic; commonly used (low cost, ease of use)
- **Fentanyl:** Synthetic opioid; more potent and shorter acting than morphine; less histamine release than morphine (ie, less potential for drug-induced hypotension)

These opioids can be administered as continuous infusions, intermittent boluses, or as part of patient-controlled analgesia (PCA) regimen. Because narcotics can cause respiratory depression, careful titration is necessary, especially when narcotics are combined with benzodiazepines. Epidural anesthesia provides good local analgesia and decreases requirements for IV narcotics.

Many critically ill patients need long-term sedation and analgesia. Current data suggest that daily interruption of sedation decreases mechanical ventilation days and ICU length of stay.

Neuromuscular paralysis is rarely indicated but may be necessary for patients with severe respiratory failure who cannot properly oxygenate or ventilate. Eliminating the muscular elastic recoil of the chest wall and ventilator dyssynchrony may improve pulmonary compliance and ventilation–oxygenation ability.

20

CARDIOVASCULAR SYSTEM

Cardiovascular instability is one of the most common problems encountered in the ICU. The first step in evaluating the cardiovascular system is a thorough physical exam.

Inspection: Jugular Venous Distention (JVD)

- Neck vein visualization (with the patient sitting at a 45-degree angle) implies CVP > 12–15 mm Hg
- JVD *plus* systemic hypotension suggests *life-threatening pathology:*
  1. Tension pneumothorax
  2. Pericardial tamponade
  3. Severe cardiac dysfunction

Inspection: Precordial Contusion

- Associated with blunt trauma from a steering wheel; injury pattern implies possible myocardial contusion. *Treatment:* Continuous ECG monitoring; correction of arrhythmias (most common: sinus tachycardia). To identify anatomic heart injury and pericardial effusion, obtain an echocardiogram if arrhythmias occur.

Inspection: Extremity Perfusion

- Check extremities for **perfusion** (pulse, color, temperature, and capillary refill)
- *Note:* Pay special attention to sites distal for:
  1. Long bone fractures
  2. Joint dislocations
  3. Indwelling arterial catheters

Blood Pressure (BP)

Over the short term, BP is considered adequate if renal perfusion is maintained (usually MAP > 70 mm Hg in young, previously healthy persons). Premorbid medical problems and aging, however, may mandate a higher MAP.

Note: If the cuff is too small for the arm (ie, the patient is obese), the measured systolic BP will be falsely elevated.

Systolic Hypertension: Systolic BP > 140 mm Hg with normal diastolic BP. In the acute setting, due to:

- Increased cardiac output
- Thyrotoxicosis
- Generalized response to stress
- Anemia
- Pain, anxiety, or both

Diastolic Hypertension: Diastolic BP > 90 mm Hg. Isolated diastolic hypertension may be associated with:

- Intrinsic renal disease
- Endocrine disorders
- Renovascular hypertension
- Neurologic disorders

20

Treatment: Hypertension is a concern after acute coronary syndromes, subarachnoid hemorrhage, and vascular anastomosis (especially carotid artery surgery). Systolic BP > 180 mm Hg usually necessitates *immediate treatment.* Commonly used agents include nitroprusside, nicardipine, metoprolol, labetalol, esmolol, hydralazine, and nitroglycerin. Use a rapid-acting and easily reversible beta-blocker (eg, esmolol) to manage hypertension associated with ruptured aortic aneurysm or blunt traumatic aortic injury. Emergency management of hypertension is discussed in Chapter 21, and the specific antihypertensive agents are discussed in Chapter 22.

Mean Arterial Pressure (MAP)

Calculated as DBP + [(SBP – DBP)/3]

Pulse Pressure (SBP – DBP)

Wide Pulse Pressure: (> 40 mm Hg) associated with:

- Thyrotoxicosis
- Arteriovenous fistula
- Aortic insufficiency

Narrow Pulse Pressure: (< 25 mm Hg) associated with:

- Significant tachycardia
- Early hypovolemic shock
- Pericarditis
- Pericardial effusion or tamponade
- Ascites
- Aortic stenosis

Paradoxical Pulse: Systolic BP changes during the respiratory cycle as a function of changes in intrathoracic pressure (see Chapter 13 for measurement technique). Normally, systolic BP falls 6–10 mm Hg with inspiration. If this variation occurs over a wider range (> 10 mm Hg), the patient is said to have a paradoxical pulse (Figure 20–1, below). Associated conditions include:

- Pericardial tamponade
- Asthma and COPD
- Ruptured diaphragm
- Pneumothorax

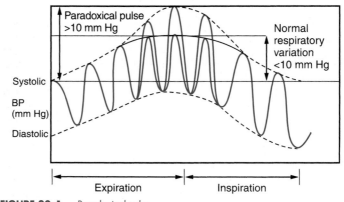

FIGURE 20–1.   Paradoxical pulse.

Auscultation: Heart Murmurs

The presence of a premorbid cardiac murmur and, more important, the interval development of a new cardiac murmur are important in the care of a critically ill patient. Characterize all new murmurs by intensity, location, and variation with position and respiration as well as whether they are systolic or diastolic. In general, diastolic murmurs are usually pathologic (see Chapter 1 for more information on heart murmurs).

CARDIOVASCULAR PHYSIOLOGY
Definitions

Cardiac Output (CO): Volume of blood pumped by the heart each minute; approximately 3.5–5.5 L/min (adult). CO is standardized to patient size by calculation of the cardiac index (CI): CI = CO/BSA; normal CI ≈ 2.8–3.2 L/min/ m^2. CI < 2.5 L/min/m^2 may require pharmacologic intervention if O_2 delivery is inadequate. CO is the product of heart rate and stroke volume. Stroke volume is a function of preload, afterload, and contractility.

Preload: Initial length of myocardial muscle fibers is proportional to left ventricular end-diastolic volume (LVEDV), which is governed by the volume of blood remaining in the left ventricle after systole. As LVEDV increases, the stretch on myocardial muscle fibers increases. Furthermore (Figure 20–2, top), as LVEDV increases (ie, stretch), the energy of contraction increases proportionally until an optimal tension develops (Starling law; Figure 20–2, middle). However, when the myocardial muscle fiber is overstretched, contractile strength decreases.

Afterload: Resistance to ventricular ejection; measured clinically with aortic BP and calculation of systemic vascular resistance (SVR).

Contractility: Ability of heart to alter its contractile force and velocity independent of fiber length (ie, the intrinsic strength of the individual muscle fiber cells). Contractility may be increased by stimulation of beta-receptors in the heart (see following section).

Review of Sympathetic Nervous System Influence on the Cardiovascular System

CO and its determinants (preload, afterload, and contractility) are influenced by the sympathetic nervous system (SNS). The SNS releases catecholamines (predominantly epinephrine and norepinephrine), which bind to end-organ receptors and exert a physiologic response. Adrenergic receptors are divided into two major classes: alpha (α) and beta (β). End-organ function after receptor activation is summarized in Table 20–1, page 411.

Adrenergic receptors are important because many of the cardiovascular drugs used in the ICU act through their sympathomimetic properties. Such drugs have a specific receptor affinity (ie, α versus β) and consequently differ in end-organ effects. For example, drugs that act on the α_1 receptors are called **vasopressors** because they cause nonspecific systemic vasoconstriction. Conversely, drugs that act on β_1 receptors are called **inotropes** because they increase myocardial contractility and heart rate.

Because each drug exerts receptor-specific effects, use of these agents provides differential activation of receptors and ultimately end-organ effects. Through tailoring pharmacologic support, physicians provide the necessary car-

20

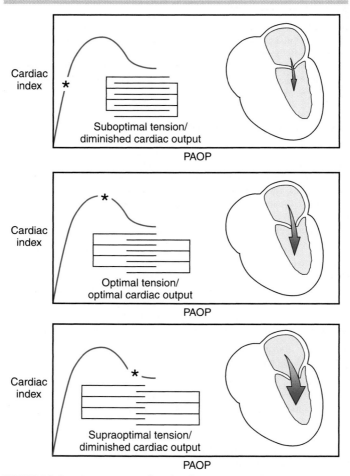

FIGURE 20–2.   Representation of Starling law. PAOP = pulmonary artery occlusion pressure.

diovascular assistance to critically ill patients. Commonly used sympathomimetics and their relative receptor affinities are listed in Table 20–2, page 411. A guide to administration of these agents appears in Table 20–11, page 450.

CENTRAL VENOUS PRESSURE (CVP)

The central venous catheter is one of two major devices used for cardiovascular instrumentation. The other, the PA catheter (also called PA catheter, Swan–Ganz catheter, and right-heart catheter), is discussed in the next section. For CVP monitoring, a 14-gauge IV catheter is inserted into the central venous circulation through the internal jugular or subclavian vein (see Chapter 13). A pressure transducer and monitor connected to the catheter provide the measurements. A CXR is required to confirm the position of the catheter in the superior vena cava. The zero point for the

TABLE 20–1
Adrenergic Receptors and Their Actions
on the Cardiovascular System

Receptor	Location	Action
Alpha $(\alpha)_1$	Peripheral arterioles	Vasoconstriction (increased SVR)
Beta $(\beta)_1$	Myocardium	Increased contractility
	SA node	Increased heart rate
Beta $(\beta)_2$	Peripheral arterioles	Vasodilatation (decreased SVR)
	Bronchiolar smooth muscle	Bronchodilatation

SVR = systemic vascular resistance; SA = sinoatrial.

transducer is the level of the right atrium in a supine patient; this phlebostatic axis is usually 5 cm caudal to the sternal notch in the midaxillary line.

The transduced CVP reflects right atrial pressure, and by association, right ventricular filling pressure or preload. Although CVP is a relatively inaccurate indicator of preload, trends in relation to volume status and hemodynamics may be clinically useful. The general implications of CVP readings are listed in Table 20–3.

CVP Limitations

1. CVP does not *entirely* reflect total blood volume or left ventricular function. CVP is altered by:

- Changes in PA resistance
- Changes in compliance of the right ventricle
- Intrathoracic pressure (eg, mechanical ventilation)

TABLE 20–2
Relative Actions of Sympathomimetic Drugs
on Adrenergic Receptors

Drug	Effect On			
	α	β_1	β_2	D
Phenylephrine	++++	0	0	
Norepinephrine	++++	++	0	
Epinephrine	++++	++++	++	
Dobutamine	+	++++	++	
Isoproterenol	0	++++	+++	
Dopamine (mcg/kg/min)	10–20	5–10		1–5

Key: + = Relative effect; 0 = no clinically significant effect; D=dopaminergic receptors.

20

TABLE 20–3
Interpretation of CVP Measurements

Reading (mm Hg)	General Description	Clinical Implications
< 3	Low	Intravenous fluids may be administered
3–10	Midrange	Probable clinical euvolemia
>10	High	Suspect fluid overload, CHF, CP, COPD, tension PTX

CVP = central venous pressure; CHF = congestive heart failure; CP = cor pulmonale; COPD = chronic obstructive pulmonary disease; PTX = pneumothorax.

2. An accurate clinical picture can be limited by conditions that radically change intrathoracic pressure:

   - Positive pressure ventilation, especially when high PEEP is used
   - Pneumothorax, hemothorax, hydrothorax, and tension pneumothorax
   - Presence of intrathoracic tumors

3. CVP can be normal in the face of sepsis or hypovolemia when accompanied by compromised myocardial function
4. Left ventricular failure can occur in the presence of normal CVP
5. Patients with COPD may need an elevated CVP to optimize CO
6. PA catheter readings more accurately reflect fluid and cardiac status, but the technique is more invasive and expensive than use of CVP catheters.

Technical Tips Regarding CVP Measurements
   - CVP readings are inaccurate if they do not fluctuate with respiration.
   - If appropriate, remove the patient from the ventilator when taking a CVP reading.
   - To ensure comparable readings, have the patient positioned in the same manner for each measurement.
   - Flatten the bed and use the same zero point for the transducer (phlebostatic axis).

PULMONARY ARTERY CATHETERS

Used for direct measurement of central cardiovascular pressures, which are calculated circulatory values used in critical care. The catheter is placed in a central vein (usually the subclavian or internal jugular) and then passed into the right atrium, across the tricuspid valve, into the right ventricle, and through the pulmonic valve. The distal end is floated into the PA (Figure 20–3). The PA catheter is used to measure PA pressure (PAP), PA occlusion pressure (PAOP, also known as pulmonary capillary wedge pressure [PCWP]), and CVP. Intravascular volume status, vascular resistance (both pulmonary and systemic), and the pumping ability of the heart (CO) are calculated, mixed venous oxygen saturation ($S\bar{v}o_2$) is monitored, and right ventricular ejection fraction (REF) and right ventricular end-diastolic volume index (RVEDVI) are measured.

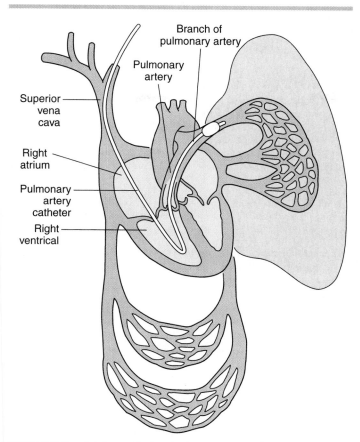

FIGURE 20–3. Relative positioning of pulmonary artery catheter.

Key point: The data obtained with a PA catheter are only as good as the initial setup and the *actual* measurements obtained (ie, pressures). If the pressure measurements are in error *or* if patient data (height, weight, etc) are incorrectly entered into the system, the subsequent calculations will be *incorrect*.

Indications

There has been debate concerning the utility of PA catheters (*JAMA* 2005;294: 1664–1670). However, many clinicians find these catheters an essential tool in the following settings:

- Acute heart failure
- Shock states
- Complex circulatory and fluid conditions (massive resuscitation)
- Complicated MI
- Intraoperative management in high-risk cardiac patients (eg, aneurysm repair, elderly patient undergoing major operation)

20

Catheter Description

The PA catheter generally consists of three (or four) lumens and a thermistor at the tip (Figure 20–4); markings are typically in 10-cm increments; the catheter is radiopaque.

Lumens

- **Balloon port:** Usually a square white port; route to inflate the balloon at the tip of the catheter; inflation of the balloon requires 1.0–1.5 mL of air
- **Proximal port:** Approximately 30 cm proximal to the tip; lies in the superior vena cava; may be used for fluid administration when not used for determination of CVP and CO
- **Distal port:** Lies in PA beyond the balloon; this port is attached to a pressure transducer for continuous PAP tracings and intermittent PAOP measurement

Thermistor: Temperature sensor that provides continuous core temperature measurements as well as measurements used in thermal dilution CO techniques (see page 419)

Additional Functions and Measurement Capabilities

- **Pacing PA catheters:** Extra ports (approximately 19 cm from the tip) through which pacing wires are passed into the right ventricle; other models contain electrodes along the surface of the catheter; capable of pacing both right atrium and right ventricle

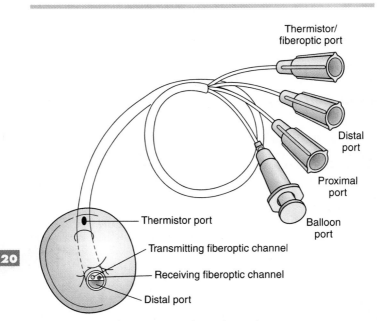

20

FIGURE 20–4. Pulmonary artery catheter. This one features an oximetric measuring feature.

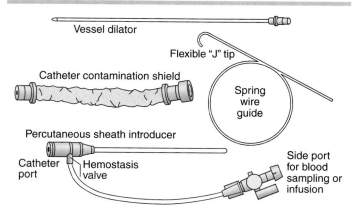

FIGURE 20–5. Additional items used for pulmonary artery catheter placement. (From: *Office & Bedside Procedures*. Chesnutt MS, et al [ed]. Appleton & Lange, Stamford, CT, 1992. Used with permission.)

- **Oximetric PA catheter:** Standard PA catheter ports with fiberoptic components; emit light impulses to and from distal end of catheter; light impulses are then reflected by hemoglobin and measured; continuous O_2 saturation monitoring (see Figure 20–4)
- **Right ventricular ejection fraction catheter:** Used to measure REF, which is then used to calculate RVEDVI (best indicator of preload)

Contraindications to PA Catheter Use: No absolute contraindications. Patients with LBBB may experience complete heart block (requiring temporary pacemaker); frequent manipulation may increase infection risk, as with any IV catheter.

Materials: There are many versions of the flow-directed, balloon-tipped PA catheter; a generic representation is in Figure 20–4. A PA catheter introducer insertion kit contains an introducer sheath (cordis catheter), flexible J-tip guidewire, vessel dilator, catheter contamination shield, and other items needed to insert the catheter (Figure 20–5 above). The monitoring system (transducers, tubing, and stopcocks) and pressurized flush system are usually set up by the nursing staff and should be operational before catheter insertion.

Pulmonary Artery Catheterization Procedure

1. Obtain informed consent from the patient or the patient's medical decision maker.
2. Make sure that emergency resuscitation medications are on hand in the event of refractory arrhythmia.
3. Choose a site. In a patient who may receive thrombolytic therapy or who has a coagulopathy, femoral and internal jugular veins may be preferred because of their compressibility if a complication occurs. The easiest sites for floating the PA catheter are the right internal jugular and the left subclavian veins. *Rationale:* The PA catheter is packaged in a coiled position; these sites tend to the natural curve of the catheter as it assists in placement.
4. Widely prep the insertion site with a topical antiinfective agent such as chlorhexidine gluconate. *Important:* Antiinfective agents must *fully dry on the skin* to be effective.

20

5. Fully drape the patient (not just the immediate site) because of the length of the tubing and guidewire. Use aseptic technique with gown, gloves, and mask to decrease the rate of line infection.

6. With the patient in Trendelenburg position, cannulate the chosen central vein (see Central Venous Catheterization, Chapter 13). Pass the flexible end of the J-wire (standard length, 45 cm) into the vein through the needle. **Never** force a guidewire, and always keep one hand on the guidewire while it is in the patient. **The flexible tip end is passed first because the stiff end can perforate the blood vessel.**

7. Mount the introducer sheath on the vessel dilator. Pass the dilator–sheath unit over the wire. Make a *full-thickness skin nick* at the wire entry site with a no. 11 blade scalpel.

8. Pass the vessel dilator–sheath unit into the vessel over the guidewire (Figure 20–6). A gentle, slight twisting motion may be necessary. Remove the guidewire and the vessel dilator. Catheter sheaths have a hemostatic valve mechanism to prevent air from entering the central system and blood from escaping. The side port does not have a valve, so cap it or clamp it. Mount a syringe on the side port and aspirate blood to confirm intravascular positioning of the sheath; flush with sterile saline solution after confirmation.

9. Prepare the PA catheter (attach to the monitor, flush lumens with sterile saline). Zero the transducer at the phlebostatic axis; ask the ICU nursing staff for help with the setup. Check balloon function and gently wave the catheter to ensure that an appropriate waveform is present on the monitor. *Note:* Never fill the balloon with fluid; use only air. The volume is typically 1.5 mL. After placing the catheter through the contamination shield, check balloon function by insufflating with 1.5 mL of air.

10. Insert the prepared catheter (flushed, transduced, contamination shield in place) into the sheath (Figure 20–7). Once you have advanced approximately 15–20 cm and a CVP tracing is visible on the monitor, gently inflate the balloon with 1.0–1.5 mL of air using the volume-limiting syringe provided with the set. There should be no resistance to balloon inflation.

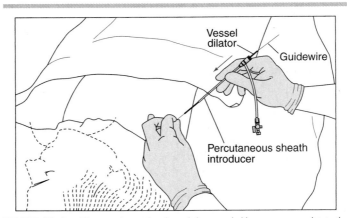

FIGURE 20–6. The introducer sheath and the vessel dilator are passed into the vessel. (From: *Office & Bedside Procedures.* Chesnutt MS, et al [ed]. Appleton & Lange, Stamford, CT, 1992. Used with permission.)

20

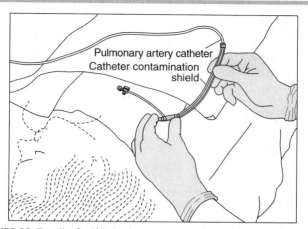

FIGURE 20-7. The fluid-filled pulmonary artery catheter is passed into the introducer sheath. (From: *Office & Bedside Procedures.* Chesnutt MS, et al [ed]. Appleton & Lange, Stamford, CT, 1992. Used with permission.)

11. Once the balloon is inflated, advance the catheter to the level of the right atrium under the guidance of the pressure waveform and the ECG. Monitor the waveform and ECG at all times while advancing the balloon catheter. Figure 20–8B, page 418 shows the normal pressures encountered as the catheter is advanced. *Important:* **Never** advance the catheter with the balloon deflated. Conversely, always withdraw the PA catheter with the balloon deflated.

12. Positioning of the PA catheter in the right atrium is probably best determined by watching for the characteristic waveform on the monitor (Figure 20–8B). The right atrium is generally approximately 30 cm from the right internal jugular or subclavian vein insertion site and approximately 35–40 cm from the left subclavian vein insertion site.

13. An abrupt change in the pressure tracing occurs as the catheter enters the right ventricle (Figure 20–8B). There is generally little ectopy on entry into the right ventricle; however, as the catheter advances into the right ventricular outflow tract, PVCs may occur.

14. Steadily advance the catheter until ectopy disappears and the PA tracing (heralded by a rise in diastolic pressure) is obtained (Figure 20–8). If this does not occur by the time 60 cm is reached, deflate the balloon, withdraw the catheter to 20 cm, and make another attempt with the balloon inflated after slightly rotating the catheter.

15. Once the catheter is in the PA, obtain the PAOP after advancing the catheter another 10–15 cm. The final position of the catheter should be such that PAOP is obtained with no less than full balloon inflation *and* the PAP tracing is present with the balloon deflated. In the ideal position, transition from PAP to PAOP (and vice versa) occurs within three or fewer heartbeats. In an adult, the typical length to the PA position is 45–60 cm. Table 20–4 shows normal PA catheter measurements important for patient evaluation and treatment.

20

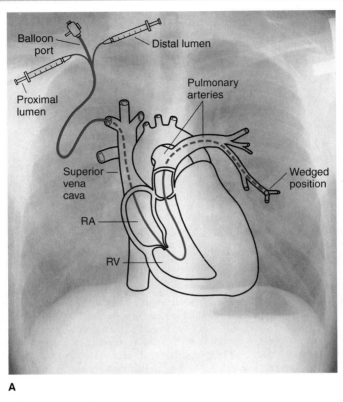

A

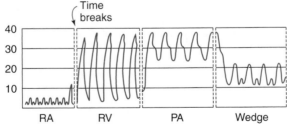

B

FIGURE 20–8. Positioning and pressure waveforms seen as the pulmonary artery catheter is advanced. RA = right atrium; RV = right ventricle; PA = pulmonary artery. (From: *Internal Medicine on Call*, 2nd ed. Haist SA, et al [ed]. Appleton & Lange, Stamford, CT, 1996. Used with permission.)

20

16. Once the position is acceptable, lock the contamination shield onto the sheath. The catheter can be readjusted after the sterile field is taken down. Suture the sheath to the skin, secure the catheter in place and dress the surgical site according to unit protocol. Connect catheters to the ports on the

sheath. The inflow port on the sheath can be used for IV fluid and medication administration.

17. Obtain a CXR to document the catheter position and to rule out pneumothorax or other complications. A properly positioned catheter should lie just beyond the vertebral bodies in the nonwedged position.

18. **Common problems:** Catheter placement is more difficult if severe PA hypertension is present. If there is significant cardiac enlargement, particularly dilatation of the right-heart structures, the catheter may coil in its path to the right ventricular outflow tract; fluoroscopy may be needed for correct positioning. Furthermore, under these conditions, the PA catheter may have difficulty holding its proper position. Because the balloon-tipped catheter depends on flow to carry it through the right-heart chambers, placement in the PA may be difficult if the patient has low CO.

19. **CO can be measured by thermal dilution (Fick equation).** Connect the thermistor to the CO computer and then rapidly inject fluid (usually 10 mL of ice-cooled NS) through the right atrial port. The computer displays a curve, and CO is calculated from the area under the thermal dilution curve. Do this two more times. If all of these values are approximately the same, average the readings and record. Continuous CO-monitoring PA catheters are used in some hospitals. Normal values for CO and CI are listed in Table 20–4.

Complications of PA Catheters

1. Most complications due to PA catheterization are related to central vein cannulation: Arterial puncture, extravascular placement, pneumothorax, hemothorax

2. Arrhythmias are common. Transient **PVCs** are most common and occur when the catheter is advanced into the right ventricular outflow tract. If a patient

TABLE 20–4
Normal Pulmonary Artery and Cardiac Performance Measurements

Parameter	Range
Right atrial pressure	1–7 mm Hg
Right ventricular pressure	
Systolic	15–25 mm Hg
Diastolic	0–8 mm Hg
PAP	
Systolic	15–25 mm Hg
Diastolic	8–15 mm Hg
Mean	10–20 mm Hg
PAOP ("wedge pressure")	6–12 mm Hg
Cardiac output	3.5–5.5 L/min
Cardiac index	2.8–3.2 L/min/m^2
Mixed venous O_2 saturation	65–85%

PAP = pulmonary artery pressure; PAOP = pulmonary artery occlusion pressure.

20

with a PA catheter suddenly develops frequent PVCs, deflate the balloon and pull back the catheter to prepare for another attempt.

3. Ventricular tachycardia and fibrillation are *rare*. If they continue after the catheter has been withdrawn, treat the patient with standard ACLS protocols (see Chapter 21).

4. Transient RBBB occurs occasionally as the catheter passes through the right ventricular outflow tract. In a patient with preexisting LBBB, complete heart block can occur. In this setting, have backup pacing readily available.

5. Pulmonary infarction and PA rupture are serious but infrequent complications of PA catheters and are usually secondary to "over wedge" or peripheral placement of the catheter. Place the patient affected-lung-down, and intubate (if not already done). Insert the ET tube into the unaffected mainstem bronchus to protect the airway. Obtain an emergency thoracic surgery consultation.

6. Complications tend to increase with the length of time the catheter is in place. The risk of bacteremia and spontaneous bacterial endocarditis (SBE) are high in severely ill patients undergoing long-term instrumentation. In the setting of unexplained fever, always remove and culture the PA catheter and sheath. Replace the catheter and sheath at a different site if a pulmonary catheter is still indicated.

PA Catheter Measurements

PA Pressure: Measured when the PA catheter is in its resting position (balloon deflated). Measurements include pulmonary systolic arterial pressure (PAS), mean pulmonary arterial pressure (MPAP), and diastolic (PAD) arterial pressure.

Pulmonary Artery Occlusion Pressure (PAOP):   Estimate of left atrial pressure (LAP). Measured while the inflated balloon at the tip of the PA catheter occludes a branch of the PA. *Important:* To avoid pulmonary infarction, fully deflate the balloon when it is not in use.

In the absence of mitral valvular disease, PAOP correlates closely with LAP and with the left ventricular end-diastolic pressure (LVEDP). This correlation exists because of the unobstructed continuity between the PA and the left side of the heart. As a result of this continuity, PAOP may never be greater than the PAD. Increased LVEDP is reflected in an increase in PAOP, which increases PAD. Therefore *if a PA catheter monitor shows a wedge pressure higher than PAD pressure, a technical error exists.*

Left Ventricular End-Diastolic Pressure: A measure of preload used to optimize fluid resuscitation and CO. For optimal stroke volume on the Starling curve, the preload must be adequate to stretch the wall of the left ventricle (see Figure 20–2). Hypovolemia results in too little tension on the muscle fibers and therefore decreased stroke volume and CO. Too much preload stretches beyond the point of maximum tension and decreases CO. Clinically, LVEDP and PAOP are used to keep preload in an optimum range. The normal PAOP varies between 6 and 12 mm Hg but may be higher for different disease states and for preexisting cardiac disease leading to decreased chamber compliance.

Right Ventricular Ejection Fraction (REF)/Right Ventricular End-Diastolic Volume Index (RVEDVI):   RVEDVI, the most accurate assessment of preload, is most helpful in patients with high intrathoracic pressure. A rapid-response thermistor and CO computer are used to calculate REF. Once REF and CO are known, RVEDVI can be calculated. RVEDVI is a more accurate assessment of volume status than PAOP. For example, a patient with severe ARDS may have markedly elevated peak inspiratory pressure. Although the CVP and PAOP may be falsely elevated, RVEDVI is a calculation of a volume, not pressure, so volume status can be determined across a variety of clinical situations. The normal range for EDVI is 80–120 mL/m^2.

Continuous CO Measurement

The specially designed PA catheter emits small pulses of energy that heat the surrounding blood for continuous CO measurement. CO is then calculated on the basis of the magnitude and rate of temperature change. This continuous measurement, along with calculated derivatives, is intermittently updated and displayed on the device.

Differential Diagnosis of PA Catheter Abnormalities

Table 20–4 and Figure 20–8 show normal PA pressures and cardiovascular measurements. Perturbations of these values indicate a disease process with the differential diagnoses shown in Table 20–5, page 422.

Clinical Applications

Estimation of volume status and myocardial performance: CO is a function of heart rate and stroke volume. Stroke volume depends on preload, afterload, and contractility.

Heart Rate: Heart rate is increased to maintain or increase CO in the face of inadequate tissue perfusion. Hence, tachycardia is an additional indicator of O$_2$ debt (ie, delivery–demand deficit). Tachycardia > 120 beats/min increases myocardial O$_2$ demand significantly and should be promptly treated. The PA catheter is used to establish adequate myocardial filling pressures such that heart rate may be clinically manipulated to maximize CO. In a patient with adequate filling pressures, slow heart rate (< 80 beats/min), and low CO, drugs that accelerate heart rate (chronotropes) can be used to increase CO. Alternatively, tachycardia > 120 beats/min with an adequate PAOP can be pharmacologically slowed to decrease strain on the heart.

Preload (Stroke Volume): Indicated by PAOP or EDVI, a reflection of LVEDV. In simple terms, preload is the amount of blood in the heart before contraction. Consequently, preload represents the stretch placed on an individual myocardial cell. When PAOP is optimized, myocardial performance is optimized according to the Starling curve.

1. **Clinical implications in a healthy heart.** Low PAOP or EDVI means suboptimal myocardial muscle stretch. CO can be increased first by administration of fluids. The result is an increase in LVEDV, an increase in myocardial muscle tension, and improved myocardial performance.
2. **Clinical implications in a failing heart.** Long-standing myocardial disease can shift the Starling curve to the right. Consequently, a markedly elevated PAOP may be needed to optimize myocardial performance. It is common for patients who have just undergone heart valve replacement to need a PAOP of 20–25 mm Hg to optimize CO (because of decreased compliance of the postoperative heart muscle). Patients with a recent MI may similarly need a PAOP of 16–18 mm Hg to optimize output.

TABLE 20-5
Differential Diagnosis by Category Based on Perturbations in Hemodynamic Parameters[a]

Diagnosis	Systemic Blood Pressure	CVP	CO	PAOP/LVEDP	PAP	PVR	SVR
Cardiogenic shock	↓	↑	↓	↑	↑	↑	↑
Cardiac tamponade	↓	↑	↓	↑	↑	—	↑
Pulmonary embolism	↓	↑	↓	— or ↓	↑	↑	↑
Hypovolemic shock	↓	↓	↓	↓	↓	↑	↑
Neurogenic shock	↓	↓	↓	↓	↓	↓	↓
Septic shock	↓	↓	↑	↓	↓	↓	↓

[a]These are the trends usually seen with the conditions noted. Clinical variables (medications, secondary conditions, etc) may vary these trends somewhat. **Highlighted areas** denote major differences between subgroups.

CVP = central venous pressure; CO = cardiac output; PAOP = pulmonary artery occlusion pressure; LVEDP = left ventricular end-diastolic pressure; PAP = pulmonary artery pressure; PVR = peripheral vascular resistance; SVR = systemic vascular resistance. ↑ = usually increased; ↓ = usually decreased; — = usually unchanged.

20

Afterload: Resistance to ventricular ejection; measured clinically by calculation of SVR. Normal SVR = 900 – 1200 dynes/s/cm^3.

$$SVR = \frac{(MAP - CVP) \times 80}{Cardiac\ output\ (L/min)}$$

1. **Indications for afterload reduction.**
   - Significant mitral regurgitation
   - An increased PAOP coincident with elevated SVR/decreased CI
2. **Treatment.** Vasodilators (eg, nitroprusside, nitrates, ACE inhibitors, hydralazine)

Contractility: The ability of the heart to alter its contractile force and velocity *independent* of fiber length. This aspect is difficult to measure directly but can be estimated with surrogate markers. Correctable metabolic causes of depressed contractility include:

- Hypoxia
- Acidosis (pH < 7.3)
- Hypophosphatemia
- Adrenal insufficiency
- Hypothermia

Improve contractility with inotropic agents such as dobutamine or milrinone.

Continuous S$\bar{v}$O$_2$ Monitoring

Oximetric PA catheters are used for direct measurement of mixed venous Hgb saturation (S$\bar{v}$O$_2$). A microprocessor then displays a continuous graph of S$\bar{v}$O$_2$ measurements. Calibration is periodically confirmed with ABG measured from heparinized blood drawn from the distal port of the oximetric catheter.

Clinical Application
- Follow trends in O$_2$ supply–demand balance.
- Because it is the best indicator of decreased peripheral O$_2$ delivery, a decrease in S$\bar{v}$O$_2$ is an early sign of organ dysfunction. Correct the problem before hemodynamic compromise occurs.
- Fix the underlying cause. The effect of interventions (eg, transfusions, fluid administration, inotropic agents) can be assessed by following S$\bar{v}$O$_2$ before changes are apparent in other hemodynamic variables.
- Clinically, S$\bar{v}$O$_2$ values between 65% and 85% represent adequate tissue O$_2$ delivery and extraction. This *generally* implies appropriate perfusion of peripheral tissues.
- If S$\bar{v}$O$_2$ drops to < 60%, *immediately* assess O$_2$ delivery. As O$_2$ delivery falls, S$\bar{v}$O$_2$ falls proportionally because there is less O$_2$ for the tissues to extract.
- If S$\bar{v}$O$_2$ is < 60% *and* O$_2$ delivery is unchanged, identify unrecognized conditions causing increased O$_2$ demand.

In summary, a decline of S$\bar{v}$O$_2$ must prompt a review of the parameters of O$_2$ delivery (ie, CO, [Hgb], SaO$_2$) and consumption (SaO$_2$ – S$\bar{v}$O$_2$). Potential treatments include:

- Correction of hypoxia
- Optimization of myocardial performance for decreased CO

20

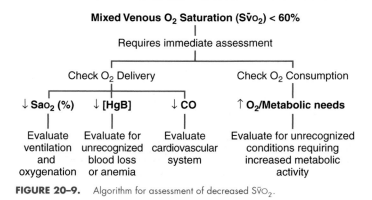

FIGURE 20–9. Algorithm for assessment of decreased $S\bar{v}o_2$.

- RBC transfusion for symptomatic anemia
- Identification and management of conditions leading to increased metabolic demands (eg, unrecognized seizures, shivering, and large tissue defects) because these conditions markedly increase in O_2 demand (Figure 20–9, above)

Continuous Spo$_2$ Monitoring (Pulse Oximetry)

The same fiberoptic technology used to measure $S\bar{v}o_2$ is used to measure Sao_2. A light-emitting external probe is placed around a well-perfused appendage such as a digit, earlobe, lip, or bridge of the nose. The light is transmitted through the appendage and reflected by hemoglobin according to its O_2 saturation (the hemoglobin molecule absorbs different wavelengths of light at different O_2 saturations). The oximeter, in addition to calculating oxyhemoglobin saturation, measures the pulse rate and is thus referred to as the pulse oximeter. The reading obtained is the Spo_2.

Spo_2 < 90% implies inadequate oxygenation and under most circumstances necessitates immediate intervention. *One exception* would be a patient with severe COPD who may have a normal O_2 saturation in the upper 80% range. Conversely, Spo_2 > 90% does not necessarily imply adequate O_2 delivery (see following section). Pulse oximetry is not useful in the setting of smoke inhalation and carbon monoxide poisoning because of the higher affinity of the hemoglobin molecule for carbon monoxide.

CLINICAL PULMONARY PHYSIOLOGY

The key to understanding pulmonary physiology and mechanical ventilation in the ICU is to know the difference between oxygenation and ventilation (Figure 20–10).

Ventilation

Ventilation is the mechanical movement of air into and out of the respiratory system. The result is the exchange of CO_2. Several parameters, such as volumes and capacities, are important in assessing the adequacy of ventilation. Spirometry

20

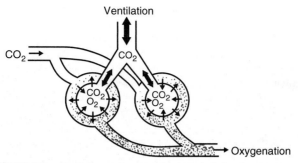

FIGURE 20–10. Ventilation and oxygenation in typical alveoli.

gives both dynamic information (ie, ability to move air into and out of the lungs) and static volume measurements. The lung volume subdivisions and capacities are shown on a spirometric graph in Figure 20–11, below.

Lung Volumes: Total lung capacity (TLC), or the amount of gas in the lung at full inspiration, comprises four basic lung volumes:

1. **Inspiratory reserve volume (IRV):** The volume of gas that can be maximally inspired beyond a normal tidal volume inspiration
2. **Tidal volume (TV):** The volume of inspired gas during a normal breath; approximately 6–8 mL/kg in resting, healthy adults
3. **Expiratory reserve volume (ERV):** The volume of gas that can be maximally expired beyond a normal tidal volume expiration
4. **Residual volume (RV):** The volume of gas that remains in the lung after a maximal expiratory effort

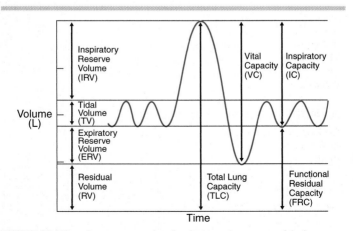

FIGURE 20–11. Spirometric graph with volumes and capacities of the lung.

Lung Capacity: The sum of two or more of these lung volumes makes up four divisions called lung capacities (see Figure 20–11).

1. **Vital capacity (VC):** The volume of gas expired after a maximal inspiration followed by maximal expiration (VC = ERV + TV + IRV)
2. **Inspiratory capacity (IC):** The volume of gas expired from maximal inspiration to the end of a normal, resting TV (IC = TV + IRV)
3. **Functional residual capacity (FRC):** The amount of gas remaining in the lung after a normal tidal volume expiration (FRC = ERV + RV); acts as a buffer against extreme changes in alveolar Po_2 and consequent dramatic changes in arterial Po_2 with each breath

Clinical Implications

These volumes and capacities are important factors in assessing ventilation because they can change under different conditions (eg, atelectasis, obstruction, consolidation, small airway collapse). For example, as ERV decreases with small airway collapse, FRC decreases (Figure 20–12, below). These alterations in lung volume affect respiratory reserve as well as oxygenation and ventilation.

Critical Closing Volume (CCV):   CCV is the minimum volume and pressure of gas necessary to prevent small airways from collapsing during expiration. When collapse occurs, blood is shunted around nonventilated alveoli. This phenomenon decreases the surface area available for gas exchange. CCV can vary as compliance changes. If CCV > FRC (air in the lung after tidal expiration), collapse tends to occur in a higher proportion of airways (see Figure 20–12, below).

One method of overcoming CCV is to increase the amount of positive end-expiratory pressure (PEEP) in the lung (see later, Ventilator Management, page 437). The effect of PEEP is to increase FRC by minimizing small airway collapse at the end of expiration. This maneuver improves alveolar ventilation, decreases shunting, and ultimately improves oxygenation (Figure 20–13).

Lung Compliance: Compliance is the *change* in lung volume (V) as a function of *change* in pressure (P) (Figure 20–14):

$$\text{Lung compliance} = \frac{\Delta V}{\Delta P}$$

This value can be measured at the bedside and is a reflection of FRC and CCV.

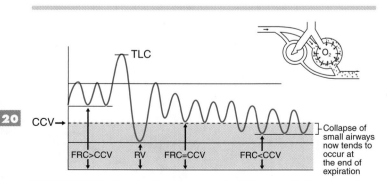

FIGURE 20–12.   Functional residual capacity (FRC) and critical closing volume (CCV). TLC = total lung capacity; RV = residual volume.

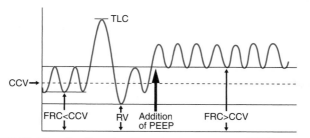

FIGURE 20-13. The effect of positive end-expiratory pressure (PEEP) is to increase functional residual capacity (FRC). CCV = critical closing volume; TLC = total lung capacity; RV = residual volume.

Dynamic Compliance: Measure tidal volume (TV) and divide it by peak inspiratory pressure (PIP):

$$\text{Dynamic compliance} = \frac{TV}{PIP - PEEP}$$

Normal: 80–100 mL/cm water

Static Compliance: Similar to dynamic compliance, except that *static* PIP is substituted for PIP. Measure static peak pressure (also called plateau pressure) by occluding the exhalation port at the beginning of exhalation (no flow = static pressure).

Comparing *dynamic* with *static* compliance may indicate the type of processes causing changes in the elasticity of the lung. Dynamic compliance is affected by both elasticity and airway resistance. Static compliance reflects elasticity and is not affected by airway resistance because there *is no flow.*

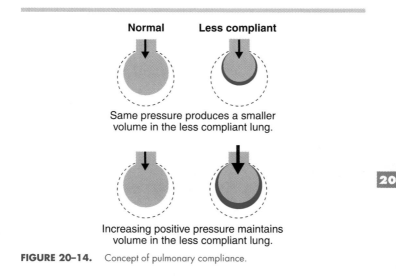

FIGURE 20-14. Concept of pulmonary compliance.

1. Reduction in dynamic compliance *without* a change in static compliance indicates an airway resistance problem (obstruction, bronchospasm, or collapse of the small airways)
2. Reduction in *both* static and dynamic compliance indicates a decrease in lung elasticity (pulmonary edema, atelectasis, or excessive PEEP)

Oxygenation

Oxygenation is the process of transporting O_2 from the alveolus across the capillary membrane into the pulmonary circulation and subsequently distributing that O_2 to the body's tissues. O_2 delivery is a function of arterial O_2 content and CO.

Arterial Oxygen Content (CaO_2): The ability of the blood to carry O_2 to the periphery depends on the O_2 content. CaO_2 is directly influenced by Hgb concentration ([Hgb]) and the saturation of Hgb with O_2 (SaO_2) (ie, $CaO_2 = SaO_2 \times 1.39$ [Hgb])

Oxygen Delivery (DO_2): Normal $DO_2 \approx 600$ mL of O_2/min with an average normal O_2 uptake of 250 mL of O_2/min. Calculate DO_2 with PA catheter data by multiplying measured CO by calculated (CaO_2).

    Note: This calculation simplifies DO_2 to three parameters: CO, SaO_2, and [Hgb]. PaO_2 has been omitted because of the *extremely small role* it plays with regard to CaO_2 (Remember: its contribution is $0.0031 \times PaO_2$).

Alveolar-to-Arterial (A–a) Gradient: Assessment of alveolar–capillary gas exchange used to indirectly quantify ventilation–perfusion abnormalities. The calculation is occasionally useful as a tool to help determine the cause of hypoxemia (eg, hypoventilation).

Shunt Fraction: Normal < 5%. Reflects the portion of CO that traverses the heart from right to left without increasing CaO_2 ($\approx$ 5% of pulmonary capillary blood leaves the lung without being oxygenated). In an ideal state, the volume of lung ventilation equals the volume of pulmonary capillary blood flow (Figure 20–15, below). Alterations in these ventilation–perfusion relationships have two causes:

- Relative obstruction of alveolar ventilation
- Relative obstruction of pulmonary blood flow

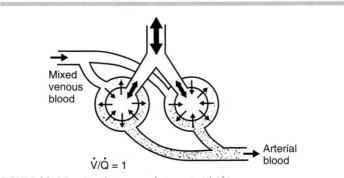

FIGURE 20–15.   Ventilation to perfusion ratio ($\dot{V}/\dot{Q}$).

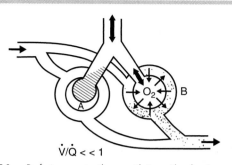

$$\dot{V}/\dot{Q} << 1$$

FIGURE 20–16. Perfusion greater than ventilation. Alveolus **A** receives no ventilation because of bronchiolar obstruction (**B**).

1. **Perfusion greater than ventilation:** A common scenario is *pulmonary consolidation* due to infection or secretions (Figure 20–16). An alveolus receives no ventilation because of bronchiolar obstruction, yet normal pulmonary capillary perfusion continues (ie, complete pulmonary A–V shunt exists with respect to that alveolus).

2. **Ventilation greater than perfusion:** Impairment of pulmonary blood flow to the alveolar level occurs after lung surgery and after pulmonary embolism (Figure 20–17, below). Uniform ventilation continues to the alveoli, but no blood flow passes some of them. This situation increases the ventilated physiologic dead space *and* increases the shunt fraction.

3. **Compensation mechanism:** Figure 20–18 represents the compensatory changes that occur when an alveolus is partially occluded. Local vasoconstriction results in diversion of blood flow to better ventilated alveoli. This mechanism is called hypoxic pulmonary vasoconstriction.

Principle: Recognize that at any given time, combinations of these situations exist *simultaneously* within the lung (remember that the normal shunt fraction is $\approx$ 5%). Therefore alterations in either ventilation or perfusion can seriously affect oxygenation.

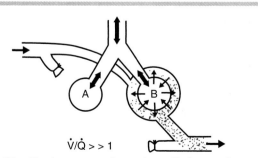

$$\dot{V}/\dot{Q} >> 1$$

FIGURE 20–17. Ventilation greater than perfusion. Uniform ventilation continues to alveoli **A** and **B**, but no blood flow passes alveolus **A**.

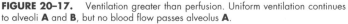

20

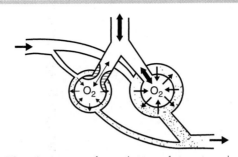

FIGURE 20–18.   Compensation for ventilation–perfusion mismatch.

1. **Decreased lung-to-blood transfer.** Associated factors include:

    - Pulmonary edema
    - ARDS
    - Bronchial secretions
    - Atelectasis
    - Pneumonia
    - Pneumonitis

2. **Decreased perfusion.** Associated factors include:

    - Massive PE
    - Continued micropulmonary embolization
    - Postoperative changes

Calculation of A–a Gradient and Shunt Fraction: The equations for determining A–a gradient and shunt fraction are in comprehensive textbooks on critical care. Online (eg, http://medcalc3000.com) and PDA-based resources are available to assist in the calculations.

INDICATIONS FOR INTUBATION

The decision to intubate is often a stress-provoking process. The primary objective of mechanical ventilation is to decrease the work of breathing and reverse life-threatening hypoxia and hypercapnia. A point-prevalence study has shown that the most common indications for intubation and mechanical ventilation are respiratory failure (66%), coma (15%), acute exacerbation of COPD (13%), and neuromuscular disorders (5%). Common indications for mechanical ventilation include:

   - **Inability to adequately ventilate** (eg, airway obstruction, severe chest trauma, excessive sedation, neuromuscular disease, paralyzed or fatigued respiratory muscles)
   - **Inability to adequately oxygenate** (eg, pneumonia, pulmonary embolism [PE], pulmonary edema, ARDS)
   - **Excessive work of breathing** (eg, severe bronchospasm, airway obstruction)
   - **Airway protection** (eg, unconsciousness, altered mental status, massive resuscitation, facial or head trauma)

20

TABLE 20–6
**Indicators of Impending Respiratory Failure Necessitating
Intubation and Mechanical Ventilation**

Condition	Normal Range (adults)
Respiratory impairment	
Tachypnea > 30 breaths/min	10–20 breaths/min
Dyspnea	
Neurologic impairment	
Loss of gag reflex	
Altered mental status (ie, patient is unable to protect airway against aspiration)	
Gas exchange impairment	
$PaCO_2$ > 60 mm Hg	35–45 mm Hg
PaO_2 < 70 mm Hg (on 50% mask)	80–100 mm Hg (on room air)
SaO_2 < 90%	

A timely decision to intubate a decompensating patient can turn an otherwise chaotic intubation into a controlled, elective procedure. Diagnostic factors that help predict impending respiratory failure are listed in Table 20–6.

SECURING THE AIRWAY

An essential treatment component of respiratory failure is securing and maintaining a patent airway (see Chapter 21). Briefly, the airway is kept open with the chin-lift or the jaw-thrust maneuver. Perform the maneuver with great care if there is a possible cervical spine injury. Use a nasopharyngeal or oropharyngeal airway to keep the patient's tongue from obstructing the oropharynx. Definitive airway management includes oral or nasal endotracheal intubation. Use a laryngeal mask airway (LMA) as a temporary measure if attempts at endotracheal intubation fail. Use the Difficult Airway Algorithm established by the American Association of Anesthesiologists (Figure 20–19) as a framework for managing a difficult airway. (See also Chapter 21, page 463.)

Confirmation of Endotracheal Tube Placement: Confirm tube placement with a colorimetric end-tidal CO_2 detector and auscultation of bilateral breath sounds.

Surgical Options:
- **Tracheostomy.** Used when long-term intubation is anticipated and for patients with severe maxillofacial injuries. This procedure is elective, unlike cricothyroidotomy. The benefits of tracheostomy are improved patient comfort and oral hygiene, ease of secretion removal, and a more secure airway.
- **Cricothyroidotomy.** *Emergency procedure* used when nonsurgical attempts to secure the airway have failed:

20

(Text continues on page 435.)

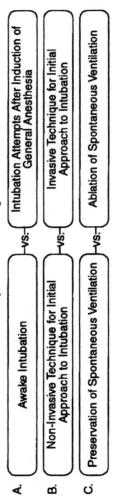

ASA AMERICAN SOCIETY OF ANESTHESIOLOGISTS

DIFFICULT AIRWAY ALGORITHM

1. Assess the likelihood and clinical impact of basic management problems:

   A. Difficult Ventilation
   B. Difficult Intubation
   C. Difficulty with Patient Cooperation or Consent
   D. Difficult Tracheostomy

2. Actively pursue opportunities to deliver supplemental oxygen throughout the process of difficult airway management

3. Consider the relative merits and feasibility of basic management choices:

   A. Awake Intubation — vs: — Intubation Attempts After Induction of General Anesthesia

   B. Non-Invasive Technique for Initial Approach to Intubation — vs: — Invasive Technique for Initial Approach to Intubation

   C. Preservation of Spontaneous Ventilation — vs: — Ablation of Spontaneous Ventilation

4. Develop primary and alternative strategies:

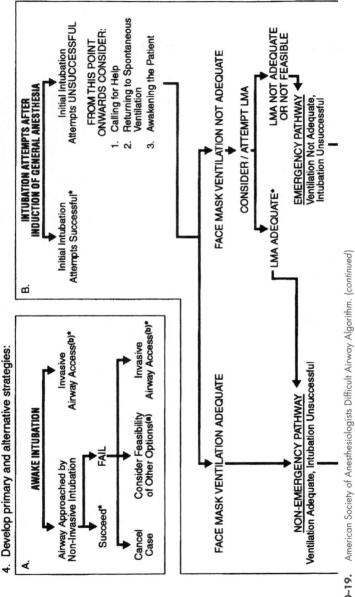

FIGURE 20-19. American Society of Anesthesiologists Difficult Airway Algorithm. (continued)

433

20

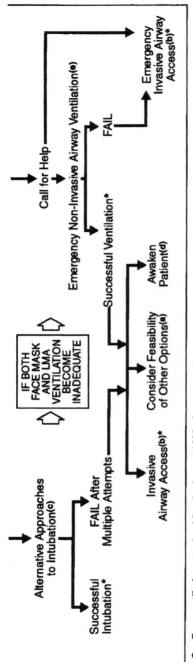

*** Confirm ventilation, tracheal intubation, or LMA placement with exhaled CO₂**

a. Other options include (but are not limited to): surgery utilizing face mask or LMA anesthesia, local anesthesia infiltration or regional nerve blockade. Pursuit of these options usually implies that mask ventilation will not be problematic. Therefore, these options may be of limited value if this step in the algorithm has been reached via the Emergency Pathway.

b. Invasive airway access includes surgical or percutaneous tracheostomy or cricothyrotomy.

c. Alternative non-invasive approaches to difficult intubation include (but are not limited to): use of different laryngoscope blades, LMA as an intubation conduit (with or without fiberoptic guidance), fiberoptic intubation, intubating stylet or tube changer, light wand, retrograde intubation, and blind oral or nasal intubation.

d. Consider re-preparation of the patient for awake intubation or canceling surgery.

e. Options for emergency non-invasive airway ventilation include (but are not limited to): rigid bronchoscope, esophageal-tracheal combitube ventilation, or transtracheal jet ventilation.

FIGURE 20–19. (Continued)

(Text continued from page 431.)

1. Extend the neck (if possible).
2. Make a midline incision with a no. 11 blade.
3. Puncture the cricothyroid membrane with the scalpel and rotate 90 degrees.
4. Keeping a finger in the cricothyroidotomy site, place a 6-0 ETT or cricoid tube into cricothyroidotomy site, and confirm placement.
5. Establish a definitive airway as soon as possible.

Complications: Esophageal intubation; pneumothorax; pneumomediastinum; recurrent laryngeal nerve injury; hemorrhage; tracheal stenosis (can be avoided by keeping cuff pressures < 25 mm Hg); ET tube dislodgement/self-extubation

MECHANICAL VENTILATION MODES (FIGURE 20–20, PAGE 436)

Controlled Mechanical Ventilation (CMV): The patient receives *only* ventilator-delivered breaths at a set rate (ie, patient cannot initiate a breath without the ventilator). This mode once was used in the care of patients who were intentionally paralyzed by drugs because of extreme illness or trauma.

Assist-Control Ventilation (AC): The ventilator delivers a full tidal volume with each inspiratory effort. The respiratory rate can be determined by the patient, although a set rate ensures adequate minute ventilation.

- *Advantages:* The patient can easily increase minute ventilation even with poor inspiratory effort. The result is a marked decrease in the work of breathing.
- *Disadvantages:* Can produce overventilation and respiratory alkalosis in tachypneic patients. Agitation can also result in breath-stacking and auto-PEEP. The reduced work of breathing with this mode comes at the expense of predisposition to diaphragmatic and intercostal muscle atrophy.

Synchronous Intermittent Mandatory Ventilation (SIMV): The ventilator delivers set tidal volume at a minimum set rate (synchronized to patient inspiratory effort) during spontaneous breathing between mandatory tidal volumes. The spontaneous tidal volumes can be augmented with pressure support (PS). As the ventilator rate is decreased, the patient assumes more and more work of breathing. This mode can either provide full support (with a high mandatory rate) or be used as a weaning mode by decreasing the rate over time.

Pressure-Controlled Ventilation: Maximal inspiratory pressure is defined. The delivered tidal volume is then a function of specified pressures and lung compliance. With volume-targeted modes, airway pressure varies with changing lung compliance. This mode requires careful monitoring because minute ventilation can decline with worsening lung compliance. Pressure control is often used in conjunction with inverse-ratio ventilation (ie, longer inspiratory times with shorter expiratory times) as another means of increasing mean airway pressure to improve oxygenation in hypoxic patients.

Pressure Support Ventilation (PSV): Flow-cycled; patient determines tidal volume and cycle length. A preset level of positive pressure boost is turned on during inspiration and is off during expiration. The higher the PS, the less work the patient expends to take a breath. Because the patient is able to control the duration of lung inflation and tidal volume, PSV tends to be comfortable for most patients. PSV is

20

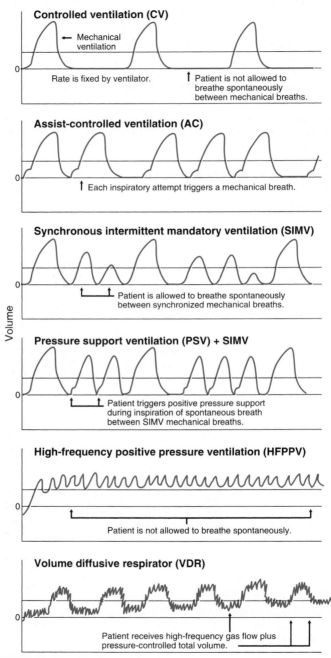

FIGURE 20–20. Ventilator modes.

useful for weaning because the PS can be turned down slowly, with changes as small as 1 cm water. Patient assumes additional work of breathing in small increments.

Pressure-Regulated Volume Control (PRVC):   Used in the setting of increased airway pressures (eg, acute lung injury, ARDS). A microprocessor in the ventilator minimizes the pressure needed to deliver the specified tidal volume by using decelerating flow during inspiration. PRVC can be thought of as dynamic pressure-controlled ventilation without the variation in tidal volumes associated with changing lung compliance.

VENTILATOR MANAGEMENT
Ventilator Orders

The following is a sample of typical initial ventilator settings for an adult:

- Mode (eg, AC, SIMV)
- FIO_2 30–100%
- Rate 10–18 breaths/min
- Tidal volume 4–6 mL/kg
- PS (5–20 cm water)
- PEEP (5 cm water or higher, if needed)

Ventilator Setting Changes

Five basic respiratory parameters (FIO_2, minute ventilation, PS, PEEP, I/E ratio) can be changed to improve ventilation, oxygenation, and compliance.

1. **FIO_2:** Choose an initial FIO_2 that ensures adequate arterial O_2 saturation ($SaO_2 > 90\%$). Increasing the level of PEEP is often a helpful means of decreasing the FIO_2 requirement while maintaining adequate oxygenation. Once adequate oxygenation is established, decrease the FIO_2 to avoid O_2 toxicity (avoid $FIO_2 > 60\%$).

    - O_2 toxicity: Damage to lungs occurs if the intraalveolar O_2 concentration is $> 60\%$ (injury actually occurs after a few hours if $FIO_2 = 1.0$). The mechanism probably involves generation of reactive O_2 species that oxidize the cell membranes. O_2 toxicity has not been documented if FIO_2 is maintained $< 60\%$.

2. **Minute ventilation:** Adjust to maintain PCO_2 within a normal range (35–45 mm Hg). Because minute ventilation is the product of rate and tidal volume, make this adjustment by varying either of these values. Once a tidal volume is chosen, set the respiratory rate (≈ 8–16 breaths/min) for adequate minute ventilation. For a spontaneously breathing patient, PS can be increased to achieve a target minute ventilation.

3. **Pressure support:** After the patient's respiratory pattern is established on SIMV, add PS at an initial level of 5–10 cm water. Increase PS to the level at which the patient can achieve reasonable tidal volume and breathe at a comfortable rate (< 30 breaths/min). Depending on the overall stability and mental status of the patient, turn down the number of SIMV backup breaths so that the patient assumes more control of ventilation. PS *rarely* has to exceed 20 cm water.

4. **PEEP:** With the addition of PEEP, the ventilator maintains positive airway pressure at the end of expiration even though net airflow is zero.

PEEP increases alveolar ventilation by preventing small-airway collapse, thereby improving lung compliance and FRC. Increasing levels of PEEP are typically used in the care of hypoxemic patients who need $FIO_2 > 50\%$. With PEEP, FIO_2 can be reduced and O_2 toxicity limited. PEEP $\approx$ 5 cm water is considered physiologic. If oxygenation remains marginal, PEEP is added in 2- to 3-cm increments until oxygenation is improved. In acute lung injury, the PEEP at which lung compliance is optimized can be determined by observation of pressure-volume loops.

High-Dose PEEP: The elevated intrathoracic pressure associated with high PEEP can compromise venous return and thus decrease stroke volume and CO, particularly in hypovolemic patients. The result is decreased oxygen delivery. Consider placement of a PA catheter. Because ICP can become elevated, titrate PEEP upward with caution in patients with intracranial hypertension.

5. **Inspiratory to expiratory (I/E) ratio:** The normal I/E ratio is 1/2 or 1/3. Inverse-ratio ventilation (eg, 2/1) results in progressive recruitment of alveoli and elevation of mean airway pressure, which improves oxygenation. This beneficial effect on oxygenation is lost if "breath stacking" or auto-PEEP occurs. *Note:* This technique may be inappropriate in the care of patients with obstructive lung disease, in which longer expiratory times are required. Inverse-ratio ventilation is poorly tolerated by awake patients and typically requires heavy sedation. Shorter expiratory times can result in hypercapnia; this "permissive hypercapnia" is sometimes accepted to improve oxygenation. Balance FIO_2 and peak pressure to keep peak pressure < 35 cm water. If unable to do so, move to pressure support ventilation.

Ventilator Weaning

Before weaning the patient from the ventilator, assess pulmonary mechanics and oxygenation (Table 20–7, page 439).

Pulmonary Mechanics: Information about the patient's ability to perform the work of respiration. Routine pulmonary mechanics consist of:

- Vital capacity
- Tidal volume
- Spontaneous respiratory rate
- Lung compliance

Inspiratory Force: The maximum negative pressure that can be exerted against a completely closed airway (a function of respiratory muscle strength). An inspiratory force between 0 and –25 cm water suggests that the patient may be incapable of generating adequate inspiratory effort for successful extubation.

Weaning Modes: Ventilators are designed to facilitate weaning. Once the preceding criteria have been met, select a ventilator mode appropriate to the clinical situation. SIMV and PSV are considered weaning modes because the patient assumes more of the workload of breathing as mechanical support is reduced.

Order of Weaning: Take the following steps to wean the patient from the ventilator:

1. Reduce FIO_2 to 40% while monitoring SpO_2.
2. Sequentially reduce the IMV rate to a level of 4–8 breaths/min. Add PS to maintain adequate minute ventilation. Closely monitor minute ventilation (on ventilator display).
3. Sequentially reduce PEEP in increments of 2- to 3-cm water while maintaining $SpO_2 > 90\%$ until a level of 5 cm water is achieved.

20

TABLE 20–7
Criteria for Extubation from Mechanical Ventilation

Parameter	Value
Pulmonary mechanics	
Vital capacity	> 10–15 mL/kg
Resting minute ventilation (tidal volume × rate)	> 10 L/min
Spontaneous respiratory rate	< 33 breaths/min
Lung compliance	> 100 mL/cm water
Negative Inspiratory force (NIF)	> –25 cm water
Oxygenation	
A–a gradient	< 300–500 mm Hg
Shunt fraction	< 15%
PO_2 (on 40% FIO_2)	> 70 mm Hg
PCO_2	< 45 mm Hg

4. Sequentially reduce PS by increments of 2–3 cm water while maintaining minute ventilation (goal: 5–10 cm water); monitor respiratory rate, work of breathing, and minute ventilation.

Checklist for Extubation
- Correction of primary problem that prompted intubation and mechanical ventilation (eg, successfully treated pneumonia, returned hemodynamic stability)
- Level of consciousness stable or improved
- Stable vital signs
- Pulmonary mechanics and oxygenation meet acceptable criteria (see Table 20–7, above)

Extubation Trials: Once weaning has been achieved, attempt trials with minimal mechanical support while the patient is still intubated. CPAP trials (with 5 cm water positive pressure) is the most commonly used method. A CPAP trial with an FIO_2 of 40% should result in a PaO_2 of > 70 mm Hg, and a respiratory rate < 25 breaths/min. One of the best predictors of successful extubation is the ratio of respiratory rate to tidal volume (f/Vt, or Tobin index). Extubation frequently is unsuccessful in patients with a rapid–shallow breathing pattern. A ratio > 100 has been shown in some studies to be predictive of extubation failure (*N Engl J Med* 1991;324:1445–1450). These trials may vary in duration from 30 min to several hours and are used primarily as the last test before extubation.

Extubation: A patient who is able to maintain a PO_2 > 70 mm Hg, a PCO_2 < 45 mm Hg, and a respiratory rate < 25 breaths/min for 1–2 h on a CPAP trial is ready for extubation.

1. Disconnect the ET tube from the ventilator or T-piece.
2. Suction the ET tube and oropharynx.
3. Have the patient take a deep breath.
4. As the patient expires forcefully, deflate the cuff and remove the tube.
5. Suction any secretions and administer O_2 through a nasal cannula at 2–4 L/min.
6. Check postextubation ABG if adequate ventilation and oxygenation are in doubt.

20

NUTRITION IN THE ICU

The nutritional support of critically ill patients is crucial to their survival. Restoring an anabolic state hastens recovery and avoids complications. Protocols for nutritional support are covered in Chapters 11 and 12. Remember the following two rules:

1. The "2-day" rule applies to most patients. If you believe the critically ill patient will not be able to take nutrition for 2 days because of conditions such as postoperative ileus and intubation, make arrangements for nutritional support.
2. "If the gut works, use it." Use enteral nutrition (oral, NG tube, jejunostomy tube) in all patients with a functioning intestinal tract (see Chapter 11).

COMPLICATIONS IN CRITICAL CARE

Acute Respiratory Distress Syndrome (ARDS)

ARDS is acute pulmonary injury manifested by marked respiratory distress and hypoxia. Pulmonary capillaries become more permeable, resulting in noncardiogenic pulmonary edema. ARDS has been defined by the American–European Consensus Conference as:

- Acute onset
- P/F ratio (PaO_2/FIO_2) $\leq$ 200 regardless of PEEP level
- Bilateral infiltrates on CXR
- PAOP < 18 if measured, or no clinical evidence of left atrial hypertension

Acute lung injury is similarly defined; it differs only in the degree of hypoxemia (P/F ratio $\leq$ 300).

Causes: The causes of ARDS are multifactorial and include but are not limited to:

- Trauma
- Sepsis
- Aspiration
- Pneumonia
- Severe pancreatitis
- Severe burns
- Transfusion-related acute lung injury
- Chemical pneumonitis or inhalational injury

Treatment: Management of ARDS is generally supportive. Focus efforts on preventing secondary insults and avoiding ventilator-associated lung injury. The ARDS Network low tidal volume approach entails use of a tidal volume of 6 mL/kg of predicted body weight with respiratory rate adjusted to achieve adequate minute ventilation. The goal is to achieve plateau pressures of $\leq$ 30 cm water. The PEEP ladder in Table 20–8 guides PEEP settings according to FIO_2.

20

Upper Gastrointestinal Hemorrhage

Critically ill patients are at increased risk of GI hemorrhage secondary to stress-induced mucosal ulceration. Head injury (**Cushing ulcers**); mechanical ventilation; NSAID use; shock, trauma, and burns (**Curling ulcers**); coagulopathy; and a history of peptic ulcer disease or portal hypertension are a few of the risk factors.

TABLE 20–8
PEEP Ladder

FiO$_2$	0.30	0.40	0.50	0.60	0.70	0.80	0.90	1.0
PEEP	5	5–8	8–10	10	10–14	14	14–18	18–22

Based on data in: The Acute Respiratory Distress Syndrome Network. *N Engl J Med* 2000;342:1301–1308.

Prophylaxis
- **Enteral feedings:** method of choice to protect the gastric mucosa
- Cardiovascular support of visceral perfusion
- Acid suppression: prophylaxis with H$_2$-blockers (eg, ranitidine, famotidine). Proton-pump inhibitors (eg, lansoprazole, omeprazole) for refractory bleeding or in patients with adverse reaction to histamine blockade.

Management of Ulceration

1. Early endoscopy for upper GI bleeding
2. Endoscopic or surgical intervention for visible bleeding vessel
3. Aggressive acid suppression for diffuse gastritis; empiric therapy for *Helicobacter pylori* infection
4. Possible surgical intervention for persistent bleeding from gastritis

Shock

Shock can be defined simply as tissue hypoperfusion. Uncorrected shock leads to cellular dysfunction, organ failure, and death. Direct the management of shock at *correcting the underlying problem.* Endogenous compensatory mechanisms directed at reversing hypotension and shock include the release of catecholamines, cortisol, and activation of the renin–angiotensin–aldosterone axis.

The morbidity and mortality of shock are related to the cause but probably more to the *degree and time of circulatory compromise.* When the causes are identified and corrected, the patient is resuscitated to restore tissue perfusion and reverse the effects of shock.

Hypovolemic Shock: Inadequate circulating blood volume (at least 20% loss) is caused by dehydration or acute hemorrhage. Hemodynamic parameters show decreased CVP, PAOP, and EDVI with a consequent decrease in CO and increase in SVR. Table 20–9 lists the current classification and physiologic changes associated with hypovolemic shock.

Treatment

1. Control the source of intravascular volume loss.
2. Rapidly replace intravascular volume with isotonic crystalloid, colloid, or blood products as appropriate.

Cardiogenic Shock: Cardiogenic shock is caused by pump failure either from intrinsic cardiac abnormalities (eg, severe valvular disease, AMI, coronary ischemia, arrhythmias) or extrinsic processes (eg, tension pneumothorax, pericardial tamponade, PE).

Treatment: Directed at improving cardiac performance

1. Resolve extrinsic processes if present.

20

TABLE 20–9
Physiologic Changes Associated with Degree of Hemorrhagic Shock

	Class I	Class II	Class III	Class IV
Blood loss (%)	< 15	15–30	30–40	> 40
Blood loss (mL)[a]	< 750	750–1500	1500–2000	> 2000
Mental status	—	Anxiety	Confusion	Lethargy
Heart rate	—	Mild ↑	Moderate ↑↑	Severe ↑↑↑
Blood pressure				
Systolic	—	—	↓	↓↓
Diastolic	—	↑	↓	↓↓
Respiratory rate(breaths/min)	—	Mild ↑	Moderate ↑↑	Severe ↑↑↑
Urine output	—	Mild ↓	Oliguria	Anuria

[a]Based on 70 kg adult.
— = No significant change; ↑ = increased; ↓ = decreased.

2. Optimize preload for CO.
3. Decrease afterload (ACE inhibitors, nitrates, etc).
4. Improve cardiac contractility with inotropic support.
5. Consider mechanical support (intraaortic balloon pump).
6. Consider aspirin and heparin therapy.

Septic Shock: Septic shock is a clinical syndrome associated with severe infection and is characterized by a systemic inflammatory response with resultant tissue injury. The following definitions have been established by a consensus conference convened by the American College of Chest Physicians and the Society of Critical Care Medicine (*Crit Care Med* 2003;31, no. 4).

Systemic inflammatory response syndrome (two or more of the following):

- Temperature > 38°C or < 36°C
- Heart rate > 90 beats/min
- Respiratory rate > 20 breaths/min or P_{CO_2} < 32 mmHg
- WBC > 12,000/μL or < 4000/μL

Sepsis: Infection with a systemic inflammatory response
Severe sepsis: Sepsis with organ dysfunction
Septic Shock: Acute circulatory failure with persistent unexplained hypotension

Surviving Sepsis Campaign Guidelines: Evidence-based recommendations for the management of sepsis and septic shock published in 2004 (*Crit Care Med* 2004;32, no. 3) call for early goal-directed therapy.

    Initial Resuscitation: Begin as soon as the syndrome is recognized. Do not wait for ICU admission. Goals for the first 6 h of resuscitation include:

- CVP 8–12 mm Hg
- MAP ≥ 65 mm Hg
- Urine output ≥ 0.5 mL/kg/h

20

- Central venous or $S\bar{v}o_2 \geq 70\%$
- If the $S\bar{v}o_2$ goal is not achieved with fluid resuscitation to the target CVP within the first 6 h, add transfusion of PRBC to a hematocrit of $\geq 30\%$, infusion of dobutamine, or both.

Diagnosis: Obtain cultures before initiating antibiotic therapy. Draw blood cultures peripherally, and from each vascular access device. Obtain appropriate imaging studies to evaluate for possible sources when possible. Remember: transport of a critically ill patient can be dangerous.

Antibiotic Therapy: Obtain cultures and initiate IV antibiotics within the first hour after recognizing severe sepsis. Consider broad-spectrum antibiotics on the basis of susceptibility patterns at the hospital. Alter antibiotics as dictated by culture results, or discontinue them if a noninfectious cause of cardiovascular collapse is identified.

Source Control: Evaluate for possible source control measures (eg, abscess drainage, debridement, removal of infected devices). Expedite source control after initial resuscitation.

Fluid Therapy: No evidence-based support exists to guide choice of resuscitation fluid (natural or artificial colloid vs isotonic crystalloid). Give fluid challenges as a bolus with careful monitoring so that hemodynamic response can be observed. Large volumes may be needed during the first 24 h of management.

Vasopressors: If fluid resuscitation does not restore adequate blood pressure and perfusion, initiate vasopressor support with dopamine or norepinephrine via a central venous catheter. Do not use "renal dose" dopamine as a protective strategy because it has no demonstrated outcome benefit. Direct measure of arterial blood pressure with arterial catheters is preferred over cuff measurements in the setting of shock. Add low-dose vasopressin (0.01–0.04 units/min) if shock is refractory to fluid resuscitation and usual vasopressor support.

Inotropic Therapy: If CO stays low despite fluid resuscitation, add dobutamine with the goal of achieving adequate O_2 delivery to peripheral tissues. If hypotension is present, use dobutamine in conjunction with vasopressors (ie, norepinephrine).

Steroids: Hydrocortisone is recommended for patients with septic shock necessitating vasopressor support (200–300 mg/d in divided doses or by continuous infusion). Higher doses are not effective and are potentially harmful. Relative adrenal insufficiency has been defined as a post-ACTH (250 mcg stimulation test) cortisol increase < 9 mcg/dL at 30–60 min. Some clinicians would discontinue steroid therapy in patients who respond appropriately to the stimulation test.

Recombinant Human Activated Protein C: Consider rhAPC (Xigris) for patients at high risk of death (APACHE II score ≥ 25, multiple organ system dysfunction, septic shock, sepsis-induced ARDS). Carefully review contraindications before starting this therapy.

Blood Product Administration: After resolution of the shock state (and in the absence of ongoing hemorrhage, coronary artery disease, etc), decrease the transfusion threshold to 7 g/dL for most patients with a target hemoglobin of 7–9 g/dL. Erythropoietin is not recommended for management of anemia associated with sepsis in the absence of other indications (eg, renal failure). FFP is not recommended for the correction of abnormal clotting times unless bleeding is present or an invasive procedure anticipated. Administration of antithrombin is not recommended. Transfuse platelets when the platelet count decreases to < 5000/μL, and consider transfusion for platelet counts of 5000–30,000/μL if there is high risk of hemorrhage.

20

Mechanical Ventilation of Sepsis-Induced Acute Lung Injury: The Surviving Sepsis Guidelines support the low tidal volume (6 mL/kg) strategy (ie, ARDS-Net) with goal plateau pressures < 30 cm water. Permissive hypercapnia is allowed if needed; PEEP is adjusted on the basis of FIO_2 requirement or is titrated to achieve optimal compliance. Consider prone positioning of patients who need high FIO_2. Elevate the head of bed to 45 degrees to reduce pneumonia risk.

Sedation, Analgesia, and Neuromuscular Blockade in Sepsis: Sedation protocols (with scales such as the RASS) and daily interruption of sedation have been shown to decrease duration of mechanical ventilation and hospital length of stay. Avoid neuromuscular blockade unless absolutely necessary.

Glucose Control: Recommended upper limit for glucose control is 150 mg/dL. (The range used in the landmark study [*N Engl J Med* 2001;345:1359–1367] of intensive insulin therapy in critically ill patients was 80–110 mg/dL). Extending the upper range of glucose control reduces hypoglycemic episodes. Tight glucose control is achieved through infusion of insulin. Assure a glucose source (eg, D_5 or D_{10} infusion). Enteral feeding is the preferred source of glucose.

Renal Replacement: If the patient is in hemodynamically stable condition, continuous venovenous hemofiltration (CVVH) and intermittent hemodialysis are equivalent therapies. CVVH is more appropriate for hemodynamically unstable patients.

Bicarbonate Therapy: Bicarbonate therapy is not recommended for the management of sepsis-related lactic acidemia for pH ≥ 7.15.

Deep Vein Thrombosis Prophylaxis: Administer DVT prophylaxis in the form of subcutaneous heparin or low-molecular-weight heparin. If contraindications are present, consider mechanical prophylaxis sequential compression devices).

Stress Ulcer Prophylaxis: H_2-receptor inhibitors are preferred.

Consideration for Limitation of Support: Communication between caregivers and families is vital, particularly with respect to end of life care and patient wishes.

Pediatric Considerations: In general, the aforementioned guidelines apply to adult patients. Refer to the Surviving Sepsis Campaign guidelines for special issues related to the care of pediatric patients (*Crit Care Med* 2004;32[11 suppl]).

Neurogenic Shock: Caused by loss of sympathetic vascular tone (eg, high thoracic or cervical spinal cord injury) producing an increase in vascular capacitance.

Treatment:

1. Optimize filling pressures by IV fluid administration.
2. Provide vasopressor support as necessary.
3. Keep fluids and room temperature warm because these patients lose the ability to thermoregulate.

Acute Renal Failure (ARF)

Sudden development of renal insufficiency resulting in retention of nitrogenous wastes (BUN, creatinine), variable effects on fluid balance, oliguria and anuria, and progressive azotemia. ARF is usually divided into prerenal, renal, and postrenal causes (see Chapter 6). Once ARF is recognized, the primary objective is to *correct the underlying cause.* The most common causes of renal failure in the ICU are acute tubular necrosis (ATN) and prerenal disease. Among the many causes of ATN are nephrotoxic medications, ischemia, and hypotension. Prerenal causes include intravascular volume depletion and CHF. Indications for hemodialysis include:

20

* Refractory fluid overload
* Severe metabolic acidosis
* Hyperkalemia
* Severe uremia
* Toxic accumulation of drugs

Contrast Nephropathy: Iatrogenic cause of ARF. If use of contrast agents is unavoidable in high-risk patients (eg, diabetic patients with chronic renal insufficiency) the following strategies may reduce the risk:

* Avoiding volume depletion and NSAIDs
* Acetylcysteine (600 mg PO bid the day before and the day of contrast administration) and prehydration (*N Engl J Med* 2000;343:180–184)
* Bicarbonate infusion (154 mEq/L at 3 mL/kg/h for 1 h) before exposure, then 1 mL/kg/h during exposure and for 6 h after exposure (*JAMA* 2004; 291:2328–2334)

Abdominal Compartment Syndrome

Consequence of intraabdominal hypertension resulting in symptomatic organ dysfunction. Caused by resuscitation-related bowel edema and fluid sequestration or retroperitoneal hemorrhage causing a mass effect. Increased intraabdominal pressure directly decreases visceral perfusion and results in organ dysfunction and respiratory compromise.

Diagnosis: Consider the diagnosis in the setting of worsening lung compliance, abdominal distention, and oliguria. Hypotension is a late finding. Measurement of bladder pressure confirms the diagnosis. Although the clinical scenarios can be highly variable, organ dysfunction may be present with pressures as low as 10 mm Hg. Consider abdominal decompression when abdominal pressure exceeds 20–25 mm Hg.

Treatment: *Early* decompressive celiotomy. Close the abdominal fascia when edema and organ dysfunction resolve.

Acalculous Cholecystitis

Cholecystitis in the absence of gallstones is common among ICU patients. Although the precise cause is not known, it is probably related to diminished blood flow to the gallbladder and to bacterial overgrowth.

Diagnosis: Signs are similar to those in noncritical patients with cholecystitis and include right upper quadrant pain, fever, and leukocytosis. Perform right upper quadrant ultrasonography. Add a HIDA scan if the sonographic findings are nondiagnostic (nonvisualization of the gallbladder is highly suggestive of acalculous cholecystitis).

Treatment: Treatment is open surgical removal of the gallbladder (cholecystectomy). Percutaneous cholecystostomy is an alternative in the care of critically ill patients who may not tolerate operative intervention. Interval cholecystectomy is performed when the patient's condition improves.

20

Acute Adrenal Insufficiency

Adrenal crisis may be precipitated in patients with primary adrenal insufficiency in the setting of severe infection or surgical stress. It may also arise as a consequence of bilateral adrenal infarction or hemorrhage. Clinical manifestations include cardiovascular collapse, hyponatremia, hyperkalemia, fever, abdominal pain, and nonspecific findings such as malaise, anorexia, nausea, and decreased mental status. Initial treatment is directed at correcting hypotension and electrolyte abnormalities, as well as cortisol replacement. Initiate resuscitation with normal saline solution; large volumes may be required. Administer IV dexamethasone (4 mg) or hydrocortisone (100 mg) first. Dexamethasone may be preferable initially because it is longer acting than hydrocortisone and does not interfere with ACTH stimulation tests. Determine the factor that precipitated the adrenal crisis (eg, infection) and correct it promptly. Once the crisis resolves, administer oral glucocorticoids and taper them over several days. Consider adding mineralocorticoid (eg, fludrocortisone) replacement.

Infection

Ventilator-Associated Pneumonia: Clinical pneumonia that develops after 48 h of mechanical ventilation. Occurs in approximately 25% of intubated ICU patients; overall mortality, 20–50%. The strongest risk factor for ICU pneumonia is mechanical ventilation (6- to 15-fold increase); others are age > 70 y, chronic lung disease, nasoenteric tubes, altered mental status, chest trauma or surgery, and frequent transportation of the patient.

Diagnosis: A positive airway culture (preferably of a bronchoalveolar lavage (BAL) specimen with quantitative cultures showing > 10^4 CFU/mL) plus three of the four following:

- New, persistent, or progressive CXR infiltrate
- Purulent tracheobronchial secretions
- Fever
- Leukocytosis

Treatment: Empiric therapy customized according to the institution's antibiogram for the particular ICU and adjusted when C&S data are available. Continue therapy for 8–12 d. Repeat BAL with cultures and special stains as needed if standard antibiotic therapy fails.

Line Sepsis: Indwelling catheters are essential, but they also act as a portal of entry for bacteria. Consider catheter-related sepsis if a fever develops in an ICU patient. The most common mechanism is entry of skin flora along the catheter track. Because prolonged use of polyurethane dressings increases the risk of infection, avoid these dressings. Some ICUs have a policy of routine line changes over a guidewire every 3–4 d. This policy, however, is not supported by evidence in the literature, and the infection rate may increase with this approach. Prevent line sepsis with meticulous aseptic technique during line placement (including full gowning, gloving, and draping) and meticulous care of the line once it is in place.

Diagnosis: If the site does not appear infected, the catheter may be exchanged over a guidewire and the intracutaneous segment and tip sent for culture. A new IV site is chosen if the catheter culture result is positive. Erythema is suggestive of catheter site infection; however, coagulase-negative staphylococci can elicit minimal inflammation.

Treatment: Remove short-term central venous catheters suspected of being infected and culture them. Start empiric antimicrobial therapy pending culture results. A catheter colony count > 15 CFU suggests catheter infection.

20

Deep Venous Thrombosis (DVT) and Pulmonary Embolism (PE)

PE causes $\approx$ 150,000 deaths annually in the United States. DVT causes most cases of PE in hospitalized patients. About 90% of cases of PE originate in the femoral–iliac–pelvic veins. DVT is promoted by the presence of the Virchow triad: endothelial injury, hypercoagulability, and blood stasis.

Prevention of DVT: Risk factors include malignant disease, obesity, history of DVT, age > 40 y, extensive abdominal or pelvic surgery, long bone or pelvic fractures, and prolonged immobilization. For surgical patients, initiate prophylaxis in the OR *before induction of anesthesia.* Use of sequential compression devices and selected heparinoids has reduced the incidence of DVT.

Physical Methods: Leg elevation, sequential compression devices, and *early postoperative ambulation* (**most important**).

Pharmacologic Methods

- **Heparin** 5000 units SQ q8h. Monitor platelet count (~= q3d) for heparin-induced thrombocytopenia.
- **Coumadin** for chronic therapy
- **Low-molecular-weight heparin** (LMWH) (eg, Enoxaparin) is the drug of choice for high-risk patients.

Diagnosis of PE

- **Signs and symptoms:** None is diagnostic; dyspnea, tachypnea, tachycardia, chest pain (usually pleuritic), and hypoxia.
- **CXRs** are not sensitive enough to be useful in the diagnosis of PE but help may rule out other causes of the symptoms (eg, pneumonia, pneumothorax).
- **Spiral CT:** The clinical validity of CT in ruling out PE equals that of pulmonary angiography (*JAMA* 2005;293:2012–2017).

Treatment

1. **Support oxygenation.** Monitor SpO_2 Intubation may be needed.
2. **Anticoagulate** with unfractionated or LMWH to prevent clot propagation, decrease inflammation, and allow intrinsic fibrinolysis to lyse the clot.
   a. Evidence-based guidelines suggest body weight–adjusted subcutaneous LMWH is the preferred initial therapy for acute nonmassive PE (*Chest* 2004;126:401s–428s). If unfractionated heparin is chosen (eg, patient with severe renal failure), administer bolus with 80 units/kg IV and start an infusion at 18 units/kg/h. Titrate the infusion to maintain the PTT at 2–2.5 × control value. Check the PTT 6 h after rate adjustments.
   b. Monitor the platelet count for heparin-induced thrombocytopenia.
   c. Start oral warfarin (Coumadin) by day 3 of heparin therapy to achieve and maintain an INR of 2–3 (see Chapter 22).
3. In massive PE, administer thrombolytic therapy (TPA) if not contraindicated.
4. Consider pulmonary embolectomy for hemodynamically unstable patients with massive PE if medical therapy is not successful.
5. If anticoagulation is contraindicated (eg, recent surgery, stroke, GI bleeding) or if PE recur despite anticoagulation, consider placement of a vena caval filter placement.

(*Text continues on page 454.*)

20

TABLE 20-10
Quick Reference to Common ICU Equations

Determination	Derivation	Normal
RAP-CVP	Measured	2-10 mm Hg
RSVP/RVDP	Measured	15-30/0-5 mm Hg
PAS/PAD	Measured	15-30/8-15 mm Hg
MPAP	$PAD + \dfrac{[PAS - PAD]}{3}$	11-18 mm Hg
PAOP (ie, PCWP)	Measured	5-16 mm Hg
MAP	$DBP \times \dfrac{(SBP - DBP)}{3}$	85-90 mm Hg
CO	$SV \times HR$ $\dfrac{Vo_2 \times 10}{[1.39[Hgb]] \times (Sao_2 - S\bar{v}o_2)}$	3.5-5.5 L/min
CI	CO/BSA	2.5-4.2 L/min/m²
SVR	$\dfrac{(MAP - CVP)}{CO} \times 80$	770-1500 dynes × s/cm⁵
SVRI	SVR/BSA	
PVR	$\dfrac{(MPAP - PAOP)}{CO} \times 80$	20-120 dynes × s/cm5
PVRI	PVR/BSA	
Alveolar O₂ estimate (PAO₂)	$FiO_2 \times (P_{atmospheric} - PH_2O) - \dfrac{(PaCO_2)}{0.8}$	

(continued)

20

TABLE 20–10
(Continued)

Determination	Derivation	Normal
A–a Gradient	$PaO_2 - PaO_2$	room air = 12–22 mm Hg 100% FiO_2 = 10–60 mm Hg
CcO_2 (pulmonary capillary O_2 content)	$(1.39[Hgb] \times ScO_2) + (PcO_2 \times 0.0031)$	18–24 mL O_2/dl blood
CaO_2 (arterial O_2 content)	$(1.39[Hgb] \times SaO_2) + (PaO_2 \times 0.0031)$	16–22 mL O_2/dl blood
$C\bar{v}O_2$ (mixed venous O_2 content)	$(1.39[Hgb] \times S\bar{v}O_2) + (P\bar{v}O_2 \times 0.0031)$	12–17 mL O_2/dl blood
$C(a-v)$ O_2 (A–v O_2 difference)	$(1.39[Hgb] \times (SaO_2 - S\bar{v}O_2)$	3.5–5.5 mL O_2/dl blood
O_2 carrying capacity (CcO_2)	$[Hgb] \times SaO_2 \times CO \times 10$	700–1400 mL/min delivery
O_2 consumption (VO_2)	$(CaO_2 - C\bar{v}O_2) \times CO \times 10$	180–280 mL/min
Qs/Qt (shunt fraction)	$(CcO_2 - C\bar{v}O_2)/(CcO_2 - C\bar{v}O_2)$	0.05
ICP	Measured	0–20 mm Hg
CPP	MAP – ICP	Ideally > 70 mm Hg

BSA = body surface area (m²) = height (cm)$^{0.427}$ × Weight (kg)$^{0.718}$ × 74.5; RAP = right atrial pressures; CVP = central venous pressure; RVSP = right ventricular systolic pressure; RVDP = right ventricular diastolic pressure; PAS = pulmonary artery systolic pressure; PAD = pulmonary artery diastolic pressure; MPAP = mean pulmonary artery pressure; PAOP = pulmonary artery occlusion pressure; PCWP = pulmonary capillary wedge pressure; MAP = mean arterial pressure; DBP = diastolic blood pressure; SBP = systolic blood pressure; CO = cardiac output; SV = stroke volume; HR = heart rate; VO_2 = oxygen consumption; Hgb = hemoglobin concentration; SaO_2 = arterial oxygen saturation; $S\bar{v}O_2$ = mixed venous oxygen saturation; CI = cardiac index; SVR = systemic vascular resistance; SVRI = systemic vascular resistance index; PVR = pulmonary vascular resistance; PVRI = pulmonary vascular resistance index; FiO_2 = inhaled O_2 concentration; $P_{atmospheric}$ = atmospheric pressure ~ 760 torr; PH_2O = water vapor pressure ~ 47 torr $PaCO_2$ = partial pressure of CO_2 in arterial blood; PaO_2 = partial pressure of O_2 in alveolus; Qs = volume of shunted blood (ie, blood shunted past nonventilated alveoli not participating in gas exchange); Qt = total cardiac output; ICP = intracranial pressure; CPP = cerebral perfusion pressure.

TABLE 20–11
Guidelines for Adult Critical Care Drug Infusions

Drug	Use/Mechanism	Dose Range	Side Effects/Cautions
Amrinone (Inocor)	Inotrope and vasodilator (systemic, pulmonary coronary); used in CHF-resistant to diuretics and afterload reduction	Load: 0.75 mg/kg over 3 min Dose: 5–20 mcg/kg/min (max 10 mg/kg/d)	Adverse effects to catecholamines and digoxin; hypotension (dose-dependent); thrombocytopenia (1–2%); increase AV and ventricular conduction; nausea/vomiting/abdominal pain
Diltiazem (Cardizem)	Slow calcium channel blocker; negative inotrope; prolongs AV node refractory time; vasodilates to lower BP without reflex tachycardia	Bolus=0.25 mg/kg over 2 min (may give second bolus 0.35 mg/kg 15 min after initial dose) Dose 5–15 mg/hr	Hypotension: AV block; drug-induced hepatitis; flushing *Contraindications:* Wide-complex tachycardia; Wolffe–Parkinson–White syndrome; existing 2nd or 3rd degree AV block; concurrent β-blockade
Dobutamine (Dobutrex)	Racemic mixture (L-isomer: α-agonist/D-isomer; β-agonist); positive inotrope/afterload reduction for circulatory failure after AMI, CHF, etc	Dose: 2–20 mcg/kg/min Max: 40 mcg/kg/min	May exacerbate ventricular arrhythmias *Contraindications:* hypertrophic cardiomyopathy
Dopamine (Inotropin)	Dopaminergic (0.5–2.0 mcg/kg/min): renal, cerebral, mesenteric vasodilation α-/β-agonist (2.0–10 g/kg/min): positive inotrope and vasopressor	α-agonist (10–20 mcg/kg/min); predominantly vasopressor Max: 40 mcg/kg/min	Enhances AV conduction, especially with atrial fibrillation; may exacerbate psychosis and arrhythmias *Caution:* Urgently treat extravasated drug with phentolamine to prevent skin necrosis

20

TABLE 20–11
(Continued)

Drug	Use/Mechanism	Dose Range	Side Effects/Cautions
Epinephrine (Adrenalin)	Nonspecific adrenergic agonist ($\beta > \alpha$); potent bronchodilator (β_2, agonist)	Shock: 2 mcg/min, then titrate Cardiac arrest: 1 mg IV q3–5 min	Increases myocardial oxygen consumption; pro-tachyarrhythmia; splanchnic vasoconstrictor (if dose < 4 mcg/min); diabetogenic; promotes hypokalemia
Esmolol (Brevibloc)	β_1-selective; very short half-life (9 min); slows AV node conduction; useful to test β-blockade in patients with potential contraindications	Load: 500 mcg/kg over 1 min Dose: 50 mcg/kg min; titrate by 50 mcg/kg min to target HR (may need to repeat load)	Bronchospasm; pallor; nausea; flushing; bradycar-dia; pulmonary edema (if heart failure occurs); asystole
Isoproterenol (Isuprel)	Nonspecific β-agonist; potent inotrope/chrono-trope for bradycardic states	Initially: 1–4 mcg/min Titrate up to 20 mcg/min based on target HR	Hypotension; tachycardia; myocardial ischemia *Contraindications:* Angina/myocardial ischemia; tachycardia; digitalis-induced bradycardia
Milrinone (Primacor)	Inotrope and vasodilator (systemic, pulmonary, coronary); used in CHF	Load: 50 mcg/kg over 10 min Dose: 0.37–75 mcg/kg/min	Renal elimination; hypotension; tachycardia; aggravates atrial, ventricular arrhythmias; head-ache

(continued)

20

451

TABLE 20–11
(Continued)

Drug	Use/Mechanism	Dose Range	Side Effects/Cautions
Nicardipine (Cardene)	Calcium channel blocker; vasodilator >> negative inotrope; short halflife and rapid hepatic elimination	Dose 5 mg/h; titrate to BP goal (increase rate by 2.5 mg/h q5–15min) Max: 15 mg/h	Delayed clearance with hepatic and renal insufficiency; may worsen portal hypertension; may cause reflex tachycardia *Contraindications:* Critical aortic stenosis; will alter cyclosporine levels
Nitroglycerin (Tridil)	Arterial/venous vasodilator (dose-dependent); coronary vasodilator; combined with dobutamine with acute coronary syndrome	Dose: 5–10 mcg/min; titrate by 10–20 mcg/min q5 min based on current dose and patient condition; hypotension at 200 mg/min	Headache, nausea, vomiting, dizziness *Contraindications:* Increased ICP; narrow-angle glaucoma; pericardial tamponade
Nitroprusside (Nipride)	Arterial/venous vasodilator; donates nitric oxide to interact with vascular smooth muscle >> visceral smooth muscle	Dose: 0.5–10 mcg/kg/min; titrate to goal BP every few min Max: 10 mcg/kg/min	Reacts with Hgb to form met-Hgb → cyanide accumulation; detoxified to thiocyanate by liver and kidney; keep met-Hgb < 10%; may shunt blood away from renal/splanchnic beds

(continued)

TABLE 20–11
(Continued)

Drug	Use/Mechanism	Dose Range	Side Effects/Cautions
Norepinephrine (Levophed)	Potent β_1/α-agonist (low- dose: $\beta > \alpha$) (high-dose: $\alpha > \beta$); use for cardiogenic/septic/neurogenic shock after volume repletion	Initial: 2 mcg/min Dose: 2–20 mg/min; titrate to response Max: 40 mg/min	Peripheral A-lines may be dampened by vasoconstriction; suspect volume depletion with hypotension; treat extravasation with phentolamine May decrease splanchnic blood flow; spares cerebral, coronary blood flow
Phenylephrine (Neo-Synephrine)	Postsynaptic α-agonist; use for hypotension shock, spinal anesthesia, or drug-induced hypotension	Bolus: 0.1–0.5 mcg IV q15min Initial: 100 mcg/min; titrate to 40–200 mcg/min	May cause reflex brachycardia (blocked by atropine); constricts coronary, cerebral, and pulmonary vessels *Contraindications:* Use reduced doses in patients taking MAO inhibitors
Vasopressin (Pitressin)	Potent vasoconstrictor; anti-diuretic; procoagulant; used for variceal hemorrhage to reduce portal pressures; emerging indications in septic shock	Dose: 0.04–0.1 units/min	Myocardial ischemia due to coronary vasoconstriction; may need to combine with nitroglycerin; hepatic/renal metabolism with renal excretion SIADH/water intoxication; abdominal cramps

ªNote: These agents must be administered in the appropriately monitored clinical setting.
CHF = congestive heart failure; AV = atrioventricular; BP = blood pressure; AMI = acute myocardial infarction; HR = heart rate; Hgb = hemoglobin; MAO = monoamine oxidase; SIADH = syndrome of inappropriate antidiuretic hormone.

20

(Text continued from page 447.)

QUICK REFERENCE FOR CRITICAL CARE FORMULAS

Table 20–10, page 448, provides a summary of commonly used formulas in the critical care setting.

GUIDELINES FOR ADULT CRITICAL CARE INFUSIONS

Table 20–11, page 450, provides key information on the use of infusions in the ICU setting.

20

COMMON MEDICAL EMERGENCIES

Overview of Emergency Cardiac Care
Cardiopulmonary Resuscitation
Advanced Cardiac Life Support (ACLS)
Emergency Airway and Ventilatory
    Support
Automatic External Defibrillation,
    Defibrillation, Cardioversion

Acute Coronary Syndromes and
    Myocardial Infarction
Stroke
Other Common Emergencies

OVERVIEW OF EMERGENCY CARDIAC CARE

The algorithms and guidelines of the American Heart Association (AHA) and International Liaison Committee on Cardiac Resuscitation (ILCOR) have been updated. The latest guidelines promote the use of automatic external defibrillator (AEDs) by emergency medical services (EMS), police, and the general public. The establishment of public access defibrillator (PAD) programs and continued development of EMS protocols make it necessary for receiving physicians in emergency departments to be knowledgeable in the current recommendations of the AHA regarding the use of the prehospital AEDs. These recommendations can be found in the most current Guidelines for Cardiopulmonary Resuscitation and Emergency Cardiovascular Care 2005.*

According to the latest AHA guidelines, if a person experiences witnessed sudden cardiac death (cardiac arrest) and a defibrillator or an AED is available, defibrillation should be performed as soon as possible. However, if a person is "found down" and may have been unresponsive for several minutes, ~ 5 cycles (~ 2 min) of CPR should be performed before initiation of defibrillation.

People who experience cardiac arrest and receive immediate defibrillation are more likely to be successfully defibrillated after the first shock. For every minute of circulatory arrest there is an ~ 10% decrease in the likelihood of successful resuscitation. Patients who are subject to delays in receiving resuscitation do not fare as well, unless there has been a brief period of CPR before defibrillation.

Many communities, organizations, and EMS systems participate in **PAD programs.** These programs facilitate early recognition and management by the use of **AEDs,** and some hospitals have AEDs available, so that a patient who "arrests" can be defibrillated before the arrival of the code team.

Many patients who experience sudden cardiac death due to ventricular fibrillation (VF) or pulseless ventricular tachycardia (VT) can be defibrillated before they arrive at the hospital. That the rescuer does not have to interpret the cardiac rhythm may increase the chance of survival by markedly decreasing time to

---

*2005 American Heart Association Guidelines for Cardiopulmonary Resuscitation and Emergency Cardiovascular Care. *Circulation* 2005;112(24 suppl). Available online at: http://circ.ahajournals.org/content/vol112/24_suppl (accessed July 8, 2006).

"first shock." New guidelines for resuscitation stress timely defibrillation and early, consistent chest compressions with minimal interruption.

Children often experience VF after respiratory arrest. It is reasonable that CPR be performed (5 cycles/2 min) before defibrillation is attempted, unless the child suddenly collapses. In that case, the AED should be applied as soon as it is available.

CARDIOPULMONARY RESUSCITATION

CPR Basics: ABCs (Airway, Breathing, Circulation)

Universal precautions dictate that protective eye wear, gloves, and when necessary, water-impervious gowns and footwear be used. All patients must have a patent **airway,** be **breathing,** and have signs of spontaneous **circulation.** Figure 21–1 shows the basic life support (BLS) algorithm. The new guidelines differentiate resuscitation by nonprofessional rescuers from resuscitation by health care providers.

CPR of Unresponsive Adult (Age > 8 y): Witnessed Collapse

If a patient becomes unresponsive (no response to verbal or tactile stimuli, ie, "shake and shout"), call for help (CODE, 911). Do not move the patient unless in immediate danger.

1. Get a defibrillator or AED to the bedside stat.
2. Stand or kneel at the patient's shoulder. Position patient on back as a unit, protecting the neck.
3. **Airway.** Open the patient's airway. If there are signs of airway compromise (apnea, stridor, coughing, use of accessory muscles), immediately open and clear the airway using the **head tilt-chin lift method** (nonprofessional rescuer) or a **jaw thrust** (health care provider) if cervical spinal injury is suspected.
4. If a foreign body is visualized in the airway, and can easily be removed, remove it. If airway care is needed, proceed according to clinical need (see later, Emergency Airway and Ventilatory Support).
5. **Breathing.** Determine whether the patient is breathing by **looking, listening, and feeling. Look** at the patient's chest to determine whether there are signs of movement. **Listen** at the patient's mouth and nose to determine whether air is being moved through (escaping) from the upper airway. **Feel** for warm, moist air coming out of the mouth and nose by placing your ear close to the patient's mouth and nose.
6. If the patient is breathing, place him or her in the **recovery position:** a stable, side-lying position in which the tongue does not block the airway and fluid can drain from the mouth. Keep the spine straight, and position the arms so that the chest is not compressed. Continue to monitor the patient for breathing. Call for assistance!
7. If the patient is not breathing, ventilate by administering two positive-pressure breaths. Allowing 1 s per breath using either a bag valve mask or a barrier device such as a pocket mask.
8. **Circulation.** To determine whether there are signs of circulation, check the neck for a carotid pulse for ≤ 10 s (health care provider). However, if there is any doubt regarding the presence or absence of a pulse, start chest compressions.

21

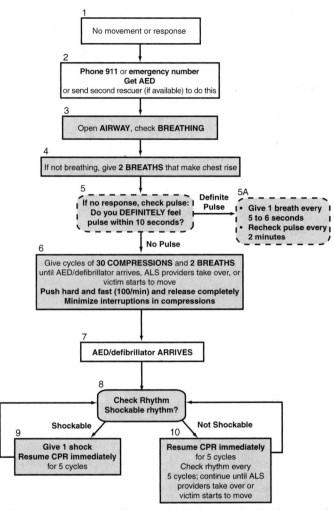

FIGURE 21-1. Adult basic life support health care provider algorithm. Boxes dotted borders indicate actions or steps performed by health care providers but not the general public. ALS = advanced life support. (Reproduced with permission from *Circulation* 2005;112:IV-19–IV-34.)

9. If there is a definite pulse, give 1 breath every 5–6 s, approximately 10–12 breaths/min, rechecking for a pulse every 2 min. If an advanced airway is placed, ventilate with 8–10 breaths/min (approximately 1 breath every 6–8 s asynchronously).

10. If there are no obvious signs of circulation, begin chest compressions: Place both hands the patient's sternum, the heel of one hand on top of the heel of the other. Push **fast** and push **hard,** to a depth of 1.5–2.0 in (4–5 cm), allowing full recoil of the chest. Continue compressions until a defibrillator or an AED is brought to the patient's side. If a defibrillator is not immediately available, continue chest compressions and ventilations at a ratio of 30/2 at a rate of approximately 100 compressions/min.

11. When the defibrillator or AED arrives, attach the two pads to the patient's bare chest. Right-sided sternal pad: right superoanterior infraclavicular position; left-sided apical pad: inferolateral left side of chest lateral to the left breast. Minimize interruption of chest compressions and compress until the pads are on the chest, if possible.

12. Stop compressions. Analyze the rhythm, and if indicated (presence of VF or pulseless VT), deliver a single shock.

13. Immediately resume CPR for another 5 cycles of 30 compressions/2 breaths (2 min). Do not check for a pulse until another 5 cycles of CPR have been performed. The defibrillated, stunned myocardium may not yet be pumping efficiently.

14. If there is no pulse, resume CPR, recharge the defibrillator and administer another single shock followed by immediate CPR.

15. If unsuccessful, proceed to the **advanced cardiac life support (ACLS) algorithms and guidelines.**

CPR of Unconscious Adult (Age > 8 y): Unknown Down Time

If an unconscious patient is encountered who is not breathing and has no apparent signs of circulation and the time of onset of symptoms is unknown, the situation is called unwitnessed arrest.

1. Perform CPR as described earlier (CPR of Unresponsive Adult: Witnessed Collapse) for 2 min (5 cycles of 30 compressions and 2 ventilations) before attempting defibrillation.

2. Resume CPR immediately after the first shock and reassess the patient after (2 min) or 5 cycles of 30 compressions and 2 breaths. If there are no signs of spontaneous circulation, ie, no carotid pulse, recharge the AED or defibrillator while doing CPR and administer another single shock.

3. If the defibrillation results in successful termination of VF, treat the patient supportively observing for changes in blood pressure, heart rate, and respiratory status. If unsuccessful, proceed to the **ACLS** algorithms and guidelines.

4. After successful defibrillation, an unstable rhythm may develop and necessitate intervention. Some patients may arrive in the emergency department with a pulseless rhythm, asystole, pulseless electrical activity, and VT or VF. Other patients may have a slow heart rate incapable of providing good perfusion pressure, ie, bradycardia (heart rate < 60 beats/min) or tachycardia (heart rate > 100 beats/min). Proceed to the appropriate ACLS algorithms and guidelines (see later).

CPR of Child (Age 1–8 y): Witnessed Cardiac Arrest

If a child becomes unresponsive and experiences respiratory arrest, the approach is similar to that for an adult: ABCs and a call for help. Get a defibrillator or AED stat.

21

1. **Airway:** Open the airway with the head-tilt chin lift maneuver or, if a cervical spinal injury is a concern, a jaw thrust.

2. **Breathing:** Determine breathlessness: **look, listen, feel. If the patient is breathing, place him or her in the recovery position. If no breathing is present, give 2 effective breaths (1 s/breath).**

3. **Circulation:** Check for signs of circulation; carotid pulse check < 10 s (health care provider). If a pulse is obviously present, perform rescue breathing at a rate of 12–20 breaths/min (1 breath every 3–5 s) or (12–20 breaths/min). If an advanced airway is present, 8–10 breaths/min (~ 1 breath/6–8 s asynchronously).

4. If no signs of circulation are present, begin chest compressions. Compress the chest with the heel of one hand at the lower half of the sternum to a depth of $1/3$ to $1/2$ of the chest. A ratio of 15 compressions/2 breaths can be assumed with two rescuers. The rate of compressions should be approximately 100/min. Avoid unnecessary interruptions in CPR.

5. As soon as a defibrillator is available, immediately apply the defibrillator or AED pads (pediatric) to the patient's bare chest with minimal interruption in chest compressions. Adult AED pads are acceptable if pediatric pads are not available; however, do not let the pads touch each other on the chest.

6. Stop CPR and allow the AED to analyze the rhythm.

7. Shock if indicated (2 J/kg if manual defibrillator).

8. Resume CPR immediately for 5 cycles and analyze the rhythm.

9. If defibrillation is unsuccessful, recharge the AED or defibrillator while resuming and continuing CPR. Reshock (4 J/kg manually) and immediately do 2 min of CPR. Reasses the patient and rhythm.

10. If unsuccessful, proceed to the pediatric advanced life support (PALS) guidelines (Table 21–1).

TABLE 21–1
Pediatric Advanced Life Support for Ventricular Fibrillation, Ventricular Tachycardia, and Pulseless Electrical Activity

ABCs		
Airway		
Breathing		
Circulation		
Chest Compressions/Ventilation	1 rescuer	30/2
	2 rescuers	15/2
Compress Hard and Fast	rate > 100 beats/ min	
Call 911/Code/EMS		
AED application 2J/kg		
Medications:	Epinephrine	0.01 mg/kg IV/IO VT/VF/pulseless OR 0.1 mg/kg (1:1000): 0.1 mL/kg per ET q3–5min
	Amiodarone	5 mg/kg IV/IO
	Lidocaine	1 mg/kg IV/IO
	Magnesium	25–50 mg/kg IV/IO Torsade de pointes

Consider ET tube administration if no vascular access.
Based on recommendations from *Circulation* 2005;112:IV-167–IV-187.
IO = intraosseous; VT = ventricular tachycardia; VF = ventricular fibrillation.

21

TABLE 21-2
Pediatric Bradycardia and Tachycardia Management

Bradycardia	Tachycardia
ABCs	
Epinephrine 0.01 mg/kg IV/IO (1:10,000:0.01 mL/kg)	Adenosine 0.1 mg/kg (max 6 mg)
Atropine 0.02 mg/kg IV/IO	Cardioversion 2 J/kg Amiodarone 5 mg/kg IV/30 min Procainamide 15 mg/kg/45 min

Based on recommendations from Circulation 2005; 122:IV-167–IV-187.

CPR of Child (Age 1–8 y): Unwitnessed Cardiac Arrest

If a child is found to be apneic (breathless) and not showing signs of spontaneous circulation (no carotid pulse when checked by health care provider) with an unknown down time, the situation is considered unwitnessed cardiac arrest.

1. Begin CPR, as described earlier (CPR of Child: Witnessed Cardiac Arrest), for 2 min (5 cycles) before attempting defibrillation using a defibrillator or AED and pediatric pads. (*Note:* Adult pads can be used if pediatric pads not available. Make sure pads are not touching each other).
2. Defibrillate with AED if child's age > 1 y (2 J/kg with manual defibrillator).
3. Immediately resume CPR for 2 min.
4. Assess patient for pulse. If the defibrillation attempt was unsuccessful, resume CPR, recharge the AED or defibrillator and provide another single shock when charged. (Use 4 J/kg for second defibrillation if a manual defibrillator is used). If unsuccessful, proceed to the appropriate PALS management (Tables 21–1 and 21–2).
5. Like adults, children may present in asystole, pulseless electrical activity, or pulseless VT or VF, or these rhythms may develop after defibrillation. Furthermore, children can present with bradycardia or tachycardia. Proceed to the PALS guidelines (Tables 21–1 and 21–2, and Figure 21–2), and attempt to correct the dysrhythmia and determine the cause of the event.

CPR of Unresponsive Infant (Age < 1 y): Witnessed or Unwitnessed Cardiac Arrest

1. **Airway:** Head tilt-chin lift or jaw thrust.
2. **Breathing:** Look, listen, and feel for breathing. If absent, give 2 effective breaths at 1 s/breath.
3. **Circulation:** Check the brachial or femoral pulse. If no pulse is present, start chest compressions. Use 2 or 3 fingers or a thumb just below the nipple line, and press to 1/2 to 1/3 the depth of the chest.
4. Use 30 compressions/2 ventilations (single rescuer) or 15 compressions/2 ventilations (2 health care providers) Rate of compressions is 100/min. Rate of ventilation is 12–20 breaths/min (or ~ 1 breath/3–5 s).
5. If an advanced airway is present, use 8–10 breaths/min (~ 1 breath/6–8 s asynchronously).
6. Perform CPR for 2 min or 5 cycles, then reassess the patient. There are no recommendations regarding defibrillation in this situation. If no success,

21

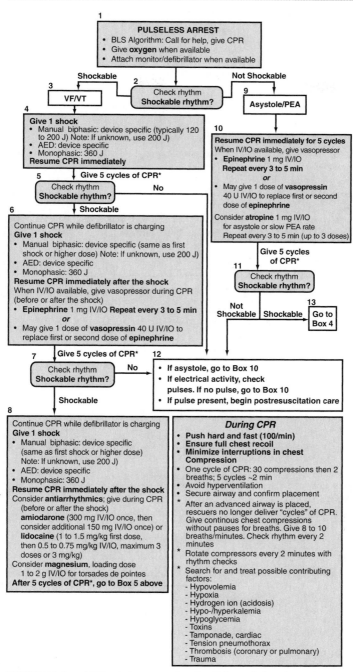

FIGURE 21–2. ACLS pulseless arrest algorithm. PEA = pulseless electrical activity; IO = intraosseous. (Reproduced with permission from *Circulation* 2005;112:IV-58–IV-66.)

proceed to the advanced algorithms and guidelines (Tables 21–1 and 21–2, and Figure 21–2).

Neonatal Resuscitation

Immediately after delivery, a neonate begins to undergo a physiologic transition. Rapid assessment can determine the need for resuscitation:

1. Was the born baby at term?
2. Is the amniotic fluid clear and free of meconium and infection?
3. Is the baby breathing or crying?
4. Does the baby have good muscle tone?

If the answer to all these questions is yes, resuscitation probably is not needed.

It is normal for amniotic fluid to be present in the upper airways of newborns, and this fluid must be cleared. Help the neonate to breath spontaneously, maintain body temperature, and adapt to new circulatory patterns. Provide an infant warmer, oxygen, neonatal airway adjuncts, and drying materials. The sequence of basic actions is summarized in Figure 21–3.

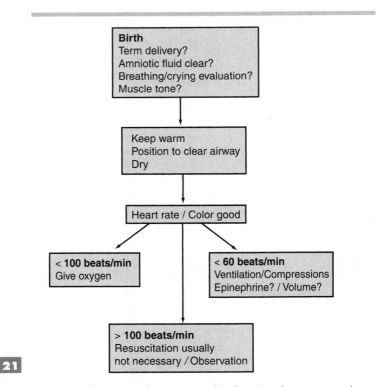

21

FIGURE 21–3. Neonatal resuscitation algorithm. (Based on recommendations from *Circulation* 2005;112:IV-188–IV-195.)

ADVANCED CARDIAC LIFE SUPPORT (ACLS)

The foundation of ACLS is sound BLS. In the advanced phase (sometimes called the "D" in the ABCDs of emergency cardiac care), specific arrhythmias are managed primarily through administration of medications. Rapid reference guides to ACLS and other commonly used emergency medications are on the inside front and back covers of this book. ECG interpretation is reviewed in Chapter 19.

Cardiac Arrest

Four rhythms can produce pulseless cardiac arrest: VF, VT, pulseless electrical activity (PEA), and asystole. (See adult ACLS pulseless arrest algorithm in Figure 21–2.)

Symptomatic Bradycardia and Tachycardia

Monitor for the development of arrhythmias in any patient with chest pain or who has undergone resuscitation. In addition to the foregoing cardiac arrest arrhythmias, patients may have bradycardia or tachycardia that requires monitoring and therapy if they become symptomatic. Management of bradycardia and tachycardia based on 2005 emergency cardiac care guidelines is outlined in Table 21–3.

EMERGENCY AIRWAY AND VENTILATORY SUPPORT

To improve oxygenation, administer 100% inspired oxygen during BLS (see also Chapter 18). Airway adjuncts are useful for this purpose and are classified as basic and advanced airway techniques. Make sure suction is readily available.

TABLE 21–3
Bradycardia and Tachycardia

Bradycardia (HR < 60 beats/min)	Tachycardia (HR > 100 beats/min)
High degree AV block II/III	Narrow complex
Transcutaneous pacing	Adenosine 6 mg, 12 mg, 12 mg IV
Atropine 0.5 mg IV (max 3 mg)	Beta blocker
Epinephrine 2–10 mcg/min IV	Wide complex
Dopamine 2–10 mcg/kg/min IV	Amiodarone 150 mg IV/10 min (max) 2.2 g/24 h
Identify and manage correctable factors	
Hypovolemia	Toxins
Hypoxia	Tamponade
Hydrogen ion	Tension pneumothorax
Hypo/hyperkalemia	Thrombosis PE/CAD
Hypoglycemia	Trauma
Hypothermia	

Consider ET tube administration if no IV access.
Based on recommendations from *Circulation* 2005;112(Suppl I):IV-6–IV-77.

21

Exhaled CO_2 detectors are useful for determining proper tube placement. High exhaled CO_2 levels confirm proper tube placement.

Basic Airway Management

Bag Mask Ventilation: Can be supplied with room air or oxygen supplementation; can also be connected to an advanced airway if present. Open the airways adequately with chin lift, lifting the jaw against the mask and maintaining a tight seal. During CPR give two ventilations during a brief 3- to 4-s pause between every 30 compressions. Deliver a tidal volume sufficient to raise the chest (~ 6–7 mL/kg or 500–600 mL in an adult) over 1 s. Can cause gastric inflation with subsequent complications (eg, aspiration).

Oropharyngeal Airway: Use only if trained in the technique and only if the patient is unconscious and has no gag reflex.

Nasopharyngeal Airway: Better tolerated by patients who are not deeply unconscious. Useful for patients with tightly clenched jaws; use with caution in craniofacial trauma.

Advanced Airways

Used only by health care providers with proper training and frequent practice. Because placement of an advanced airway may require interruption of basic CPR the risk/benefit ratio must be considered. The bag mask can be connected to an advanced airway for delivery of ventilation.

Esophagotracheal Airway (Combitube or ETC): A multilumen airway that consists of a single, dual-lumen tube with two cuffs. After placement, port 1 (blue pilot balloon) is inflated with 100 mL air, then port 2 (white pilot balloon) is inflated with 15 mL air. Ventilate through the longer blue tube 1; if breath sounds are heard, and auscultation of gastric insufflation is negative, continue ventilation. If auscultation of breath sounds is negative and auscultation of gastric insufflation positive, ventilate through the shorter clear tube 2.

Laryngeal Mask Airway (LMA): Inflatable silicone mask and rubber connecting tube. Inserted blindly into the pharynx, a cuff is inflated that forms a low-pressure seal around the laryngeal inlet, allowing gentle positive-pressure ventilation. *Note:* The black line on the airway tube must be oriented toward the upper lip, and a bite block must be in place. Aspiration may be less common with an LMA than with a bag mask.

Endotracheal Tube (ET): Technique is reviewed in Chapter 13. Unskilled providers can cause more harm than good in attempting ET intubation during resuscitation. Indicated when the rescuer cannot ventilate an unconscious patient with a bag mask and in the absence of airway reflexes.

AUTOMATIC EXTERNAL DEFIBRILLATION, DEFIBRILLATION, CARDIOVERSION

In addition to familiarizing yourself with the location of the code cart, airway supplies, emergency numbers, etc, on each new rotation, become familiar with the defibrillator and AED. AEDs are small, free-standing, battery-operated defibrillators, equipped with computer hardware and software. They are designed to "recognize" lethal, nonperfusing, "shockable" dysrhythmias such as VF and VT. More complicated AEDs can actually "cardiovert." When it recognizes lethal dysrhyth-

21

mia, the AED gives visual or voice prompts for the rescuer to press a button and defibrillate the patient. Some models of AED automatically shock the patient after emitting an audible or visual warning to the rescuer to "stand clear." There are monophasic and biphasic defibrillators and AEDs in hospitals. In addition, there are biphasic, and probably some older monophasic, AEDs in public places as part of public access defibrillation programs.

General AED Instructions

1. Place the AED near the patient in such a way that access to the airway and chest is unimpeded.
2. Turn on the AED unit. Most AEDs give auditory or visual prompts such as:

   - "Connect electrodes to AED."
   - "Place electrodes to patient's bare chest." (*Note:* Do not allow the pads to touch each other.)
   - "Do not touch the patient!"
   - "Analyzing rhythm."
   - "Shock advised—Do not touch the patient!"
   - "Push [flashing button] to shock patient."

3. The AED then prompts for patient evaluation, pulse check, etc. Some AEDs still have the 2000 guidelines algorithms on them. **The 2005 guidelines call for delivery of only 1 shock, followed immediately by CPR for 2 min before assessment of circulation.**
4. Repeat as clinically indicated.

Defibrillation

When defibrillating a patient, follow the updated algorithms.

1. Place pads securely on patient's chest: one to the right of the patient's sternum, just below the clavicle, the other on the left anterior axillary line. (Most pads and paddles are labeled to facilitate placement.) Make sure there is good contact to decrease resistance. (Most pads can be used for ECG monitoring, defibrillation, cardioversion, and pacing.)
2. If using paddles, use electrode gel or paste and use at least 25 lb of downward force to enhance contact with the chest. Most paddles can be used to "quick-look" the rhythm.
3. Charge the defibrillator to the appropriate energy (measured in joules).
4. Shout "CLEAR—SHOCKING PATIENT!" Verify that no one (including yourself) is in contact with the patient.
5. Depress both buttons on the paddles to deliver the shock.

Cardioversion

There are rapid rhythms (eg, atrial fibrillation with uncontrolled rates, supraventricular tachycardia [SVT], Wolff–Parkinson–White [WPW]) that render a patient's condition unstable with a decrease in blood pressure, change in mentation, etc. These circumstances may necessitate that the rhythm be electrically terminated with cardioversion. For **cardioversion,** the control knob **synchronizes** the shock automatically with the peak of the R wave on the ECG strip. This step prevents shock delivery during the vulnerable period of the cardiac cycle, which can promote development of a lethal nonperfusing rhythm such as VF. The defibrillator hardware and software control the dis-

21

charge of the shock after the "Shock" button is pressed. The procedure is otherwise as described for defibrillation. Because cardioversion is done with the patient conscious, consider sedation with a drug such as midazolam if clinically feasible.

ACUTE CORONARY SYNDROMES AND MYOCARDIAL INFARCTION

Perform a 12-lead ECG on any patients experiencing chest pain (see Chapters 13 and 19). If the patient has signs of ischemia or has had an AMI (shown in 2 contiguous leads), a quick decision must be made to administer thrombolytics (within 30 min of patient presentation), if appropriate. Review the contraindications. Absolute contraindications include CNS abnormalities (eg, A–V malformation, tumor, history of intracranial hemorrhage, recent head trauma) and bleeding diathesis. Relative contraindications include pregnancy, history of poorly controlled hypertension, and recent (2–4 wk) internal bleeding (see *Circulation* 2005;112:IV-89–IV-110, Table 1). If the patient is not a candidate for thrombolysis, prepare to take the him or her to the cardiac catheterization lab (balloon inflation within 90 min of patient presentation), if available. The appropriate sequence of acute coronary syndrome management is shown in Figure 21–4. **Remember: "Time is muscle!"**

STROKE

Stroke is also called "brain attack." A similar caveat as for the heart holds true: **"Time is brain."** Signs and symptoms of a stroke include:

- Facial droop
- Change in mental status
- Pronator drift
- Unilateral motor weakness
- Slurred speech
- Syncope
- Difficulty swallowing
- Confusion

In the field, EMS personnel use the Cincinnati Prehospital Stroke Scale or the Los Angeles Prehospital Stroke Screen to determine the likelihood that a patient may have a stroke (Table 21–4). Carefully determine time of symptom onset. This step is crucial in decision making regarding the use of thrombolytics in a stroke patient without bleeding. Measure a fingerstick glucose level to detect possible hypoglycemia. If hypoglycemia is present, correct it immediately. Perform a neurologic screening exam, draw samples for lab work, order an emergency CT scan, obtain a 12-lead ECG, and take the patient to the CT suite. **Activate the stroke team.** The AHA stroke algorithm is in Figure 21–5.

OTHER COMMON EMERGENCIES

Anaphylaxis

Allergic Reaction with Systolic BP < 90 mm Hg or Airway Failure

Epinephrine   Drug of choice **Dose: *Adults.*** IV bolus: 100 mcg of 1:100,000 over 5–10 min (mix 0.1 mL of 1:1,000 epi in 10 mL NS). IV inf: 1–4 mcg/min. ***Peds.*** IV inf: 0.1–0.3 mcg/kg/min, max 1.5 mcg/kg/min

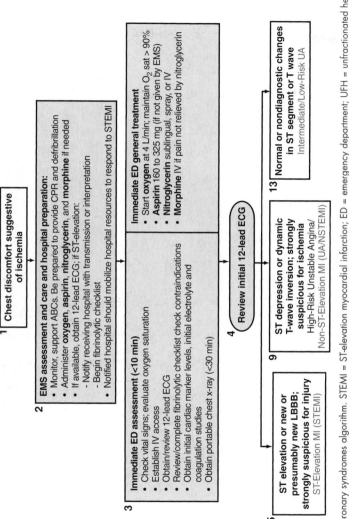

FIGURE 21–4. Acute coronary syndromes algorithm. STEMI = ST-elevation myocardial infarction; ED = emergency department; UFH = unfractionated heparin; PCI = percutaneous coronary intervention. (Reproduced with permission from *Circulation* 2005;112:IV-89–IV-110.) *(continued)*

1 Chest discomfort suggestive of ischemia

2 EMS assessment and care and hospital preparation:
- Monitor, support ABCs. Be prepared to provide CPR and defibrillation
- Administer **oxygen, aspirin, nitroglycerin,** and **morphine** if needed
- If available, obtain 12-lead ECG; if ST-elevation:
  - Notify receiving hospital with transmission or interpretation
  - Begin fibrinolytic checklist
- Notified hospital should mobilize hospital resources to respond to STEMI

3 Immediate ED assessment (<10 min)
- Check vital signs; evaluate oxygen saturation
- Establish IV access
- Obtain/review 12-lead ECG
- Review/complete fibrinolytic checklist check contraindications
- Obtain initial cardiac marker levels, initial electrolyte and coagulation studies
- Obtain portable chest x-ray (<30 min)

Immediate ED general treatment
- Start **oxygen** at 4 L/min; maintain O₂ sat > 90%
- **Aspirin** 160 to 325 mg (if not given by EMS)
- **Nitroglycerin** sublingual, spray, or IV
- **Morphine** IV if pain not relieved by nitroglycerin

4 Review initial 12-lead ECG

5 ST elevation or new or presumably new LBBB; strongly suspicious for injury
ST-Elevation MI (STEMI)

9 ST depression or dynamic T-wave inversion; strongly suspicious for ischemia
High-Risk Unstable Angina/Non-ST-Elevation MI (UA/NSTEMI)

13 Normal or nondiagnostic changes in ST segment or T wave
Intermediate/Low-Risk UA

21

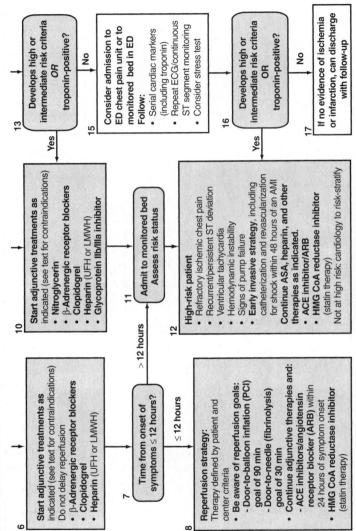

6

Start adjunctive treatments as indicated (see text for contraindications)
Do not delay reperfusion
- β-Adrenergic receptor blockers
- Clopidogrel
- Heparin (UFH or LMWH)

7

Time from onset of symptoms ≤ 12 hours?

≤12 hours

>12 hours

8

Reperfusion strategy:
Therapy defined by patient and center criteria
- Be aware of reperfusion goals:
  - Door-to-balloon inflation (PCI) goal of 90 min
  - Door-to-needle (fibrinolysis) goal of 30 min
- Continue adjunctive therapies and:
  - ACE inhibitors/angiotensin receptor blocker (ARB) within 24 hours of symptom onset
- HMG CoA reductase inhibitor (statin therapy)

10

Start adjunctive treatments as indicated (see text for contraindications)
- Nitroglycerin
- β-Adrenergic receptor blockers
- Clopidogrel
- Heparin (UFH or LMWH)
- Glycoprotein IIb/IIIa inhibitor

11

Admit to monitored bed
Assess risk status

12

High-risk patient
- Refractory ischemic chest pain
- Recurrent/persistent ST deviation
- Ventricular tachycardia
- Hemodynamic instability
- Signs of pump failure
- **Early invasive strategy,** including catheterization and revascularization for shock within 48 hours of an AMI
  Continue ASA, heparin, and other therapies as indicated.
  - ACE inhibitor/ARB
- HMG CoA reductase inhibitor (statin therapy)
  Not at high risk: cardiology to risk-stratify

13

Develops high or intermediate risk criteria **OR** troponin-positive?

No

Yes

15

Consider admission to ED chest pain unit or to monitored bed in ED
Follow:
- Serial cardiac markers (including troponin)
- Repeat ECG/continuous ST segment monitoring
- Consider stress test

16

Develops high or intermediate risk criteria **OR** troponin-positive?

No

Yes

17

If no evidence of ischemia or infarction, can discharge with follow-up

FIGURE 21-4. Continued.

TABLE 21–4
Two Systems for Field Evaluations of Stroke Risk

Cincinnati Prehospital Stroke Scale
If any of these signs are present, the probability of a stroke is 72%:
   Facial droop: Ask patient to smile; sign is present if one side does
      not move as well as the other
   Arm drift: Ask patient to close eyes and hold arms out for 10 s; sign
      is present if one arm does not move or drifts downward
   Abnormal speech: Sign is present if the patient slurs speech or uses
      wrong words

Los Angeles Prehospital Stroke Screen
If any of these factors are present, there is high likelihood of a stroke in
a patient with a nontraumatic neurologic complaint:
   Age > 45 y
   No seizure or epilepsy history
   Symptoms present < 24 h
   Patient not wheelchair bound or bedridden at baseline
   Blood glucose 60–400 mg/dL
   Asymmetry of face, grip, or arm strength

Based on data from *Circulation* 2005;112:IV-111–IV-120.

Allergic Reaction with Systolic BP > 90 mm Hg

Epinephrine   Dose: *Adults.* 0.3–0.5 mL (1:1000) SQ. *Peds.* 0.01 mL/kg
(1:1000), max 0.5 mL
   Supplemental drugs for anaphylaxis include:

Diphenhydramine   Dose: *Adults.* IV/IM/PO 50 mg. *Peds.* IV/IM/PO 1 mg/kg

Methylprednisolone   Dose: 1–2 mg/kg IV

Ranitidine (Zantac)   Dose: *Adults.* IV 50 mg over 5 min. *Peds.* IV 0.5 mg/
kg over 5 min

Albuterol   Dose: *Adults.* 2.5 mg nebulized. *Peds.* 1.25 mg nebulized

Asthma Attack: Mild

Albuterol (Nebulized)   Dose: *Adults.* 2.5–5.0 mg at 20 min for up to 3
doses in first hour. *Peds.* 1.25–2.5 mg at 20 min for up to 3 doses in first hour.
Supplemental oxygen to keep sats > 90%

Asthma Attack: Moderate to Severe

Ipratropium Bromide (Nebulized)   Dose: *Adults.* 0.5 mg combined
with first albuterol treatment. *Peds.* 250 mcg with first albuterol treatment. Give
continuously or every 20 min for first hour.

Levalbuterol (Xopenex)   Dose: 0.63–1.25 mg nebulized q6–8h

21

Methylprednisolone   Dose: *Adults.* 60–125 mg IV. *Peds.* 2 mg/kg IV
Supplemental oxygen to keep sats > 90%

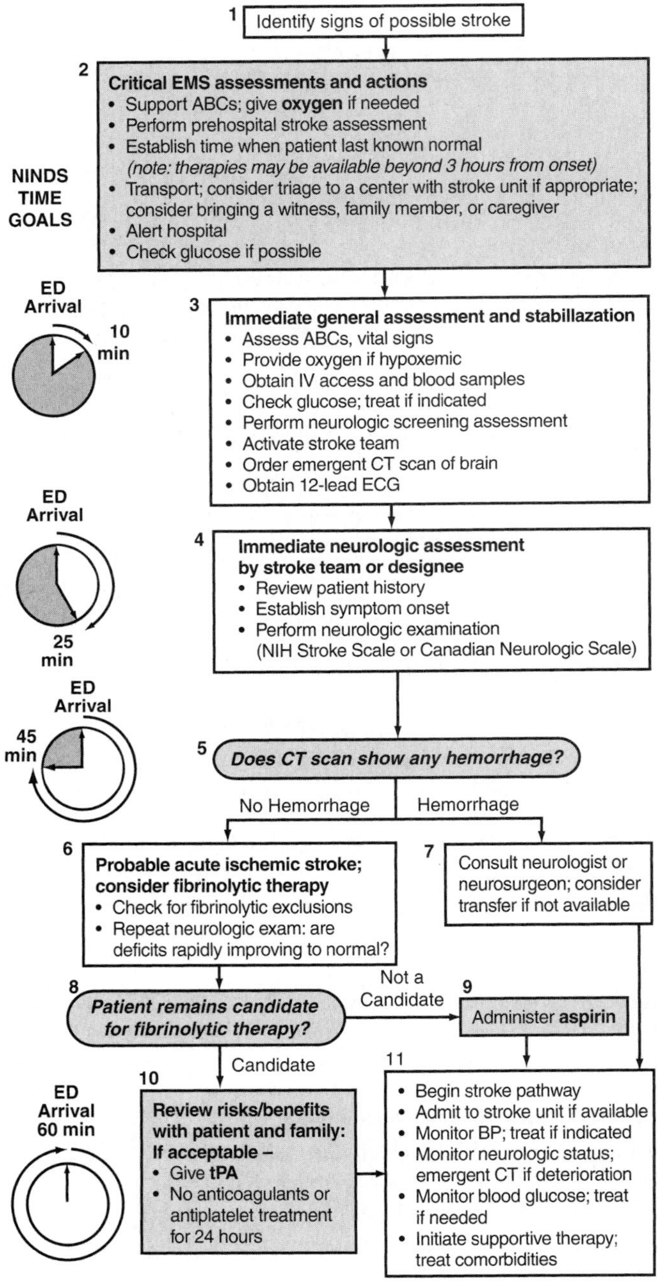
1 Identify signs of possible stroke
NINDS TIME GOALS
2 Critical EMS assessments and actions
• Support ABCs; give oxygen if needed
• Perform prehospital stroke assessment
• Establish time when patient last known normal (note: therapies may be available beyond 3 hours from onset)
• Transport; consider triage to a center with stroke unit if appropriate; consider bringing a witness, family member, or caregiver
• Alert hospital
• Check glucose if possible
ED Arrival 10 min
3 Immediate general assessment and stabilazation
• Assess ABCs, vital signs
• Provide oxygen if hypoxemic
• Obtain IV access and blood samples
• Check glucose; treat if indicated
• Perform neurologic screening assessment
• Activate stroke team
• Order emergent CT scan of brain
• Obtain 12-lead ECG
ED Arrival 25 min
4 Immediate neurologic assessment by stroke team or designee
• Review patient history
• Establish symptom onset
• Perform neurologic examination (NIH Stroke Scale or Canadian Neurologic Scale)
ED Arrival 45 min
5 Does CT scan show any hemorrhage?
No Hemorrhage
Hemorrhage
6 Probable acute ischemic stroke; consider fibrinolytic therapy
• Check for fibrinolytic exclusions
• Repeat neurologic exam: are deficits rapidly improving to normal?
7 Consult neurologist or neurosurgeon; consider transfer if not available
8 Patient remains candidate for fibrinolytic therapy?
Not a Candidate
9 Administer aspirin
Candidate
ED Arrival 60 min
10 Review risks/benefits with patient and family: If acceptable –
• Give tPA
• No anticoagulants or antiplatelet treatment for 24 hours
11
• Begin stroke pathway
• Admit to stroke unit if available
• Monitor BP; treat if indicated
• Monitor neurologic status; emergent CT if deterioration
• Monitor blood glucose; treat if needed
• Initiate supportive therapy; treat comorbidities

FIGURE 21–5. Algorithm for management of suspected stroke. NINDS = National Institute of Neurological Disorders and Stroke. (Reproduced with permission from *Circulation* 2005;112:IV-111–IV-120.)

Asthma Attack: Severe

Administer aerosolized beta-agonists with anticholinergic continuously. Intubate and ventilate with 100% oxygen if impending or actual respiratory arrest. Administer IV corticosteroid.

Methylprednisolone Dose: *Adults.* 60–125 mg IV. *Peds.* 2 mg/kg IV

Anticholinergic Toxicity

Usually related to drug overdose. Patients present "Hot as Hades, Blind as a Bat, Dry as a Bone, Red as a Beet, Mad as a Hatter."

Physostigmine Controversial; use only when seizures, coma, hypotension, agitation are refractory to conventional therapy **Dose:** 0.5–2.0 mg IV *Note:* Administer S-L-O-W-L-Y (can cause seizures if given rapidly). Have cardiac monitor attached and resuscitation equipment at the bedside. **Use only in consultation with the poison control center or a toxicologist**

Coma

1. Establish and secure airway (protect cervical spine if trauma has occurred).
2. Assess for respiratory failure and shock; use BLS and ACLS techniques as appropriate.
3. Supply oxygen, IV access, cardiac monitor, and pulse oximetry.
4. Administer 1 amp (50 mL) of D_{50} IV manually; consider checking a stat glucose first. If not hypoglycemic, can worsen stroke outcomes.
5. Administer 100 mg thiamine IV.
6. Give 0.4 mg naloxone (Narcan) IV (see later, Opioid Overdose).
7. Obtain fingerstick glucose, SMA, CBC, urinalysis, and ABG. Consider ECG, CT of head (see later, Seizures, Status Epilepticus).

Dental Emergencies

Not including facial fractures, there are generally two major categories of dental emergencies: toothaches with associated abscesses and avulsed (knocked-out) teeth. Most toothaches can be managed with antibiotics (usually penicillin-V 500 mg, q6h) and analgesics until proper dental attention can be obtained. Drain fluctuant abscesses if convenient. The exception to this rule is submandibular or infraorbital swelling. With submandibular infections, Ludwig angina, a life-threatening occurrence, can develop. Hold these patients for observation with special attention to maintaining the airway until a dental consult can be obtained. Infraorbital infections can lead to cavernous sinus thrombosis if allowed to progress.

Avulsed teeth may or may not have an associated dentoalveolar fracture. Reposition the displaced tooth in the socket within 30 min or as soon as possible. If the tooth root is dirty, wash it gently with sterile saline solution. Do not scrub or scrape the root. Obtain a dental consult to arrange to have the tooth splinted back in the socket.

Hypercalcemia

See Chapter 9, page 189.

Hyperkalemia

See Chapter 9, page 187.

21

Hypertensive Crisis

Treat only if signs of end organ damage are present.
  Do not reduce MAP > 20–25% over 30–60 min.

Labetalol **Dose:** 20 mg IV bolus then 2 mg/min IV to target BP *or*

Sodium Nitroprusside **Dose:** 0.5 mcg/kg/min to max (10 mcg/kg/min)

Hypoglycemia

1. Draw a stat serum glucose. **Do not wait for result before treating if hypoglycemia is suspected.** A finger Dextro stick can usually be quickly checked.
2. Give orange juice with sugar if the patient is awake and alert; if not, give *Adults.* 1 amp of D_{50} IV *Peds.* 1 mL/kg (D_{10} for newborn).
3. If IV access is not possible, give glucagon 1 mg IM or SC.

Opioid Overdose

Naloxone (Narcan) **Dose:** *Adults.* 0.4–2.0 mg IV or IM, repeat as needed. *Note:* If you suspect the patient is addicted to narcotics, give 0.4 mg and repeat PRN to avoid severe withdrawal. *Peds.* 0.01–0.02 mg/kg IV or IM, repeat PRN.

1. Observe patient for at least 6 h after treatment.
2. Manage airway by intubation if airway failure not immediately responsive to naloxone. (See Coma, page 471.)

Poisoning (Common Agents)

1. Support airway, respiration, and circulation, as needed. *Note:* Do not use Ipecac syrup to induce vomiting; it is no longer a recommended treatment.
2. Determine ingested substance; give specific antidote, if available. **Call Regional Poison Center for assistance (1-800-222-1222).** Some common poisons with their antidotes (Adult, unless specified) are in Table 21–5, page 473.
3. Prevent further absorption as described for consciousness level.

Unconscious Patient

1. Protect airway with an endotracheal tube.
2. Consider lavage with an Ewald tube or 28 Fr or larger NG tube, if ingestion has occurred within the last hour.
3. Use a series of 300-mL NS boluses through the NG or Ewald tube for adults and 20-mL/kg boluses for children.
4. Consider using activated charcoal with sorbitol unless an oral antidote is to be given.

Conscious Patient

1. Consider giving activated charcoal 1 g/kg; contraindicated for iron, lithium, lead, alkali, acid. Also give 70% sorbitol solution (2 mL/kg body weight). Monitor any patient given sorbitol for hypokalemia and hypomagnesemia.
2. Attempt to promote excretion through IV hydration.
3. Administer alkalinization (0.5–1 mEq/kg/L in IV fluids) for salicylates, barbiturates, tricyclics.

21

TABLE 21–5
Antidotes for Common Poisoning Emergencies

Acetaminophen	N-acetylcysteine, 140 mg/kg PO, then 70 mg/kg × 17
Anticholinesterases	Atropine 0.5–2 mg IV; may need up to 5 mg IV every 15 min if severe poisoning
Benzodiazepines	Flumazenil 0.2 mg IV (see page 536)
Beta-blockers	Glucagon 0.05 mg/kg IV bolus for BP <90, then infusion of 75–150 mg/kg/h
Carbon monoxide	High-flow oxygen or hyperbaric oxygen
Calcium channel blockers	Calcium chloride 10–20 mL/kg of 1% solution then 20 mg/kg/h
Cyanide	Amyl nitrate pearls, inhale every 2 min then sodium nitrite 10 mL 3% IV over 3 min (0.33 mL/kg of 3% solution in children) or sodium thiosulfate 50 mL of 25% solution over 10 min or 1.65 mL/kg in children
Cyclic antidepressants	NaHCO$_3$ 3 amps (50 mg/50 mL) in 1 L D$_5$W at 2–3 mL/kg/h
Digoxin	Digoxin-specific Fab Number of vials = Serum digoxin levels $\times \dfrac{\text{Patient's weight (kg)}}{100}$
Ethylene glycol	Fomepizole 15 mg/kg slow infusion
Methanol	Fomepizole (see above) or ethanol–loading dose 1 g/kg of a 10% solution slowly IV, followed by an infusion of 130 mg/kg/h to keep serum level of 100–150 mg/dL
Opiates	Naloxone, see page 572

Seizures, Status Epilepticus

Status epilepticus refers to 30 min or more of continuous seizure activity or two or more seizures without recovery of consciousness between seizures.

Initial Supportive Care

1. Maintain airway with cervical spine precautions.
2. Deliver oxygen by nasal cannula.
3. Monitor ECG and blood pressure.
4. Maintain normal temperature.

Pharmacologic Therapy (Table 21–6, page 474).

21

1. Establish IV, administer thiamine 100 mg IV.
2. Administer 1 amp of D$_{50}$ IV in an adult (2 mL/kg D$_{25}$ in children) unless obviously hyperglycemic.

TABLE 21–6
Drugs for the Management of Status Epilepticus

Drug	Pediatric Dose (mg/kg)	Adult Dose	Maximum Rate (mg/min)
Diazepam (Valium)	0.10–0.20 IV	5–10 mg IV (up to 30 mg)	3–5
Fosphenytoin	NA	20 mg/kg IV	150
Paraldehyde[a]	0.15–0.3 mL/kg PR	30 mL PR	NA
Phenytoin (Dilantin)[b]	15 IV	Same as for child	50
Phenobarbital[c]	10 IV or IM	120–140 mg IV	100

NA = not applicable.
[a]When given rectally, mix 2:1 with cottonseed or olive oil.
[b]When given IV, use a maximum dose of 50 mg/min and monitor ECG and vital signs closely. Can cause severe hypotension and bradycardia. Mix with NS to prevent precipitation.
[c]Indicated when the patient is allergic to phenytoin, patients may need intubation.

3. Administer IV lorazepam or diazepam initially (midazolam 0.2 mg/kg); can be given IM in children if no IV.
4. If seizures persist, give fosphenytoin or phenytoin.
5. If seizures persist, give phenobarbital, paraldehyde.
6. If still no response, obtain emergency neurosurgery and anesthesiology consultations.

COMMONLY USED MEDICATIONS

Medication Key
Controlled Substance Classification
FDA Fetal Risk Categories
Breast Feeding

Generic Drug Data
Natural and Herbal Agents
Drug Tables

This chapter is a directory of key information on some of the most commonly used or important medications available in the United States. Our editorial board has extracted this information from the package inserts, FDA advisories, and relevant publications. Medications are listed in alphabetical order by generic name. Some of the more commonly recognized trade names are listed for each medication (in parentheses after the generic name). The information provided is to be used as a general prescribing guideline AND IS NOT MEANT AS A REPLACEMENT FOR THE COMPLETE PRESCRIBING INFORMATION FOUND ON THE PACKAGE LABELING.

MEDICATION KEY

Generic Drug Name (Selected Common Brand Names [Controlled Substance Class])

WARNING: Summarized version of the "Black Box" precautions deemed necessary by the FDA. These are significant precautions and contraindications concerning the individual medication. **Uses:** Both *FDA-labeled indications* bracketed by asterisks and "off label" uses of the medication. Many medications are used to treat various conditions on the basis of results in the medical literature, and these conditions are not listed in the package insert. On the basis of input from our editorial board, we list common uses of the medication rather than just the official "labeled indications" (FDA approved). **Action:** How the drug works. This information is helpful in comparing classes of drugs and understanding side effects and contraindications. **Spectrum:** Activity against selected microbes **Dose:** *Adults.* Where no specific pediatric dose is given, the implication is that this drug is not commonly used or indicated in that age group. At the end of the dosing line, important dosing modifications may be noted (eg, take with food, avoid antacids) **Caution:** (Pregnancy/fetal risk categories, breast feeding [see symbols in the Breast Feeding section]) Cautions concerning the use of the drug in specific settings **Contra:** Contraindications **Supplied:** Common dosing forms **SE:** Common or significant side effects **Notes:** Other key information about the drug

22

CONTROLLED SUBSTANCE CLASSIFICATION

Medications under the control of the US Drug Enforcement Agency (Schedule I–V controlled substances) are indicated by the symbol [C]. Most medications are "uncontrolled" and do not require a DEA prescriber number on the prescription. Drugs available without a prescription are indicated [OTC]. The following is a general description of the schedules of DEA controlled substances:

Schedule I (C-I):   All nonresearch use forbidden (eg, heroin, LSD, mescaline)

Schedule II (C-II):   High addictive potential; medical use accepted. No telephone call-in prescriptions; no refills. Some states require special prescription form (eg, cocaine, morphine, methadone).

Schedule III (C-III):   Low to moderate risk of physical dependence, high risk of psychological dependence; prescription must be rewritten after 6 mo or five refills (eg, acetaminophen plus codeine)

Schedule IV (C-IV):   Limited potential for dependence; prescription rules same as for schedule III (eg, benzodiazepines, propoxyphene)

Schedule V (C-V):   Very limited abuse potential; prescribing regulations often same as for uncontrolled medications; some states have additional restrictions

FDA FETAL RISK CATEGORIES

Category A: Adequate studies in pregnant women have not shown risk to the fetus in the first trimester of pregnancy; no evidence of risk in the last two trimesters

Category B: Animal studies have not shown risk to the fetus, but no adequate studies have been done with pregnant women

   or

   Animal studies have shown an adverse effect, but adequate studies with pregnant women have not shown risk to the fetus during the first trimester and there is no evidence of risk in the last two trimesters

Category C: Animal studies have shown an adverse effect on the fetus, but no adequate studies have been done with humans. The benefits from the use of the drug by pregnant women may be acceptable despite its potential risks

   or

   No animal reproduction studies and no adequate studies with humans have been done

Category D: Evidence of human fetal risk, but the potential benefits of the use of the drug by pregnant women may be acceptable despite the risks

Category X: Studies in animals or humans or adverse reaction reports, or both, have shown fetal abnormalities. Risk of use by pregnant women clearly outweighs any possible benefit.

Category ?:   No data available (not a formal FDA classification; included to provide complete data set)

BREAST FEEDING

22   No formally recognized classification exists for drugs and breast feeding. The following shorthand was developed for the *Clinician's Pocket Drug Reference.*

+	Compatible with breast feeding
M	Monitor patient or use with caution
±	Excreted, or likely excreted, with unknown effects or at unknown concentration
?/–	Unknown excretion, but effects likely to be of concern
–	Contraindicated in breast feeding
?	No data available

GENERIC DRUG DATA

Abacavir (Ziagen) **WARNING:** Allergy (fever, rash, fatigue, GI, resp) reported; stop drug immediately & do not rechallenge; lactic acidosis & hepatomegaly/steatosis reported **Uses:** *HIV Infxn* **Action:** Nucleoside RT inhibitor **Dose:** *Adults.* 300 mg PO bid *Peds.* 8 mg/kg bid **Caution:** [C, –] CDC recommends HIV-infected mothers not breast feed because of risk of infant transmission **Supplied:** Tabs 300 mg; soln 20 mg/mL **SE:** See Warning, ↑ LFTs, fat redistribution **Notes:** Numerous drug interactions

Abciximab (ReoPro) **Uses:** *Prevent acute ischemic complications in PTCA,* MI **Action:** ↓ plt aggregation (glycoprotein IIb/IIIa inhibitor) **Dose:** 0.25 mg/kg bolus 10–60 min pre PTCA, then 0.125 mcg/kg/min (max = 10 mcg/min) cont inf × 12 h **Caution:** [C, ?/–] **Contra:** Active or recent (w/in 6 wk) internal hemorrhage, CVA w/in 2 y or CVA w/significant neurologic deficit, bleeding diathesis or PO anticoagulants use w/in 7 d (unless PT ≥ 2 × control), thrombocytopenia (< 100,000 cells/µL), recent trauma or major surgery (w/in 6 wk), CNS tumor, A–V malformation, aneurysm, severe uncontrolled HTN, vasculitis, use of dextran before or during PTCA, allergy to murine proteins **Supplied:** Inj 2 mg/mL **SE:** Allergic Rxns, bleeding, thrombocytopenia possible **Notes:** Use w/heparin

Acamprosate (Campral) **Uses:** *Maint abstinence from ETOH* **Action:** Blocks glutamatergic transmission; modulates neuronal hyperexcitability; related to GABA **Dose:** 666 mg PO tid; CrCl 30–50 mL/min: 333 mg PO tid **Caution:** [C; ?/–] **Contra:** CrCl < 30 mL/min **Supplied:** Tabs 333 mg **SE:** N/D, depression, anxiety **Notes:** Does not eliminate ETOH withdrawal Sx; continue even if relapse occurs

Acarbose (Precose) **Uses:** *Type 2 DM* **Action:** α-Glucosidase inhibitor; delays digestion of carbohydrates to ↓ glucose **Dose:** 25–100 mg PO tid (w/1st bite each meal) **Caution:** [B, ?] Avoid if CrCl < 25 mL/min **Contra:** IBD, cirrhosis **Supplied:** Tabs 25, 50, 100 mg **SE:** Abdominal pain, D, flatulence, ↑ LFTs **Notes:** OK w/sulfonylureas; can affect digoxin levels; LFTs q3mo for 1st y

Acebutolol (Sectral) **Uses:** *HTN, arrhythmias* **Action:** Blocks β-adrenergic receptors, β_1, & ISA **Dose:** 200–800 mg/d, ↓ if CrCl < 50 mL/min **Caution:** [B, D in 2nd & 3rd tri, +] Can exacerbate ischemic heart Dz, do not D/C abruptly **Contra:** 2nd-, 3rd-degree heart block **Supplied:** Caps 200, 400 mg **SE:** Fatigue, HA, dizziness, bradycardia

Acetaminophen, APAP, *N*-acetyl-*p*-aminophenol (Tylenol, other generic) [OTC] **Uses:** *Mild–moderate pain, HA, fever* **Action:** Nonnarcotic analgesic; ↑ CNS synthesis of prostaglandins acts on hypothalamic heat-regulating center **Dose:** *Adults.* 650 mg PO or PR q4–6h or 1000 mg PO q6h; max 4 g/24 h *Peds. < 12 y.* 10–15 mg/kg/dose PO or PR q4–6h; max 2.6 g/24 h.

22

Quick dosing Table 22–1 (page 627). Administer q6h if CrCl 10–50 mL/min & q8h if CrCl < 10 mL/min **Caution:** [B, +] Hepatotoxic in elderly & w/EtOH use w/> 4 g/d; alcoholic liver Dz **Contra:** G6PD deficiency **Supplied:** Tabs 160, 325, 500, 650 mg; chew tabs 80, 160 mg; liq 100 mg/mL, 120 mg/2.5 mL, 120 mg/5 mL, 160 mg/5 mL, 167 mg/5 mL, 325 mg/5 mL, 500 mg/15 mL; gtt 48 mg/mL, 60 mg/0.6 mL; supp 80, 120, 125, 300, 325, 650 mg **SE:** OD hepatotox at 10 g; 15 g is potentially lethal; Rx w/*N*-acetylcysteine **Notes:** No antiinflammatory or plt-inhibiting action; avoid EtOH

Acetaminophen + Butalbital ± Caffeine (Fioricet, Medigesic, Repan, Sedapap-10, Two-Dyne, Triaprin, Axocet, Phrenilin Forte) [C-III]

Uses: *Tension HA,* mild pain **Action:** Nonnarcotic analgesic w/barbiturate **Dose:** 1–2 tabs or caps PO q4/6h PRN; ↓ in renal/hepatic impair; 4 g/24 h APAP max **Caution:** [D, +] Alcoholic liver Dz **Contra:** G6PD deficiency **Supplied:** Caps *Medigesic, Repan, Two-Dyne:* butalbital 50 mg, caffeine 40 mg, + APAP 325 mg. Caps *Axocet, Phrenilin Forte:* butalbital 50 mg + APAP 650 mg; *Triapin:* butalbital 50 mg + APAP 325 mg. Tabs *Medigesic, Fioricet, Repan:* butalbital 50 mg, caffeine 40 mg, + APAP 325 mg; *Phrenilin:* butalbital 50 mg + APAP 325 mg; *Sedapap-10:* butalbital 50 mg + APAP 650 mg **SE:** Drowsiness, dizziness, "hangover" effect **Notes:** Butalbital habit-forming; avoid EtOH

Acetaminophen + Codeine (Tylenol No. 1, No. 2, No. 3, No. 4) [C-III, C-V]

Uses: *Mild–moderate pain (No. 1, 2, 3); moderate–severe pain (No. 4)* **Action:** Combined APAP & narcotic analgesic **Dose:** *Adults.* 1–2 tabs q3–4h PRN (max dose APAP = 4 g/d). *Peds.* APAP 10–15 mg/kg/dose; codeine 0.5–1 mg/kg dose q4–6h (dosing guide: 3–6 y, 5 mL/dose; 7–12 y, 10 mL/dose); ↓ in renal/hepatic impair **Caution:** [C, +] Alcoholic liver Dz **Contra:** G6PD deficiency **Supplied:** Tabs 300 mg APAP + codeine; caps 325 mg APAP + codeine; helix, susp (C-V) APAP 120 mg + codeine 12 mg/5 mL **SE:** Drowsiness, dizziness, N/V **Notes:** Codeine in No. 1 = 7.5 mg, No. 2 = 15 mg, No. 3 = 30 mg, No. 4 = 60 mg

Acetazolamide (Diamox)

Uses: *Diuresis, glaucoma, prevent high-altitude sickness, refractory epilepsy* **Action:** Carbonic anhydrase inhibitor; ↓ renal excretion of hydrogen & ↑ renal excretion of Na^+, K^+, HCO_3^-, & H_2O **Dose:** *Adults.* Diuretic: 250–375 mg IV or PO q24h. Glaucoma: 250–1000 mg PO q24h in ÷ doses. Epilepsy: 8–30 mg/kg/d PO in ÷ doses. Altitude sickness: 250 mg PO q8–12h or SR 500 mg PO q12–24h start 24–48 h before & 48 h after highest ascent. *Peds.* Epilepsy: 8–30 mg/kg/24 h PO in ÷ doses; max 1 g/d. Diuretic: 5 mg/kg/24 h PO or IV. Alkalinization of urine: 5 mg/kg/dose PO bid–tid. Glaucoma: 5–15 mg/kg/24 h PO in ÷ doses; max 1 g/d; adjust in renal impair; avoid if CrCl < 10 mL/min **Caution:** [C, +] **Contra:** Renal/hepatic failure, sulfa allergy **Supplied:** Tabs 125, 250 mg; SR caps 500 mg; inj 500 mg/vial **SE:** Malaise, metallic taste, drowsiness, photosensitivity, hyperglycemia **Notes:** Follow Na^+ & K^+; watch for metabolic acidosis; SR forms not for epilepsy

Acetic Acid & Aluminum Acetate (Otic Domeboro)

Uses: *Otitis externa* **Action:** Antiinfective **Dose:** 4–6 gtt in ear(s) q2–3h **Caution:** [C, ?] **Contra:** Perforated tympanic membranes **Supplied:** 2% otic soln **SE:** Local irritation

Acetylcysteine (Acetadote, Mucomyst)

Uses: *Mucolytic* adjuvant Rx for chronic bronchopulmonary Dzs & CF; *antidote to APAP hepatotox*

22

Action: Splits disulfide linkages between mucoprotein molecular complexes; protects liver by restoring glutathione in APAP OD **Dose:** *Adults & Peds.* Nebulizer: 3–5 mL of 20% soln diluted w/equal vol of H_2O or NS tid–qid. *Antidote:* PO or NG: 140 mg/kg load, then 70 mg/kg q4h for 17 doses. (Dilute 1:3 in carbonated beverage or orange juice). *Acetadote:* load 150 mg/kg over 15 min, then 50 mg/kg over 4h, then 100 mg/kg over 16h **Caution:** [C, ?] **Supplied:** Soln 10%, 20%; Acetadote IV soln **SE:** Bronchospasm (inhal), N/V, drowsiness; anaphylactoid Rxns w/IV **Notes:** Activated charcoal adsorbs acetylcysteine if given PO for APAP ingestion; start Rx for APAP overdose w/in 6–8 h

Acitretin (Soriatane) WARNING: Must not be used by women who are pregnant or intend to become pregnant during therapy or for up to 3 y after D/C of therapy; EtOH must not be ingested during therapy or for 2 mo after cessation of therapy; do not donate blood for 3 y after cessation **Uses:** *Severe psoriasis*; other keratinization disorders (eg, lichen planus) **Action:** Retinoid-like activity **Dose:** 25–50 mg/d PO, w/main meal; if no response by 4 wk ↑ to 75 mg/d **Caution:** [X, –] Renal/hepatic impair; in women of reproductive potential **Contra:** See Warning **Supplied:** Caps 10, 25 mg **SE:** Cheilitis, skin peeling, alopecia, pruritus, rash, arthralgia, GI upset, photosensitivity, thrombocytosis, hypertriglyceridemia **Notes:** Follow LFTs; response often takes 2–3 mo; pt agreement/informed consent before use

Acyclovir (Zovirax) **Uses:** *Herpes simplex & zoster Infxns* **Action:** Interferes w/viral DNA synthesis **Dose:** *Adults.* PO: Initial genital herpes: 200 mg PO q4h while awake, 5 caps/d × 10 d or 400 mg PO tid × 7–10 d. *Chronic suppression:* 400 mg PO bid. *Intermittent Rx:* As for initial Rx, except treat for 5 d, or 800 mg PO bid, at prodrome. *Herpes zoster:* 800 mg PO 5×/d for 7–10 d. *IV:* 5–10 mg/kg/dose IV q8h. *Topical: Initial herpes genitalis:* Apply q3h (6×/d) for 7 d. *Peds.* 5–10 mg/kg/dose IV or PO q8h or 750 mg/m²/24 h ÷ q8h. *Chickenpox:* 20 mg/kg/dose PO qid; ↓ for CrCl < 50 mL/min **Caution:** [B, +] **Supplied:** Caps 200 mg; tabs 400, 800 mg; susp 200 mg/5 mL; inj 500 mg/vial; oint 5% **SE:** Dizziness, lethargy, confusion, rash, inflammation at IV site **Notes:** PO better than topical for herpes genitalis

Adalimumab (Humira) WARNING: Cases of TB have been observed; check TB skin test before use **Uses:** *Moderate–severe RA w/inadequate response to one or more DMARDs* **Action:** TNF-α inhibitor **Dose:** 40 mg SQ qowk; may ↑ 40 mg qwk if not on MTX **Caution:** [B, ?/–] Serious Infxns & sepsis reported **Supplied:** Prefilled 1 mL (40 mg) syringe **SE:** Inj site Rxns, serious Infxns, neurologic events, malignancies **Notes:** Refrigerate prefilled syringe, rotate inj sites, OK w/other DMARDs

Adefovir (Hepsera) WARNING: Acute exacerbations of hepatitis may occur after therapy (monitor LFTs); chronic use may lead to nephrotox, especially in pts w/underlying renal impair (monitor renal Fxn); HIV resistance may emerge; lactic acidosis & severe hepatomegaly w/steatosis reported when used alone or in combo w/other antiretrovirals **Uses:** *Chronic active hepatitis B virus* **Action:** Nucleotide analog **Dose:** CrCl > 50 mL/min: 10 mg PO qd; CrCl 20–49 mL/min: 10 mg PO q48h; CrCl 10–19 mL/min: 10 mg PO q72h; HD: 10 mg PO q7d postdialysis; adjust w/CrCl < 50 mL/min **Caution:** [C, –] **Supplied:** Tabs 10 mg **SE:** Asthenia, HA, abdominal pain; see Warning

Adenosine (Adenocard) **Uses:** *PSVT*; including associated w/WPW **Action:** Class IV antiarrhythmic; slows AV node conduction **Dose:** *Adults.* 6

22

mg IV bolus; may repeat in 1–2 min; max 12 mg IV. *Peds.* 0.05 mg/kg IV bolus; may repeat q1–2 min to 0.25 mg/kg max **Caution:** [C, ?] **Contra:** 2nd- or 3rd-degree AV block or SSS (w/o pacemaker); recent MI or cerebral hemorrhage **Supplied:** Inj 6 mg/2 mL **SE:** Facial flushing, HA, dyspnea, chest pressure, ↓ BP **Notes:** Doses > 12 mg not OK; can cause momentary asystole when administered; caffeine, theophylline antagonize effects

Albumin (Albuminar, Buminate, Albutein)
Uses: *Plasma volume expansion for shock* (eg, burns, hemorrhage) **Action:** Maint of plasma colloid oncotic pressure **Dose:** *Adults.* Initial 25 g IV; subsequent dose based on response; 250 g/48h max. *Peds.* 0.5–1 g/kg/dose; inf at 0.05–0.1 g/min **Caution:** [C, ?] Severe anemia; cardiac, renal, or hepatic insuff due to added protein load & possible hypervolemia **Contra:** Cardiac failure **Supplied:** Soln 5%, 25% **SE:** Chills, fever, CHF, tachycardia, ↓ BP, hypervolemia **Notes:** Contains 130–160 mEq Na+/L; may precipitate pulmonary edema

Albuterol (Proventil, Ventolin, Volmax)
Uses: *Asthma; prevent exercise-induced bronchospasm* **Action:** β-Adrenergic sympathomimetic bronchodilator; relaxes bronchial smooth muscle **Dose:** *Adults.* Inhaler: 2 inhal q4–6h PRN; 1 Rotacap inhaled q4–6h. *PO:* 2–4 mg PO tid–qid. *Neb:* 1.25–5 mg (0.25–1 mL of 0.5% soln in 2–3 mL of NS) tid–qid. *Peds.* Inhaler: 2 inhal q4–6h. *PO:* 0.1–0.2 mg/kg/dose PO; max 2–4 mg PO tid *Neb:* 0.05 mg/kg (max 2.5 mg) in 2–3 mL of NS tid–qid **Caution:** [C, +] **Supplied:** Tabs 2, 4 mg; XR tabs 4, 8 mg; syrup 2 mg/5 mL; 90 mcg/dose met-dose inhaler; Rotacaps 200 mcg (Withdrawn from market); soln for neb 0.083, 0.5% **SE:** Palpitations, tachycardia, nervousness, GI upset

Albuterol & Ipratropium (Combivent)
Uses: *COPD* **Action:** Combo of β-adrenergic bronchodilator & quaternary anticholinergic **Dose:** 2 inhal qid **Caution:** [C, +] **Contra:** Peanut/soybean allergy **Supplied:** Met-dose inhaler, 18 mcg ipratropium/103 mcg albuterol/puff **SE:** Palpitations, tachycardia, nervousness, GI upset, dizziness, blurred vision

Aldesleukin, IL-2 (Proleukin)
WARNING: Use restricted to pts w/nl pulmonary & cardiac Fxn **Uses:** *Metastatic RCC, melanoma* **Action:** Acts via IL-2 receptor; numerous immunomodulatory effects **Dose:** 600,000 IU/kg q8h × 14 doses (FDA-approved dose/schedule for RCC). Multiple cont inf & alternate schedules (including "high dose" using 24×10^6 IU/m^2 IV q8h on d 1–5 & 12–16) **Caution:** [C, ?/–] **Contra:** Organ allografts **Supplied:** Inj 1.1 mg/mL (22×10^6 IU) **SE:** Flu-like syndrome (malaise, fever, chills), N/V/D, ↑ bilirubin; capillary leak syndrome w/↓ BP, pulmonary edema, fluid retention & weight gain; renal & mild hematologic tox (anemia, thrombocytopenia, leukopenia) & secondary eosinophilia; cardiac tox (ischemia, atrial arrhythmias); neurologic tox (CNS depression, somnolence, rarely coma, delirium). Pruritic rashes, urticaria & erythroderma common. **Notes:** Cont inf less likely to cause severe ↓ BP & fluid retention

Alefacept (Amevive)
WARNING: Must monitor CD4 before each dose; w/hold if < 250; D/C if < 250 × 1 month **Uses:** *Moderate/severe chronic plaque psoriasis* **Action:** Fusion protein inhibitor **Dose:** 7.5 mg IV or 15 mg IM once weekly × 12 wk **Caution:** [B, ?/–] PRG registry; associated w/serious Infxn **Contra:** Lymphopenia **Supplied:** 7.5-, 15-mg vials **SE:** Pharyngitis, myalgia, inj site Rxn, malignancy **Notes:** IV or IM different formulations; may repeat course 12 wk later if CD4 OK

22

Alendronate (Fosamax) Uses: *Rx & prevention of osteoporosis, Rx of steroid-induced osteoporosis & Paget Dz* **Action:** ↓ nl & abnormal bone resorption **Dose:** *Osteoporosis: Rx:* 10 mg/d PO or 70 mg qwk. *Steroid-induced osteoporosis: Rx:* 5 mg/d PO. *Prevention:* 5 mg/d PO or 35 mg qwk. *Paget Dz:* 40 mg/d PO **Caution:** [C, ?] Not OK if CrCl < 35 mL/min, w/NSAID use **Contra:** Esophageal anomalies, inability to sit/stand upright for 30 min, ↓ Ca^{2+} **Supplied:** Tabs 5, 10, 35, 40, 70 mg soln **SE:** GI disturbances, HA, pain, jaw osteonecrosis (w/dental procedures, chemo) **Notes:** Take 1st thing in AM w/H_2O (8 oz) > 30 min before 1st food/beverage of the day. Do not lie down for 30 min after. Use Ca^{2+} & vitamin D supl; Fosamax Plus D has 2,800 IU vitamin D; give one weekly

Alfentanil (Alfenta) [C-II] Uses: *Adjunct in the maint of anesthesia; analgesia* **Action:** Short-acting narcotic analgesic **Dose:** *Adults & Peds > 12 y.* 3–75 mcg/kg IV inf; total depends on duration of procedure **Caution:** [C, +/–] ↑ ICP, resp depression **Supplied:** Inj 500 mcg/mL **SE:** Bradycardia, ↓ BP arrhythmias, peripheral vasodilation, ↑ ICP, drowsiness, resp depression

Alfuzosin (Uroxatral) WARNING: May prolong QTc interval Uses: *BPH* **Action:** α-Blocker **Dose:** 10 mg PO daily immediately after the same meal **Caution:** [B, –] **Contra:** W/CYP3A4 inhibitors; moderate–severe hepatic impair **Supplied:** Tabs 10 mg **SE:** Postural ↓ BP, dizziness, HA, fatigue **Notes:** XR tablet—do not cut or crush; fewest reports of ejaculatory disorders compared w/other drugs in class

Alginic Acid + Aluminum Hydroxide & Magnesium Trisilicate (Gaviscon) [OTC] Uses: *Heartburn*; pain from hiatal hernia **Action:** Protective layer blocks gastric acid **Dose:** 2–4 tabs or 15–30 mL PO qid followed by H_2O; **Caution:** [B, –] Avoid in renal impair or Na^+-restricted diet **Supplied:** Tabs, susp **SE:** D, constipation

Allopurinol (Zyloprim, Lopurin, Aloprim) Uses: *Gout, hyperuricemia of malignancy, uric acid urolithiasis* **Action:** Xanthine oxidase inhibitor; ↓ uric acid production **Dose:** *Adults.* *PO:* Initial 100 mg/d; usual 300 mg/d; max 800 mg/d. *IV:* 200–400 mg/m^2/d (max 600 mg/24 h); (after meal w/plenty of fluid). *Peds.* Only for hyperuricemia of malignancy if < 10 y: 10 mg/kg/24 h PO or 200 mg/m^2/d IV ÷ q6–8h (max 600 mg/24 h); ↓ in renal impair **Caution:** [C, M] **Supplied:** Tabs 100, 300 mg; inj 500 mg/30 mL (Aloprim) **SE:** Rash, N/V, renal impair, angioedema **Notes:** Aggravates acute gout; begin after acute attack resolves; IV dose of 6 mg/mL final conc as single daily inf or ÷ 6, 8, or 12–h intervals

Almotriptan (Axert) See Table 22–11 (page 645)

Alosetron (Lotronex) WARNING: Serious GI side effects, some fatal, including ischemic colitis reported. May be prescribed only through participation in the prescribing program for Lotronex Uses: *Severe diarrhea-predominant IBS in women after failed conventional therapy* **Action:** Selective 5-HT_3 receptor antagonist **Dose:** *Adults.* 1 mg PO qd × 4 wk; titrate to 1 mg bid max; D/C after 4 wk at max dose if Sxs not controlled **Caution:** [B, ?/–] **Contra:** Hx chronic/severe constipation, GI obstruction, strictures, toxic megacolon, GI perforation, adhesions, ischemic colitis, Crohn Dz, ulcerative colitis, diverticulitis, thrombophlebitis, or hypercoagulable state. **Supplied:** Tabs 1 mg **SE:** Constipation, abdominal pain, nausea **Notes:** D/C immediately if constipation or Sxs of ischemic colitis develop; pt must sign informed consent before use

22

Alpha₁-Protease Inhibitor (Prolastin) **Uses:** *α₁-Antitrypsin deficiency*; panacinar emphysema **Action:** Replace human α₁-protease inhibitor **Dose:** 60 mg/kg IV once/wk **Caution:** [C, ?] **Contra:** Selective IgA deficiencies w/ known IgA antibodies **Supplied:** Inj 500 mg/20 mL, 1000 mg/40 mL **SE:** Fever, dizziness, flu-like Sxs, allergic Rxns

Alprazolam (Xanax) [C-IV] **Uses:** *Anxiety & panic disorders,* anxiety w/depression **Action:** Benzodiazepine; antianxiety agent **Dose:** *Anxiety:* Initial, 0.25–0.5 mg tid; ↑ to a max of 4 mg/d in ÷ doses. *Panic:* Initial, 0.5 mg tid; may gradually ↑ to response; ↓ in elderly, debilitated & hepatic impair **Caution:** [D, –] **Contra:** NAG, w/itra-/ketoconazole **Supplied:** Tabs 0.25, 0.5, 1, 2 mg; soln 1 mg/mL **SE:** Drowsiness, fatigue, irritability, memory impair, sexual dysfunction **Notes:** Avoid abrupt D/C after prolonged use

Alprostadil [Prostaglandin E₁] (Prostin VR) **Uses:** *Conditions where blood flow must be maintained in ductus arteriosus* sustain pulmonary/systemic circulation until surgery (eg, pulmonary atresia/stenosis, tricuspid atresia, transposition, severe tetralogy of Fallot) **Action:** Vasodilator, plt inhibitor; ductus arteriosus smooth muscle is especially sensitive **Dose:** 0.05 mcg/kg/min IV; ↓ to lowest that maintains response **Caution:** [X, –] **Contra:** Neonatal resp distress syndrome **Supplied:** Injectable forms **SE:** Cutaneous vasodilation, Sz-like activity, jitteriness, ↑ temp, ↓ Ca²⁺, apnea, thrombocytopenia, ↓ BP; may cause apnea **Notes:** Keep intubation kit at bedside if pt is not intubated

Alprostadil, Intracavernosal (Caverject, Edex) **Uses:** *Erectile dysfunction* **Action:** Relaxes smooth muscles, dilates cavernosal arteries, ↑ lacunar spaces and blood entrapment by compressing venules against tunica **Dose:** 2.5–60 mcg intracavernosal; titrate at physician's office **Caution:** [X, –] **Contra:** Predisposition to priapism (eg, sickle cell); penile deformities/implants; men in whom sexual activity is inadvisable **Supplied:** *Caverject:* 6–5, 6–10, 6–20, 6–49 mcg vials ± diluent syringes. *Caverject Impulse:* Self-contained syringe (29 gauge) 10 & 20 mcg. *Edex cartridges:* 10, 20, 40 mcg **SE:** Local pain w/inj **Notes:** Counsel about priapism, penile fibrosis & hematoma risks, titrate w/Obs

Alprostadil, Urethral Suppository (Muse) **Uses:** *Erectile dysfunction* **Action:** Urethral mucosal absorption; vasodilator, smooth muscle relaxant of corpus cavernosa **Dose:** 125–1000 mcg system 5–10 min before sexual activity; titrate at physician's office **Caution:** [X, –] **Contra:** Predisposition to priapism (eg, sickle cell) penile deformities/implants; men for whom sexual activity is inadvisable **Supplied:** 125, 250, 500, 1000 mcg w/transurethral delivery system **SE:** ↓ BP, dizziness, syncope, penile/testicular pain, urethral burning/bleeding, priapism **Notes:** Supervision, titrate w/Obs

Alteplase, Recombinant [tPA] (Activase) **Uses:** *AMI, PE, acute ischemic stroke & CV cath occlusion* **Action:** Thrombolytic; binds to fibrin in the thrombus, initiates local fibrinolysis **Dose:** *AMI & PE:* 100 mg IV over 3 h (10 mg over 2 min, then 50 mg over 1 h, then 40 mg over 2 h). *Stroke:* 0.9 mg/kg (max 90 mg) inf over 60 min. *Cath occlusion:* 10–29 kg 1 mg/mL, ≥ 30 kg 2 mg/mL **Caution:** [C, ?] **Contra:** Active internal bleeding; uncontrolled HTN (systolic BP = > 185 mm Hg/diastolic = > 110 mm Hg); recent (w/in 3 mo) CVA, GI bleed, trauma, surgery, prolonged external cardiac massage; intracranial neoplasm, suspected aortic dissection, AVM/aneurysm/subarachnoid hemorrhage, bleeding/hemostatic defects, Sz at the time of stroke **Supplied:** Powder for inj 50, 100 mg **SE:** Bleeding, bruising (eg, venipuncture sites), ↓ BP **Notes:** Give heparin to prevent reocclusion; in AMI, doses of > 150 mg associated w/ intracranial bleeding

Altretamine (Hexalen) **Uses:** *Epithelial ovarian CA* **Action:** Unknown; cytotoxic agent, unknown alkylating agent; ↓ nucleotide incorporation into DNA/RNA **Dose:** 260 mg/m^2/d in 4 ÷ doses for 14–21 d of a 28-d Rx cycle; dose ↑ to 150 mg/m^2/d for 14 d in multiagent regimens (per protocols) **Caution:** [D, ?/–]. **Contra:** Preexisting BM depression or neurologic tox **Supplied:** Caps 50 mg **SE:** V/D, cramps; neurologic (peripheral neuropathy, CNS depression); minimally myelosuppressive

Aluminum Hydroxide (Amphojel, AlternaGEL) [OTC] **Uses:** *Relief of heartburn, upset or sour stomach, acid indigestion*; supl to Rx of hyperphosphatemia **Action:** Neutralizes gastric acid; binds PO_4^{-2} **Dose:** *Adults.* 10–30 mL or 2 tabs PO q4–6h. *Peds.* 5–15 mL PO q4–6h or 50–150 mg/kg/24 h PO ÷ q4–6h (hyperphosphatemia) **Caution:** [C, ?] **Supplied:** Tabs 300, 600 mg; chew tabs 500 mg; susp 320, 600 mg/5 mL **SE:** Constipation **Notes:** OK in renal failure

Aluminum Hydroxide + Magnesium Carbonate (Gaviscon) [OTC] **Uses:** *Relief of heartburn, acid indigestion* **Action:** Neutralizes gastric acid **Dose:** *Adults.* 15–30 mL PO pc & hs. *Peds.* 5–15 mL PO qid or PRN; avoid in renal impair **Caution:** [C, ?] **Supplied:** Liq w/aluminum hydroxide 95 mg + magnesium carbonate 358 mg/15 mL **SE:** May cause ↑ Mg^{2+} (w/renal insuff), constipation, D **Notes:** Doses qid are best given pc & hs; may affect absorption of some drugs

Aluminum Hydroxide + Magnesium Hydroxide (Maalox) [OTC] **Uses:** *Hyperacidity* (peptic ulcer, hiatal hernia, etc) **Action:** Neutralizes gastric acid **Dose:** *Adults.* 10–60 mL or 2–4 tabs PO qid or PRN. *Peds.* 5–15 mL PO qid or PRN **Caution:** [C, ?] **Supplied:** Tabs, susp **SE:** May cause ↑ Mg^{2+} in renal insuff, constipation, D **Notes:** Doses qid best given pc & hs

Aluminum Hydroxide + Magnesium Hydroxide & Simethicone (Mylanta, Mylanta II, Maalox Plus) [OTC] **Uses:** *Hyperacidity w/ bloating* **Action:** Neutralizes gastric acid & defoaming **Dose:** *Adults.* 10–60 mL or 2–4 tabs PO qid or PRN. *Peds.* 5–15 mL PO qid or PRN; avoid in renal impair **Caution:** [C, ?] **Supplied:** Tabs, susp **SE:** ↑ Mg^{2+} in renal insuff, D, constipation **Notes:** Mylanta II contains 2× aluminum & magnesium hydroxide of Mylanta; may affect absorption of some drugs

Aluminum Hydroxide + Magnesium Trisilicate (Gaviscon, Gaviscon-2) [OTC] **Uses:** *Relief of heartburn, upset or sour stomach, or acid indigestion* **Action:** Neutralizes gastric acid **Dose:** Chew 2–4 tabs qid; avoid in renal impair **Caution:** [C, ?] **Contra:** Mg^{2+}, sensitivity **Supplied:** *Gaviscon:* Aluminum hydroxide 80 mg & magnesium trisilicate 20 mg; *Gaviscon-2:* Aluminum hydroxide 160 mg & magnesium trisilicate 40 mg **SE:** ↑ Mg^{2+} in renal insuff, constipation, D **Notes:** May affect absorption of some drugs

Amantadine (Symmetrel) **Uses:** *Rx or prophylaxis influenza A viral Infxns, parkinsonism & drug-induced EPS* **Action:** Prevents release of infectious viral nucleic acid into host cell; releases dopamine from intact dopaminergic terminals **Dose:** *Adults.* Influenza A: 200 mg/d PO or 100 mg PO bid. *Parkinsonism:* 100 mg PO qd–bid. *Peds. 1–9 y:* 4.4–8.8 mg/kg/24 h to 150 mg/ 24 h max ÷ doses daily bid. *10–12 y:* 100–200 mg/d in 1–2 ÷ doses; ↓ in renal

22

impair **Caution:** [C, M] **Supplied:** Caps 100 mg; tabs 100 mg; soln 50 mg/5 mL **SE:** Orthostatic ↓ BP, edema, insomnia, depression, irritability, hallucinations, dream abnormalities

Amifostine (Ethyol) **Uses:** *Xerostomia prophylaxis during RT (head, neck, ovarian, non-small-cell lung CA). ↓ renal tox associated w/repeated administration of cisplatin* **Action:** Prodrug, dephosphorylated by alkaline phosphatase to active thiol metabolite **Dose:** 910 mg/m²/d 15-min IV inf 30 min before chemo **Caution:** [C, +/−] **Supplied:** 500-mg vials lyophilized w/500 mg of mannitol, reconstitute in sterile NS **SE:** Transient ↓ BP (> 60%), N/V, flushing w/hot or cold chills, dizziness, ↓ Ca²⁺, somnolence, sneezing. **Notes:** Does not ↓ effectiveness of cyclophosphamide plus cisplatin chemo

Amikacin (Amikin) **Uses:** *Serious gram(−) bacterial Infxns* & mycobacteria Infxn **Action:** Aminoglycoside; ↓ protein synthesis *Spectrum:* Good gram(−) bacterial coverage: *Pseudomonas* sp; *Mycobacterium* sp **Dose:** *Adults & Peds.* 5–7.5 mg/kg/dose ÷ q8–24h based on renal Fxn. *Neonates < 1200 g, 0–4 wk:* 7.5 mg/kg/dose q12h–18h. *Postnatal age < 7 d, 1200–2000 g:* 7.5 mg/kg/dose q12h. *> 2000 g:* 10 mg/kg/dose q12h. *Postnatal age > 7 d, 1200–2000 g:* 7 mg/kg/dose q8h. *> 2000 g:* 7.5–10 mg/kg/dose q8h **Caution:** [C, +/−] **Supplied:** Inj 100, 500 mg/2 mL **SE:** Nephro/oto/neurotox; avoid use w/diuretics **Notes:** May be effective against gram(−) bacteria resistant to gentamicin & tobramycin; monitor renal Fxn for dosage adjustments; monitor levels (Table 22–2, page 628)

Amiloride (Midamor) **Uses:** *HTN, CHF & thiazide-induced ↓ K⁺* **Action:** K⁺-sparing diuretic; interferes w/K⁺/Na⁺ exchange in distal tubule **Dose:** *Adults.* 5–10 mg PO daily. *Peds.* 0.625 mg/kg/d; ↓ in renal impair **Caution:** [B, ?] **Contra:** ↑ K⁺, SCr > 1.5, BUN > 30 **Supplied:** Tabs 5 mg **SE:** ↑ K⁺ possible; monitor K⁺; HA, dizziness, dehydration, impotence

Amino Acid Cervical Cream (Amino-Cerv pH 5.5 Cream) **Uses:** *Mild cervicitis,* postpartum cervicitis/cervical tears, postcauterization, postcryosurgery & postconization **Action:** Hydrating agent; removes excess keratin in hyperkeratotic conditions **Dose:** 1 Applicatorful intravag hs for 2–4 wk **Caution:** [C, ?] Use in viral skin Infxn **Supplied:** Vaginal cream **SE:** Transient stinging, local irritation **Notes:** AKA carbamide or urea; contains 8.34% urea, 0.5% sodium propionate, 0.83% methionine, 0.35% cystine, 0.83% inositol & benzalkonium chloride

Aminocaproic Acid (Amicar) **Uses:** *Excessive bleeding from systemic hyperfibrinolysis & urinary fibrinolysis* **Action:** ↓ fibrinolysis via inhibition of TPA substances **Dose:** *Adults.* 5 g IV or PO (1st h) followed by 1–1.25 g/h IV or PO (max dose/d: 30 g) *Peds.* 100 mg/kg IV (1st h) then 1 g/m²/h; max 18 g/m²/d; ↓ in renal failure **Caution:** [C, ?] Upper urinary tract bleeding **Contra:** DIC **Supplied:** Tabs 500 mg; syrup 250 mg/mL; inj 250 mg/mL **SE:** ↓ BP, bradycardia, dizziness, HA, fatigue, rash, GI disturbance, ↓ plt Fxn **Notes:** Administer for 8 h or until bleeding controlled; not for upper urinary tract bleeding

Aminoglutethimide (Cytadren) **Uses:** Adrenocortical carcinoma, *Cushing syndrome,* breast CA & CAP **Action:** ↓ adrenal steroidogenesis & conversion of androgens to estrogens **Dose:** 750–1500 mg/d in divided doses plus hydrocortisone 20–40 mg/d; ↓ in renal insuff **Caution:** [D, ?] **Supplied:** Tabs 250 mg **SE:** Adrenal insuff ("medical adrenalectomy"), hypothyroidism, masculinization, ↓ BP, V, rare hepatotox, rash, myalgia, fever

22

Aminophylline Uses: *Asthma, COPD* & bronchospasm **Action:** Relaxes smooth muscle (bronchi, pulmonary vessels); stimulates diaphragm **Dose:** *Adults.* *Acute asthma:* Load 6 mg/kg IV, then 0.4–0.9 mg/kg/h IV cont inf. *Chronic asthma:* 24 mg/kg/24 h PO or PR ÷ q6h. *Peds.* Load 6 mg/kg IV, then 1 mg/kg/h IV cont inf; ↓ in hepatic insuff & w/certain drugs (macrolide & quinolone antibiotics, cimetidine & propranolol) **Caution:** [C, +] Uncontrolled arrhythmias/Sz disorder, hyperthyroidism, peptic ulcers **Supplied:** Tabs 100, 200 mg; soln 105 mg/5 mL; supp 250, 500 mg; inj 25 mg/mL **SE:** N/V, irritability, tachycardia, ventricular arrhythmias, Szs **Notes:** Individualize dosage; follow levels (as theophylline, Table 22–2, page 628); aminophylline ≈85% theophylline; erratic rectal absorption

Amiodarone (Cordarone, Pacerone) Uses: *Recurrent VF or hemodynamically unstable VT,* supraventricular arrhythmias, AF **Action:** Class III antiarrhythmic (see Table 22–12, page 646) **Dose:** *Adults.* *Ventricular arrhythmias: IV:* 15 mg/min for 10 min, then 1 mg/min for 6 h, then maint 0.5 mg/min cont inf or *PO:* Load: 800–1600 mg/d PO for 1–3 wk. Maint: 600–800 mg/d PO for 1 mo, then 200–400 mg/d. *Supraventricular arrhythmias: IV:* 300 mg IV over 1 h, then 20 mg/kg for 24 h, then 600 mg PO qd for 1 wk, then maint 100–400 mg qd or *PO:* Load: 600–800 mg/d PO for 1–4 wk. Maint: Gradually ↓ to 100–400 mg q d. *Peds.* 10–15 mg/kg/24 h ÷ q12h PO for 7–10 d, then 5 mg/kg/24 h ÷ q12h or daily (infants/neonates need higher loading); ↓ in liver insuff **Caution:** [D, –] **Contra:** Sinus node dysfunction, 2nd- or 3rd-degree AV block, sinus bradycardia (w/o pacemaker) **Supplied:** Tabs 200 mg; inj 50 mg/mL **SE:** Pulmonary fibrosis, exacerbation of arrhythmias, prolongs QT interval; CHF, hypo-/hyperthyroidism, ↑ LFTs, liver failure, corneal microdeposits, optic neuropathy/neuritis, peripheral neuropathy, photosensitivity **Notes:** Half-life 53 d; IV conc of > 0.2 mg/mL via a central catheter; may require ↓ digoxin and warfarin dose

Amitriptyline (Elavil) WARNING: Antidepressants may ↑ risk of suicidality; consider risks and benefits of use. Monitor patients closely Uses: *Depression,* peripheral neuropathy, chronic pain, tension HA **Action:** TCA; ↓ reuptake of serotonin & norepinephrine by presynaptic neurons **Dose:** *Adults.* Initial, 30–50 mg PO hs; may ↑ to 300 mg hs. *Peds.* Not OK < 12 y unless for chronic pain; initial 0.1 mg/kg PO hs, ↑ over 2–3 wk to 0.5–2 mg/kg PO hs; taper when D/C **Caution:** [D, +/–] NAG, hepatic impair **Contra:** W/MAOIs, during AMI recovery **Supplied:** Tabs 10, 25, 50, 75, 100, 150 mg; inj 10 mg/mL **SE:** Strong anticholinergic SEs; OD may be fatal; urine retention, sedation, ECG changes, photosensitivity

Amlodipine (Norvasc) Uses: *HTN, stable or unstable angina* **Action:** CCB; relaxes coronary vascular smooth muscle **Dose:** 2.5–10 mg/d PO **Caution:** [C, ?] **Supplied:** Tabs 2.5, 5, 10 mg **SE:** Peripheral edema, HA, palpitations, flushing **Notes:** Take w/o regard to meals

Amlodipine/Atorvastatin (Caduet) Uses: *HTN, chronic stable/vasospastic angina, control cholesterol & triglycerides* **Action:** CCB & HMG-CoA reductase inhibitor **Dose:** Amlodipine 2.5–10 mg PO qd/Atorvastatin 10–80 mg PO qd **Caution:** [X, –] **Contra:** Active liver Dz, ↑ serum transaminases **Supplied:** Tabs amlodipine/atorvastatin: 2.5/10, 2.5/20, 2.5/40, 5/10, 5/20, 5/40, 5/80, 10/10, 10/20, 10/40, 10/80 mg **SE:** Peripheral edema, HA, palpitations, flushing, myopathy, arthralgia, myalgia, GI upset **Notes:** Monitor LFTs

22

Ammonium Aluminum Sulfate [Alum] [OTC] Uses: *Hemorrhagic cystitis when saline bladder irrigation fails* Action: Astringent Dose: 1–2% soln w/constant NS bladder irrigation Caution: [+/–] Supplied: Powder for reconstitution SE: Encephalopathy possible; obtain aluminum levels, especially in renal insuff; can precipitate & occlude catheters Notes: Safe to use w/o anesthesia & w/vesicoureteral reflux

Amoxicillin (Amoxil, Polymox) Uses: *Ear, nose & throat, lower resp, skin, urinary tract Infxns resulting from susceptible gram(+) bacteria* endocarditis prophylaxis Action: β-Lactam antibiotic; ↓ cell wall synthesis *Spectrum:* Gram(+) (*Strep* sp, *Enterococcus* sp); some gram(–) (*H. influenzae, E. coli, N. gonorrhoeae, H. pylori* & *P. mirabilis*) Dose: *Adults.* 250–500 mg PO tid or 500–875 mg bid. *Peds.* 25–100 mg/kg/24 h PO ÷ q8h. 200–400 mg PO bid (equivalent to 125–250 mg tid); ↓ in renal impair Caution: [B, +] Supplied: Caps 250, 500 mg; chew tabs 125, 200, 250, 400 mg; susp 50 mg/mL, 125, 200, 250 & 400 mg/5 mL; tabs 500, 875 mg SE: D; rash common Notes: Cross hypersensitivity PCN; many strains of *E. coli* resistant

Amoxicillin & Clavulanic Acid (Augmentin, Augmentin 600 ES, Augmentin XR) Uses: *Ear, lower resp, sinus, urinary tract, skin Infxns caused by β-lactamase-producing H. influenzae, S. aureus & E. coli* Action: Combo β-lactam antibiotic & β-lactamase inhibitor. *Spectrum:* Gram(+) same as amox alone, MSSA; gram(–) as w/amox alone, β-lactamase–producing *H. influenzae, Klebsiella* sp, *M. catarrhalis* Dose: *Adults.* 250–500 mg PO q8h or 875 mg q12h; XR 2000 mg PO Q12H. *Peds.* 20–40 mg/kg/d as amoxicillin PO ÷ q8h or 45 mg/kg/d ÷ q12h; ↓ in renal impair; take w/food Caution: [B, ?] Supplied (as amoxicillin/clavulanic acid): Tabs 250/125, 500/125, 875/125 mg; chew tabs 125/31.25, 200/28.5, 250/62.5, 400/57 mg; susp 125/31.25, 250/62.5, 200/28.5, 400/57 mg/5 mL; 600-ES 600/42.9 mg tab; XR tab 1000/62.5 mg SE: Abdominal discomfort, N/V/D, allergic Rxn, vaginitis Notes: Do not substitute two 250-mg tabs for one 500-mg tab (OD of clavulanic acid)

Amphotericin B (Fungizone) Uses: *Severe, systemic fungal Infxns; oral & cutaneous candidiasis* Action: Binds ergosterol in the fungal membrane to alter permeability Dose: *Adults & Peds.* Test dose: 1 mg IV adults or 0.1 mg/kg to 1 mg IV in children; then 0.25–1.5 mg/kg/24 h IV over 2–6 h (range 25–50 mg/d or qod). Total dose varies w/indication. *PO:* 1 mL qid. *Topical:* Apply bid–qid for 1–4 wk depending on Infxn; ↓ in renal impair Caution: [B, ?] Supplied: Powder for inj 50 mg/vial; PO susp 100 mg/mL; cream, lotion, oint 3% SE: ↓ K⁺/Mg²⁺ from renal wasting; anaphylaxis reported, HA, fever, chills, nephrotoxicity, ↓ BP, anemia Notes: Monitor renal Fxn/LFTs; pretreatment w/APAP & antihistamines (Benadryl) minimizes adverse IV effects (eg, fever, chills)

Amphotericin B Cholesteryl (Amphotec) Uses: *Aspergillosis in pts intolerant or refractory to conventional amphotericin B,* systemic candidiasis Action: Binds sterols in the cell membrane, alters permeability Dose: *Adults & Peds.* Test dose 1.6–8.3 mg, over 15–20 min, then 3–4 mg/kg/d; 1 mg/kg/h inf; ↓ in renal insuff Caution: [B, ?] Supplied: Powder for inj 50 mg, 100 mg/vial (final = 0.6 mg/mL) SE: Anaphylaxis reported; fever, chills, HA, ↓ K⁺, ↓ Mg²⁺, nephrotox, ↓ BP, anemia Notes: Do not use in-line filter; monitor LFT & electrolytes

Amphotericin B Lipid Complex (Abelcet) Uses: *Refractory invasive fungal Infxn in pts intolerant to conventional amphotericin B* Action: Binds sterols in cell membrane, alters permeability Dose: *Adults & Peds.* 5 mg/kg/d IV single daily dose; 2.5 mg/kg/h inf **Caution:** [B, ?] **Supplied:** Inj 5 mg/mL **SE:** Anaphylaxis; fever, chills, HA, ↓ K+, ↓ Mg2+, nephrotox, ↓ BP, anemia **Notes:** Filter soln w/5-mm filter needle; do not mix in electrolyte-containing solns; if inf > 2 h, manually mix bag

Amphotericin B Liposomal (AmBisome) Uses: *Refractory invasive fungal Infxn in pts intolerant to conventional amphotericin B, cryptococcal meningitis in HIV, empiric Rx of febrile neutropenia, visceral leishmaniasis* **Action:** Binds to sterols in cell membrane, changes membrane permeability **Dose:** *Adults & Peds.* 3–5 mg/kg/d, inf 60–120 min; ↓ in renal insuff **Caution:** [B, ?] **Supplied:** Powder for inj 50 mg **SE:** Anaphylaxis reported; fever, chills, HA, ↓ K+, ↓ Mg2+ nephrotox, ↓ BP, anemia **Notes:** Use no less than 1-μm filter

Ampicillin (Amcill, Omnipen) Uses: *Resp, GU, or GI tract Infxns, meningitis due to gram(–) & gram(+) bacteria; endocarditis prophylaxis* **Action:** β-Lactam antibiotic; ↓ cell wall synthesis. *Spectrum:* Gram(+) (*Streptococcus* sp, *Staphylococcus* sp, *Listeria*); gram(–) (*Klebsiella* sp, *E. coli, H. influenzae, P. mirabilis, Shigella* sp, *Salmonella* sp) **Dose:** *Adults.* 500 mg–2 g IM or IV q6h or 250–500 mg PO q6h. *Peds. Neonates < 7 d:* 50–100 mg/kg/24 h ÷ q8h. *Term infants:* 75–150 mg/kg/24 h ÷ q6–8h IV or PO. *Children > 1 mo:* 100–200 mg/kg/24 h ÷ q4–6h IM or IV; 50–100 mg/kg/24 h ÷ q6h PO up to 250 mg/dose. *Meningitis:* 200–400 mg/kg/24 h ÷ q4–6h IV; ↓ in renal impair; take on empty stomach **Caution:** [B, M] Cross hypersensitivity w/PCN **Supplied:** Caps 250, 500 mg; susp 100 mg/mL (reconstituted as drops), 125 mg/5 mL, 250 mg/5 mL, 500 mg/5 mL; powder for inj 125 mg, 250 mg, 500 mg, 1 g, 2 g, 10 g/ vial **SE:** D, rash, allergic Rxn **Notes:** Many strains of *E. coli* resistant

Ampicillin–Sulbactam (Unasyn) Uses: *Gynecologic, intraabdominal, skin Infxns caused by β-lactamase–producing strains of *S. aureus, Enterococcus, H. influenzae, P. mirabilis* & *Bacteroides* sp* **Action:** Combo β-lactam antibiotic & β-lactamase inhibitor. *Spectrum:* Gram(+) & gram(–) as for amp alone; also *Enterobacter, Acinetobacter, Bacteroides* **Dose:** *Adults.* 1.5–3 g IM or IV q6h. *Peds.* 100–200 mg ampicillin/kg/d (150–300 mg Unasyn) q6h; ↓ in renal failure **Caution:** [B, M] **Supplied:** Powder for inj 1.5, 3.0 g/vial **SE:** Allergy Rxns, rash, D, pain at injection site **Notes:** 2:1 ratio ampicillin:sulbactam

Amprenavir (Agenerase) WARNING: PO soln contra in children < 4 y (potential tox from large volume of polypropylene glycol in formulation) **Uses:** *HIV Infxn* **Action:** Protease inhibitor; prevents the maturation of virion to mature virus **Dose:** *Adults.* 1200 mg bid. *Peds.* 20 mg/kg bid or 15 mg/kg tid up to 2400 mg/d **Caution:** [C, ?] CDC recommends HIV-infected mothers not breast feed (risk of HIV transmission); Hx sulfonamides allergy **Contra:** CYP450 3A4 substrates (ergot derivatives, midazolam, triazolam, etc); soln < 4 y, PRG, hepatic or renal failure, disulfiram, or metronidazole **Supplied:** Caps 50, 150 mg; soln 15 mg/mL **SE:** Life-threatening rash, hyperglycemia, hypertriglyceridemia, fat redistribution, N/V/D, depression **Notes:** Caps & soln contain vitamin E exceeding RDA; avoid high-fat meals; many drug interactions

Anakinra (Kineret) WARNING: Associated w/↑ incidence of serious Infxn; D/C w/serious Infxn **Uses:** *Reduce signs & Sxs of moderate/severe active RA, failed 1 or more DMARD * **Action:** Human IL-1 receptor antagonist **Dose:** 100 mg SQ qd **Caution:** [B, ?] **Contra:** Allergy to *E. coli*–derived proteins, active Infxn, < 18 y **Supplied:** 100-mg prefilled syringes **SE:** Neutropenia, especially when used w/TNF-blocking agents, inj site Rxn, Infxn

22

Anastrozole (Arimidex) Uses: *Breast CA: postmenopausal w/metastatic breast CA, adjuvant Rx of postmenopausal w/early hormone-receptor(+) breast CA* **Action:** Selective nonsteroidal aromatase inhibitor, ↓ circ estradiol **Dose:** 1 mg/d **Caution:** [C, ?] **Contra:** PRG **Supplied:** Tabs 1 mg **SE:** May ↑ cholesterol; D, HTN, flushing, ↑ bone & tumor pain, HA, somnolence **Notes:** No effect on adrenal corticosteroids or aldosterone

Anistreplase (Eminase) Uses: *AMI* **Action:** Thrombolytic; activates conversion of plasminogen to plasmin, ↑ thrombolysis **Dose:** 30 units IV over 2–5 min **Caution:** [C, ?] **Contra:** Active internal bleeding, Hx CVA, recent (< 2 mo) intracranial or intraspinal surgery/trauma, intracranial neoplasm, A–V malformation, aneurysm, bleeding diathesis, severe uncontrolled HTN **Supplied:** Vials w/30 units **SE:** Bleeding, ↓ BP, hematoma **Notes:** Ineffective if readministered > 5 d after previous dose of anistreplase or streptokinase, or streptococcal Infxn (production of antistreptokinase Ab)

Anthralin (Anthra-Derm) Uses: *Psoriasis* **Action:** Keratolytic **Dose:** Apply qd **Caution:** [C, ?] **Contra:** Acutely inflamed psoriatic eruptions, erythroderma **Supplied:** Cream, oint 0.1, 0.2, 0.25, 0.4, 0.5, 1% **SE:** Irritation; hair/fingernails/skin discoloration

Antihemophilic Factor, AHF, Factor VIII (Monoclate) Uses: *Classic hemophilia A, von Willebrand Dz* **Action:** Provides factor VIII needed to convert prothrombin to thrombin **Dose:** *Adults & Peds.* 1 AHF unit/kg ↑ factor VIII level ≈2%. Units required = (kg) (desired factor VIII ↑ as % nl) × (0.5). Prevent spontaneous hemorrhage = 5% nl. Hemostasis after trauma/surgery = 30% nl. Head injuries, major surgery, or bleeding = 80–100% nl. Determine pt's % of nl factor VIII before dosing **Caution:** [C, ?] **Supplied:** Check each vial for units contained **SE:** Rash, fever, HA, chills, N/V

Antithymocyte Globulin. See Lymphocyte Immune Globulin, page 562

Apomorphine (Apokyn) WARNING: Do not administer IV Uses: *Acute, intermittent hypomobility ("off") episodes of Parkinson Dz* **Action:** Dopamine agonist **Dose:** *Adults.* 0.2–mL SQ test dose under medical supervision; if BP OK, initial 0.2 mL SQ during "off" periods; only 1 dose per "off" period; requires careful titration; 0.6 mL max single doses; requires concomitant antiemetic; ↓ in renal impair **Caution:** [C, +/−] Avoid EtOH; antihypertensives, vasodilators, cardio or cerebrovascular Dz, hepatic impair **Contra:** $5HT_3$ antagonists, sulfite allergy **Supplied:** Inj 10 mg/mL, 3-mL prefilled pen cartridges; 2–mL amp **SE:** Emesis, syncope, QT prolongation, orthostatic ↓ BP, somnolence, ischemia, injection site Rxn, abuse potential, dyskinesia, fibrotic conditions, priapism **Notes:** Potential for daytime somnolence may limit activities; trimethobenzamide 300 mg tid PO or other non-$5HT_3$ antagonist antiemetic given 3 d before & up to 2 mo after initiation

Apraclonidine (Iopidine) Uses: *Glaucoma, postop intraocular HTN* **Action:** α_2-Adrenergic agonist **Dose:** 1–2 gtt of 0.5% tid **Caution:** [C, ?] **Contra:** MAOI use **Supplied:** 0.5, 1% soln **SE:** Ocular irritation, lethargy, xerostomia

Aprepitant (Emend) Uses: *Prevents N/V assoc w/emetogenic CA chemo (eg, cisplatin) (use in combo w/other antiemetics)* **Action:** Substance P/neurokinin 1 (NK_1) receptor antagonist **Dose:** 125 mg PO d 1, 1 h before chemo, then 80 mg PO q AM on d 2 & 3 **Caution:** [B, ?/−]; substrate & moderate inhibitor of CYP3A4; inducer of CYP2C9 **Contra:** Use w/pimozide **Supplied:** Caps 80,

125 mg **SE:** Fatigue, asthenia, hiccups **Notes:** ↓ Effectiveness of PO contraceptives; ↓ effect of warfarin

Aprotinin (Trasylol) **Uses:** *↓/Prevents blood loss during CABG* **Action:** Protease inhibitor, antifibrinolytic **Dose:** 1-mL IV test dose. *High dose:* 2 million KIU load, 2 million KIU to prime pump, then 500,000 KIU/h until surgery ends. *Low dose:* 1 million KIU load, 1 million KIU to prime pump, then 250,000 KIU/h until surgery ends; 7 million KIU max total **Caution:** [B, ?] Thromboembolic Dz requiring anticoagulants or blood factor administration; FDA Advisory 2/2006: may be associated with ↑ risk of kidney problems, MI and stroke **Supplied:** Inj 1.4 mg/mL (10,000 KIU/mL) **SE:** AF, MI, heart failure, dyspnea, postop renal dysfunction **Notes:** 1000/KIU = 0.14 mg of aprotinin

Ardeparin (Normiflo) (Withdrawn from market)

Argatroban (Acova) **Uses:** *Prophylaxis or Rx of thrombosis in HIT, PCI in pts w/risk of HIT* **Action:** Anticoagulant, direct thrombin inhibitor **Dose:** 2 mcg/kg/min IV; adjust until aPTT 1.5–3 × baseline not to exceed 100 s; 10 mcg/kg/min max; ↓ in hepatic impair **Caution:** [B, ?] Avoid PO anticoagulants, ↑ bleeding risk; avoid concomitant use of thrombolytics **Contra:** Overt major bleed **Supplied:** Inj 100 mg/mL **SE:** AF, cardiac arrest, cerebrovascular disorder, ↓ BP, VT, N/V/D, sepsis, cough, renal tox, ↓ Hgb **Note:** Steady state in 1–3h

Aripiprazole (Abilify) **WARNING:** Increased mortality in elderly with dementia-related psychosis **Uses:** *Schizophrenia* **Action:** Dopamine & serotonin antagonist **Dose:** *Adults.* 10–15 mg PO qd; ↓ when used w/potent CYP3A4 or CYP2D6 inhibitors (page 647); ↑ when used w/inducer of CYP3A4 **Caution:** [C, –] **Supplied:** Tabs 5, 10, 15, 20, 30 mg; soln 1 mg/ml **SE:** Neuroleptic malignant syndrome, tardive dyskinesia, orthostatic ↓ BP, cognitive & motor impair, hyperglycemia

Artificial Tears (Tears Naturale) [OTC] **Uses:** *Dry eyes* **Action:** Ocular lubricant **Dose:** 1–2 gtt tid–qid **Supplied:** OTC soln

L-Asparaginase (Elspar, Oncaspar) **Uses:** *ALL* (in combo w/other agents) **Action:** Protein synthesis inhibitor **Dose:** 500–20,000 IU/m^2/d for 1–14 d (per protocols) **Caution:** [C, ?] **Contra:** Active/Hx pancreatitis **Supplied:** Inj 10,000 IU **SE:** Allergy 20–35% (from urticaria to anaphylaxis test dose recommended); rare GI tox (mild nausea/anorexia, pancreatitis)

Aspirin (Bayer, Ecotrin, St. Joseph's) [OTC] **Uses:** *Angina, CABG, PTCA, carotid endarterectomy, ischemic stroke, TIA, MI, arthritis, pain,* *HA,* *fever,* inflammation, Kawasaki Dz **Action:** Prostaglandin inhibitor **Dose:** *Adults. Pain, fever:* 325–650 mg q4–6h PO or PR. *RA:* 3–6 g/d PO in ÷ doses. *Plt inhibitor:* 81–325 mg PO qd. *Prevent MI:* 81–325 mg PO qd. *Peds. Antipyretic:* 10–15 mg/kg/dose PO or PR q4h up to 80 mg/kg/24 h. *RA:* 60–100 mg/kg/24 h PO ÷ q4–6h (keep levels between 15 & 30 mg/dL); avoid w/CrCl < 10 mL/min, in severe liver Dz **Caution:** [C, M] Use linked to Reye syndrome; avoid w/viral illness in children **Contra:** Allergy to ASA, chickenpox/flu Sxs, syndrome of nasal polyps, asthma, rhinitis **Supplied:** Tabs 325, 500 mg; chew tabs 81 mg; EC tabs 165, 325, 500, 650, 975 mg; SR tabs 650, 800 mg; effervescent tabs 325, 500 mg; supp 120, 200, 300, 600 mg **SE:** GI upset & erosion **Notes:** D/C 1 wk before surgery to ↓ bleeding; avoid/limit EtOH

22

Aspirin & Butalbital Compound (Fiorinal) [C-III]   Uses: *Tension HA,* pain **Action:** Combo barbiturate & analgesic **Dose:** 1–2 PO q4h PRN, max 6 tabs/d; avoid w/CrCl < 10 mL/min & severe liver Dz **Caution:** [C (D if prolonged use or high doses at term), ?] **Contra:** ASA allergy, GI ulceration, bleeding disorder, porphyria, syndrome of nasal polyps, angioedema & bronchospasm to NSAIDs **Supplied:** Caps (Fiorgen PF, Fiorinal) Tabs (Fiorinal, Lanorinal) ASA 325 mg/butalbital 50 mg/caffeine 40 mg **SE:** Drowsiness, dizziness, GI upset, ulceration, bleeding **Notes:** Butalbital habit-forming; avoid or limit EtOH intake

Aspirin + Butalbital, Caffeine & Codeine (Fiorinal + Codeine) [C-III]   Uses: Mild *pain,* HA, especially when associated w/stress **Action:** Sedative analgesic, narcotic analgesic **Dose:** 1–2 tabs (caps) PO q4–6h PRN **Caution:** [D, ?] **Contra:** Allergy to ASA **Supplied:** Cap/tab contains 325 mg ASA, 40 mg caffeine, 50 mg of butalbital, 30 mg of codeine **SE:** Drowsiness, dizziness, GI upset, ulceration, bleeding

Aspirin + Codeine (Empirin No. 2, No. 3, No. 4) [C-III]   Uses: Mild to *moderate pain* **Action:** Combined effects of ASA & codeine **Dose:** *Adults.* 1–2 tabs PO q4–6h PRN. *Peds.* ASA 10 mg/kg/dose; codeine 0.5–1 mg/kg/dose q4h **Caution:** [D, M] **Contra:** Allergy to ASA/codeine, PUD, bleeding, anticoagulant Rx, children w/chickenpox or flu Sxs **Supplied:** Tabs 325 mg of ASA & codeine (codeine in No. 2 = 15 mg, No. 3 = 30 mg, No. 4 = 60 mg) **SE:** Drowsiness, dizziness, GI upset, ulceration, bleeding

Atazanavir (Reyataz)   WARNING: Hyperbilirubinemia may require drug D/C **Uses:** *HIV-1 Infxn* **Action:** Protease inhibitor **Dose:** 400 mg PO qd w/food; when given w/efavirenz 600 mg, administer atazanavir 300 mg + ritonavir 100 mg once/d; separate doses from buffered didanosine administration; ↓ in hepatic impair **Caution:** [B, –]; ↑ levels of statins, sildenafil, antiarrhythmics, warfarin, cyclosporine, TCAs; atazanavir ↓ by St. John's wort **Contra:** Use w/midazolam, triazolam, ergots, cisapride, pimozide **Supplied:** Caps 100, 150, 200 mg **SE:** HA, N/V/D, rash, abdominal pain, DM, photosensitivity, ↑ PR interval **Notes:** May have less adverse effect on cholesterol

Atenolol (Tenormin)   Uses: *HTN, angina, MI* **Action:** Competitively blocks β-adrenergic receptors, β₁ **Dose:** *HTN & angina:* 50–100 mg/d PO. *AMI:* 5 mg IV × 2 over 10 min, then 50 mg PO bid if tolerated; ↓ in renal impair **Caution:** [D, M] DM, bronchospasm; abrupt D/C can exacerbate angina & ↑ MI risk **Contra:** Bradycardia, cardiogenic shock, cardiac failure, 2nd- or 3rd- degree AV block **Supplied:** Tabs 25, 50, 100 mg; inj 5 mg/10 mL **SE:** Bradycardia, ↓ BP, 2nd- or 3rd-degree AV block, dizziness, fatigue

Atenolol & Chlorthalidone (Tenoretic)   Uses: *HTN* **Action:** β-Adrenergic blockade w/diuretic **Dose:** 50–100 mg/d PO; ↓ in renal impair **Caution:** [D, M] DM, bronchospasm **Contra:** See atenolol; anuria **Supplied:** *Tenoretic 50:* Atenolol 50 mg/chlorthalidone 25 mg; *Tenoretic 100:* Atenolol 100 mg/ chlorthalidone 25 mg **SE:** Bradycardia, ↓ BP, 2nd- or 3rd-degree AV block, dizziness, fatigue, ↓ K⁺, photosensitivity

Atomoxetine (Strattera)   WARNING: Severe liver injury may occur in rare cases. D/C w/jaundice or ↑ LFT; ↑ risk suicidal thinking **Uses:** * ADHD* **Action:** Selective norepinephrine reuptake inhibitor **Dose:** *Adults & Peds > 70 kg.* 40 mg × 3 d, ↑ to 80–100 mg ÷ daily–bid. *Peds < 70 kg.* 0.5 mg/kg × 3 d, then ↑ 1.2 mg/kg max daily or bid **Caution:** [C, ? /–] **Contra:** NAG, use w/or w/in 2 wk of D/C of MAOI **Supplied:** Caps 10, 18, 25, 40, 60 mg **SE:** ↑ BP, tachycardia, weight loss, sexual dysfunction **Notes:** ↓ dose w/hepatic insuff, ↓ in combo w/inhibitors of CYP2D6 (page 647)

Atorvastatin (Lipitor) Uses: *↑ cholesterol & triglycerides* **Action:** HMG-CoA reductase inhibitor **Dose:** Initial 10 mg/d, may ↑ to 80 mg/d **Caution:** [X, –] **Contra:** Active liver Dz, unexplained ↑ of transaminases **Supplied:** Tabs 10, 20, 40, 80 mg **SE:** Myopathy, HA, arthralgia, myalgia, GI upset **Notes:** monitor LFTs

Atovaquone (Mepron) Uses: *Rx & prevention PCP* **Action:** ↓ nucleic acid & ATP synthesis **Dose:** *Rx:* 750 mg PO bid for 21 d. *Prevention:* 1500 mg PO once/d (w/meals) **Caution:** [C, ?] **Supplied:** Suspension 750 mg/5 mL **SE:** Fever, HA, anxiety, insomnia, rash, N/V

Atovaquone/Proguanil (Malarone) Uses: *Prevention or Rx *P. falciparum* malaria* **Action:** Antimalarial **Dose:** *Adults.* Prevention: 1 tab PO 2 d before, during & 7 d after leaving endemic region; *Rx:* 4 tabs PO single dose qd × 3 d. *Peds.* See insert **Caution:** [C, ?] **Contra:** CrCl < 30 mL/min **Supplied:** Tab atovaquone 250 mg/proguanil 100 mg; peds 62.5/25 mg **SE:** HA, fever, myalgia

Atracurium (Tracrium) Uses: *Anesthesia adjunct to facilitate ET intubation* **Action:** Nondepolarizing neuromuscular blocker **Dose:** *Adults & Peds.* 0.4–0.5 mg/kg IV bolus, then 0.08–0.1 mg/kg q20–45 min PRN **Caution:** [C, ?] **Supplied:** Inj 10 mg/mL **SE:** Flushing **Notes:** Pt must be intubated & on controlled ventilation; use adequate amounts of sedation & analgesia

Atropine Uses: *Preanesthetic; symptomatic bradycardia & asystole* **Action:** Antimuscarinic agent; blocks acetylcholine at parasympathetic sites **Dose:** *Adults.* ECC: 0.5–1 mg IV q3–5min. *Preanesthetic:* 0.3–0.6 mg IM. *Peds.* ECC: 0.01–0.03 mg/kg IV q2–5min, max 1 mg, min dose 0.1 mg. *Preanesthetic:* 0.01 mg/kg/dose SC/IV (max 0.4 mg) **Caution:** [C, +] **Contra:** Glaucoma **Supplied:** Tabs 0.3, 0.4, 0.6 mg; inj 0.05, 0.1, 0.3, 0.4, 0.5, 0.8, 1 mg/mL; ophth 0.5, 1, 2% **SE:** Blurred vision, urinary retention, constipation, dried mucous membranes

Azathioprine (Imuran) Uses: *Adjunct to prevent renal transplant rejection, RA,* SLE **Action:** Immunosuppressive; antagonizes purine metabolism **Dose:** *Adults & Peds.* 1–3 mg/kg/d IV or PO (↓ in renal failure) **Caution:** [D, ?] **Contra:** PRG **Supplied:** Tabs 50 mg; inj 100 mg/20 mL **SE:** GI intolerance, fever, chills, leukopenia, thrombocytopenia; chronic use may ↑ neoplasia **Notes:** Handle inj w/cytotoxic precautions; interaction w/allopurinol; do not administer live vaccines to a pt taking azathioprine

Azelastine (Astelin, Optivar) Uses: *Allergic rhinitis (rhinorrhea, sneezing, nasal pruritus); allergic conjunctivitis* **Action:** Histamine H$_1$-receptor antagonist **Dose:** *Nasal:* 2 sprays/nostril bid. *Ophth:* 1 gt into each affected eye bid **Caution:** [C, ?/–] **Contra:** Component sensitivity **Supplied:** Nasal 137 mcg/spray; ophth soln 0.05% **SE:** Somnolence, bitter taste

Azithromycin (Zithromax) Uses: *Community-acquired pneumonia, pharyngitis, otitis media, skin Infxns, nongonococcal urethritis & PID; Rx & prevention of MAC in HIV* **Action:** Macrolide antibiotic; ↓ protein synthesis. *Spectrum:* Chlamydia, H. ducreyi, H. influenzae, Legionella, M. catarrhalis, M. pneumoniae,

22

M. hominis, N. gonorrhoeae, S. aureus, S. agalactiae, S. pneumoniae, S. pyogenes
Dose: *Adults.* PO: Resp tract Infxn: 500 mg d 1, then 250 mg/d PO × 4 d; 500 mg/d PO × 3 d; or 2g PO × 1. *Nongonococcal urethritis:* 1 g PO single dose. *Prevention of MAC:* 1200 mg PO once/wk. IV: 500 mg × 2 d, then 500 mg PO × 7–10 d. *Peds. Otitis media:* 10 mg/kg PO d 1, then 5 mg/kg/d d 2–5. *Pharyngitis:* 12 mg/kg/d PO × 5 d (take susp on an empty stomach; tabs may be taken w/wo food) **Caution:** [B, +] **Supplied:** Tabs 250, 600 mg; Z-Pack (5-d); Tri-Pak (500-mg tabs × 3); susp 1-g; single-dose packet Zmax (2 g); susp 100, 200 mg/5 mL; inj 500 mg **SE:** GI upset

Aztreonam (Azactam) Uses: *Aerobic gram(–) UTI, lower resp, intraabdominal, skin, gynecologic Infxns & septicemia* **Action:** Monobactam. ↓ Cell wall synthesis. *Spectrum:* Gram(–) (*Pseudomonas, E. coli, Klebsiella, H. influenzae, Serratia, Proteus, Enterobacter, Citrobacter*) **Dose:** *Adults.* 1–2 g IV/IM q6–12h. *Peds. Premature:* 30 mg/kg/dose IV q12h. *Term & children:* 30 mg/kg/ dose q6–8h; ↓ in renal impair **Caution:** [B, +] **Supplied:** Inj 500 mg, 1 g, 2 g **SE:** N/V/D, rash, pain at injection site **Notes:** No gram(+) or anaerobic activity; OK in PCN-allergic pts

Baclofen (Lioresal) Uses: *Spasticity due to severe chronic disorders (eg, MS, ALS, spinal cord lesions),* trigeminal neuralgia, hiccups **Action:** Centrally acting skeletal muscle relaxant; ↓ transmission of both monosynaptic & polysynaptic cord reflexes **Dose:** *Adults.* Initial, 5 mg PO tid; ↑ q3d to effect; max 80 mg/d. *Intrathecal:* Via implantable pump *Peds.* 2–7 y: 10–15 mg/d ÷ q8h; titrate, max 40 mg/d. > 8 y: Max 60 mg/d. *IT:* Via implantable pump; ↓ in renal impair; w/food or milk **Caution:** [C, +] Epilepsy, neuropsychiatric disturbances; withdrawal may occur w/abrupt D/C **Supplied:** Tabs 10, 20 mg; IT inj 10 mg/20 mL, 10 mg/5 mL **SE:** Dizziness, drowsiness, insomnia, ataxia, weakness, ↓ BP

Balsalazide (Colazal) Uses: *Ulcerative colitis* **Action:** 5-ASA derivative, antiinflammatory, ↓ leukotriene synthesis **Dose:** 2.25 g (3 caps) tid × 8–12 wk **Caution:** [B, ?] Severe renal/hepatic failure **Contra:** Mesalamine or salicylates hypersensitivity **Supplied:** Caps 750 mg **SE:** Dizziness, HA, nausea, agranulocytosis, pancytopenia, renal impair, allergic Rxns **Notes:** Daily dose of 6.75 g = 2.4 g mesalamine

Basiliximab (Simulect) Uses: *Prevent acute organ transplant rejection* **Action:** IL-2 receptor antagonists **Dose:** *Adults.* 20 mg IV 2 h before transplant, then 20 mg IV 4 d posttransplant. *Peds.* 12 mg/m^2 ↑ to max of 20 mg 2 h before transplant; the same dose IV 4 d posttransplant **Caution:** [B, ?/–] **Contra:** Hypersensitivity to murine proteins **Supplied:** Inj 20 mg **SE:** Edema, HTN, HA, dizziness, fever, pain, Infxn, GI effects, electrolyte disturbances **Notes:** Murine/ human MoAb

BCG [Bacillus Calmette-Guérin] (TheraCys, Tice BCG) Uses: *Bladder carcinoma (superficial),* TB prophylaxis **Action:** Immunomodulator **Dose:** Bladder CA, 1 vial prepared & instilled in bladder for 2 h. Repeat once/wk for 6 wk; then maint 3/wk at 3, 6, 12, 18 & 24 mo after initial therapy **Caution:** [C, ?] Asthma, do not administer w/traumatic catheterization or UTI **Contra:** Immunosuppression, UTI, steroid use, acute illness, fever of unknown origin **Supplied:** Inj 81 mg (10.5 ± 8.7 × 10^8 CFU vial) (TheraCys), 1–8 × 10^8 CFU/vial (Tice BCG) **SE:** *Intravesical:* Hematuria, urinary frequency, dysuria, bacterial UTI, rare BCG sepsis **Notes:** Routine adult BCG immunization not OK in US; occasionally used in high-risk children who are PPD(–) & cannot take INH

Becaplermin (Regranex Gel) **Uses:** Adjunct to local wound care w/
diabetic foot ulcers **Action:** Recombinant PDGF, enhances granulation tissue
Dose: Based on lesion; $1^1/3$-in ribbon from 2–g tube, $^2/3$-in ribbon from 7.5- or
15-g tube/in^2 of ulcer; apply & cover w/moist gauze; rinse after 12h; do not
reapply; repeat in 12 h **Caution:** [C, ?] **Contra:** Neoplasm/or active site Infxn
Supplied: 0.01% gel in 2-, 7.5-, 15-g tubes **SE:** Erythema, local pain **Notes:**
Use w/good wound care; wound must be vascularized

Beclomethasone (Beconase, Vancenase Nasal Inhaler) **Uses:**
Allergic rhinitis refractory to antihistamines & decongestants; *nasal polyps*
Action: Inhaled steroid **Dose:** *Adults.* 1 spray intranasal bid–qid. *Aqueous
inhal:* 1–2 sprays/nostril daily. *Peds 6–12 y.* 1 spray intranasal tid **Caution:** [C,
?] **Supplied:** Nasal met-dose inhaler **SE:** Local irritation, burning, epistaxis
Notes: Nasal spray delivers 42 mcg/dose & 84 mcg/dose

Beclomethasone (Qvar) **Uses:** Chronic *asthma* **Action:** Inhaled corticosteroid **Dose:** *Adults & Peds.* 1–4 inhal bid (rinse mouth/throat after) **Caution:** [C, ?] **Contra:** Acute asthma **Supplied:** PO met-dose inhaler; 40, 80 mcg/
inhal **SE:** HA, cough, hoarseness, oral candidiasis **Notes:** Not effective for acute
asthma

Belladonna & Opium Suppositories (B & O Supprettes) [C-II]
Uses: *Bladder spasms; moderate/severe pain* **Action:** Antispasmodic, analgesic **Dose:** 1 supp PR q6h PRN; 15A = 30 mg powdered opium/16.2 mg belladonna extract; 16A = 60 mg powdered opium/16.2 mg belladonna extract
Caution: [C, ?] **Supplied:** Supp 15A, 16A **SE:** Anticholinergic (sedation, urinary retention, constipation)

Benazepril (Lotensin) **Uses:** *HTN,* DN, CHF **Action:** ACE inhibitor
Dose: 10–40 mg/d PO **Caution:** [C (1st tri), D (2nd & 3rd tri), +] **Contra:**
Angioedema, Hx edema **Supplied:** Tabs 5, 10, 20, 40 mg **SE:** Symptomatic ↓
BP w/diuretics; dizziness, HA, ↓ K$^+$, nonproductive cough

Benzocaine & Antipyrine (Auralgan) **Uses:** *Analgesia in severe otitis media* **Action:** Anesthetic w/local decongestant **Dose:** Fill ear & insert a
moist cotton plug; repeat 1–2 h PRN **Caution:** [C, ?] **Contra:** W/perforated ear-
drum **Supplied:** Soln **SE:** Local irritation

Benzonatate (Tessalon Perles) **Uses:** Symptomatic relief of *cough*
Action: Anesthetizes the stretch receptors in the resp passages **Dose:** *Adults &
Peds > 10 y.* 100 mg PO tid **Caution:** [C, ?] **Supplied:** Caps 100 mg **SE:** Seda-
tion, dizziness, GI upset **Notes:** Do not chew or puncture the caps

Benztropine (Cogentin) **Uses:** *Parkinsonism & drug-induced extrapyramidal disorders* **Action:** Partially blocks striatal cholinergic receptors **Dose:**
Adults. 0.5–6 mg PO, IM, or IV in ÷ doses/d. *Peds > 3 y.* 0.02–0.05 mg/kg/dose
1–2/d **Caution:** [C, ?] **Contra:** < 3 y **Supplied:** Tabs 0.5, 1, 2 mg; inj 1 mg/mL
SE: Anticholinergic side effects **Notes:** Physostigmine 1–2 mg SC/IV to reverse
severe Sxs

Beractant (Survanta) **Uses:** *Prevention & Rx of RDS in premature
infants* **Action:** Replaces pulmonary surfactant **Dose:** 100 mg/kg via ET tube;
may repeat 3× q6h; max 4 doses/48 h **Supplied:** Susp 25 mg of phospholipid/
mL **SE:** Transient bradycardia, desaturation, apnea **Notes:** Administer via 4-
quadrant method

22

Betaxolol (Kerlone) Uses: *HTN* Action: Competitively blocks β-adrenergic receptors, $β_1$ Caution: [C (1st tri), D (2nd or 3rd tri), +/–] Contra: Sinus bradycardia, AV conduction abnormalities, cardiac failure Dose: 10–20 mg/d Supplied: Tabs 10, 20 mg SE: Dizziness, HA, bradycardia, edema, CHF

Betaxolol, Ophthalmic (Betoptic) Uses: Glaucoma Action: Competitively blocks β-adrenergic receptors, $β_1$ Dose: 1 gt bid Caution: [C (1st tri), D (2nd or 3rd tri), ?/–] Supplied: Soln 0.5%; susp 0.25% SE: Local irritation, photophobia

Bethanechol (Urecholine, Duvoid, others) Uses: *Neurogenic bladder atony w/retention,* acute *postop* & postpartum functional *(nonobstructive) urinary retention* Action: Stimulates cholinergic smooth muscle receptors in bladder & GI tract Dose: *Adults.* 10–50 mg PO tid–qid or 2.5–5 mg SQ tid–qid & PRN. *Peds.* 0.6 mg/kg/24 h PO ÷ tid–qid or 0.15–2 mg/kg/d SQ ÷ 3–4× (take on empty stomach) Caution: [C, ?/–] Contra: BOO, PUD, epilepsy, hyperthyroidism, bradycardia, COPD, AV conduction defects, parkinsonism, ↓ BP, vasomotor instability Supplied: Tabs 5, 10, 25, 50 mg; inj 5 mg/mL SE: Abdominal cramps, D, salivation, ↓ BP Notes: Do not use IM/IV

Bevacizumab (Avastin) WARNING: Associated w/GI perforation, wound dehiscence & fatal hemoptysis Uses: *Colorectal metastatic carcinoma, w/5-FU* Nonsquamous NSCLC w/paclitaxel and carboplatin Action: Vascular endothelial GF inhibitor Dose: *Adults.* 5 mg/kg IV q14d; 1st dose over 90 min; 2nd over 60 min, 3rd over 30 min if tolerated Caution: [C, –] Do not use w/in 28 d of surgery if time for separation of drug & anticipated surgical procedure is unknown; D/C w/ serious adverse events Supplied: 100 mg/4 mL, 400 mg/16 mL vials SE: Wound dehiscence, GI perforation, hemoptysis, hemorrhage, HTN, proteinuria, CHF, inf Rxns, D, leukopenia, thromboembolism Notes: Monitor for ↑ BP & proteinuria

Bicalutamide (Casodex) Uses: *Advanced CAP (metastatic)* (w/GnRH agonists [eg, leuprolide, goserelin]) Action: Nonsteroidal antiandrogen Dose: 50 mg/d Caution: [X, ?] Contra: Women Supplied: Caps 50 mg SE: Hot flashes, loss of libido, impotence, D/N/V, gynecomastia & LFT elevation

Bicarbonate (See Sodium Bicarbonate, page 601)

Bisacodyl (Dulcolax) [OTC] Uses: *Constipation; preop bowel prep* Action: Stimulates peristalsis Dose: *Adults.* 5–15 mg PO or 10 mg PR PRN. *Peds.* < 2 y: 5 mg PR PRN. > 2 y: 5 mg PO or 10 mg PR PRN (do not chew tabs or give w/in 1 h of antacids or milk) Caution: [B, ?] Contra: Acute abdomen or bowel obstruction, appendicitis, gastroenteritis Supplied: EC tabs 5 mg; supp 10 mg SE: Abdominal cramps, proctitis & inflammation w/suppositories

Bismuth Subsalicylate (Pepto-Bismol) [OTC] Uses: Indigestion, nausea & *D*; combo for Rx of *H. pylori* Infxn* Action: Antisecretory & antiinflammatory effects Dose: *Adults.* 2 tabs or 30 mL PO PRN (max 8 doses/24 h). *Peds.* 3–6 y: 1/3 tab or 5 mL PO PRN (max 8 doses/24 h). 6–9 y: 2/3 tab or 10 mL PO PRN (max 8 doses/24 h). 9–12 y: 1 tab or 15 mL PO PRN (max 8 doses/24 h) Caution: [C, D (3rd tri), –] Avoid in renal failure Contra: Influenza or chickenpox (↑ risk of Reye syndrome), ASA allergy Supplied: Chew tabs 262 mg; liq 262, 524 mg/15 mL SE: May turn tongue & stools black

Bisoprolol (Zebeta) Uses: *HTN* Action: Competitively blocks $β_1$-adrenergic receptors Dose: 5–10 mg/d (max dose 20 mg/d); ↓ in renal impair Cau-

tion: [C (D 2nd & 3rd tri), +/–] **Contra:** Sinus bradycardia, AV conduction abnormalities, cardiac failure **Supplied:** Tabs 5, 10 mg **SE:** Fatigue, lethargy, HA, bradycardia, edema, CHF **Notes:** Not dialyzed

Bitolterol (Tornalate) **Uses:** Prophylaxis & Rx of *asthma* & reversible bronchospasm **Action:** Sympathomimetic bronchodilator; stimulates pulmonary β_2-adrenergic receptors **Dose:** *Adults & Peds.* 2 inhal q8h **Caution:** [C, ?] **Supplied:** Aerosol 0.8% **SE:** Dizziness, nervousness, trembling, HTN, palpitations

Bivalirudin (Angiomax) **Uses:** *Anticoagulant w/ASA in unstable angina undergoing PTCA* **Action:** Anticoagulant, thrombin inhibitor **Dose:** 1 mg/kg IV bolus, then 2.5 mg/kg/h over 4 h; PRN, use 0.2 mg/kg/h for up to 20 h (give w/aspirin 300–325 mg/d; start pre-PTCA) **Caution:** [B, ?] **Contra:** Major bleeding **Supplied:** Powder for inj **SE:** Bleeding, back pain, nausea, HA

Bleomycin Sulfate (Blenoxane) **Uses:** *Testis CA; Hodgkin Dz & NHL; cutaneous lymphoma; & squamous cell CA (head & neck, larynx, cervix, skin, penis); sclerosing agent for malignant pleural effusion* **Action:** Induces breakage (scission) of DNA **Dose:** 10–20 mg (units)/m^2 1–2/wk (per protocols); ↓ in renal impair **Caution:** [D, ?] Severe pulmonary Dz **Supplied:** Inj 15 mg (15 U) **SE:** Hyperpigmentation (skin staining) & allergy (rash to anaphylaxis); fever in 50%; lung tox (idiosyncratic & dose related); pneumonitis may progress to fibrosis; Raynaud phenomenon, N/V **Notes:** Test dose 1 mg (U) OK, especially in lymphoma pts; lung tox w/total dose > 400 mg (U)

Bortezomib (Velcade) WARNING: May worsen preexisting neuropathy **Uses:** *Progression of multiple myeloma despite two previous Rxs* **Action:** Proteasome inhibitor **Dose:** 1.3 mg/m^2 bolus IV 2×/wk × 2 wk, w/10-day rest period (= 1 cycle); ↓ dose w/hematologic tox, neuropathy **Caution:** [D, ?/–] **Supplied:** 3.5-mg vial **SE:** Asthenia, GI upset, anorexia, dyspnea, HA, orthostatic ↓ BP, edema, insomnia, dizziness, rash, pyrexia, arthralgia, neuropathy **Notes:** May interact w/drugs metabolized via CYP450 (page 647)

Brimonidine (Alphagan) **Uses:** *Open-angle glaucoma, ocular HTN* **Action:** α_2-Adrenergic agonist **Dose:** 1 gt in eye(s) tid (wait 15 min to insert contacts) **Caution:** [B, ?] **Contra:** MAOI therapy **Supplied:** 0.2% soln **SE:** Local irritation, HA, fatigue

Brinzolamide (Azopt) **Uses:** *Open-angle glaucoma, ocular HTN* **Action:** Carbonic anhydrase inhibitor **Dose:** 1 gt in eye(s) tid **Caution:** [C, ?] **Supplied:** 1% susp **SE:** Blurred vision, dry eye, blepharitis, taste disturbance

Bromocriptine (Parlodel) **Uses:** *Parkinson Dz, hyperprolactinemia, acromegaly, pituitary tumors* **Action:** Direct-acting on the striatal dopamine receptors; ↓ prolactin secretion **Dose:** Initial, 1.25 mg PO bid; titrate to effect **Caution:** [C, ?] **Contra:** Severe ischemic heart Dz or PVD **Supplied:** Tabs 2.5 mg; caps 5 mg **SE:** ↓ BP, Raynaud phenomenon, dizziness, nausea, hallucinations

Budesonide (Rhinocort, Pulmicort) **Uses:** *Allergic & nonallergic rhinitis, asthma* **Action:** Steroid **Dose:** *Intranasal:* 2 sprays/nostril bid or 4 sprays/nostril/d. *Aqueous:* 1 spray/nostril/d. *PO inhaled:* 1–4 inhal bid. *Peds.* 1–2 inhal bid (rinse mouth after PO use) **Caution:** [C, ?/–] **Supplied:** Met-dose Turbuhaler, nasal inhaler & aqueous spray **SE:** HA, cough, hoarseness, *Candida* Infxn, epistaxis

22

Bumetanide (Bumex) Uses: *Edema from CHF, hepatic cirrhosis & renal Dz* Action: Loop diuretic; ↓ reabsorption of Na⁺ & Cl–, in the ascending loop of Henle & the distal tubule Dose: *Adults.* 0.5–2 mg/d PO; 0.5–1 mg IV q8–24h (max 10 mg/d). *Peds.* 0.015–0.1 mg/kg/d PO, IV, or IM ÷ q6–24h Caution: [D, ?] Contra: Anuria, hepatic coma, severe electrolyte depletion Supplied: Tabs 0.5, 1, 2 mg; inj 0.25 mg/mL SE: ↓ K⁺, ↓ Na⁺, ↑ creatinine, ↑ uric acid, dizziness, ototox Notes: Monitor fluid & electrolytes

Bupivacaine (Marcaine) Uses: *Local, regional & spinal anesthesia, local & regional analgesia* Action: Local anesthetic Dose: *Adults & Peds.* Dose dependent on procedure (eg, tissue vascularity, depth of anesthesia) (Table 22–3, page 632) Caution: [C, ?] Contra: Severe bleeding, ↓ BP, shock & arrhythmias, local Infxns at anesthesia site, septicemia Supplied: Inj 0.25, 0.5, 0.75% SE: ↓ BP, bradycardia, dizziness, anxiety

Buprenorphine (Buprenex) [C-V] Uses: *Moderate/severe pain* Action: Opiate agonist–antagonist Dose: 0.3–0.6 mg IM or slow IV push q6h PRN Caution: [C, ?/–] Supplied: Inj 0.324 mg/mL (= 0.3 mg of buprenorphine) SE: Sedation, ↓ BP, resp depression Notes: Withdrawal if opioid-dependent

Bupropion (Wellbutrin, Wellbutrin SR, Wellbutrin XL, Zyban) WARNING: Closely monitor for worsening depression or emergence of suicidality Uses: *Depression, adjunct to smoking cessation* Action: Weak inhibitor of neuronal uptake of serotonin & norepinephrine; ↓ neuronal dopamine reuptake Dose: *Depression:* 100–450 mg/d ÷ bid–tid; SR 100–200 mg bid; XL 150–300 mg qd. *Smoking cessation:* 150 mg/d × 3 d, then 150 mg bid ×8–12 wk; ↓ in renal/ hepatic impair Caution: [B, ?/–] Contra: Sz disorder, Hx anorexia nervosa or bulimia, MAOI, abrupt D/C of EtOH or sedatives Supplied: Tabs 75, 100 mg; SR tabs 100, 150, 200 mg; XL tabs 150, 300 mg SE: Associated w/Szs; agitation, insomnia, HA, tachycardia Notes: Avoid EtOH & other CNS depressants

Buspirone (BuSpar) WARNING: Closely monitor for worsening depression or emergence of suicidality Uses: Short-term relief of *anxiety* Action: Antianxiety; antagonizes CNS serotonin receptors Dose: 5–10 mg PO tid; ↑ to effect; usual 20–30 mg/d; max 60 mg/d; ↓ in severe hepatic/renal insuff Caution: [B, ?/–] Supplied: Tabs 5, 10, 15, 30 mg dividose SE: Drowsiness, dizziness; HA, N Notes: No abuse potential or physical/psychological dependence

Busulfan (Myleran, Busulfex) Uses: *CML,* preparative regimens for allogeneic & ABMT in high doses Action: Alkylating agent Dose: 4–12 mg/d for several wk; 16 mg/kg once or 4 mg/kg/d for 4 d w/another agent in BMT (per protocol) Caution: [D, ?] Supplied: Tabs 2 mg, inj 60 mg/10 mL SE: Myelosuppression, pulmonary fibrosis, nausea (high-dose therapy), gynecomastia, adrenal insuff & skin hyperpigmentation

Butorphanol (Stadol) [C-IV] Uses: *Anesthesia adjunct, pain* & migraine HA Action: Opiate agonist–antagonist w/central analgesic actions Dose: 1–4 mg IM or IV q3–4h PRN. *HA:* 1 spray in 1 nostril; may repeat ×1 if pain not relieved in 60–90 min; ↓ in renal impair Caution: [C (D if high doses or prolonged periods at term), +] Supplied: Inj 1, 2 mg/mL; nasal spray 10 mg/ mL SE: Drowsiness, dizziness, nasal congestion Notes: May induce withdrawal in opioid dependency

Calcipotriene (Dovonex) Uses: *Plaque psoriasis* Action: Keratolytic Dose: Apply bid Caution: [C, ?] Contra: ↑ Ca²⁺; vitamin D tox; do not apply to face Supplied: Cream; oint; soln 0.005% SE: Skin irritation, dermatitis

22

Calcitonin (Cibacalcin, Miacalcin) Uses: *Paget Dz of bone, $\uparrow$ Ca^{2+},* osteogenesis imperfecta, *postmenopausal osteoporosis* **Action:** Polypeptide hormone **Dose:** *Paget Dz salmon form:* 100 units/d IM/SC initial, 50 units/d or 50–100 units q1–3d maint. *Paget Dz human form:* 0.5 mg/d initial; maint 0.5 mg 2–3 ×/wk or 0.25 mg/d, max 0.5 mg bid. $\uparrow$ Ca^{2+} salmon calcitonin: 4 units/kg IM/SC q12h; $\uparrow$ to 8 units/kg q12h, max q6h. *Osteoporosis salmon calcitonin:* 100 units/d IM/SQ; intranasal 200 units = 1 nasal spray/d **Caution:** [C, ?] **Supplied:** Spray, nasal 200 units/activation; inj, human (Cibacalcin) 0.5 mg/vial, salmon 200 units/mL (2 mL) **SE:** Facial flushing, nausea, injection site edema, nasal irritation, polyuria **Notes:** Human (Cibacalcin) & salmon forms; human only approved for Paget bone Dz

Calcitriol (Rocaltrol) Uses: *Reduction of $\uparrow$ PTH levels, $\downarrow$ Ca^{2+} on dialysis* **Action:** 1,25-Dihydroxycholecalciferol (vitamin D analog) **Dose:** *Adults. Renal failure:* 0.25 mcg/d PO, $\uparrow$ 0.25 mcg/d q4–6wk PRN; 0.5 mcg 3×/wk IV, $\uparrow$ PRN. *Hyperparathyroidism:* 0.5–2 mcg/d. *Peds. Renal failure:* 15 ng/kg/d, $\uparrow$ PRN; maint 30–60 ng/kg/d. *Hyperparathyroidism:* < 5 y, 0.25–0.75 mcg/d. > 6 y, 0.5–2 mcg/d **Caution:** [C, ?] **Contra:** $\uparrow$ Ca^{2+}; vitamin D tox **Supplied:** Inj 1, 2 mcg/mL (in 1-mL); caps 0.25, 0.5 mcg **SE:** $\uparrow$ Ca^{2+} possible **Notes:** Monitor to keep Ca^{2+} WNL

Calcium Acetate (Calphron, Phos-Ex, PhosLo) Uses: *ESRD-associated hyperphosphatemia* **Action:** Ca^{2+} supl w/o aluminum to $\downarrow$ PO_4^{2-} **Dose:** 2–4 tabs PO w/meals **Caution:** [C, ?] **Contra:** $\uparrow$ Ca^{2+} **Supplied:** Caps Phos-Ex 500 mg (125 mg Ca); tabs Calphron & PhosLo 667 mg (169 mg Ca) **SE:** Can $\uparrow$ Ca^{2+}, hypophosphatemia, constipation **Notes:** Monitor Ca^{2+}

Calcium Carbonate (Tums, Alka-Mints) [OTC] Uses: *Hyperacidity associated w/peptic ulcer Dz, hiatal hernia,* etc **Action:** Neutralizes gastric acid **Dose:** 500 mg–2 g PO PRN; $\downarrow$ in renal impair **Caution:** [C, ?] **Supplied:** Chew tabs 350, 420, 500, 550, 750, 850 mg; susp **SE:** $\uparrow$ Ca^{2+}, hypophosphatemia, constipation

Calcium Glubionate (Neo-Calglucon) [OTC] Uses: *Rx & prevent calcium deficiency* **Action:** Ca^{2+} supl **Dose:** *Adults.* 6–18 g/d ÷ doses. *Peds.* 600–2000 mg/kg/d ÷ qid (9 g/d max); $\downarrow$ in renal impair **Caution:** [C, ?] **Contra:** $\uparrow$ Ca^{2+} **Supplied:** OTC syrup 1.8 g/5 mL = Ca 115 mg/5 mL **SE:** $\uparrow$ Ca^{2+}, hypophosphatemia, constipation

Calcium Salts (Chloride, Gluconate, Gluceptate) Uses: *Ca^{2+} replacement,* VF, Ca^{2+} blocker tox, Mg^{2+} intox, tetany, *hyperphosphatemia in ESRD* **Action:** Ca^{2+} supl/replacement **Dose:** *Adults.* Replacement: 1–2 g/d PO. *Cardiac emergencies:* CaCl 0.5–1 g IV q 10 min or Ca gluconate 1–2 g IV q 10 min. *Tetany:* 1 g CaCl over 10–30 min; repeat in 6 h PRN. *Peds.* Replacement: 200–500 mg/kg/ 24 h PO or IV ÷ qid. *Cardiac emergency:* 100 mg/kg/dose IV gluconate salt q 10 min. *Tetany:* 10 mg/kg CaCl over 5–10 min; repeat in 6 h or use inf (200 mg/kg/d max). *Adult & Peds.* $\downarrow$ Ca^{2+} due to citrated blood inf: 0.45 mEq Ca/100 mL citrated blood inf ($\downarrow$ in renal impair) **Caution:** [C, ?] **Contra:** $\uparrow$ Ca^{2+} **Supplied:** CaCl inj 10% = 100 mg/mL = Ca 27.2 mg/mL = 10-mL amp; Ca gluconate inj 10% = 100 mg/mL = Ca 9 mg/mL; tabs 500 mg = 45 mg Ca, 650 mg = 58.5 mg Ca, 975 mg = 87.75 mg Ca, 1 g = 90 mg Ca; Ca gluceptate inj 220 mg/mL = 18 mg/mL Ca **SE:** Bradycardia, cardiac arrhythmias, $\uparrow$ Ca^{2+} **Notes:** CaCl 270 mg (13.6 mEq) elemental Ca/g & calcium gluconate 90 mg (4.5 mEq) Ca/g. *RDA for Ca:* Adults = 800 mg/d; Peds = < 6 mo 360 mg/d, 6 mo–1 y 540 mg/d, 1–10 y 800 mg/d, 10–18 y 1200 mg/d

22

Calfactant (Infasurf) Uses: *Prevention & Rx of RDS in infants* **Action:** Exogenous pulmonary surfactant **Dose:** 3 mL/kg instilled into lungs. Can retreat for a total of 3 doses given 12 h apart **Caution:** [?, ?] **Supplied:** Intratracheal susp 35 mg/mL **SE:** Monitor for cyanosis, airway obstruction, bradycardia during administration

Candesartan (Atacand) Uses: *HTN,* DN, CHF **Action:** Angiotensin II receptor antagonist **Dose:** 2–32 mg/d (usual 16 mg/d) **Caution:** [X, –] **Contra:** Primary hyperaldosteronism; bilateral renal artery stenosis **Supplied:** Tabs 4, 8, 16, 32 mg **SE:** Dizziness, HA, flushing, angioedema

Capsaicin (Capsin, Zostrix, others) [OTC] Uses: Pain due to *postherpetic neuralgia,* chronic neuralgia, *arthritis, diabetic neuropathy,* postop pain, psoriasis, intractable pruritus **Action:** Topical analgesic **Dose:** Apply tid–qid **Caution:** [?, ?] **Supplied:** OTC creams; gel; lotions; roll-ons **SE:** Local irritation, neurotox, cough

Captopril (Capoten, others) Uses: *HTN, CHF, MI,* LVD, DN **Action:** ACE inhibitor **Dose:** *Adults.* HTN: Initial, 25 mg PO bid–tid; ↑ to maint q1–2wk by 25-mg increments/dose (max 450 mg/d) to effect. *CHF:* Initial, 6.25–12.5 mg PO tid; titrate PRN *LVD:* 50 mg PO tid. *DN:* 25 mg PO tid. *Peds.* Infants < 2 mo: 0.05–0.5 mg/kg/dose PO q8–24h. *Children:* Initial, 0.3–0.5 mg/kg/dose PO; ↑ to 6 mg/kg/dose max (1 h before meals) **Caution:** [C (1st tri); D (2nd & 3rd tri); unknown effects in renal impair +] **Contra:** Hx angioedema **Supplied:** Tabs 12.5, 25, 50, 100 mg **SE:** Rash, proteinuria, cough, ↑ K+

Carbamazepine (Tegretol) WARNING: Aplastic anemia & agranulocytosis have been reported w/carbamazepine Uses: *Epilepsy, trigeminal neuralgia,* EtOH withdrawal **Action:** Anticonvulsant **Dose:** *Adults.* Initial, 200 mg PO bid; ↑ by 200 mg/d; usual 800–1200 mg/d ÷ doses. *Peds.* < 6 y: 5 mg/kg/d, ↑ to 10–20 mg/kg/d ÷ in 2–4 doses. *6–12 y:* Initial, 100 mg PO bid or 10 mg/kg/24 h PO ÷ qd–bid; ↑ to maint 20–30 mg/kg/24 h ÷ tid–qid; ↓ in renal impair (take w/food) **Caution:** [D, +] **Contra:** MAOI use, Hx BM suppression **Supplied:** Tabs 200 mg; chew tabs 100 mg; XR tabs 100, 200, 400 mg; susp 100 mg/5 mL **SE:** Drowsiness, dizziness, blurred vision, N/V, rash, ↓ Na+, leukopenia, agranulocytosis **Notes:** Monitor CBC & serum levels (Table 22–2, page 628), generic products not interchangeable

Carbidopa/Levodopa (Sinemet) Uses: *Parkinson Dz* **Action:** ↑ CNS dopamine levels **Dose:** 25/100 mg bid–qid; ↑ as needed (max 200/2000 mg/d) **Caution:** [C, ?] **Contra:** NAG, suspicious skin lesion (may activate melanoma), melanoma, MAOI use **Supplied:** Tabs (mg carbidopa/mg levodopa) 10/100, 25/100, 25/250; tabs SR (mg carbidopa/mg levodopa) 25/100, 50/200 **SE:** Psychiatric disturbances, orthostatic ↓ BP, dyskinesia, cardiac arrhythmia

Carboplatin (Paraplatin) Uses: *Ovarian, lung, head & neck, testicular, urothelial,* & brain *CA, NHL* & allogeneic & ABMT in high doses **Action:** DNA cross-linker; forms DNA-platinum adducts **Dose:** 360 mg/m² (ovarian carcinoma); AUC dosing 4–7 mg/mL (Culvert formula: mg = AUC × [25 + calculated GFR]); adjust based on pretreatment plt count, CrCl & BSA (Egorin formula); up to 1500 mg/m² used in ABMT setting (per protocols) **Caution:** [D, ?] **Contra:** Severe BM suppression, excessive bleeding **Supplied:** Inj 50, 150, 450 mg **SE:** Myelosuppression, N/V/D, nephrotox, hematuria, neurotox, ↑ LFTs **Notes:** Physiologic dosing based on either Culvert or Egorin formula allows ↑ doses w/↓ tox

Carisoprodol (Soma) Uses: *Adjunct to sleep & physical therapy to relieve painful musculoskeletal conditions* **Action:** Centrally acting muscle relaxant **Dose:** 350 mg PO tid–qid **Caution:** [C, M] Tolerance may result; w/ renal/hepatic impair **Contra:** Allergy to meprobamate; acute intermittent porphyria **Supplied:** Tabs 350 mg **SE:** CNS depression, drowsiness, dizziness, tachycardia **Notes:** Avoid EtOH & other CNS depressants; available in combo w/ASA or codeine.

Carmustine, BCNU (BiCNU, Gliadel) Uses: *Primary brain tumors, melanoma, Hodgkin lymphoma & NHL, multiple myeloma & induction for allogeneic & ABMT in high doses; adjunct to surgery in pts w/recurrent glioblastoma* **Action:** Alkylating agent; nitrosourea forms DNA cross-links to inhibit DNA **Dose:** 150–200 mg/m^2 q6–8wk single or ÷ dose qd inj over 2 d; 20–65 mg/m^2 q4–6wk; 300–900 mg/m^2 in BMT (per protocols); ↓ in hepatic impair **Caution:** [D, ?] ↓ WBC, RBC, plt counts, renal/hepatic impair **Contra:** Myelosuppression, PRG **Supplied:** Inj 100 mg/vial; wafer: 7.7 mg **SE:** ↓ BP, N/V, myelosuppression (WBC & plt), phlebitis, facial flushing, hepatic/renal dysfunction, pulmonary fibrosis, optic neuroretinitis; hematologic tox may persist 4–6 wk after dose **Notes:** Do not give course more frequently than q6wk (cumulative tox); baseline PFTs OK

Carteolol (Cartrol, Ocupress Ophthalmic) Uses: *HTN, ↑ intraocular pressure, chronic open-angle glaucoma* **Action:** Blocks β-adrenergic receptors (β$_1$, β$_2$), mild ISA **Dose:** PO 2.5–5 mg/d; ophth 1 gt in eye(s) bid; ↓ in renal impair **Caution:** [C (1st tri); D (2nd & 3rd tri), ?/–] Cardiac failure, asthma **Contra:** Sinus bradycardia; heart block > 1st degree; bronchospasm **Supplied:** Tabs 2.5, 5 mg; ophth soln 1% **SE:** Drowsiness, sexual dysfunction, bradycardia, edema, CHF *Ocular:* Conjunctival hyperemia, anisocoria, keratitis, eye pain **Notes:** No value in CHF

Carvedilol (Coreg) Uses: *HTN, CHF, MI* **Action:** Blocks adrenergic receptors, β$_1$, β$_2$, α **Dose:** *HTN:* 6.25–12.5 mg bid. *CHF:* 3.125–25 mg bid; w/ food to minimize ↓ BP **Caution:** [C (1st tri); D (2nd & 3rd tri), ?/–] Bradycardia, asthma, diabetes **Contra:** Decompensated cardiac failure, 2nd-/3rd-degree heart block, SSS, severe hepatic impair **Supplied:** Tabs 3.125, 6.25, 12.5, 25 mg **SE:** Dizziness, fatigue, hyperglycemia, bradycardia, edema, hypercholesterolemia **Notes:** Do not D/C abruptly; ↑ digoxin levels

Caspofungin (Cancidas) Uses: *Invasive aspergillosis refractory/intolerant to standard therapy, esophageal candidiasis* **Action:** An echinocandin; ↓ fungal cell wall synthesis; highest activity in regions of active cell growth **Dose:** 70 mg IV load day 1, 50 mg/d IV; slow inf; ↓ in hepatic impair **Caution:** [C, ?/–] Do not use w/cyclosporine; not studied as initial therapy **Contra:** Allergy to any component **Supplied:** IV inf **SE:** Fever, HA, N/V, thrombophlebitis at site, ↑ LFTs **Notes:** Monitor during inf; limited experience beyond 2 wk of therapy

Cefaclor (Ceclor) Uses: *Bacterial Infxns of the upper & lower resp tract, skin, bone, urinary tract, abdomen, gynecologic system* **Action:** 2nd-gen cephalosporin; ↓ cell wall synthesis. *Spectrum:* More gram(–) activity than 1st-gen cephalosporins; effective against gram(+) (*S. aureus*); good gram(–) coverage against *H. influenzae*) **Dose:** *Adults.* 250–500 mg PO tid; XR 375–500 mg bid. *Peds.* 20–40 mg/kg/d PO ÷ 8–12h; ↓ renal impair **Caution:** [B, +] **Contra:** Cephalosporin allergy **Supplied:** Caps 250, 500 mg; XR tabs 375, 500 mg; susp 125, 187, 250, 375 mg/5 mL SE: D, rash, eosinophilia, ↑ transaminases

22

500   Clinician's Pocket Reference, 11th Edition

Cefadroxil (Duricef, Ultracef)   Uses: *Infxns of skin, bone, upper & lower resp tract, urinary tract* Action: 1st-gen cephalosporin; ↓ cell wall synthesis. *Spectrum:* Good gram(+) coverage (group A b-hemolytic *Strep, Staph*); gram(−) (*E. coli, Proteus, Klebsiella*) **Dose: Adults.** 1–2 g/d PO, 2 ÷ doses **Peds.** 30 mg/kg/d ÷ bid; ↓ in renal impair **Caution:** [B, +] **Contra:** Cephalosporin allergy **Supplied:** Caps 500 mg; tabs 1 g; susp 125, 250, 500 mg/5 mL **SE:** N/V/ D, rash, eosinophilia, ↑ transaminases

Cefazolin (Ancef, Kefzol)   Uses: *Infxns of skin, bone, upper & lower resp tract, urinary tract* **Action:** 1st-gen cephalosporin; ↓ cell wall synthesis. *Spectrum:* Good coverage gram(+) bacilli & cocci, (*Strep, Staph* (except *Enterococcus*); some gram(−) (*E. coli, Proteus, Klebsiella*) **Dose: Adults.** 1–2 g IV q8h **Peds.** 25–100 mg/kg/d IV ÷ q6–8h; ↓ in renal impair **Caution:** [B, +] **Contra:** Cephalosporin allergy **Supplied:** Inj **SE:** D, rash, eosinophilia, elevated transaminases, pain at inj site **Notes:** Widely used for surgical prophylaxis

Cefdinir (Omnicef)   Uses: *Infxns of the resp tract, skin, bone & urinary tract* **Action:** 3rd-gen cephalosporin; ↓ cell wall synthesis *Spectrum:* Active against wide range of gram(+) & gram(−) organisms; more active than cefaclor & cephalexin against *Streptococcus, Staphylococcus;* active against some anaerobes **Dose: Adults.** 300 mg PO bid or 600 mg/d PO. **Peds.** 7 mg/kg PO bid or 14 mg/ kg/d PO; ↓ in renal impair **Caution:** [B, +] In PCN-sensitive pts, serum sickness-like Rxns reported **Contra:** Hypersensitivity to cephalosporins **Supplied:** Caps 300 mg; susp 125 mg/5 mL **SE:** Anaphylaxis, D, rare pseudomembranous colitis

Cefditoren (Spectracef)   Uses: *Acute exacerbations of chronic bronchitis, pharyngitis, tonsillitis; skin Infxns* **Action:** 3rd-gen cephalosporin; ↓ cell wall synthesis. Spectrum: Good gram(+) (Strep & Staph); gram(−) (H. influenzae & M. catarrhalis) **Dose: Adults & Peds > 12 y.** Skin: 200 mg PO bid × 10 d. Chronic bronchitis, pharyngitis, tonsillitis: 400 mg PO bid × 10 d; avoid antacids w/in 2 h; take w/meals; ↓ in renal impair **Caution:** [B, ?] Renal/hepatic impair **Contra:** Cephalosporin/PCN allergy, milk protein, or carnitine deficiency **Supplied:** 200-mg tabs **SE:** HA, N/V/D, colitis, nephrotox, hepatic dysfunction, Stevens–Johnson syndrome, toxic epidermal necrolysis, allergy Rxns **Notes:** Causes renal excretion of carnitine; tablets contain milk protein

Cefepime (Maxipime)   Uses: *UTI, pneumonia, febrile neutropenia, skin/ soft tissue Infxns* **Action:** 4th-gen cephalosporin; ↓ cell wall synthesis. *Spectrum:* gram(+) *S. pneumoniae, S. aureus,* gram(−) *K. pneumoniae, E. coli, P. aeruginosa,* & *Enterobacter* sp **Dose: Adults.** 1–2 g IV q12h. **Peds.** 50 mg/kg q8h for febrile neutropenia; 50 mg/kg bid for skin/soft tissue Infxns; ↓ in renal impair **Caution:** [B, +] **Contra:** Cephalosporin allergy **Supplied:** Inj 500 mg, 1, 2 g **SE:** Rash, pruritus, N/V/D, fever, HA, (+) Coombs' test w/o hemolysis **Notes:** Administered IM or IV

Cefixime (Suprax)   Uses: *Infxns of the resp tract, skin, bone & urinary tract* **Action:** 3rd-gen cephalosporin; ↓ cell wall synthesis. *Spectrum: S. pneumoniae, S. pyogenes, H. influenzae* & enterobacteria. **Dose: Adults.** 400 mg PO qd–bid. **Peds.** 8 mg/kg/d PO ÷ qd–bid; ↓ in renal impair **Caution:** [B, +] **Contra:** Cephalosporin allergy **Supplied:** Tabs 200, 400 mg; susp 100 mg/5 mL **SE:** N/V/D, flatulence & abdominal pain **Notes:** Monitor renal & hepatic Fxn; use susp for otitis media

Cefmetazole (Zefazone)   Uses: *Rx Infxns of the upper & lower resp tract, skin, bone, urinary tract, abdomen & gynecologic system* **Action:** 2ndgen cephalosporin; ↓ cell wall synthesis. *Spectrum:* Gram(+) against *S. aureus;* gram(−) activity & some anaerobic activity; use in mixed aerobic–anaerobic Infxns where *B. fragilis* likely **Dose: *Adults.*** 2 g IV q6–12h; ↓ in renal impair **Caution:** [B, +] **Contra:** Cephalosporin allergy **Supplied:** Inj 1, 2 g **SE:** Eosinophilia, leukopenia, N/V/D, ↑ LFTs, bleeding risk, rash, pseudomembranous colitis, disulfiram Rxn **Notes:** Avoid EtOH; safety not established in children

Cefonicid (Monocid) Uses: *Rx bacterial Infxns (resp tract, skin, bone & joint, urinary tract, gynecologic; sepsis)* **Action:** 2nd-gen cephalosporin; ↓ bacterial cell wall synthesis. *Spectrum:* Gram(+) including MSSA & many streptococci; gram(−) bacilli including *E. coli, Klebsiella, P. mirabilis, H. influenzae,* & *Moraxella* **Dose:** 0.5–2 g/24 h IM/IV; ↓ in renal impair **Caution:** [B, +] **Contra:** Cephalosporin allergy **Supplied:** Powder for inj 500 mg, 1 g, 10 g **SE:** D, rash, ↑ plts, eosinophilia, ↑ transaminases

Cefoperazone (Cefobid) Uses: *Rx Infxns of the resp, skin, urinary tract, sepsis* **Action:** 3rd-gen cephalosporin; ↓ bacterial cell wall synthesis. *Spectrum:* Gram(−) (eg, *E. coli, Klebsiella*); variable against *Streptococcus* & *Staphylococcus* sp; active *P. aeruginosa* but < ceftazidime **Dose: *Adults.*** 2–4 g/d IM/IV ÷ q 8–12h (12 g/d max). ***Peds.*** (not approved) 100–150 mg/kg/d IM/IV ÷ bid–tid (12 g/d max); ↓ in renal/hepatic impair **Caution:** [B, +] May ↑ risk of bleeding **Contra:** Cephalosporin allergy **Supplied:** Powder for inj 1, 2 g **SE:** D, rash, eosinophilia, ↑ LFTs, hypoprothrombinemia & bleeding (due to MTT side chain) **Notes:** May interfere w/warfarin

Cefotaxime (Claforan) Uses: *Rx Infxns of resp tract, skin, bone, urinary tract, meningitis, sepsis* **Action:** 3rd-gen cephalosporin; ↓ cell wall synthesis. *Spectrum:* Most gram(−) (not *Pseudomonas*), some gram(+) cocci (not *Enterococcus*); many PCN-resistant pneumococci **Dose: *Adults.*** 1–2 g IV q4–12h. ***Peds.*** 50–200 mg/kg/d IV ÷ q 4–12h; ↓ dose renal/hepatic impair **Caution:** [B, +] Arrhythmia associated w/rapid inj; caution in colitis **Contra:** Cephalosporin allergy **Supplied:** Powder for inj 500 mg, 1, 2, 10 g **SE:** D, rash, pruritus, colitis, eosinophilia, ↑ transaminases

Cefotetan (Cefotan) Uses: *Rx Infxns of the upper & lower resp tract, skin, bone, urinary tract, abdomen & gynecologic system* **Action:** 2nd-gen cephalosporin; ↓ cell wall synthesis. *Spectrum:* Less active against gram(+); anaerobes including *B. fragilis;* gram(−), including *E. coli, Klebsiella* & *Proteus* **Dose: *Adults.*** 1–2 g IV q12h. ***Peds.*** 20–40 mg/kg/d IV ÷ q12h; ↓ in renal impair **Caution:** [B, +] May ↑ bleeding risk; Hx of PCN allergies **Contra:** Cephalosporin allergy **Supplied:** Powder for inj 1, 2, 10 g **SE:** D, rash, eosinophilia, ↑ transaminases, hypoprothrombinemia & bleeding (due to MTT side chain) **Notes:** Caution w/other nephrotoxic drugs; may interfere w/warfarin

Cefoxitin (Mefoxin) Uses: *Rx Infxns of the upper & lower resp tract, skin, bone, urinary tract, abdomen & gynecologic system* **Action:** 2nd-gen cephalosporin; ↓ cell wall synthesis. *Spectrum:* Good gram(−) against enteric bacilli (ie, *E. coli, Klebsiella* & *Proteus*); anaerobic activity against *B. fragilis* **Dose: *Adults.*** 1–2 mg IV q6–8h. ***Peds.*** 80–160 mg/kg/d ÷ q4–6h; ↓ in renal impair **Caution:** [B, +] **Contra:** Cephalosporin allergy **Supplied:** Powder for inj 1, 2, 10 g **SE:** D, rash, eosinophilia, ↑ transaminases

Cefpodoxime (Vantin) Uses: *Rx resp, skin & urinary tract Infxns* **Action:** 3rd-gen cephalosporin; ↓ cell wall synthesis. *Spectrum: S. pneumoniae*

and non-β-lactamase-producing *H. influenzae;* acute uncomplicated *N. gonorrhoeae;* some uncomplicated gram(–) (*E. coli, Klebsiella, Proteus*) **Dose:** *Adults.* 200–400 mg PO q12h. *Peds.* 10 mg/kg/d PO ÷ bid; ↓ in renal impair, take w/food **Caution:** [B, +] **Contra:** Cephalosporin allergy **Supplied:** Tabs 100, 200 mg; susp 50, 100 mg/5 mL **SE:** D, rash, HA, eosinophilia, elevated transaminases **Notes:** Drug interactions w/agents that ↑ gastric pH

Cefprozil (Cefzil) **Uses:** *Rx resp tract, skin & urinary tract Infxns* **Action:** 2nd-gen cephalosporin; ↓ cell wall synthesis. *Spectrum:* Active against MSSA, strep & gram(–) bacilli (*E. coli, Klebsiella, P. mirabilis, H. influenzae, Moraxella*) **Dose:** *Adults.* 250–500 mg PO daily–bid. *Peds.* 7.5–15 mg/kg/d PO ÷ bid; ↓ in renal impair **Caution:** [B, +] **Contra:** Cephalosporin allergy **Supplied:** Tabs 250, 500 mg; susp 125, 250 mg/5 mL **SE:** D, dizziness, rash, eosinophilia, ↑ transaminases **Notes:** Use higher doses for otitis & pneumonia

Ceftazidime (Fortaz, Ceptaz, Tazidime, Tazicef) **Uses:** *Rx resp tract, skin, bone, urinary tract Infxns, meningitis & septicemia* **Action:** 3rd-gen cephalosporin; ↓ cell wall synthesis. *Spectrum: P. aeruginosa* sp, good gram(–) activity **Dose:** *Adults.* 500–2 g IV q8–12h. *Peds.* 30–50 mg/kg/dose IV q8h; ↓ in renal impair **Caution:** [B, +] **Contra:** Cephalosporin allergy **Supplied:** Powder for inj 1, 2, 10 g **SE:** D, rash, eosinophilia, ↑ transaminases

Ceftibuten (Cedax) **Uses:** *Rx resp tract, skin, urinary tract Infxns & otitis media* **Action:** 3rd-gen cephalosporin; ↓ cell wall synthesis. *Spectrum: H. influenzae & M. catarrhalis;* weak against *S. pneumoniae* **Dose:** *Adults.* 400 mg/d PO. *Peds.* 9 mg/kg/d PO; ↓ in renal impair; take on empty stomach **Caution:** [B, +] **Contra:** Cephalosporin allergy **Supplied:** Caps 400 mg; susp 90, 180 mg/5 mL **SE:** D, rash, eosinophilia, ↑ transaminases

Ceftizoxime (Cefizox) **Uses:** *Rx resp tract, skin, bone & urinary tract Infxns, meningitis, septicemia* **Action:** 3rd-gen cephalosporin; ↓ cell wall synthesis. *Spectrum:* Good gram(–) bacilli (not *Pseudomonas*), some gram(+) cocci (not *Enterococcus*) & some anaerobes **Dose:** *Adults.* 1–2 g IV q8–12h. *Peds.* 150–200 mg/kg/d IV ÷ q6–8h; ↓ in renal impair **Caution:** [B, +] **Contra:** Cephalosporin allergy **Supplied:** Inj 500 mg, 1, 2, 10 g **SE:** D, fever, rash, eosinophilia, thrombocytosis, ↑ transaminases

Ceftriaxone (Rocephin) **Uses:** *Resp tract (pneumonia), skin, bone, urinary tract Infxns, meningitis & septicemia;* **Action:** 3rd-gen cephalosporin; ↓ cell wall synthesis. *Spectrum:* Moderate gram(+); excellent against β-lactamase producers **Dose:** *Adults.* 1–2 g IV q12–24h. *Peds.* 50–100 mg/kg/d IV ÷ q12–24h; ↓ in renal impair **Caution:** [B, +] **Contra:** Cephalosporin allergy; hyperbilirubinemic neonates (displaces bilirubin from binding sites) **Supplied:** Powder for inj 250 mg, 500 mg, 1, 2 g **SE:** D, rash, leukopenia, thrombocytosis, eosinophilia, ↑ transaminases

Cefuroxime (Ceftin PO, Zinacef Parenteral) **Uses:** *Upper & lower resp tract, skin, bone, urinary tract, abdomen, gynecologic Infxns* **Action:** 2nd-gen cephalosporin; ↓ cell wall synthesis *Spectrum:* Staphylococci, group B streptococci, *H. influenzae, E. coli, Enterobacter, Salmonella & Klebsiella* **Dose:** *Adults.* 750 mg–1.5 g IV q8h or 250–500 mg PO bid. *Peds.* 100–150 mg/kg/d IV ÷ q8h or 20–30 mg/kg/d PO ÷ bid; ↓ in renal impair; take w/food **Caution:** [B, +] **Contra:** Cephalosporin allergy **Supplied:** Tabs 125, 250, 500 mg; susp 125, 250 mg/5 mL; powder for inj 750 mg, 1.5, 7.5 g **SE:** D, rash, eosin-

22

ophilia, ↑ LFTs **Notes:** Cefuroxime film-coated tablets & PO susp not bioequivalent; do not substitute on a mg/mg basis; IV crosses blood–brain barrier

Celecoxib (Celebrex) WARNING: ↑ Risk of serious CV thrombotic events, MI & stroke, which can be fatal; ↑ risk of serious GI adverse events including bleeding, ulceration & perforation of the stomach or intestines, which can be fatal. **Uses:** *Osteoarthritis & RA, ankylosing spondylitis*; acute pain, primary dysmenorrhea; preventive in familial adenomatous polyposis **Action:** NSAID; ↓ the COX-2 pathway **Dose:** 100–200 mg/d or bid; ↓ in hepatic impair; take w/food/milk **Caution:** [C/D (3rd tri), ?] Caution in renal impair **Contra:** Allergy to sulfonamides, periop CABG **Supplied:** Caps 100, 200 mg **SE:** see Warning; GI upset, HTN, edema, renal failure, HA **Notes:** Watch for Sxs of GI bleeding; no effect on plt/bleeding time; can affect drugs metabolized by P-450 pathway

Cephalexin (Keflex, Keftab) **Uses:** *Skin, bone, upper/lower resp tract, urinary tract Infxns* **Action:** 1st-gen cephalosporin; ↓ cell wall synthesis. *Spectrum: Strep, Staph, E. coli, Proteus, Klebsiella* **Dose:** *Adults.* 250–500 mg PO qid. *Peds.* 25–100 mg/kg/d PO ÷ qid; ↓ in renal impair; on empty stomach **Caution:** [B, +] **Contra:** Cephalosporin allergy **Supplied:** Caps 250, 500 mg; tabs 250, 500, 1000 mg; susp 125, 250 mg/5 mL **SE:** D, rash, eosinophilia, ↑ LFTs

Cephradine (Velosef) **Uses:** *Respiratory, GU, GI, skin, soft tissue, bone & joint Infxns* **Action:** 1st-gen cephalosporin; ↓ cell wall synthesis. *Spectrum:* Gram(+) bacilli & cocci (not *Enterococcus*); some gram(–) bacilli (*E. coli, Proteus & Klebsiella*) **Dose:** *Adults.* 250–500 mg q6–12h (8 g/d max). *Peds > 9 mo.* 25–100 mg/kg/d ÷ bid–qid (4 g/d max); ↓ in renal impair **Caution:** [B, +] **Contra:** Cephalosporin allergy **Supplied:** Caps: 250, 500 mg; powder for susp 125, 250 mg/5 mL, inj **SE:** Rash, eosinophilia, ↑ LFTs, N/V/D

Cetirizine (Zyrtec, Zyrtec D) **Uses:** *Allergic rhinitis & other allergic Sxs including urticaria* **Action:** Nonsedating antihistamine **Dose:** *Adults & Children > 6 y.* 5–10 mg/d. Zyrtec D 5/120 mg PO bid whole *Peds.* 6–11 mo: 2.5 mg qd. *12–23 mo:* 2.5 mg qd–bid; ↓ in renal/hepatic impair **Caution:** [B, ?/–] Elderly & nursing mothers; > 10 mg/d may cause drowsiness **Contra:** Allergy to cetirizine, hydroxyzine **Supplied:** Tabs 5, 10 mg; syrup 5 mg/5 mL; Zyrtec D: Tab 5/120 mg (cetirizine/pseudoephedrine) **SE:** HA, drowsiness, xerostomia

Cetuximab (Erbitux) WARNING: Severe inf Rxns including rapid onset of airway obstruction (bronchospasm, stridor, hoarseness), urticaria & hypotension. Permanent D/C is required. **Uses:** EGFR-expressing metastatic colorectal CA w/wo irinotecan **Action:** Human/mouse recombinant MoAb; binds EGFR, ↓ tumor cell growth **Dose:** Per protocol; load 400 mg/m^2 IV over 2 h; 250 mg/m^2 given over 1 h × 1 wk **Caution:** [C, –] **Supplied:** Inj 100 mg/ 50 mL **SE:** Acneform rash, asthenia/malaise, N/V/D, abdominal pain, alopecia, inf Rxn, dermatologic tox, interstitial lung disease, fever, sepsis, dehydration, kidney failure, PE **Notes:** Assess tumor for EGFR before Rx; pretreat w/diphenhydramine; w/ mild SE ↓ inf rate by 50%; limit sun exposure

Charcoal, Activated (Superchar, Actidose, Liqui-Char) **Uses:** *Emergency Rx in poisoning by most drugs & chemicals* **Action:** Adsorbent detoxicant **Dose:** Give w/70% sorbitol (2 mL/kg); repeated use of sorbitol not OK *Adults.* Acute intox: 30–100 g/dose. *GI dialysis:* 20–50 g q6h for 1–2 d.

22

Peds 1–12 y. Acute intox: 1–2 g/kg/dose. *GI dialysis:* 5–10 g/dose q4–8h **Caution:** [C, ?] May cause vomiting (hazardous in petroleum distillate & caustic ingestions); do not mix w/milk, ice cream, or sherbet **Contra:** Not effective for cyanide, mineral acids, caustic alkalis, organic solvents, iron, EtOH, methanol poisoning, Li; do not use sorbitol in pts w/fructose intolerance **Supplied:** Powder, liq, caps **SE:** Some liq dosage forms in sorbitol base (a cathartic); V/D, black stools, constipation **Notes:** Charcoal w/sorbitol not OK in children < 1 y; monitor for ↓ K⁺ & Mg²⁺; protect airway in lethargic or comatose pts

Chloral Hydrate (Aquachloral, Supprettes) [C-IV] Uses: *Short-term nocturnal & preop sedation* **Action:** Sedative hypnotic; active metabolite trichloroethanol **Dose:** ***Adults.*** *Hypnotic:* 500 mg–1 g PO or PR 30 min hs or before procedure. *Sedative:* 250 mg PO or PR tid. ***Peds.*** *Hypnotic:* 20–50 mg/kg/24 h PO or PR 30 min hs or before procedure. *Sedative:* 5–15 mg/kg/dose q8h; avoid w/CrCl < 50 mL/min or severe hepatic impair **Caution:** [C, +] Porphyria & neonates **Contra:** Allergy to components; severe renal, hepatic or cardiac Dz **Supplied:** Caps 500 mg; syrup 250, 500 mg/5 mL; supp 324, 500, 648 mg **SE:** GI irritation, drowsiness, ataxia, dizziness, nightmares, rash **Notes:** May accumulate; tolerance may develop > 2 wk; taper dose; mix syrup in H₂O or fruit juice; avoid EtOH & CNS depressants

Chlorambucil (Leukeran) Uses: *CLL, Hodgkin Dz, Waldenström macroglobulinemia* **Action:** Alkylating agent **Dose:** 0.1–0.2 mg/kg/d for 3–6 wk or 0.4 mg/kg/dose q2wk (per protocol) **Caution:** [D, ?] Sz disorder & BM suppression; affects human fertility **Contra:** Previous resistance; alkylating agent allergy **Supplied:** Tabs 2 mg **SE:** Myelosuppression, CNS stimulation, N/V, drug fever, rash, chromosomal damage can cause secondary leukemia, alveolar dysplasia, pulmonary fibrosis, hepatotox **Notes:** Monitor LFTs, CBC, leukocyte counts, plts, serum uric acid; ↓ initial dosage if pt has received radiation

Chlordiazepoxide (Librium, Mitran, Libritabs) [C-IV] Uses: *Anxiety, tension, EtOH withdrawal,* & preop apprehension **Action:** Benzodiazepine; antianxiety agent **Dose:** ***Adults.*** *Mild anxiety:* 5–10 mg PO tid–qid or PRN. *Severe anxiety:* 25–50 mg IM, IV, or PO q6–8h or PRN. *EtOH withdrawal:* 50–100 mg IM or IV; repeat in 2–4 h if needed, up to 300 mg in 24 h; gradually taper daily dose. ***Peds > 6 y.*** 0.5 mg/kg/24 h PO or IM ÷ q6–8h; ↓ in renal impair, elderly **Caution:** [D, ?] Resp depression, CNS impair, Hx of drug dependence; avoid in hepatic impair **Contra:** Preexisting CNS depression **Supplied:** Caps 5, 10, 25 mg; tabs 10, 25 mg; inj 100 mg **SE:** Drowsiness, CP, rash, fatigue, memory impair, xerostomia, weight gain **Notes:** Erratic IM absorption

Chlorothiazide (Diuril) Uses: *HTN, edema* **Action:** Thiazide diuretic **Dose:** ***Adults.*** 500 mg–1 g PO daily–bid; 100–500 mg/d IV (for edema only). ***Peds > 6 mo.*** 20–30 mg/kg/24 h PO ÷ bid; 4 mg/kg/d IV **Caution:** [D, +] Do not administer inj IM or SQ **Contra:** Cross-sensitivity to thiazides/sulfonamides, anuria **Supplied:** Tabs 250, 500 mg; susp 250 mg/5 mL; inj 500 mg/vial **SE:** ↓ K⁺, Na⁺, dizziness, hyperglycemia, hyperuricemia, hyperlipidemia, photosensitivity **Notes:** May be taken w/food/milk; take early in the day to avoid nocturia; use sun block; monitor electrolytes

Chlorpheniramine (Chlor-Trimeton, others) [OTC] Uses: *Allergic Rxns; common cold* **Action:** Antihistamine **Dose:** ***Adults.*** 4 mg PO q4–6h or 8–12 mg PO bid of SR ***Peds.*** 0.35 mg/kg/24 h PO ÷ q4–6h or 0.2 mg/kg/24 h SR **Caution:** [C, ?/–] BOO; NAG; hepatic insuff **Contra:** Allergy **Supplied:**

Tabs 4 mg; chew tabs 2 mg; SR tabs 8, 12 mg; syrup 2 mg/5 mL; inj 10, 100 mg/mL **SE:** Anticholinergic SE & sedation common, postural ↓ BP, QT changes, extrapyramidal Rxns, photosensitivity

Chlorpromazine (Thorazine) Uses: *Psychotic disorders, N/V,* apprehension, intractable hiccups **Action:** Phenothiazine antipsychotic; antiemetic **Dose:** *Adults. Psychosis:* 10–25 mg PO or PR bid–tid (usual 30–800 mg/d in ÷ doses). *Severe Sxs:* 25 mg IM/IV initial; may repeat in 1–4 h; then 25–50 mg PO or PR tid. *Hiccups:* 25–50 mg PO bid–tid. *Peds > 6 mo.* Psychosis & N/V: 0.5–1 mg/kg/dose PO q4–6h or IM/IV q6–8h; avoid in severe hepatic impair **Caution:** [C, ?/–] Safety in children < 6 mo not established; Szs, BM suppression **Contra:** Cross-sensitivity w/phenothiazines; NAG **Supplied:** Tabs 10, 25, 50, 100, 200 mg; SR caps 30, 75, 150 mg; syrup 10 mg/5 mL; conc 30, 100 mg/mL; supp 25, 100 mg; inj 25 mg/mL **SE:** Extrapyramidal SE & sedation; α-adrenergic blocking properties; ↓ BP; prolongs QT interval **Notes:** Do not D/C abruptly; dilute PO conc in 2–4 oz liq

Chlorpropamide (Diabinese) Uses: *Type 2 DM* **Action:** Sulfonylurea; ↑ pancreatic insulin release; ↑ peripheral insulin sensitivity; ↓ hepatic glucose output **Dose:** 100–500 mg/d; w/food **Caution:** [C, ?/–] CrCl < 50 mL/min; ↓ in hepatic impair **Contra:** Cross-sensitivity w/sulfonamides **Supplied:** Tabs 100, 250 mg **SE:** HA, dizziness, rash, photosensitivity, hypoglycemia, SIADH **Notes:** Avoid EtOH (disulfiram-like Rxn)

Chlorthalidone (Hygroton, others) Uses: *HTN* **Action:** Thiazide diuretic **Dose:** *Adults.* 50–100 mg PO daily. *Peds.* (Not approved) 2 mg/kg/dose PO 3×/wk or 1–2 mg/kg/d PO; ↓ in renal impair **Caution:** [D, +] **Contra:** Cross-sensitivity w/thiazides or sulfonamides; anuria **Supplied:** Tabs 15, 25, 50, 100 mg **SE:** ↓ K⁺, dizziness, photosensitivity, hyperglycemia, hyperuricemia, sexual dysfunction **Notes:** May take w/food/milk

Chlorzoxazone (Paraflex, Parafon Forte DSC, others) Uses: *Adjunct to rest & physical therapy to relieve discomfort associated w/acute, painful musculoskeletal conditions* **Action:** Centrally acting skeletal muscle relaxant **Dose:** *Adults.* 250–500 mg PO tid–qid. *Peds.* 20 mg/kg/d in 3–4 ÷ doses **Caution:** [C, ?] Avoid EtOH & CNS depressants **Contra:** Severe liver Dz **Supplied:** Tabs 250; caps 250, 500 mg **SE:** Drowsiness, tachycardia, dizziness, hepatotox, angioedema

Cholecalciferol, Vitamin D₃ (Delta D) Uses: Dietary supl to Rx vitamin D deficiency **Action:** Enhances intestinal Ca^{2+} absorption **Dose:** 400–1000 IU/d PO **Caution:** [A (D doses above RDA), +] **Contra:** ↑ Ca^{2+}, hypervitaminosis, allergy **Supplied:** Tabs 400, 1000 IU **SE:** Vitamin D tox (renal failure, HTN, psychosis) **Notes:** 1 mg cholecalciferol = 40,000 IU vitamin D activity

Cholestyramine (Questran, LoCHOLEST) Uses: *Hypercholesterolemia; Rx pruritus associated w/partial biliary obstruction; diarrhea associated w/excess fecal bile acids* **Action:** Binds intestinal bile acids, forms insoluble complexes **Dose:** *Adults.* Individualize: 4 g/d–bid (↑ to max 24 g/d & 6 doses/d). *Peds.* 240 mg/kg/d in 3 ÷ doses **Caution:** [C, ?] Constipation, phenylketonuria **Contra:** Complete biliary obstruction; hypolipoproteinemia types III, IV, V **Supplied:** 4 g of cholestyramine resin/9 g powder; w/aspartame: 4 g resin/5 g powder **SE:** Constipation, abdominal pain, bloating, HA, rash **Notes:** OD may result in GI obstruction; mix 4 g in 2–6 oz of noncarbonated beverage; take other meds 1–2 h before or 6 h after

Ciclopirox (Loprox) Uses: *Tinea pedis, tinea cruris, tinea corporis, cutaneous candidiasis, tinea versicolor* **Action:** Antifungal antibiotic in vitro cellular depletion of essential substrates &/or ions **Dose:** *Adults & Peds > 10 y.* Massage into affected area bid **Caution:** [B, ?] **Contra:** Component sensitivity **Supplied:** Cream, gel, lotion 1% **SE:** Pruritus, local irritation, burning **Notes:** D/C if irritation occurs; avoid dressings; gel best for athlete's foot

Cidofovir (Vistide) **WARNING:** Renal impair is major tox. Follow administration instructions **Uses:** *CMV retinitis in pts w/HIV* **Action:** Selective inhibition of viral DNA synthesis **Dose:** *Rx:* 5 mg/kg IV over 1 h once/wk for 2 wk w/probenecid. *Maint:* 5 mg/kg IV once/2 wk w/probenecid. *Probenecid:* 2 g PO 3 h before cidofovir, then 1 g PO at 2 h & 8 h after cidofovir; ↓ in renal impair **Caution:** [C, –] SCr > 1.5 mg/dL or CrCl = 55 mL/min or urine protein > 100 mg/dL; w/other nephrotoxic drugs **Contra:** Probenecid or sulfa allergy **Supplied:** Inj 75 mg/mL **SE:** Renal tox, chills, fever, HA, N/V/D, thrombocytopenia, neutropenia **Notes:** Hydrate w/NS before each inf

Cilostazol (Pletal) Uses: *Reduce Sxs of intermittent claudication* **Action:** Phosphodiesterase III inhibitor; ↑ cAMP in plts & blood vessels, vasodilation & inhibit plt aggregation **Dose:** 100 mg PO bid, 1/2 h before or 2 h after breakfast & evening meal **Caution:** [C, +/–] ↓ dose when used w/other drugs that inhibit CYP3A4 & CYP2C19 (page 647) **Contra:** CHF **Supplied:** Tabs 50, 100 mg **SE:** HA, palpitation, D

Cimetidine (Tagamet, Tagamet HB) [OTC] Uses: *Duodenal ulcer; ulcer prophylaxis in hypersecretory states (eg, trauma, burns); & GERD* **Action:** H₂ receptor antagonist **Dose:** *Adults.* Active ulcer: 2400 mg/d IV cont inf or 300 mg IV q6h; 400 mg PO bid or 800 mg hs. *Maint:* 400 mg PO hs. *GERD:* 300–600 mg PO q6h; maint 800 mg PO hs. *Peds.* Infants: 10–20 mg/kg/24 h PO or IV ÷ q6–12h. *Children:* 20–40 mg/kg/24 h PO or IV ÷ q6h; ↑ interval w/renal insuff; ↓ dose in the elderly **Caution:** [B, +] Many drug interactions (P-450 system) **Contra:** Component sensitivity **Supplied:** Tabs 200, 300, 400, 800 mg; liq 300 mg/5 mL; inj 300 mg/2 mL **SE:** Dizziness, HA, agitation, thrombocytopenia, gynecomastia **Notes:** Take 1 h before or 2 h after antacids; avoid EtOH

Cinacalcet (Sensipar) Uses: *Secondary hyperparathyroidism in CRF; ↑ Ca²⁺ in parathyroid carcinoma* **Action:** ↓ PTH by ↑ calcium-sensing receptor sensitivity **Dose:** *Secondary hyperparathyroidism:* 30 mg PO daily. *Parathyroid carcinoma:* 30 mg PO bid; titrate q2–4wk based on calcium & PTH levels; swallow whole; take w/food **Caution:** [C, ?/–] Dose adjust w/addition/deletion of CYP3A4 inhibitors **Supplied:** Tabs 30, 60, 90 mg **SE:** N/V/D, myalgia, dizziness, ↓ Ca²⁺ **Notes:** Monitor Ca²⁺, PO₄²⁻, PTH

Ciprofloxacin (Cipro) Uses: *Rx lower resp tract, sinuses, skin & skin structure, bone/joints & UT Infxns including prostatitis* **Action:** Quinolone antibiotic; ↓ DNA gyrase. *Spectrum:* Broad-spectrum gram(+) & gram(–) aerobics; little against *Strep;* good *Pseudomonas, E. coli, B. fragilis, P. mirabilis, K. pneumoniae, C. jejuni,* & *Shigella* **Dose:** *Adults.* 250–750 mg PO q12h; XR 500–1000 mg PO q24h; or 200–400 mg IV q12h; ↓ in renal impair **Caution:** [C, ?/–] Peds < 18 y **Contra:** Component sensitivity **Supplied:** Tabs 100, 250, 500, 750 mg; tabs XR 500, 1000 mg; susp 5 g/100 mL, 10 g/100 mL; inj 200, 400 mg **SE:** Restlessness, N/V/D, rash, ruptured tendons, ↑ LFTs **Notes:** Avoid antacids; reduce/restrict caffeine intake; interactions w/theophylline, caffeine, sucralfate, warfarin, antacids

22

Ciprofloxacin, Ophthalmic (Ciloxan) Uses: *Rx & prevention of ocular Infxns (conjunctivitis, blepharitis, corneal abrasions)* **Action:** Quinolone antibiotic; ↓ DNA gyrase **Dose:** 1–2 gtt in eye(s) q2h while awake for 2 d, then 1–2 gtt q4h while awake for 5 d **Caution:** [C, ?/–] **Contra:** Component sensitivity **Supplied:** Soln 3.5 mg/mL **SE:** Local irritation

Ciprofloxacin, Otic (Cipro HC Otic) Uses: *Otitis externa* **Action:** Quinolone antibiotic; ↓ DNA gyrase **Dose:** *Adult & Peds > 1 mo.* 1–2 gtt in ear(s) bid for 7 d **Caution:** [C, ?/–] **Contra:** Perforated tympanic membrane, viral Infxns of the external canal **Supplied:** Susp ciprofloxacin 0.2% & hydrocortisone 1% **SE:** HA, pruritus

Cisplatin (Platinol, Platinol AQ) Uses: *Testicular, small-cell & non-small-cell lung, bladder, ovarian, breast, head & neck & penile CAs; osteosarcoma; ped brain tumors* **Action:** DNA-binding; denatures double helix; intrastrand cross-linking; formation of DNA adducts **Dose:** 10–20 mg/m^2/d for 5 d q3wk; 50–120 mg/m^2 q3–4wk; (per protocols); ↓ in renal impair **Caution:** [D, –] Cumulative renal tox may be severe; monitor Mg^{2+}, electrolytes before & w/in 48 h after cisplatin **Contra:** Allergy to platinum-containing compounds; preexisting renal insuff, myelosuppression, hearing impair **Supplied:** Inj 1 mg/mL **SE:** Allergic Rxns, N/V, nephrotox (worse w/administration of other nephrotoxic drugs; minimize by NS inf & mannitol diuresis), high-frequency hearing loss in 30%, peripheral "stocking glove"-type neuropathy, cardiotox (ST-, T-wave changes), ↓ Mg^{2+}, mild myelosuppression, hepatotox; renal impair dose-related & cumulative **Notes:** Give taxanes before platinum derivatives

Citalopram (Celexa) WARNING: Closely monitor for worsening depression or emergence of suicidality, particularly in ped pts Uses: *Depression* **Action:** SSRI **Dose:** Initial 20 mg/d, may ↑ to 40 mg/d; ↓ in elderly & hepatic/renal insuff **Caution:** [C, +/–] Hx of mania, Szs & pts at risk for suicide **Contra:** MOAI or w/in 14 d of MAOI use **Supplied:** Tabs 10, 20, 40 mg; soln 10 mg/5 mL **SE:** Somnolence, insomnia, anxiety, xerostomia, diaphoresis, sexual dysfunction **Notes:** May cause ↓ Na$^+$/SIADH

Cladribine (Leustatin) Uses: *HCL, CLL, NHL, progressive MS* **Action:** Induces DNA strand breakage; interferes w/DNA repair/synthesis; purine nucleoside analogue **Dose:** 0.09–0.1 mg/kg/d cont IV inf for 1–7 d (per protocols) **Caution:** [D, ?/–] Causes neutropenia & Infxn **Contra:** Component sensitivity **Supplied:** Inj 1 mg/mL **SE:** Myelosuppression, T-lymphocyte suppression may be prolonged (26–34 wk), fever in 46% (may cause tumor lysis), Infxns (especially lung & IV sites), rash (50%), HA, fatigue **Notes:** Consider prophylactic allopurinol; monitor CBC

Clarithromycin (Biaxin, Biaxin XL) Uses: *Upper/lower resp tract, skin/skin structure Infxns, H. pylori Infxns & Infxns caused by nontuberculosis (atypical) Mycobacterium; prevention of MAC Infxns in HIV-Infxn* **Action:** Macrolide antibiotic, ↓ protein synthesis. *Spectrum: H. influenzae, M. catarrhalis, S. pneumoniae, M. pneumoniae, H. pylori* **Dose:** *Adults.* 250–500 mg PO bid or 1000 mg (2 × 500 mg XR tab)/d. *Mycobacterium:* 500–1000 mg PO bid *Peds > 9 mo.* 7.5 mg/kg/dose PO bid; ↓ in renal/hepatic impair **Caution:** [C, ?] Antibiotic-associated colitis; rare QT prolongation & ventricular arrhythmias, including torsade de pointes **Contra:** Allergy to macrolides; combo w/ranitidine in pts w/Hx of porphyria or CrCl < 25 mL/min **Supplied:** Tabs 250, 500 mg; susp 125, 250 mg/5 mL; 500 mg XR tab **SE:** Prolongs QT interval, causes

22

metallic taste, N/D, abdominal pain, HA, rash **Notes:** Multiple drug interactions, ↑ theophylline & carbamazepine levels; do not refrigerate suspension

Clemastine Fumarate (Tavist, Tavist-1) [OTC] **Uses:** *Allergic rhinitis & Sxs of urticaria* **Action:** Antihistamine **Dose:** *Adults & Peds > 12 y.* 1.34 mg bid–2.68 mg tid; max 8.04 mg/d *Peds < 12 y:* 0.4 PO bid **Caution:** [C, M] BOO **Contra:** NAG **Supplied:** Tabs 1.34, 2.68 mg; syrup 0.67 mg/5 mL **SE:** Drowsiness, dyscoordination, epigastric distress, urinary retention **Notes:** Avoid EtOH

Clindamycin (Cleocin, Cleocin-T) **Uses:** *Rx aerobic & anaerobic Infxns; topical for severe acne & vaginal Infxns* **Action:** Bacteriostatic; interferes w/protein synthesis. *Spectrum:* Streptococci, pneumococci, staphylococci & gram(+) & gram(–) anaerobes; no activity against gram(–) aerobes & bacterial vaginosis **Dose:** *Adults.* PO: 150–450 mg PO q6–8h. *IV:* 300–600 mg IV q6h or 900 mg IV q8h. *Vaginal:* 1 applicator hs for 7 d. *Topical:* Apply 1% gel, lotion, or soln bid. *Peds.* Neonates: (Avoid use; contains benzyl alcohol) 10–15 mg/kg/24 h ÷ q8–12h. *Peds > 1 mo:* 10–30 mg/kg/24 h ÷ q6–8h, to a max of 1.8 g/d PO or 4.8 g/d IV. *Topical:* Apply 1%, gel, lotion, or soln bid; ↓ in severe hepatic impair **Caution:** [B, +] Can cause fatal colitis **Contra:** Hx pseudomembranous colitis **Supplied:** Caps 75, 150, 300 mg; susp 75 mg/5 mL; inj 300 mg/2 mL; vaginal cream 2% **SE:** Diarrhea may be pseudomembranous colitis caused by *C. difficile*, rash, ↑ LFTs **Notes:** D/C drug if significant diarrhea, evaluate for *C. difficile*

Clofarabine (Clolar) **Uses:** Rx relapsed/refractory ALL after at least 2 regimens in children 1–21 y **Action:** Antimetabolite; ↓ ribonucleotide reductase w/false nucleotide base-inhibiting DNA synthesis **Dose:** 52 mg/m² IV over 2 h qd × 5 d (repeat q2–6wk); Per protocol **Caution:** [D, –] **Supplied:** Inj 20 mg/20 mL **SE:** N/V/D, anemia, leukopenia, thrombocytopenia, neutropenia, Infxn, ↑ AST/ALT **Notes:** Monitor for tumor lysis syndrome & SIRS/capillary leak syndrome

Clofazimine (Lamprene) **Uses:** *Leprosy & combo therapy for MAC in AIDS* **Action:** Bactericidal; ↓ DNA synthesis. *Spectrum:* Multibacillary dapsone-sensitive leprosy; erythema nodosum leprosum; *M. avium-intracellulare* **Dose:** *Adults.* 100–300 mg PO qd. *Peds.* 1 mg/kg/d in combo w/dapsone & rifampin; take w/meals **Caution:** [C, +/–] w/GI problems; use dosages > 100 mg/d for as short a duration as possible **Contra:** Component hypersensitivity **Supplied:** Caps 50 mg **SE:** Pink/brownish-black discoloration of the skin & conjunctiva, dry skin, GI intolerance **Notes:** Orphan drug for the Rx of dapsone-resistant leprosy; monitor for GI complaints

Clonazepam (Klonopin) [C-IV] **Uses:** *Lennox–Gastaut syndrome, akinetic & myoclonic Szs, absence Szs, panic attacks,* restless legs syndrome, neuralgia, parkinsonian dysarthria, bipolar disorder **Action:** Benzodiazepine; anticonvulsant **Dose:** *Adults.* 1.5 mg/d PO in 3 ÷ doses; ↑ by 0.5–1 mg/d q3d PRN up to 20 mg/d. *Peds.* 0.01–0.03 mg/kg/24 h PO ÷ tid; ↑ to 0.1–0.2 mg/kg/24 h ÷ tid; avoid abrupt withdrawal **Caution:** [D, M] Elderly pts, resp Dz, CNS depression, severe hepatic impair, NAG **Contra:** Severe liver Dz, acute NAG **Supplied:** Tabs 0.5, 1, 2 mg **SE:** CNS side effects, including drowsiness, dizziness, ataxia, memory impair **Notes:** Can cause retrograde amnesia; CYP3A4 substrate

Clonidine, Oral (Catapres) **Uses:** *HTN*; opioid, EtOH & tobacco withdrawal **Action:** Centrally acting α-adrenergic stimulant **Dose:** *Adults.* 0.1 mg PO bid adjust daily by 0.1- to 0.2–mg increments (max 2.4 mg/d). *Peds.* 5–

10 mcg/kg/d ÷ q8–12h (max 0.9 mg/d); ↓ in renal impair **Caution:** [C, +/–] Avoid w/β-blocker; withdraw slowly **Contra:** Component sensitivity **Supplied:** Tabs 0.1, 0.2, 0.3 mg **SE:** Rebound HTN w/abrupt cessation of doses > 0.2 mg bid; drowsiness, orthostatic ↓ BP, xerostomia, constipation, bradycardia, dizziness **Notes:** More effective for HTN if combined w/diuretics

Clonidine, Transdermal (Catapres TTS) Uses: *HTN* **Action:** Centrally acting α-adrenergic stimulant **Dose:** Apply 1 patch q7d to hairless area (upper arm/torso); titrate to effect; ↓ in severe renal impair; do not D/C abruptly (rebound HTN) **Caution:** [C, +/–] Avoid w/β-blocker, withdraw slowly **Contra:** Component sensitivity **Supplied:** TTS-1, TTS-2, TTS-3 (delivers 0.1, 0.2, 0.3 mg, respectively, of clonidine/d for 1 wk) **SE:** Drowsiness, orthostatic ↓ BP, xerostomia, constipation, bradycardia **Notes:** Doses > 2 TTS-3 usually not associated w/↑ efficacy; steady state in 2–3 d

Clopidogrel (Plavix) Uses: *Reduction of atherosclerotic events* **Action:** ↓ Plt aggregation **Dose:** 75 mg/d **Caution:** [B, ?] Active bleeding; risk of bleeding from trauma & other causes; TTP; liver Dz **Contra:** Active bleeding; intracranial bleeding **Supplied:** Tabs 75 mg **SE:** Prolongs bleeding time, GI intolerance, HA, dizziness, rash, thrombocytopenia, leukopenia **Notes:** Plt aggregation returns to baseline ~5 d after D/C; plt transfusion reverses effects acutely; 300 mg PO × 1 dose can be used to load pts

Clorazepate (Tranxene) [C-IV] Uses: *Acute anxiety disorders, acute EtOH withdrawal Sxs, adjunctive therapy in partial Szs* **Action:** Benzodiazepine; antianxiety agent **Dose:** *Adults.* 15–60 mg/d PO single or ÷ doses. *Elderly & debilitated pts:* Initial 7.5–15 mg/d in ÷ doses. *EtOH withdrawal:* Day 1: Initial 30 mg; then 30–60 mg in ÷ doses; day 2: 45–90 mg in ÷ doses; day 3: 22.5–45 mg in ÷ doses; day 4: 15–30 mg in ÷ doses. *Peds.* 3.75–7.5 mg/dose bid to 60 mg/d max ÷ bid–tid **Caution:** [D, ?/–] Not OK for < 9 y of age; elderly; Hx depression **Contra:** NAG **Supplied:** Tabs 3.75, 7.5, 15 mg; Tabs-SD (once-daily) 11.25, 22.5 mg **SE:** CNS depressant effects (drowsiness, dizziness, ataxia, memory impair), ↓ BP **Notes:** Monitor pts w/renal/hepatic impair (drug may accumulate); avoid abrupt D/C; may cause dependence

Clotrimazole (Lotrimin, Mycelex) [OTC] Uses: *Candidiasis & tinea Infxns* **Action:** Antifungal; alters cell wall permeability. *Spectrum:* Oropharyngeal candidiasis, dermatophytoses, superficial mycosis, cutaneous candidiasis & vulvovaginal candidiasis **Dose:** *PO: Prophylaxis:* One troche dissolved in mouth tid *Rx:* One troche dissolved in mouth 5 × d for 14 d. *Vaginal 1% Cream:* 1 applicatorful hs for 7 d. *2% Cream:* 1 applicatorful hs for 3 d *Tabs:* 100 mg vaginally hs for 7 d or 200 mg (2 tabs) vaginally hs for 3 d or 500-mg tabs vaginally hs once. *Topical:* Apply bid 10–14 d **Caution:** [B, (C if PO), ?] Not for systemic fungal Infxn; safety in children < 3 y not established **Contra:** Component allergy **Supplied:** 1% cream; soln; lotion; troche 10 mg; vaginal tabs 100, 500 mg; vaginal cream 1%, 2% **SE:** *Topical:* Local irritation; *PO:* N/V, ↑ LFTs **Notes:** PO prophylaxis used for immunosuppressed pts

Clotrimazole & Betamethasone (Lotrisone) Uses: *Fungal skin Infxns* **Action:** Imidazole antifungal & antiinflammatory. *Spectrum:* Tinea pedis, cruris & corpora **Dose:** *Pts ≥ 17 y.* Apply & massage into area bid for 2–4 wk **Caution:** [C, ?] Varicella Infxn **Contra:** Children < 12 y **Supplied:** Cream 15, 45 g; lotion 30 mL **SE:** Local irritation, rash **Notes:** Not for diaper dermatitis or under occlusive dressings

22

Clozapine (Clozaril) **WARNING:** Myocarditis, agranulocytosis, Szs & orthostatic ↓ BP associated w/clozapine; ↑ mortality in elderly w/dementia-related psychosis **Uses:** *Refractory severe schizophrenia*; childhood psychosis **Action:** "Atypical" TCA **Dose:** 25 mg daily–bid initial; ↑ to 300–450 mg/d over 2 wk. Maintain at lowest dose possible; do not D/C abruptly **Caution:** [B, +/–] Monitor for psychosis & cholinergic rebound **Contra:** Uncontrolled epilepsy; comatose state; WBC ≤ 3500 cells/μL before Rx or < 3000 cells/μL during Rx **Supplied:** Tabs 25, 100 mg **SE:** Tachycardia, drowsiness, weight gain, constipation, incontinence, rash, Szs, CNS stimulation, hyperglycemia **Notes:** Benign, self-limiting temperature elevations may occur during the 1st 3 wk of Rx, weekly CBC mandatory 1st 6 mo, then qowk

Cocaine [C-II] **Uses:** *Topical anesthetic for mucous membranes* **Action:** Narcotic analgesic, local vasoconstrictor **Dose:** Lowest amount of topical soln that provides relief; 1 mg/kg max **Caution:** [C, ?] **Contra:** PRG **Supplied:** Topical soln & viscous preparations 4%, 10%; powder, soluble tabs (135 mg) for soln **SE:** CNS stimulation, nervousness, loss of taste/smell, chronic rhinitis **Notes:** Use only on PO, laryngeal & nasal mucosa; do not use on extensive areas of broken skin

Codeine [C-II] **Uses:** *Mild–moderate pain; symptomatic relief of cough* **Action:** Narcotic analgesic; depresses cough reflex **Dose:** *Adults.* Analgesic: 15–60 mg PO or IM qid PRN. *Antitussive:* 10–20 mg PO q4h PRN; max 120 mg/d. *Peds.* Analgesic: 0.5–1 mg/kg/dose PO q4–6h PRN. *Antitussive:* 1–1.5 mg/kg/24 h PO ÷ q4h; max 30 mg/24 h; ↓ in renal/hepatic impair **Caution:** [C, (D if prolonged use or high doses at term), +] **Contra:** Component sensitivity **Supplied:** Tabs 15, 30, 60 mg; soln 15 mg/5 mL; inj 30, 60 mg/mL **SE:** Drowsiness, constipation **Notes:** Usually combined w/APAP for pain or w/agents (eg, terpin hydrate) as an antitussive; 120 mg IM = 10 mg IM morphine

Colchicine **Uses:** *Acute gouty arthritis & prevention of recurrences; familial Mediterranean fever*; primary biliary cirrhosis **Action:** ↓ migration of leukocytes; ↓ leukocyte lactic acid production **Dose:** *Initial:* 0.5–1.2 mg PO, then 0.5–0.6 mg q1–2h until relief or GI SE develop (max 8 mg/d); do not repeat for 3 d. *IV:* 1–3 mg, then 0.5 mg q6h until relief (max 4 mg/d); do not repeat for 7 d. *Prophylaxis:* PO: 0.5–0.6 mg/d or 3–4 d/wk; ↓ renal impair; caution in elderly **Caution:** [D, +] In elderly **Contra:** Serious renal, GI, hepatic, or cardiac disorders; blood dyscrasias **Supplied:** Tabs 0.5, 0.6 mg; inj 1 mg/2 mL **SE:** N/V/D, abdominal pain, BM suppression, hepatotox; severe local irritation can occur following SQ/IM **Notes:** Colchicine 1–2 mg IV w/in 24–48 h of an acute attack diagnostic/therapeutic in monoarticular arthritis

Colesevelam (Welchol) **Uses:** *Reduction of LDL & total cholesterol alone or in combo w/an HMG-CoA reductase inhibitor* **Action:** Bile acid sequestrant **Dose:** 3 tabs PO bid w/meals **Caution:** [B, ?] Severe GI motility disorders; safety & efficacy not established in peds **Contra:** Bowel obstruction **Supplied:** Tabs 625 mg **SE:** Constipation, dyspepsia, myalgia, weakness **Notes:** May ↓ absorption of fat-soluble vitamins

Colestipol (Colestid) **Uses:** *Adjunct to ↓ serum cholesterol in primary hypercholesterolemia* **Action:** Binds intestinal bile acids to form insoluble complex **Dose:** Granules: 5–30 g/d ÷ 2–4 doses; tabs: 2–16 g/d daily–bid **Caution:** [C, ?] Avoid w/high triglycerides, GI dysfunction **Contra:** Bowel obstruction **Supplied:** Tabs 1 g; granules 5, 300, 500 g **SE:** Constipation, abdominal pain, bloating, HA **Notes:** Do not use dry powder; mix w/beverage, soup, cereal, etc; may ↓ absorption of other medications; may ↓ absorption of fat-soluble vitamins

Colfosceril Palmitate (Exosurf Neonatal) (Discontinued)

Cortisone See Steroids, Tables 22–4 & 22–5 (pages 633 and 634)

Cromolyn Sodium (Intal, NasalCrom, Opticrom) **Uses:** *Adjunct to the Rx of asthma; prevent exercise-induced asthma; allergic rhinitis; ophth allergic manifestations*; food allergy **Action:** Antiasthmatic; mast cell stabilizer **Dose:** *Adults & Children > 12 y.* Inhal: 20 mg (as powder in caps) inhaled qid or met-dose inhaler 2 puffs qid. *PO:* 200 mg qid 15–20 min ac, up to 400 mg qid. *Nasal instillation:* Spray once in each nostril 2–6×/d. *Ophth:* 1–2 gtt in each eye 4–6×/d. *Peds. Inhal:* 2 puffs qid of met-dose inhaler. *PO: Infants < 2 y:* (not OK) 20 mg/kg/d in 4 ÷ doses. *2–12 y:* 100 mg qid ac **Caution:** [B, ?] **Contra:** Acute asthmatic attacks **Supplied:** PO conc 100 mg/5 mL; soln for neb 20 mg/2 mL; met-dose inhaler; nasal soln 40 mg/mL; ophth soln 4% **SE:** Unpleasant taste, hoarseness, coughing **Notes:** No benefit in acute Rx; 2–4 wk for maximal effect in perennial allergic disorders

Cyanocobalamin, Vitamin B$_{12}$ **Uses:** *Pernicious anemia & other vitamin B$_{12}$ deficiency states; ↑ requirements due to PRG; thyrotoxicosis; liver or kidney Dz* **Action:** Dietary vitamin B$_{12}$ supl **Dose:** *Adults.* 100 mcg IM or SQ qd for 5–10 d, then 100 mcg IM 2×/wk for 1 mo, then 100 mcg IM monthly. *Peds.* 100 mcg/d IM or SQ for 5–10 d, then 30–50 mcg IM q4wk **Caution:** [A (C if dose exceeds RDA), +] **Contra:** Allergy to cobalt; hereditary optic nerve atrophy; Leber Dz **Supplied:** Tabs 50, 100, 250, 500, 1000 mcg; inj 100, 1000 mcg/mL; gel 500 mcg/0.1 mL **SE:** Itching, D, HA, anxiety **Notes:** PO absorption erratic, altered by many drugs & not recommended; for use w/hyperalimentation

Cyclobenzaprine (Flexeril) **Uses:** *Relief of muscle spasm* **Action:** Centrally acting skeletal muscle relaxant; reduces tonic somatic motor activity **Dose:** 10 mg PO bid–qid (2–3 wk max) **Caution:** [B, ?] Shares the toxic potential of TCAs; urinary hesitancy or angle-closure glaucoma **Contra:** Do not use concomitantly or w/in 14 d of MAOIs; hyperthyroidism; heart failure; arrhythmias **Supplied:** Tabs 10 mg **SE:** Sedation & anticholinergic effects **Notes:** May inhibit mental alertness or physical coordination

Cyclopentolate (Cyclogyl) **Uses:** *Diagnostic procedures requiring cycloplegia & mydriasis* **Action:** Cycloplegic & mydriatic agent (can last up to 24 h) **Dose:** 1 gt then another in 5 min **Caution:** [C, ?] **Contra:** NAG **Supplied:** Soln, 0.5, 1, 2% **SE:** Blurred vision, ↑ sensitivity to light, tachycardia, restlessness

Cyclophosphamide (Cytoxan, Neosar) **Uses:** *Hodgkin Dz & NHL; multiple myeloma; small-cell lung, breast & ovarian CAs; mycosis fungoides; neuroblastoma; retinoblastoma; acute leukemia; allogeneic & ABMT in high doses; severe rheumatologic disorders* **Action:** Converted to acrolein & phosphoramide mustard, the active alkylating moieties **Dose:** 500–1500 mg/m^2 single dose at 2–4-wk intervals; 1.8 g/m^2 to 160 mg/kg (or ≈12 g/m^2 in 75-kg individual) in the BMT setting (per protocols); ↓ renal/hepatic impair **Caution:** [D, ?] w/BM suppression **Contra:** Component sensitivity **Supplied:** Tabs 25, 50 mg; inj 100 mg **SE:** Myelosuppression (leukopenia & thrombocytopenia); hemorrhagic cystitis, SIADH, alopecia, anorexia; N/V; hepatotox; rare interstitial pneumonitis; irreversible testicular atrophy possible; cardiotox rare; 2nd malignancies (bladder,

22

acute leukemias), risk 3.5% at 8 y, 10.7% at 12 y **Notes:** Hemorrhagic cystitis prophylaxis: continuous bladder irrigation & mesna uroprotection; encourage hydration, long-term bladder screening

Cyclosporine (Sandimmune, NeOral) **Uses:** *Organ rejection in kidney, liver, heart & BMT w/steroids; RA; psoriasis* **Action:** Immunosuppressant; reversible inhibition of immunocompetent lymphocytes **Dose:** *Adults & Peds.* PO: 15 mg/kg/d 12 h pretransplant; after 2 wk, taper by 5 mg/wk to 5–10 mg/kg/d. *IV:* If NPO, give ¹/₃ PO dose IV; ↓ in renal/hepatic impair **Caution:** [C, ?] Dose-related risk of nephrotox/hepatotox; live, attenuated vaccines may be less effective **Contra:** Abnormal renal Fxn; uncontrolled HTN **Supplied:** Caps 25, 50, 100 mg; PO soln 100 mg/mL; inj 50 mg/mL **SE:** May ↑ BUN & Cr & mimic transplant rejection; HTN; HA; hirsutism **Notes:** Administer in glass container; many drug interactions; NeOral & Sandimmune not interchangeable; interaction w/St. John's wort. Follow levels (see Table 22–2, page 628)

Cyclosporine Ophthalmic (Restasis) **Uses:** *↑ Tear production suppressed due to ocular inflammation* **Action:** Immune modulator, antiinflammatory **Dose:** 1 gt bid each eye 12 h apart. OK w/artificial tears, allow 15 min between **Caution:** [C, –] **Contra:** Ocular Infxn, component allergy **Supplied:** Single-use vial 0.05% **SE:** Ocular burning/hyperemia **Notes:** Mix vial well

Cyproheptadine (Periactin) **Uses:** *Allergic Rxns; itching* **Action:** Phenothiazine antihistamine; serotonin antagonist **Dose:** *Adults.* 4–20 mg PO ÷ q8h; max 0.5 mg/kg/d. *Peds.* 2–6 y: 2 mg bid–tid (max 12 mg/24 h). *7–14 y:* 4 mg bid–tid; ↓ in hepatic impair **Caution:** [B, ?] BPH **Contra:** Neonates or < 2 y; NAG; BOO; acute asthma; GI obstruction **Supplied:** Tabs 4 mg; syrup 2 mg/5 mL **SE:** Anticholinergic, drowsiness, **Notes:** May stimulate appetite

Cytarabine, ARA-C (Cytosar-U) **Uses:** *Acute leukemia, CML, NHL; IT for leukemic meningitis or prophylaxis* **Action:** Antimetabolite; interferes w/DNA synthesis **Dose:** 100–150 mg/m²/d for 5–10 d (low dose); 3 g/m² q12h for 8–12 doses (high dose); 1 mg/kg 1–2/wk (SQ maint); 5–70 mg/m² up to 3/wk IT (per protocols); ↓ in renal/hepatic impair **Caution:** [D, ?] w/marked BM suppression, ↓ dosage by ↓ the number of days of administration **Contra:** Component sensitivity **Supplied:** Inj 100, 500 mg, 1, 2 g **SE:** Myelosuppression, N/V/D, stomatitis, flu-like syndrome, rash on palms/soles, hepatic dysfunction, cerebellar dysfunction, noncardiogenic pulmonary edema, neuropathy **Notes:** Little use in solid tumors; high-dose tox limited by corticosteroid ophth soln

Cytarabine Liposome (DepoCyt) **Uses:** *Lymphomatous meningitis* **Action:** Antimetabolite; interferes w/DNA synthesis **Dose:** 50 mg IT q14d for 5 doses, then 50 mg IT q28d × 4 doses; use dexamethasone prophylaxis **Caution:** [D, ?] May cause neurotox; blockage to CSF flow may ↑ risk of neurotox; use in peds not established **Contra:** Active meningeal Infxn **Supplied:** IT inj 50 mg/5 mL **SE:** Neck pain/rigidity, HA, confusion, somnolence, fever, back pain, N/V, edema, neutropenia, thrombocytopenia, anemia **Notes:** Cytarabine liposomes are similar in microscopic appearance to WBC; caution in interpreting CSF studies

Cytomegalovirus Immune Globulin, CMV-IG IV (CytoGam) **Uses:** *Attenuation CMV Dz associated w/transplantation* **Action:** Exogenous IgG antibodies to CMV **Dose:** 150 mg/kg/dose w/in 72 h of transplant, for 16 wk posttransplant; see insert for schedule **Caution:** [C, ?] Anaphylactic Rxns; renal dysfunction **Contra:** Allergy to immunoglobulins; IgA deficiency **Supplied:** Inj 50 mg/mL **SE:** Flushing, N/V, muscle cramps, wheezing, HA, fever **Notes:** IV only; administer by separate line; do not shake

Dacarbazine (DTIC) Uses: *Melanoma, Hodgkin Dz, sarcoma* **Action:** Alkylating agent; antimetabolite as a purine precursor; ↓ protein synthesis, RNA & especially DNA **Dose:** 2–4.5 mg/kg/d for 10 consecutive d or 250 mg/m²/d for 5 d (per protocols); ↓ in renal impair **Caution:** [C, ?] In BM suppression; renal/hepatic impair **Contra:** Component sensitivity **Supplied:** Inj 100, 200, 500 mg **SE:** Myelosuppression, severe N/V, hepatotox, flu-like syndrome, ↓ BP, photosensitivity, alopecia, facial flushing, facial paresthesias, urticaria, phlebitis at inj site **Notes:** Avoid extravasation

Daclizumab (Zenapax) Uses: *Prevent acute organ rejection* **Action:** IL-2 receptor antagonist **Dose:** 1 mg/kg/dose IV; 1st dose pretransplant, then 4 doses 14 d apart posttransplant **Caution:** [C, ?] **Contra:** Component sensitivity **Supplied:** Inj 5 mg/mL **SE:** Hyperglycemia, edema, HTN, ↓ BP, constipation, HA, dizziness, anxiety, nephrotox, pulmonary edema, pain **Notes:** Administer w/in 4 h of preparation

Dactinomycin (Cosmegen) Uses: *Choriocarcinoma, Wilms tumor, Kaposi sarcoma, Ewing sarcoma, rhabdomyosarcoma, testicular CA* **Action:** DNA intercalating agent **Dose:** 0.5 mg/d for 5 d; 2 mg/wk for 3 consecutive wk; 15 mcg/kg or 0.45 mg/m²/d (max 0.5 mg) for 5 d q3–8wk in ped sarcoma (per protocols); ↓ in renal impair **Caution:** [C, ?] **Contra:** concurrent/recent chickenpox or herpes zoster; infants < 6 mo **Supplied:** Inj 0.5 mg **SE:** Myelo/immunosuppression, severe N/V, alopecia, acne, hyperpigmentation, radiation recall phenomenon, tissue damage w/extravasation, hepatotox

Dalteparin (Fragmin) Uses: *Unstable angina, non-Q-wave MI, prevention of ischemic complications due to clot formation in pts on concurrent ASA, prevent & Rx DVT following surgery* **Action:** LMWH **Dose:** *Angina/MI:* 120 IU/kg (max 10,000 IU) SQ q12h w/ASA. *DVT prophylaxis:* 2500–5000 IU SC 1–2 h preop, then qd for 5–10 d. *Systemic anticoagulation:* 200 IU/kg/d SQ or 100 IU/kg bid SQ **Caution:** [B, ?] in renal/hepatic impair, active hemorrhage, cerebrovascular Dz, cerebral aneurysm, severe HTN **Contra:** HIT; pork product allergy **Supplied:** Inj 2500 IU (16 mg/0.2 mL), 5000 IU (32 mg/0.2 mL), 10,000 IU (64 mg/mL) **SE:** Bleeding, pain at site, thrombocytopenia **Notes:** Predictable effects eliminates lab monitoring; not for IM/IV use

Dantrolene (Dantrium) Uses: *Rx spasticity due to upper motor neuron disorders, (eg, spinal cord injuries, stroke, CP, MS); malignant hyperthermia* **Action:** Skeletal muscle relaxant **Dose:** *Adults. Spasticity:* 25 mg PO daily; ↑ 25 mg to effect to 100 mg max PO qid PRN. *Peds.* 0.5 mg/kg/dose bid; ↑ by 0.5 mg/kg to effect, to 3 mg/kg/dose max qid PRN. *Adults & Peds. Malignant hyperthermia:* Rx: Continuous rapid IV, start 1 mg/kg until Sxs subside or 10 mg/kg is reached. *Postcrisis F/U:* 4–8 mg/kg/d in 3–4 ÷ doses for 1–3 d to prevent recurrence **Caution:** [C, ?] Impaired cardiac/pulmonary Fxn **Contra:** Active hepatic Dz; when spasticity needed to maintain posture or balance **Supplied:** Caps 25, 50, 100 mg; powder for inj 20 mg/vial **SE:** Hepatotox w/↑ LFTs, drowsiness, dizziness, rash, muscle weakness, pleural effusion w/pericarditis, D, blurred vision, hepatitis **Notes:** Monitor transaminases; avoid sunlight/EtOH/CNS depressants

Dapsone (Avlosulfon) Uses: *Rx & prevent PCP; toxoplasmosis prophylaxis; leprosy* **Action:** Unknown; bactericidal **Dose:** *Adults. PCP prophylaxis*

50–100 mg/d PO; Rx PCP 100 mg/d PO w/TMP 15–20 mg/kg/d for 21 d. *Peds.* *Prophylaxis of PCP* 1–2 mg/kg/24 h PO daily; max 100 mg/d **Caution:** [C, +] G6PD deficiency; severe anemia **Contra:** Component sensitivity **Supplied:** Tabs 25, 100 mg **SE:** Hemolysis, methemoglobinemia, agranulocytosis, rash, cholestatic jaundice **Notes:** Absorption ↑ by acidic environment; for leprosy, combine w/rifampin & other agents

Daptomycin (Cubicin) Uses: *Complicated skin/skin structure Infxns due to gram(+) organisms* **Action:** Cyclic lipopeptide; rapid membrane depolarization & bacterial death *Spectrum:* S. aureus (including MRSA), S. pyogenes, S. agalactiae, S. dysgalactiae subsp Equisimilis & E. faecalis (vancomycin-susceptible strains only) **Dose:** 4 mg/kg IV daily × 7–14 d (over 30 min); w/CrCl < 30 mL/min/dialysis: 4 mg/kg q48h **Caution:** [B, ?] Monitor CPK weekly **Supplied:** Inj 250, 500 mg/10 mL **SE:** Constipation, N/V/D, HA, rash, site Rxn, muscle pain/weakness, edema, cellulitis, hypo/hyperglycemia, ↑ alkaline phosphatase, cough, back pain, abdominal pain, ↓ K+, anxiety, chest pain, sore throat, cardiac failure, confusion, *Candida* Infxns **Notes:** Consider D/C HMG-CoA reductase inhibitors ↓ myopathy risk

Darbepoetin Alfa (Aranesp) Uses: *Anemia associated w/CRF* **Action:** ↑ Erythropoiesis, recombinant erythropoietin variant **Dose:** 0.45 mcg/kg single IV or SQ qwk; titrate, do not exceed target Hgb of 12 g/dL; see insert to convert from Epogen **Caution:** [C, ?] May ↑ risk of CV &/or neurologic SE in renal failure; HTN; w/Hx Szs **Contra:** Uncontrolled HTN, component allergy **Supplied:** 25, 40, 60, 100 mcg/mL, in polysorbate or albumin excipient **SE:** May ↑ cardiac risk, CP, hypo/hypertension, N/V/D, myalgia, arthralgia, dizziness, edema, fatigue, fever, ↑ risk Infxn **Notes:** Longer half-life than Epogen; weekly CBC until stable

Darifenacin (Enablex) Uses: OAB **Action:** Muscarinic receptor antagonist **Dose:** 7.5 mg/d PO; 15 mg/d max (7.5 mg/d w/moderate hepatic impair or w/ CYP3A4 inhibitors); w/drugs metabolized by CYP2D (flecainide, thioridazine, TCAs); swallow whole **Caution:** [C, ?/–] **Contra:** Urinary/gastric retention, uncontrolled NAG **Supplied:** Tabs ER 7.5 mg **SE:** Xerostomia/eyes, constipation, dyspepsia, abdominal pain, retention, abnormal vision, dizziness, asthenia

Daunorubicin (Daunomycin, Cerubidine) WARNING: Cardiac Fxn should be monitored due to potential risk for cardiac tox & CHF Uses: Acute leukemia **Action:** DNA intercalating agent; ↓ topoisomerase II; generates oxygen free radicals **Dose:** 45–60 mg/m^2/d for 3 consecutive d; 25 mg/m^2/wk (per protocols); ↓ in renal/hepatic impair **Caution:** [D, ?] **Contra:** Component sensitivity **Supplied:** Inj 20 mg **SE:** Myelosuppression, mucositis, N/V, alopecia, radiation recall phenomenon, hepatotox (hyperbilirubinemia), tissue necrosis w/extravasation, cardiotox (1–2% CHF risk w/550 mg/m^2 cumulative dose) **Notes:** Prevent cardiotox w/dexrazoxane; give allopurinol before Rx to prevent hyperuricemia

Delavirdine (Rescriptor) Uses: *HIV Infxn* **Action:** Nonnucleoside RT inhibitor **Dose:** 400 mg PO tid **Caution:** [C, ?] CDC recommends HIV-infected mothers not breast feed owing to risk of HIV transmission; renal/hepatic impair **Contra:** Concomitant use w/drugs highly dependent on CYP3A for clearance (eg, alprazolam, midazolam, pimozide, triazolam) **Supplied:** Tabs 100 mg **SE:** HA, fatigue, rash, ↑ transaminases, N/V/D **Notes:** Avoid antacids; ↓ cytochrome P-450 enzymes; numerous drug interactions; monitor LFTs

Demeclocycline (Declomycin) Uses: SIADH **Action:** Antibiotic, antagonizes ADH action on renal tubules **Dose:** 300–600 mg PO q12h on empty stomach; ↓ in renal failure; avoid antacids **Caution:** [D, +] Avoid in hepatic/renal dysfunction & children **Contra:** Tetracycline allergy **Supplied:** Tabs 150, 300 mg **SE:** D, abdominal cramps, photosensitivity, DI **Notes:** Avoid sunlight

Desipramine (Norpramin) **WARNING:** Closely monitor for worsening depression or emergence of suicidality **Uses:** *Endogenous depression,* chronic pain, peripheral neuropathy **Action:** TCA; ↑ synaptic serotonin or norepinephrine in CNS **Dose:** 25–200 mg/d single or ÷ dose; usually single hs dose (max 300 mg/d) **Caution:** [C, ?/–] CV Dz, Sz disorder, hypothyroidism **Contra:** MAOIs w/in 14 d; during AMI recovery phase **Supplied:** Tabs 10, 25, 50, 75, 100, 150 mg; caps 25, 50 mg **SE:** Anticholinergic (blurred vision, urinary retention, xerostomia); orthostatic ↓ BP; prolongs QT interval, arrhythmias **Notes:** Numerous drug interactions; blue-green urine; avoid sunlight

Desloratadine (Clarinex) Uses: *Seasonal & perennial allergic rhinitis; chronic idiopathic urticaria* **Action:** Active metabolite of Claritin, H₁-antihistamine, blocks inflammatory mediators **Dose:** *Adults & Peds > 12 y.* 5 mg PO qd; in hepatic/renal impair 5 mg PO qod **Caution:** [C, ?/–] RediTabs contain phenylalanine; safety not established for < 12 y **Supplied:** Tabs & RediTabs (rapid dissolving) 5 mg **SE:** Allergy, anaphylaxis, somnolence, HA, dizziness, fatigue, pharyngitis, xerostomia, nausea, dyspepsia, myalgia

Desmopressin (DDAVP, Stimate) Uses: *DI (intranasal & parenteral); bleeding due to uremia, hemophilia A & type I von Willebrand Dz (parenteral), nocturnal enuresis* **Action:** Synthetic analogue of vasopressin (human ADH); ↑ factor VIII **Dose:** *DI: Intranasal: Adults.* 0.1–0.4 mL (10–40 mcg/d in 1–4 ÷ doses. *Peds 3 mo–12 y.* 0.05–0.3 mL/d in 1 or 2 doses. *Parenteral: Adults.* 0.5–1 mL (2–4 mcg/d in 2 ÷ doses); converting from nasal to parenteral, use ¹/10 nasal dose. *PO: Adults.* 0.05 mg bid; ↑ to max of 1.2 mg. *Hemophilia A & von Willebrand Dz (type I): Adults & Peds > 10 kg.* 0.3 mcg/kg in 50 mL NS, inf over 15–30 min. *Peds < 10 kg.* As above w/dilution to 10 mL w/NS. *Nocturnal enuresis: Peds > 6 y.* 20 mcg intranasally hs **Caution:** [B, M] Avoid overhydration **Contra:** Hemophilia B; severe classic von Willebrand Dz; pts w/factor VIII antibodies **Supplied:** Tabs 0.1, 0.2 mg; inj 4 mcg/mL; nasal soln 0.1, 1.5 mg/mL **SE:** Facial flushing, HA, dizziness, vulval pain, nasal congestion, pain at inj site, ↓ Na⁺, H₂O intox **Notes:** In very young & old pts, ↓ fluid intake to avoid H₂O intox & ↓ Na⁺

Dexamethasone, Nasal (Dexacort Phosphate Turbinaire) Uses: *Chronic nasal inflammation or allergic rhinitis* **Action:** Antiinflammatory corticosteroid **Dose:** *Adult & Peds > 12 y.* 2 sprays/nostril bid–tid, max 12 sprays/d. *Peds 6–12 y.* 1–2 sprays/nostril bid, max 8 sprays/d **Caution:** [C, ?] **Contra:** Untreated Infxn **Supplied:** Aerosol, 84 mcg/activation **SE:** Local irritation

Dexamethasone, Ophthalmic (AK-Dex Ophthalmic, Decadron Ophthalmic) Uses: *Inflammatory or allergic conjunctivitis* **Action:** Antiinflammatory corticosteroid **Dose:** Instill 1–2 gtt tid–qid **Caution:** [C, ?/–] **Contra:** Active untreated bacterial, viral & fungal eye Infxns **Supplied:** Susp & soln 0.1%; oint 0.05% **SE:** Long-term use associated w/cataracts

Dexamethasone Systemic, Topical (Decadron) See Steroids, Systemic, page 603 & Table 22–4, page 633 & Steroids, Topical, Table 22–5, page 634

22

Dexpanthenol (Ilopan-Choline PO, Ilopan) Uses: *Minimize paralytic ileus, Rx postop distention* **Action:** Cholinergic agent **Dose:** *Adults. Relief of gas:* 2–3 tabs PO tid. *Prevent postop ileus:* 250–500 mg IM stat, repeat in 2 h, then q6h PRN. *Ileus:* 500 mg IM stat, repeat in 2 h, then q6h, PRN **Caution:** [C, ?] **Contra:** Hemophilia, mechanical obstruction **Supplied:** Inj; tabs 50 mg; cream **SE:** GI cramps

Dexrazoxane (Zinecard) Uses: *Prevent anthracycline-induced (eg, doxorubicin) cardiomyopathy* **Action:** Chelates heavy metals; binds intracellular iron & prevents anthracycline-induced free radicals Dose: 10:1 ratio dexrazoxane: doxorubicin 30 min before each dose **Caution:** [C, ?] **Contra:** Component sensitivity **Supplied:** Inj 10 mg/mL **SE:** Myelosuppression (especially leukopenia), fever, Infxn, stomatitis, alopecia, N/V/D; mild ↑ transaminase, pain at inj site

Dextran 40 (Rheomacrodex) Uses: *Shock, prophylaxis of DVT & thromboembolism, adjunct in peripheral vascular surgery* **Action:** Expands plasma volume; ↓ blood viscosity **Dose:** *Shock:* 10 mL/kg inf rapidly; 20 mL/kg max 1st 24 h; beyond 24 h 10 mL/kg max; D/C after 5 d. *Prophylaxis of DVT & thromboembolism:* 10 mL/kg IV day of surgery, then 500 mL/d IV for 2–3 d, then 500 mL IV q2–3d based on risk for up to 2 wk **Caution:** [C, ?] Inf Rxns; pts receiving corticosteroids **Contra:** Major hemostatic defects; cardiac decompensation; renal Dz w/severe oliguria/anuria **Supplied:** 10% dextran 40 in 0.9% NaCl or 5% dextrose **SE:** Allergy/anaphylactoid Rxn (observe during 1st min of inf), arthralgia, cutaneous Rxns, ↓ BP, fever **Notes:** Monitor Cr & electrolytes; keep well hydrated

Dextromethorphan (Mediquell, Benylin DM, PediaCare 1, others) [OTC] Uses: *Control nonproductive cough* **Action:** Depresses the cough center in the medulla **Dose:** *Adults.* 10–30 mg PO q4h PRN (max 120 mg/24 h). *Peds.* 7 mo–1 y: 2–4 mg q6–8h. 2–6 y: 2.5–7.5 mg q4–8h (max 30 mg/24 h). 7–12 y: 5–10 mg q4–8h (max 60 mg/24/h) **Caution:** [C, ?/–] Not for persistent or chronic cough **Supplied:** Caps 30 mg; lozenges 2.5, 5, 7.5, 15 mg; syrup 15 mg/15 mL, 10 mg/5 mL; liq 10 mg/15 mL, 3.5, 7.5, 15 mg/5 mL; sustained-action liq 30 mg/5 mL **SE:** GI disturbances **Notes:** Found in combo OTC products w/guaifenesin

Diazepam (Valium) [C-IV] Uses: *Anxiety, EtOH withdrawal, muscle spasm, status epilepticus, panic disorders, amnesia, preop sedation* **Action:** Benzodiazepine **Dose:** *Adults. Status epilepticus:* 5–10 mg q10–20min to 30 mg max in 8-h period. *Anxiety, muscle spasm:* 2–10 mg PO bid–qid or IM/IV q3–4h PRN. *Preop:* 5–10 mg PO or IM 20–30 min or IV just before procedure. *EtOH withdrawal:* Initial 2–5 mg IV, then 5–10 mg q5–10min, 100 mg in 1 h max. May require up to 1000 mg in 24-h period for severe withdrawal. Titrate to agitation; avoid excessive sedation; may lead to aspiration or resp arrest. *Peds. Status epilepticus:* < 5 y: 0.05–0.3 mg/kg/dose IV q15–30min up to a max of 5 mg. > 5 y: Give up to max of 10 mg. *Sedation, muscle relaxation:* 0.04–0.3 mg/kg/dose q2–4h IM or IV to max of 0.6 mg/kg in 8 h, or 0.12–0.8 mg/kg/24 h PO ÷ tid–qid; ↓ in hepatic impair; avoid abrupt withdrawal **Caution:** [D, ?/–] **Contra:** Coma, CNS depression, resp depression, NAG, severe uncontrolled pain, PRG **Supplied:** Tabs 2, 5, 10 mg; soln 1, 5 mg/mL; inj 5 mg/mL; rectal gel 5 mg/mL **SE:** Sedation, amnesia, bradycardia, ↓ BP, rash, ↓ resp rate **Notes:** Do not exceed 5 mg/min IV in adults or 1–2 mg/min in peds (resp arrest possible); IM absorption erratic

22

Diazoxide (Hyperstat, Proglycem) Uses: *Hypoglycemia due to hyperinsulinism (Proglycem); hypertensive crisis (Hyperstat)* **Action:** ↓ Pancreatic insulin release; antihypertensive **Dose:** *Hypertensive crisis:* 1–3 mg/kg IV (150 mg max in single inj); repeat in 5–15 min until BP controlled; repeat every 4–24 h; monitor BP closely. *Hypoglycemia:* **Adults & Peds.** 3–8 mg/kg/ 24 h PO ÷ q8–12h. *Neonates.* 8–15 mg/kg/24 h ÷ in 3 equal doses; maint 8–10 mg/kg/24 h PO in 2–3 equal doses **Caution:** [C, ?] ↓ effect w/phenytoin; ↑ effect w/diuretics, warfarin **Contra:** Allergy to thiazides or other sulfonamide-containing products; HTN associated w/aortic coarctation, AV shunt, or pheo-chromocytoma **Supplied:** Inj 15 mg/mL; caps 50 mg; PO susp 50 mg/mL **SE:** Hyperglycemia, ↓ BP, dizziness, Na⁺ & H₂O retention, N/V, weakness **Notes:** Can give false-negative insulin response to glucagons; treat extravasation w/ warm compress

Dibucaine (Nupercainal)   **Uses:** *Hemorrhoids & minor skin conditions* **Action:** Topical anesthetic **Dose:** Insert PR w/applicator bid & after each bowel movement; apply sparingly to skin **Caution:** [C, ?] **Contra:** Component sensitivity **Supplied:** 1% Oint w/rectal applicator; 0.5% cream **SE:** Local irritation, rash

Diclofenac (Cataflam, Voltaren)   **WARNING:** May ↑ risk of CV events & GI bleeding **Uses:** *Arthritis & pain* **Action:** NSAID **Dose:** 50–75 mg PO bid; w/food or milk **Caution:** [B (D 3rd tri or near delivery), ?] CHF, HTN, renal/hepatic dysfunction & Hx PUD **Contra:** NSAID/aspirin allergy; porphyria **Supplied:** Tabs 50 mg; tabs DR 25, 50, 75, 100 mg; XR tabs 100 mg; ophthal soln 0.1% **SE:** Abdominal cramps, heartburn, GI ulceration, rash, inter-stitial nephritis **Notes:** Do not crush; watch for GI bleed

Dicloxacillin (Dynapen, Dycill)   **Uses:** *Rx of pneumonia, skin & soft tissue Infxns & osteomyelitis caused by penicillinase-producing staphylococci* **Action:** Bactericidal; ↓ cell wall synthesis. *Spectrum: S. aureus & Strep* **Dose:** **Adults.** 250–500 mg qid **Peds < 40 kg.** 12.5–25 mg/kg/d ÷ qid; take on empty stomach **Caution:** [B, ?] **Contra:** Component or PCN sensitivity **Supplied:** Caps 125, 250, 500 mg; soln 62.5 mg/5 mL **SE:** N/D, abdominal pain **Notes:** Monitor PTT if pt on warfarin

Dicyclomine (Bentyl)   **Uses:** *Functional IBS* **Action:** Smooth muscle relaxant **Dose:** **Adults.** 20 mg PO qid; ↑ to 160 mg/d max or 20 mg IM q6h **Peds.** *Infants > 6 mo:* 5 mg/dose tid–qid. *Children:* 10 mg/dose tid–qid **Caution:** [B, –] **Contra:** Infants < 6 mo, NAG, MyG, severe UC, BOO **Supplied:** Caps 10, 20 mg; tabs 20 mg; syrup 10 mg/5 mL; inj 10 mg/mL **SE:** Anticholin-ergic SEs may limit dose **Notes:** Take 30–60 min before meal; avoid EtOH

Didanosine, ddl (Videx)   **WARNING:** Allergy manifested as fever, rash, fatigue, GI/resp Sxs reported; stop drug immediately & do not rechallenge; lactic acidosis & hepatomegaly/steatosis reported **Uses:** *HIV Infxn in zidovudine-intoler-ant pts* **Action:** Nucleoside antiretroviral agent **Dose:** **Adults** > 60 kg: 400 mg/d PO or 200 mg PO bid. < 60 kg: 250 mg/d PO or 125 mg PO bid; adults should take 2 tabs/administration. **Peds.** Dose by following table; ↓ in renal impair:

BSA (m²)	Tablets (mg)	Powder (mg)
1.1–1.4	100 bid	125 bid
0.8–1	75 bid	94 bid
0.5–0.7	50 bid	62 bid
<0.4	25 bid	31 bid

22

Caution: [B, –] CDC recommends HIV-infected mothers not breast feed owing to risk of HIV transmission **Contra:** Component sensitivity **Supplied:** Chew tabs 25, 50, 100, 150, 200 mg; powder packets 100, 167, 250, 375 mg; powder for soln 2, 4 g **SE:** Pancreatitis, peripheral neuropathy, D, HA **Notes:** Do not take w/meals; thoroughly chew tablets, do not mix w/fruit juice or acidic beverages; reconstitute powder w/H_2O

Diflunisal (Dolobid) **WARNING:** May ↑ risk of CV events & GI bleeding **Uses:** *Mild–moderate pain; osteoarthritis* **Action:** NSAID **Dose:** Pain: 500 mg PO bid. Osteoarthritis: 500–1500 mg PO in 2–3 ÷ doses; ↓ in renal impair, take w/ food/milk **Caution:** [C (D 3rd tri or near delivery), ?] CHF, HTN, renal/hepatic dysfunction & Hx PUD. **Contra:** Allergy to NSAIDs or aspirin, active GI bleed **Supplied:** Tabs 250, 500 mg **SE:** May ↑ bleeding time; HA, abdominal cramps, heartburn, GI ulceration, rash, interstitial nephritis, fluid retention

Digoxin (Lanoxin, Lanoxicaps) **Uses:** *CHF, AF & flutter & PAT* **Action:** Positive inotrope; ↑ AV node refractory period **Dose:** *Adults.* PO digitalization: 0.5–0.75 mg PO, then 0.25 mg PO q6–8h to total 1–1.5 mg. *IV or IM digitalization:* 0.25–0.5 mg IM or IV, then 0.25 mg q4–6h to total ≈ 1 mg. *Daily maint:* 0.125–0.5 mg/d PO, IM, or IV (average daily dose 0.125–0.25 mg). *Peds. Preterm infants: Digitalization:* 30 mcg/kg PO or 25 mcg/kg IV; give ¹/₂ of dose initial, then ¹/₄ of dose at 8–12-h intervals for 2 doses. *Maint:* 5–7.5 mcg/kg/24 h PO or 4–6 mcg/ kg/24 h IV ÷ q12h. *Term infants: Digitalization:* 25–35 mcg/kg PO or 20–30 mcg/kg IV; give ¹/₂ the dose initial, then ¹/₃ of dose at 8–12 h. *Maint:* 6–10 mcg/kg/24 h PO or 5–8 mcg/kg/24 h ÷ q12h. *1 mo–2 y: Digitalization:* 35–60 mcg/kg PO or 30–50 mcg/kg IV; give ¹/₂ the initial dose, then ¹/₃ dose at 8–12-h intervals for 2 doses. *Maint:* 10–15 mcg/kg/24 h PO or 7.5–15 mcg/kg/24 h IV ÷ q12h. *2–10 y: Digitalization:* 30–40 mcg/kg PO or 25 mcg/kg IV; give ¹/₂ initial dose, then ¹/₃ of the dose at 8–12-h intervals for 2 doses. *Maint:* 8–10 mcg/kg/24 h PO or 6–8 mcg/kg/24 h IV ÷ q12h. *7–10 y:* Same as for adults; ↓ in renal impair, follow serum levels **Caution:** [C, +] **Contra:** AV block; idiopathic hypertrophic subaortic stenosis; constrictive pericarditis **Supplied:** Caps 0.05, 0.1, 0.2 mg; tabs 0.125, 0.25, 0.5 mg; elixir 0.05 mg/mL; inj 0.1, 0.25 mg/mL **SE:** Can cause heart block; ↓ K+ potentiates tox; N/V, HA, fatigue, visual disturbances (yellow-green halos around lights), cardiac arrhythmias **Notes:** Multiple drug interactions; IM inj painful, has erratic absorption & should not be used; Levels, Table 22–2, page 628.

Digoxin Immune Fab (Digibind) **Uses:** *Life-threatening digoxin intox* **Action:** Antigen-binding fragments bind & inactivate digoxin **Dose:** *Adults & Peds.* Based on serum level & pt's weight; see charts provided w/drug **Caution:** [C, ?] **Contra:** Sheep product allergy **Supplied:** Inj 38 mg/vial **SE:** Worsening of cardiac output or CHF, ↓ K^+, facial swelling & redness **Notes:** Each vial binds ≈ 0.6 mg of digoxin; renal failure may require redosing in several days

Diltiazem (Cardizem, Cardizem CD, Cardizem SR, Cartia XT, Dilacor XR, Diltia XT, Tiamate, Tiazac) **Uses:** *Angina, prevention of reinfarction, HTN, AF or flutter & PAT* **Action:** CCB **Dose:** PO: Initial, 30 mg PO qid; ↑ to 180–360 mg/d in 3–4 ÷ doses PRN. *SR:* 60–120 mg PO bid; ↑ to 360 mg/d max. *CD or XR:* 120–360 mg/d (max 480 mg/d). *IV:* 0.25 mg/kg IV bolus over 2 min; may repeat in 15 min at 0.35 mg/kg; begin inf of 5–15 mg/h **Caution:** [C, +] ↑ effect w/amiodarone, cimetidine, fentanyl, lithium, cyclosporine, digoxin, β-blockers, cisapride, theophylline **Contra:** SSS,

AV block, ↓ BP, AMI, pulmonary congestion **Supplied:** *Cardizem CD:* Caps 120, 180, 240, 300, 360 mg; *Cardizem SR:* Caps 60, 90, 120 mg; *Cardizem:* Tabs 30, 60, 90, 120 mg; *Cartia XT:* Caps 120, 180, 240, 300 mg; *Dilacor XR:* Caps 180, 240 mg; *Diltia XT:* Caps 120, 180, 240 mg; *Tiazac:* Caps 120, 180, 240, 300, 360, 420 mg; *Tiamate (XR):* Tabs 120, 180, 240 mg; inj 5 mg/mL **SE:** Gingival hyperplasia, bradycardia, AV block, ECG abnormalities, peripheral edema, dizziness, HA **Notes:** Cardizem CD, Dilacor XR & Tiazac not interchangeable

Dimenhydrinate (Dramamine, others)   Uses:
Prevention & Rx of N/V, dizziness, or vertigo of motion sickness **Action:** Antiemetic **Dose:** *Adults.* 50–100 mg PO q4–6h, max 400 mg/d; 50 mg IM/IV PRN. *Peds.* 5 mg/kg/24 h PO or IV ÷ qid (max 300 mg/d) **Caution:** [B, ?] **Contra:** Component sensitivity **Supplied:** Tabs 50 mg; chew tabs 50 mg; liq 12.5 mg/4 mL, 12.5 mg/5 mL, 15.62 mg/5 mL; inj 50 mg/mL **SE:** Anticholinergic side effects

Dimethyl Sulfoxide, DMSO (Rimso-50)   Uses:
Interstitial cystitis **Action:** Unknown **Dose:** Intravesical, 50 mL, retain for 15 min; repeat q2wk until relief **Caution:** [C, ?] **Contra:** Component sensitivity **Supplied:** 50% soln in 50 mL SE: Cystitis, eosinophilia, GI & taste disturbance

Dinoprostone (Cervidil Vaginal Insert, Prepidil Vaginal Gel)
Uses: *Induce labor; terminate PRG (12–28 wk); evacuate uterus in missed abortion or fetal death* **Action:** Prostaglandin, changes consistency, dilatation & effacement of the cervix; induces uterine contraction **Dose:** *Gel*: 0.5 mg; if no cervical/uterine response, repeat 0.5 mg q6h (max 24-h dose 1.5 mg). *Vaginal insert:* 1 insert (10 mg = 0.3 mg dinoprostone/h over 12 h); remove w/onset of labor or 12 h after insertion. *Vaginal supp:* 20 mg repeated every 3–5 h; adjust PRN supp: 1 high in vagina, repeat at 3–5-h intervals until abortion (240 mg max) **Caution:** [X, ?] **Contra:** Ruptured membranes, allergy to prostaglandins, placenta previa or unexplained vaginal bleeding, when oxytocic drugs contraindicated or if prolonged uterine contractions are inappropriate (Hx C-section, cephalopelvic disproportion, etc) **Supplied:** *Endocervical gel:* 0.5 mg in 3-g syringes (w/10-mm & 20-mm shielded catheter) *Vaginal gel:* 0.5 mg/3 g *Vaginal supp:* 20 mg *Vaginal insert, CR:* 0.3 mg/h SE: N/V/D, dizziness, flushing, HA, fever

Diphenhydramine (Benadryl) [OTC]   Uses:
Rx & prevent allergic Rxns, motion sickness, potentiate narcotics, sedation, cough suppression & Rx of extrapyramidal Rxns **Action:** Antihistamine, antiemetic **Dose:** *Adults.* 25–50 mg PO, IV, or IM bid–tid. *Peds.* 5 mg/kg/24 h PO or IM ÷ q6h (max 300 mg/d); ↑ dosing interval in moderate–severe renal failure **Caution:** [B, –] **Contra:** W/acute asthma attack **Supplied:** Tabs & caps 25, 50 mg; chew tabs 12.5 mg; elixir 12.5 mg/5 mL; syrup 12.5 mg/5 mL; liq 6.25 mg/5 mL, 12.5 mg/5 mL; inj 50 mg/mL **SE:** Anticholinergic (xerostomia, urinary retention, sedation)

Diphenoxylate + Atropine (Lomotil) [C-V]   Uses:
D **Action:** Constipating meperidine congener, ↓ GI motility **Dose:** *Adults.* Initial, 5 mg PO tid–qid until under control, then 2.5–5 mg PO bid. *Peds > 2 y:* 0.3–0.4 mg/kg/24 h (of diphenoxylate) bid–qid **Caution:** [C, +] **Contra:** Obstructive jaundice, diarrhea due to bacterial Infxn; children < 2 y **Supplied:** Tabs 2.5 mg diphenoxylate/0.025 mg atropine; liq 2.5 mg diphenoxylate/0.025 mg atropine/5 mL **SE:** Drowsiness, dizziness, xerostomia, blurred vision, urinary retention, constipation

22

Diphtheria, Tetanus Toxoids & Acellular Pertussis Adsorbed, Hepatitis B Recombinant & Inactivated Poliovirus Vaccine IPV Combined (Pediarix) Uses: *Vaccine against diphtheria, tetanus, pertussis, HBV, polio (types 1, 2, 3) as a 3-dose primary series in infants & children < 7, born to HBsAg(–) mothers* Action: Active immunization Dose: *Peds. Infants:* Three 0.5-mL doses IM, at 6–8-wk intervals, start at 2 mo; child given 1 dose of hep B vaccine, same; child previously vaccinated w/one or more doses IPV, use to complete series Caution: [C, N/A] Contra: If HbsAG(+) mother, adults, children > 7 y, immunosuppressed, allergy to yeast, neomycin, or polymyxin B, Hx allergy to any component, encephalopathy, or progressive neurologic disorders; caution in bleeding disorders. Supplied: Single-dose vials 0.5 mL SE: Drowsiness, restlessness, fever, fussiness, ↓ appetite, nodule redness, inj site pain/swelling Notes: Give IM only

Dipivefrin (Propine) Uses: *Open-angle glaucoma* Action: α-Adrenergic agonist Dose: 1 gt in eye q12h Caution: [B, ?] Contra: Closed-angle glaucoma Supplied: 0.1% soln SE: HA, local irritation, blurred vision, photophobia, HTN

Dipyridamole (Persantine) Uses: *Prevent postop thromboembolic disorders, often in combo w/ASA or warfarin (eg, CABG, vascular graft); w/warfarin after artificial heart valve; chronic angina; w/ASA to prevent coronary artery thrombosis; dipyridamole IV used in place of exercise stress test for CAD* Action: Antiplt activity; coronary vasodilator Dose: *Adults.* 75–100 mg PO tid–qid; stress test 0.14 mg/kg/min (max 60 mg over 4 min). *Peds > 12 y.* 3–6 mg/kg/d divided tid Caution: [B, ?/–] Caution w/other drugs that affect coagulation Contra: Component sensitivity Supplied: Tabs 25, 50, 75 mg; inj 5 mg/mL SE: HA, ↓ BP, nausea, abdominal distress, flushing rash, dyspnea Notes: IV use can worsen angina

Dipyridamole & Aspirin (Aggrenox) Uses: *↓ Reinfarction after MI; prevent occlusion after CABG; ↓ risk of stroke* Action: ↓ Plt aggregation (both agents) Dose: 1 cap PO bid Caution: [C, ?] Contra: Ulcers, bleeding diathesis Supplied: Dipyridamole (XR) 200 mg/aspirin 25 mg SE: ASA component: allergic Rxns, skin Rxns, ulcers/GI bleed, bronchospasm; dipyridamole component: dizziness, HA, rash Notes: Swallow capsule whole

Dirithromycin (Dynabac) Uses: *Bronchitis, community-acquired pneumonia & skin & skin structure Infxns* Action: Macrolide antibiotic. *Spectrum: M. catarrhalis, S. pneumoniae, Legionella, H. influenzae, S. pyogenes, S. aureus* Dose: 500 mg/d PO; w/food; swallow whole Caution: [C, M] Contra: w/ pimozide Supplied: Tabs 250 mg SE: Abdominal discomfort, HA, rash, ↑ K$^+$

Disopyramide (Norpace, NAPamide) Uses: *Suppression & prevention of VT* Action: Class 1A antiarrhythmic Dose: *Adults.* 400–800 mg/d ÷ q6h for regular & q12h for SR. *Peds.* < 1 y: 10–30 mg/kg/24 h PO (÷ qid). *1–4 y:* 10–20 mg/kg/24 h PO (÷ qid). *4–12 y:* 10–15 mg/kg/24 h PO (÷ qid). *12–18 y:* 6–15 mg/kg/24 h PO (÷ qid); ↓ in renal/hepatic impair Caution: [C, +] Contra: AV block, cardiogenic shock Supplied: Caps 100, 150 mg; SR caps 100, 150 mg SE: Anticholinergic SEs; negative inotrope, may induce CHF Notes: See Drug Levels, Table 22–2, page 628.

Dobutamine (Dobutrex) Uses: *Short-term in cardiac decompensation secondary to depressed contractility* Action: Positive inotrope Dose: *Adults &*

Peds. Cont IV inf of 2.5–15 mcg/kg/min; rarely, 40 mcg/kg/min required; titrate **Caution:** [C, ?] **Contra:** Sensitivity to sulfites, IHSS **Supplied:** Inj 250 mg/20 mL **SE:** Chest pain, HTN, dyspnea **Notes:** Monitor PWP & cardiac output if possible; check ECG for ↑ heart rate, ectopic activity; follow BP

Docetaxel (Taxotere) **Uses:** *Breast (anthracycline-resistant), ovarian, lung CAs & CAP* **Action:** Antimitotic agent; promotes microtubular aggregation; semisynthetic taxoid **Dose:** 100 mg/m^2 over 1 h IV q3wk (per protocols); dexamethasone 8 mg bid prior & continue for 3–4 d; ↓ dose w/↑ bilirubin levels **Caution:** [D, –] **Contra:** Component sensitivity **Supplied:** Inj 20, 40, 80 mg/mL **SE:** Myelosuppression, neuropathy, N/V, alopecia, fluid retention syndrome; cumulative doses of 300–400 mg/m^2 w/o steroid prep & posttreatment & 600–800 mg/m^2 w/steroid prep; allergy possible (rare w/steroid prep)

Docusate Calcium (Surfak)/Docusate Potassium (Dialose)/Docusate Sodium (DOSS, Colace) **Uses:** *Constipation; adjunct to painful anorectal conditions (hemorrhoids)* **Action:** Stool softener **Dose:** *Adults.* 50–500 mg PO ÷ daily–qid. *Peds.* Infants–3 y: 10–40 mg/24 h ÷ daily–qid. *3–6 y:* 20–60 mg/24 h ÷ daily–qid. *6–12 y:* 40–150 mg/24 h ÷ daily–qid **Dose:** [C, ?] **Contra:** Use w/mineral oil; intestinal obstruction, acute abdominal pain, N/V **Supplied:** *Ca:* Caps 50, 240 mg. *K:* Caps 100, 240 mg. *Na:* Caps 50, 100 mg; syrup 50, 60 mg/15 mL; liq 150 mg/15 mL; soln 50 mg/mL **SE:** Rare abdominal cramping, D **Notes:** Take w/full glass of H$_2$O; no laxative action; do not use > 1 wk

Dofetilide (Tikosyn) **WARNING:** To minimize the risk of induced arrhythmia, pts initiated or reinitiated on Tikosyn should be placed for a minimum of 3 d in a facility that can provide calculations of CrCl, continuous ECG monitoring & cardiac resuscitation **Uses:** *Maintain normal sinus rhythm in AF/A flutter after conversion* **Action:** Type III antiarrhythmic **Dose:** 125–500 mcg PO bid based on CrCl & QTc (see insert) **Caution:** [C, –] **Contra:** Baseline QTc is > 440 ms (500 ms w/ventricular conduction abnormalities) or CrCl < 20 mL/min; concomitant use of verapamil, cimetidine, trimethoprim, or ketoconazole **Supplied:** Caps 125, 250, 500 mcg **SE:** Ventricular arrhythmias, HA, CP, dizziness **Notes:** Avoid w/other drugs that prolong the QT interval; hold class I or III antiarrhythmics for at least 3 half-lives before dofetilide; amiodarone level should be < 0.3 mg/L before dosing

Dolasetron (Anzemet) **Uses:** *Prevent chemo-associated N/V* **Action:** 5-HT$_3$ receptor antagonist **Dose:** *Adults & Peds.* IV: 1.8 mg/kg IV as single dose 30 min before chemo *Adults.* PO: 100 mg PO as a single dose 1 h before chemo *Peds.* PO: 1.8 mg/kg PO to max 100 mg as single dose **Caution:** [B, ?] **Contra:** Component sensitivity **Supplied:** Tabs 50, 100 mg; inj 20 mg/mL **SE:** Prolongs QT interval, HTN, HA, abdominal pain, urinary retention, transient ↑ LFTs

Dopamine (Intropin) **Uses:** *Short-term use in cardiac decompensation secondary to ↓ contractility; ↑ organ perfusion (at low dose)* **Action:** Positive inotropic agent w/dose response: 2–10 mcg/kg/min β-effects (↑ CO & renal perfusion); 10–20 mcg/kg/min β-effects (peripheral vasoconstriction, pressor); > 20 mcg/kg/min peripheral & renal vasoconstriction **Dose:** *Adults & Peds.* 5 mcg/kg/min by cont inf, ↑ by 5 mcg/kg/min to 50 mcg/kg/min max to effect **Caution:** [C, ?] **Contra:** Pheochromocytoma, VF, sulfite sensitivity **Supplied:** Inj 40, 80, 160 mg/mL **SE:** Tachycardia, vasoconstriction, ↓ BP, HA, N/V, dyspnea **Notes:** Dosage > 10 mcg/kg/min may ↓ renal perfusion; monitor urinary output;

22

monitor ECG for ↑ heart rate, BP & ectopy; monitor PCWP & cardiac output if possible

Dornase Alfa (Pulmozyme) Uses: *↓ Frequency of resp Infxns in CF* **Action:** Enzyme that selectively cleaves DNA **Dose:** Inhal 2.5 mg/d w/recommended nebulizer **Caution:** [B, ?] **Contra:** Chinese hamster product allergy **Supplied:** Soln for inhal 1 mg/mL **SE:** Pharyngitis, voice alteration, CP, rash

Dorzolamide (Trusopt) Uses: *Glaucoma* **Action:** Carbonic anhydrase inhibitor **Dose:** 1 gt in eye(s) tid **Caution:** [C, ?] **Contra:** Component sensitivity **Supplied:** 2% soln **SE:** Local irritation, bitter taste, superficial punctate keratitis, ocular allergic Rxn

Dorzolamide & Timolol (Cosopt) Uses: *Glaucoma* **Action:** Carbonic anhydrase inhibitor w/β-adrenergic blocker **Dose:** 1 gt in eye(s) bid **Caution:** [C, ?] **Contra:** Component sensitivity **Supplied:** Soln dorzolamide 2% & timolol 0.5% **SE:** Local irritation, bitter taste, superficial punctate keratitis, ocular allergic Rxn

Doxazosin (Cardura) Uses: *HTN & symptomatic BPH* **Action:** α_1-Adrenergic blocker; relaxes bladder neck smooth muscle **Dose:** *HTN:* Initial 1 mg/d PO; may be ↑ to 16 mg/d PO. *BPH:* Initial 1 mg/d PO, may ↑ to 8 mg/d **Caution:** [B, ?] **Contra:** Component sensitivity **Supplied:** Tabs 1, 2, 4, 8 mg **SE:** Dizziness, HA, drowsiness, sexual dysfunction, doses > 4 mg ↑ postural ↓ BP risk **Notes:** First dose hs; syncope may occur w/in 90 min of initial dose

Doxepin (Sinequan, Adapin) WARNING: Closely monitor for worsening depression or emergence of suicidality Uses: *Depression, anxiety, chronic pain* **Action:** TCA; ↑ synaptic CNS serotonin or norepinephrine **Dose:** 25–150 mg/d PO, usually hs but can be in ÷ doses; ↓ in hepatic impair **Caution:** [C, ?/–] **Contra:** NAG **Supplied:** Caps 10, 25, 50, 75, 100, 150 mg; PO conc 10 mg/mL **SE:** Anticholinergic SEs, ↓ BP, tachycardia, drowsiness, photosensitivity

Doxepin, Topical (Zonalon) Uses: *Short-term Rx pruritus (atopic dermatitis or lichen simplex chronicus)* **Action:** Antipruritic; H_1– & H_2–receptor antagonism **Dose:** Apply thin coating qid, 8 d max **Caution:** [C, ?/–] **Contra:** Component sensitivity **Supplied:** 5% cream **SE:** ↓ BP, tachycardia, drowsiness, photosensitivity **Notes:** Limit application area to avoid systemic tox

Doxorubicin (Adriamycin, Rubex) Uses: *Acute leukemia; Hodgkin Dz & NHL; soft tissue & osteosarcomas; Ewing sarcoma; Wilms tumor; neuroblastoma; bladder, breast, ovarian, gastric, thyroid & lung CAs* **Action:** Intercalates DNA; ↓ DNA topoisomerases I & II **Dose:** 60–75 mg/m² q3wk; ↓ cardiotox w/weekly (20 mg/m²/wk) or cont inf (60–90 mg/m² over 96 h); per protocols **Caution:** [D, ?] **Contra:** Severe CHF, cardiomyopathy, preexisting myelosuppression, previous Rx w/complete cumulative doses of doxorubicin, idarubicin, daunorubicin **Supplied:** Inj 10, 20, 50, 75, 200 mg **SE:** Myelosuppression, venous streaking & phlebitis, N/V/D, mucositis, radiation recall phenomenon, cardiomyopathy rare (dose-related); limit of 550 mg/m² cumulative dose (400 mg/m² w/previous mediastinal irradiation) **Notes:** Dexrazoxane may limit cardiac tox; tissue damage w/extravasation; discolors urine red/orange

Doxycycline (Vibramycin) Uses: *Broad-spectrum antibiotic* **Action:** Tetracycline; interferes w/protein synthesis. *Spectrum: Rickettsia sp, Chlamydia & M. pneumoniae* **Dose:** *Adults.* 100 mg PO q12h on 1st day, then 100 mg PO daily–bid or 100 mg IV q12h. *Peds > 8 y.* 5 mg/kg/24 h PO, to a max of 200 mg/d ÷ daily–bid **Supplied:** Tabs 50, 100 mg; caps 20, 50, 100 mg; syrup 50 mg/5 mL; susp 25 mg/5 mL; inj 100, 200 mg/vial **Caution:** [D, +] **Contra:** Children < 8 y, severe hepatic dysfunction **SE:** D, GI disturbance, photosensitivity **Notes:** ↓ effect w/antacids; tetracycline of choice in renal impair

Dronabinol (Marinol) [C-II] **Uses:** *N/V associated w/CA chemo; appetite stimulation* **Action:** Antiemetic; ↓ vomiting center in the medulla **Dose:** *Adults & Peds.* Antiemetic: 5–15 mg/m²/dose q4–6h PRN. *Adults.* Appetite stimulant: 2.5 mg PO before midday & evening meals **Caution:** [C, ?] **Contra:** Hx schizophrenia **Supplied:** Caps 2.5, 5, 10 mg **SE:** Drowsiness, dizziness, anxiety, mood change, hallucinations, depersonalization, orthostatic ↓ BP, tachycardia **Notes:** Principal psychoactive substance present in marijuana

Droperidol (Inapsine) **Uses:** *N/V; anesthetic premedication* **Action:** Tranquilizer, sedation, antiemetic **Dose:** *Adults.* Nausea: 2.5–5 mg IV or IM q3–4h PRN. *Premed:* 2.5–10 mg IV, 30–60 min preop. *Peds.* Premed: 0.1–0.15 mg/kg/dose **Caution:** [C, ?] **Contra:** Component sensitivity **Supplied:** Inj 2.5 mg/mL **SE:** Drowsiness, ↓ BP, occasional tachycardia & extrapyramidal Rxns, ↑ QT interval, arrhythmias **Notes:** Give IVP slowly over 2–5 min

Drotrecogin Alfa (Xigris) **Uses:** *↓ Mortality in adults w/severe sepsis (associated w/acute organ dysfunction) at high risk of death (eg, determined by APACHE II)* **Action:** Recombinant human activated protein C; mechanism unknown **Dose:** 24 mcg/kg/h, total of 96 h **Caution:** [C, ?] **Contra:** Active bleeding, recent stroke/CNS surgery, head trauma or CNS lesion w/herniation risk, epidural catheter **Supplied:** 5-, 20-mg vials **SE:** Bleeding **Notes:** W/single organ dysfunction & recent surgery may not be at high risk of death irrespective of APACHE II score & therefore not among the indicated population. *Percutaneous procedures:* Stop inf 2 h before the procedure & resume 1 h after. *Major surgery:* Stop inf 2 h before surgery & resume 12 h after surgery in absence of bleeding

Duloxetine (Cymbalta) **WARNING:** Antidepressants may ↑ risk of suicidality; consider risks/benefits of use. Closely monitor for clinical worsening, suicidality, or behavior changes **Uses:** *Depression, DM peripheral neuropathic pain* **Action:** Selective serotonin & norepinephrine reuptake inhibitor **Dose:** *Depression:* 40–60 mg/d PO ÷ bid. *DM neuropathy:* 60 mg/d PO; **Caution:** [C, ?/–]; use in 3rd tri; avoid if CrCl < 30 mL/min; w/fluvoxamine, inhibitors of CYP2D6, TCAs, phenothiazines, type 1C antiarrhythmics **Contra:** MAOI use w/in 14 d, w/thioridazine, NAG, hepatic insuff **Supplied:** Caps delayed-release 20, 30, 60 mg **SE:** N, dizziness, somnolence, fatigue, sweating, xerostomia, constipation, decreased appetite, sexual dysfunction, urinary hesitancy, ↑ LFTs, HTN **Notes:** Swallow whole; monitor BP; avoid abrupt D/C

Dutasteride (Avodart) **Uses:** *Symptomatic BPH* **Action:** 5α-Reductase inhibitor **Dose:** 0.5 mg PO daily **Caution:** [X, –] Hepatic impair; pregnant women should not handle pills **Contra:** Women & children **Supplied:** Caps 0.5 mg **SE:** ↓ PSA levels, impotence, ↓ libido, gynecomastia **Notes:** No blood donation until 6 mo after stopping

Echothiophate Iodine (Phospholine Ophthalmic) **Uses:** *Glaucoma* **Action:** Cholinesterase inhibitor **Dose:** 1 gt eye(s) bid w/one dose hs **Caution:** [C, ?] **Contra:** Active uveal inflammation or any inflammatory Dz of iris/ciliary

22

body **Supplied:** Powder to reconstitute 1.5 mg/0.03%; 3 mg/ 0.06%; 6.25 mg/ 0.125%; 12.5 mg/0.25% **SE:** Local irritation, myopia, blurred vision, ↓ BP, bradycardia

Econazole (Spectazole)   **Uses:** *Tinea, cutaneous *Candida* & tinea versicolor Infxns* **Action:** Topical antifungal **Dose:** Apply to areas bid (qd for tinea versicolor) for 2–4 wk **Caution:** [C, ?] **Contra:** Component sensitivity **Supplied:** Topical cream 1% **SE:** Local irritation, pruritus, erythema **Notes:** *Early* symptom/clinical improvement; complete course to avoid recurrence

Edrophonium (Tensilon)   **Uses:** *Diagnosis of MyG; acute MyG crisis; curare antagonist* **Action:** Anticholinesterase **Dose:** *Adults.* Test for MyG: 2 mg IV in 1 min; if tolerated, give 8 mg IV; (+) test is brief ↑ in strength. *Peds.* Test for MyG: Total dose 0.2 mg/kg; 0.04 mg/kg test dose; if no Rxn, give remainder in 1-mg increments to 10 mg max; ↓ in renal impair **Caution:** [C, ?] **Contra:** GI or GU obstruction; allergy to sulfite **Supplied:** Inj 10 mg/mL **SE:** N/V/D, excessive salivation, stomach cramps, ↑ aminotransferases **Notes:** Can cause severe cholinergic effects; keep atropine available

Efalizumab (Raptiva)   **WARNING:** Associated w/serious Infxns, malignancy, thrombocytopenia **Uses:** Chronic moderate–severe plaque psoriasis **Action:** MoAb **Dose:** *Adults.* 0.7 mg/kg SQ conditioning dose, followed by 1 mg/kg/wk; single doses should not exceed 200 mg **Caution:** [C, +/–] **Contra:** Admin of most vaccines **Supplied:** 125-mg vial **SE:** First-dose Rxn, HA, worsening psoriasis, ↑ LFT, immunosuppression-related Rxns (see warning) **Notes:** Minimize 1st-dose Rxn by conditioning dose; plts monthly, then every 3 mo & w/dose ↑; pts may be trained in self-admin

Efavirenz (Sustiva)   **Uses:** *HIV Infxns* **Action:** Antiretroviral; NRTI **Dose:** *Adults.* 600 mg/d PO qhs. *Peds.* See insert; avoid high-fat meals **Caution:** [C, ?] CDC recommends HIV-infected mothers not breast feed (risk of HIV transmission) **Contra:** Component sensitivity **Supplied:** Caps 50, 100, 200 mg **SE:** Somnolence, vivid dreams, dizziness, rash, N/V/D **Notes:** Monitor LFT, cholesterol

Eletriptan (Relpax)   **Uses:** Acute Rx of migraine **Action:** Selective serotonin receptor (5-HT$_1$B/$_1$D) agonist **Dose:** 20–40 mg PO, may repeat in 2 h; 80 mg/24h max **Caution:** [C, +] **Contra:** Hx ischemic heart Dz, coronary artery spasm, stroke, TIA, peripheral vascular Dz, IBD, uncontrolled HTN, hemiplegic or basilar migraine, severe hepatic impair, w/in 24 h of another 5-HT$_1$ agonist or ergot, w/in 72 h of CYP3A4 inhibitors **Supplied:** Tabs 20, 40 mg **SE:** Dizziness, somnolence, N, asthenia, xerostomia, paresthesias; pain, pressure, or tightness in chest, jaw or neck; serious cardiac events

Emedastine (Emadine)   **Uses:** *Allergic conjunctivitis* **Action:** Antihistamine; selective H$_1$-antagonist **Dose:** 1 gt in eye(s) up to qid **Caution:** [B, ?] **Contra:** Allergy to ingredients (preservatives benzalkonium, tromethamine) **Supplied:** 0.05% soln **SE:** HA, blurred vision, burning/stinging, corneal infiltrates/staining, dry eyes, foreign body sensation, hyperemia, keratitis, tearing, pruritus, rhinitis, sinusitis, asthenia, bad taste, dermatitis, discomfort **Notes:** Do not use contact lenses if eyes are red

22   **Emtricitabine (Emtriva)**   **WARNING:** Class warning for lipodystrophy, lactic acidosis & severe hepatomegaly **Uses:** HIV-1 Infxn **Action:** NRTI **Dose:**

200 mg PO daily; ↓ dose in renal impair **Caution:** [B, –] **Contra:** Component sensitivity **Supplied:** 200 mg caps **SE:** HA, D, N, rash, rare hyperpigmentation of feet & hands, posttreatment exacerbation of hepatitis **Notes:** First one-daily NRTI

Enalapril (Vasotec) **Uses:** *HTN, CHF, LVD,* DN **Action:** ACE inhibitor **Dose:** *Adults.* 2.5–40 mg/d PO; 1.25 mg IV q6h. **Peds.** 0.05–0.08 mg/kg/dose PO q12–24h; ↓ in renal impair **Caution:** [C (1st tri; D 2nd & 3rd tri), +] w/ NSAIDs, K⁺ supls **Contra:** Bilateral renal artery stenosis, angioedema **Supplied:** Tabs 2.5, 5, 10, 20 mg; IV 1.25 mg/mL (1, 2 mL) **SE:** ↓ BP with initial dose (especially with concomitant diuretics), ↑ K⁺, nonproductive cough, angioedema **Notes:** Monitor Cr; D/C diuretic for 2–3 d before initiation

Enfuvirtide (Fuzeon) WARNING: Rarely causes allergy; never rechallenge **Uses:** *W/antiretroviral agents for HIV-1 Infxn in treatment-experienced pts with evidence of viral replication despite ongoing antiretroviral therapy* **Action:** Viral fusion inhibitor **Dose:** 90 mg (1 mL) SQ bid in upper arm, anterior thigh, or abdomen; rotate site **Caution:** [B, –] **Contra:** Previous allergy to drug **Supplied:** 90 mg/mL reconstituted; pt convenience kit w/monthly supplies **SE:** Inj site Rxn (in nearly all pts); pneumonia, D, nausea, fatigue, insomnia, peripheral neuropathy **Notes:** available only via restricted distribution system; use immediately on reconstitution or refrigerate (24 h max)

Enoxaparin (Lovenox) WARNING: Recent or anticipated epidural/spinal anesthesia ↑ risk of spinal/epidural hematoma w/subsequent paralysis **Uses:** *Prevention & Rx of DVT; Rx PE; unstable angina & non-Q-wave MI* **Action:** LMWH **Dose:** *Adults. Prevention:* 30 mg SQ bid or 40 mg SQ q24h. *DVT/PE Rx:* 1 mg/kg SQ q12h or 1.5 mg/kg SQ q24h. *Angina:* 1 mg/kg SQ q12h. **Peds.** Prevention: 0.5 mg/kg SQ q12h. *DVT/PE Rx:* 1 mg/kg SQ q12h; ↓ dose w/CrCl < 30 mL/min **Caution:** [B, ?] Not for prophylaxis in prosthetic heart valves **Contra:** Active bleeding, HIT Ab(+) **Supplied:** Inj 10 mg/0.1 mL (30-, 40-, 60-, 80-, 100-, 120- & 150-mg syringes) **SE:** Bleeding, hemorrhage, bruising, thrombocytopenia, pain/hematoma at site, ↑ AST/ALT **Notes:** No effect on bleeding time, plt Fxn, PT, or aPTT; monitor plt (HIT), clinical bleeding; may monitor anti-factor Xa

Entacapone (Comtan) **Uses:** *Parkinson Dz* **Action:** Selective & reversible carboxymethyl transferase inhibitor **Dose:** 200 mg w/each levodopa/carbidopa dose; max 1600 mg/d; ↓ levodopa/carbidopa dose by 25% if levodopa dose > 800 mg **Caution:** [C, ?] Hepatic impair **Contra:** Use w/MAOI **Supplied:** Tabs 200 mg **SE:** Dyskinesia, hyperkinesia, N, D, dizziness, hallucinations, orthostatic ↓ BP, brown-orange urine **Notes:** Monitor LFT; do not D/C abruptly

Ephedrine **Uses:** *Acute bronchospasm, bronchial asthma, nasal congestion,* ↓ BP, narcolepsy, enuresis & MyG **Action:** Sympathomimetic; stimulates α- & β-receptors; bronchodilator **Dose:** *Adults.* 25–50 mg IM or IV q10min to 150 mg/d max or 25–50 mg PO q3–4h PRN. **Peds.** 0.2–0.3 mg/kg/dose IM/IV q4–6h PRN **Caution:** [C, ?/–] **Contra:** Arrhythmias; closed-angle glaucoma **Supplied:** Inj 50 mg/mL; caps 25 mg; nasal spray 0.25% **SE:** CNS stimulation (nervousness, anxiety, trembling), tachycardia, arrhythmia, HTN, xerostomia, painful urination **Notes:** Protect from light; monitor BP, HR, urinary output; can cause false(+) amphetamine EMIT; take last dose 4–6h before hs

22

Epinastine (Elestat) Uses: Itching w/allergic conjunctivitis **Action:** Antihistamine **Dose:** 1 gt bid **Caution:** [C, ?/–] **Supplied:** Soln 0.05% **SE:** Burning, folliculosis, hyperemia, pruritus, URI, HA, rhinitis, sinusitis, cough, pharyngitis **Notes:** Remove contacts before, reinsert in 10 min

Epinephrine (Adrenalin, Sus-Phrine, EpiPen, others) Uses: *Cardiac arrest, anaphylactic Rxn, bronchospasm, open-angle glaucoma* **Action:** β-adrenergic agonist, some α-effects **Dose:** *Adults.* ACLS: 0.5–1 mg (5–10 mL of 1:10,000) IV q 5 min to response. *Anaphylaxis:* 0.3–0.5 mL SQ of 1:1000 dilution, may repeat q5–15min to a max of 1 mg/dose & 5 mg/d. *Asthma:* 0.1–0.5 mL SQ of 1:1000 dilution, repeat 20-min to 4-h intervals or 1 inhal (met-dose) repeat in 1–2 min or susp 0.1–0.3 mL SQ for extended effect. *Peds.* ACLS: 1st dose 0.1 mL/kg IV of 1:10,000 dilution, then 0.1 mL/kg IV of 1:1000 dilution q3–5min to response. *Anaphylaxis:* 0.001 mg/kg SQ q15min × 2 doses, then q4h PRN. *Asthma:* 0.01 mL/kg SQ of 1:1000 dilution q8–12h. **Caution:** [C, ?] ↓ bronchodilation with β-blockers **Contra:** Cardiac arrhythmias, closed-angle glaucoma **Supplied:** Inj 1:1000, 1:2000, 1:10,000, 1:100,000; susp for inj 1:200; aerosol 220 mcg/spray; 1% inhal soln **SE:** CV (tachycardia, HTN, vasoconstriction), CNS stimulation (nervousness, anxiety, trembling), ↓ renal blood flow **Notes:** Can give via ET tube if no central line (use 2–2.5 × IV dose)

Epirubicin (Ellence) Uses: *Adjuvant therapy for + axillary nodes after resection of primary breast CA* **Actions:** Anthracycline cytotoxic agent **Dose:** per protocols; ↓ dose w/hepatic impair. **Caution:** [D, –] **Contra:** Baseline neutrophil count < 1500 cells/μL, severe myocardial insuff, recent MI, severe arrhythmias, severe hepatic dysfunction, previous anthracyclines Rx to max cumulative dose **Supplied:** Inj 50 mg/25 mL, 200 mg/100 mL **SE:** Mucositis, N/V/D, alopecia, myelosuppression, cardiotox, secondary AML, tissue necrosis w/extravasation

Eplerenone (Inspra) Uses: *HTN* **Action:** Selective aldosterone antagonist **Dose:** *Adults.* 50 mg PO daily–bid, doses > 100 mg/d no benefit w/↑ K⁺; ↓ to 25 mg PO qd if giving w/CYP3A4 inhibitors **Caution:** [B, +/–] Use of CYP3A4 inhibitors (ketoconazole, itraconazole, erythromycin, fluconazole, verapamil, saquinavir); monitor K⁺ with ACE inhibitor, ARBs, NSAIDs, K⁺-sparing diuretics; grapefruit juice, St. John's wort **Contra:** K⁺ > 5.5 mEq/L; NIDDM w/microalbuminuria; SCr > 2 mg/dL (men), > 1.8 mg/dL (women); CrCl < 50 mL/min; concurrent K⁺ supls/K⁺-sparing diuretics **Supplied:** Tabs 25, 50, 100 mg **SE:** Hypertriglyceridemia, ↑ K⁺, HA, dizziness, gynecomastia, hypercholesterolemia, D, orthostatic ↓ BP **Notes:** May take 4 wk for full effect

Epoetin Alfa [Erythropoietin, EPO] (Epogen, Procrit) Uses: * CRF associated anemia* zidovudine Rx in HIV-infected pts, CA chemo; ↓ transfusions associated w/surgery **Action:** Induces erythropoiesis **Dose:** *Adults & Peds.* 50–150 units/kg IV/SQ 3×/wk; adjust dose q4–6wk PRN. *Surgery:* 300 units/kg/ d × 10 d before surgery to 4 d after; ↓ dose if Hct approaches 36% or Hgb, ↑ > 4 points in 2–wk period **Caution:** [C, +] **Contra:** Uncontrolled HTN **Supplied:** Inj 2000, 3000, 4000, 10,000, 20,000, 40,000 units/mL **SE:** HTN, HA, fatigue, fever, tachycardia, N/V **Notes:** Refrigerate; monitor baseline & posttreatment Hct/Hgb, BP, ferritin

Epoprostenol (Flolan) Uses: *Pulmonary HTN* **Action:** Dilates pulmonary/systemic arterial vascular beds; ↓ plt aggregation **Dose:** Initial 2 ng/kg/ min; ↑ by 2 ng/kg/min q15min until dose-limiting SE (CP, dizziness, N/V, HA,

↓ BP, flushing); IV cont inf 4 ng/kg/min < max-tolerated rate; adjust according to response; see package insert **Caution:** [B, ?] ↑ tox w/diuretics, vasodilators, acetate in dialysis fluids, anticoagulants **Contra:** Chronic use in CHF 2nd-deg severe LVSD **Supplied:** Inj 0.5, 1.5 mg **SE:** Flushing, tachycardia, CHF, fever, chills, nervousness, HA, N/V/D, jaw pain, flu-like Sxs **Notes:** Abrupt D/C can cause rebound pulmonary HTN; monitor bleeding if using other antiplatelet/anticoagulants; watch ↓ BP effects with other vasodilators/diuretics

Eprosartan (Teveten) Uses: *HTN,* DN, CHF **Action:** ARB **Dose:** 400–800 mg/d single dose or bid **Caution:** [C (1st tri); D (2nd & 3rd tri), –] Lithium, ↑ K^+ with K^+-sparing diuretics/supls/high-dose trimethoprim **Contra:** Bilateral renal artery stenosis, 1st-deg aldosteronism **Supplied:** Tabs 400, 600 mg **SE:** Fatigue, depression, hypertriglyceridemia, URI, UTI, abdominal pain, rhinitis/pharyngitis/cough

Eptifibatide (Integrilin) Uses: *ACS, PCI* **Action:** Glycoprotein IIb/IIIa inhibitor **Dose:** 180 mcg/kg IV bolus, then 2 mcg/kg/min cont inf; ↓ in renal impair (SCr > 2 mg/dL, < 4 mg/dL: 135 mcg/kg bolus & 0.5 mcg/kg/min inf) **Caution:** [B, ?] Monitor bleeding with other anticoagulants **Contra:** Other GPIIb/IIIa inhibitors, Hx abnormal bleeding, hemorrhagic stroke (within 30 d), severe HTN, major surgery (within 6 wk), plt count < 100,000 cells/μL, renal dialysis **Supplied:** Inj 0.75, 2 mg/mL **SE:** Bleeding, ↓ BP, inj site Rxn, thrombocytopenia **Notes:** Monitor bleeding, coags, plts, SCr, ACT with prothrombin consumption index (maintain ACT 200–300 s)

Erlotinib (Tarceva) Uses: *NSCLC after 1 chemo agent fails* **Action:** HER1/EGFR tyrosine kinase inhibitor **Dose:** 150 mg/d PO 1 h ac or 2 h pc; ↓ (in 50-mg decrements) w/severe Rxn or w/CYP3A4 inhibitors (page 647); per protocols **Caution:** [D, ?/–]; use w/CYP3A4 (page 647) inhibitors **Supplied:** Tabs 25, 100, 150 mg **SE:** Rash, N/V/D, anorexia, abdominal pain, fatigue, cough, dyspnea, stomatitis, conjunctivitis, pruritus, dry skin, Infxn, ↑ LFT, interstitial lung disease **Notes:** May ↑ INR w/warfarin, monitor INR

Ertapenem (Invanz) Uses: *Complicated intraabdominal, acute pelvic & skin Infxns, pyelonephritis, community-acquired pneumonia* **Action:** Carbapenem; β-lactam antibiotic, ↓ cell wall synthesis. *Spectrum: Good gram(+/–) &* anaerobic coverage, but not *Pseudomonas,* PCN-resistant pneumococci, MRSA, *Enterococcus,* β-lactamase(+) *H. influenza, Mycoplasma, Chlamydia* **Dose:** *Adults.* 1 g IM/IV qd; 500 mg/d in CrCl < 30 mL/min **Caution:** [C, ?/–] Probenecid ↓ renal clearance **Contra:** < 18 y, PCN allergy **Supplied:** Inj 1 g/vial **SE:** HA, N/V/D, inj site Rxns, thrombocytosis, ↑ LFTs **Notes:** Can give IM × 7 d, IV × 14 d; 137 mg Na^+(6 mEg)/g ertapenem

Erythromycin (E-Mycin, E.E.S., Ery-Tab, EryPed, Ilotycin) Uses: *Bacterial Infxns; bowel prep*; ↑ GI motility (prokinetic); *acne vulgaris* **Action:** Bacteriostatic; interferes w/protein synthesis. *Spectrum: Group A streptococci (S. pyogenes), S. pneumoniae, N. meningitides, N. gonorrhoeae* (if PCN-allergic), *Legionella, M. pneumoniae* **Dose:** *Adults.* Base 250–500 mg PO q6–12h or ethylsuccinate 400–800 mg q6–12h; 500 mg–1 g IV q6h. *Prokinetic:* 250 mg PO tid 30 min ac. *Peds.* 30–50 mg/kg/d PO ÷ q6–8h or 20–40 mg/kg/d IV ÷ q6h, max 2 g/d **Caution:** [B, +] ↑ tox of carbamazepine, cyclosporine, digoxin, methylprednisolone, theophylline, felodipine, warfarin, simvastatin/lovastatin; ↓ sildenafil dose w/use **Contra:** Hepatic impair, preexisting liver Dz (estolate), use with pimozide **Supplied:** *Lactobionate (Ilotycin) powder for inj:* 500 mg, 1 g. *Base:* Tabs 250, 333, 500

22

mg; caps 250 mg. *Estolate (Ilosone):* Susp 125, 250 mg/5 mL. *Stearate (Erythrocin):* Tabs 250, 500 mg. *Ethylsuccinate (E.E.S, EryPed):* Chew tabs 200 mg; tabs 400 mg; susp 200, 400 mg/5 mL **SE:** HA, abdominal pain, N/V/D; QT prolongation, torsade de pointes, ventricular arrhythmias/tachycardias (rarely); cholestatic jaundice (estolate) **Notes:** 400 mg ethylsuccinate = 250 mg base/estolate; w/food minimizes GI upset; lactobionate contains benzyl alcohol (caution in neonates)

Erythromycin, Ophthalmic (Ilotycin Ophthalmic) Uses: *Conjunctival/corneal Infxns* **Action:** Macrolide antibiotic **Dose:** $^1/2$ in 2–6 ×/d **Caution:** [B, +] **Contra:** Erythromycin hypersensitivity **Supplied:** 0.5% oint **SE:** Local irritation

Erythromycin, Topical (A/T/S, EryDerm, Erycette, T-Stat) Uses: *Acne vulgaris* **Action:** Macrolide antibiotic **Dose:** Wash & dry area, apply 2% product over area bid **Caution:** [B, +] **Contra:** Component sensitivity **Supplied:** Soln 1.5%, 2%; gel 2%; pads & swabs 2% **SE:** Local irritation

Erythromycin & Benzoyl Peroxide (Benzamycin) Uses: Topical Rx of *acne vulgaris* **Action:** Macrolide antibiotic w/keratolytic **Dose:** Apply bid (AM & PM) **Caution:** [C, ?] **Contra:** Component sensitivity **Supplied:** Gel erythromycin 30 mg/benzoyl peroxide 50 mg/g **SE:** Local irritation, dryness

Erythromycin & Sulfisoxazole (Eryzole, Pediazole) Uses: *Upper & lower resp tract; bacterial Infxns; otitis media in children due to H. influenzae*; Infxns in PCN-allergic pts **Action:** Macrolide antibiotic w/sulfonamide **Dose:** Based on erythromycin content. *Adults.* 400 mg erythromycin/1200 mg sulfisoxazole PO q6h. *Peds > 2 mo.* 40–50 mg/kg/d erythromycin & 150 mg/kg/d sulfisoxazole PO ÷ q6h; max 2 g/d erythromycin or 6 g/d sulfisoxazole × 10 d; ↓ in renal impair **Caution:** [C (D if near term), +] PO anticoagulants, MTX, hypoglycemics, phenytoin, cyclosporine **Contra:** Infants < 2 mo **Supplied:** Susp erythromycin ethylsuccinate 200 mg/sulfisoxazole 600 mg/5 mL (100, 150, 200 mL) **SE:** GI disturbance

Escitalopram (Lexapro) WARNING: Closely monitor for worsening depression or emergence of suicidality, particularly in ped pts **Uses:** Depression, anxiety **Action:** SSRI **Dose:** *Adults.* 10–20 mg PO qd; 10 mg/d in elderly & hepatic impair **Caution:** [C, +/–] ↑ Risk of serotonin syndrome with other SSRI, tramadol, linezolid, sumatriptan **Contra:** W/or w/in 14 d of MAOI **Supplied:** Tabs 5, 10, 20 mg; soln 1 mg/mL **SE:** N/V/D, sweating, insomnia, dizziness, xerostomia, sexual dysfunction **Notes:** Full effects may take 3 wk

Esmolol (Brevibloc) Uses: *SVT & noncompensatory sinus tachycardia, AF/flutter* **Action:** β_1-Adrenergic blocker; class II antiarrhythmic **Dose:** *Adults & Peds.* Initial 500 mcg/kg load over 1 min, then 50 mcg/kg/min × 4 min; if inadequate response, repeat the load & maint inf of 100 mcg/kg/min × 4 min; titrate by repeating load, then incremental ↑ in the maint dose of 50 mcg/kg/min for 4 min until desired heart rate reached or ↓ BP; average dose 100 mcg/kg/min **Caution:** [C (1st tri; D 2nd or 3rd tri), ?] **Contra:** Sinus bradycardia, heart block, uncompensated CHF, cardiogenic shock, ↓ BP **Supplied:** Inj 10, 250 mg/mL; premix inf 10 mg/mL **SE:** ↓ BP; bradycardia, diaphoresis, dizziness, pain on inj **Notes:** Hemodynamic effects back to baseline w/in 30 min after D/C inf

Esomeprazole (Nexium) Uses: *Short-term (4–8 wk) for erosive esophagitis/GERD; H. pylori Infxn in combo with antibiotics* **Action:** Proton pump inhibitor, ↓ gastric acid **Dose:** *Adults.* GERD/erosive gastritis: 20–40 mg/d PO × 4–8 wk; *Maint:* 20 mg/d PO. *H. pylori Infxn:* 40 mg/d PO, plus clarithromycin

500 mg PO bid & amoxicillin 1000 mg/bid for 10 d **Caution:** [B, ?/–] **Contra:** Component sensitivity **Supplied:** Caps 20, 40 mg **SE:** HA, D, abdominal pain **Notes:** Do not chew; may open capsule & sprinkle on applesauce

Estazolam (ProSom) [C-IV] **Uses:** *Short-term management of insomnia* **Action:** Benzodiazepine **Dose:** 1–2 mg PO qhs PRN; ↓ in hepatic impair/ elderly/debilitated **Caution:** [X, –] ↑ effects w/CNS depressants **Contra:** PRG **Supplied:** Tabs 1, 2 mg **SE:** Somnolence, weakness, palpitations **Notes:** May cause psychological/physical dependence; avoid abrupt D/C after prolonged use

Esterified Estrogens (Estratab, Menest) **WARNING:** Do not use in the prevention of CV Dz **Uses:** *Vasomotor Sxs or vulvar/vaginal atrophy associated with menopause;* female hypogonadism **Action:** Estrogen supl **Dose:** *Menopause:* 0.3–1.25 mg/d, cyclically 3 wk on, 1 wk off. *Hypogonadism:* 2.5–7.5 mg/d PO × 20 d, off × 10 d **Caution:** [X, –] **Contra:** Genital bleeding of unknown cause, breast CA, estrogen-dependent tumors, thromboembolic disorders, thrombophlebitis, recent MI, PRG, severe hepatic Dz **Supplied:** Tabs 0.3, 0.625, 1.25, 2.5 mg **SE:** N, HA, bloating, breast enlargement/tenderness, edema, venous thromboembolism, hypertriglyceridemia, gallbladder Dz **Notes:** Use lowest dose for shortest time (refer to WHI data)

Esterified Estrogens + Methyltestosterone (Estratest, Estratest HS) **Uses:** *Vasomotor Sxs*; postpartum breast engorgement **Action:** Estrogen & androgen supl **Dose:** 1 tab/d × 3 wk, 1 wk off **Caution:** [X, –] **Contra:** Genital bleeding of unknown cause, breast CA, estrogen-dependent tumors, thromboembolic disorders, thrombophlebitis, recent MI, PRG **Supplied:** Tabs (estrogen/ methyltestosterone) 0.625 mg/1.25 mg hs, 1.25 mg/2.5 mg **SE:** Nausea, HA, bloating, breast enlargement/tenderness, edema, ↑ triglycerides, venous thromboembolism, gallbladder Dz **Notes:** Use lowest dose for shortest time

Estradiol (Estrace) **Uses:** *Atrophic vaginitis, vasomotor Sxs associated w/menopause, osteoporosis* **Action:** Estrogen supl **Dose:** *PO:* 1–2 mg/d, adjust PRN to control Sxs. *Vaginal cream:* 2–4 g/d × 2 wk, then 1 g 1–3 × /wk **Caution:** [X, –] **Contra:** Genital bleeding of unknown cause, breast CA, estrogen-dependent tumors, thromboembolic disorders, thrombophlebitis; recent MI; hepatic impair **Supplied:** Tabs 0.5, 1, 2 mg; vaginal cream 0.1 mg/g **SE:** Nausea, HA, bloating, breast enlargement/tenderness, edema, ↑ triglycerides, venous thromboembolism, gallbladder Dz

Estradiol, Transdermal (Estraderm, Climara, Vivelle) **Uses:** *Severe menopausal vasomotor Sxs; female hypogonadism* **Action:** Estrogen supl **Dose:** 0.1 mg/d patch 1–2 × wk based on product; adjust PRN to control Sxs **Caution:** [X, –] (See estradiol) **Contra:** PRG, undiagnosed genital bleeding, carcinoma of breast, estrogen-dependent tumors, Hx thrombophlebitis, thrombosis, **Supplied:** TD patches (deliver mg/24 h) 0.025, 0.0375, 0.05, 0.075, 0.1 **SE:** Nausea, bloating, breast enlargement/tenderness, edema, HA, hypertriglyceridemia, gallbladder Dz **Notes:** Do not apply to breasts; place on trunk & rotate sites

Estradiol Cypionate & Medroxyprogesterone Acetate (Lunelle) **WARNING:** Cigarette smoking ↑ risk of serious CV side effects from contraceptives containing estrogen. This risk ↑ with age & with heavy smoking (> 15 cigarettes/d) & is quite marked in women > 35 y. Women who use Lunelle should be strongly advised not to smoke **Uses:** *Contraceptive* **Action:** Estrogen & progestin **Dose:** 0.5 mL IM (deltoid, ant thigh, buttock) monthly, do not

22

exceed 33 d **Caution:** [X, M] HTN, gallbladder Dz, ↑ lipids, migraines, sudden HA, valvular heart Dz with complications **Contra:** PRG, heavy smokers > 35 y, DVT, PE, cerebro/CV Dz, estrogen-dependent neoplasm, undiagnosed abnormal uterine bleeding, hepatic tumors, cholestatic jaundice **Supplied:** Estradiol cypionate (5 mg), medroxyprogesterone acetate (25 mg) single-dose vial or prefilled syringe (0.5 mL) **SE:** Arterial thromboembolism, HTN, cerebral hemorrhage, MI, amenorrhea, acne, breast tenderness **Notes:** Start w/in 5 d of menstruation

Estramustine Phosphate (Estracyt, Emcyt) Uses: *Advanced CAP* **Action:** Antimicrotubule agent; weak estrogenic & antiandrogenic activity **Dose:** 14 mg/kg/d in 3–4 ÷ doses on empty stomach, do not take with milk/milk products **Caution:** [Not used in women] **Contra:** Active thrombophlebitis or thromboembolic disorders **Supplied:** Caps 140 mg **SE:** N/V, exacerbation of preexisting CHF, thrombophlebitis, MI, PE, gynecomastia in 20–100%

Estrogen, Conjugated (Premarin) WARNING: Should not be used for the prevention of CV Dz. WHI reported ↑ risk of MI, stroke, breast CA, PE & DVT when combined with methoxyprogesterone over 5 y of Rx; ↑ risk of endometrial CA **Uses:** *Moderate–severe menopausal vasomotor Sxs; atrophic vaginitis; palliative for advanced prostatic CA; prevention & Rx of estrogen deficiency osteoporosis* **Action:** Estrogen hormonal replacement **Dose:** 0.3–1.25 mg/d PO cyclically; prostatic CA 1.25–2.5 mg PO tid **Caution:** [X, –] **Contra:** Severe hepatic impair, genital bleeding of unknown cause, breast CA, estrogen-dependent tumors, thromboembolic disorders, thrombosis, thrombophlebitis, recent MI **Supplied:** Tabs 0.3, 0.625, 0.9, 1.25, 2.5 mg; inj 25 mg/mL **SE:** ↑ Risk of endometrial carcinoma, gallbladder Dz, thromboembolism, HA & possibly breast CA; generic products not equivalent

Estrogen, Conjugated + Medroxyprogesterone (Prempro, Premphase) WARNING: Should not be used for the prevention of CV Dz; the WHI study reported ↑ risk of MI, stroke, breast CA, PE & DVT over 5 y of Rx **Uses:** *Moderate–severe menopausal vasomotor Sxs; atrophic vaginitis; prevent postmenopausal osteoporosis* **Action:** Hormonal replacement **Dose:** Prempro 1 tab PO daily; Premphase 1 tab PO daily **Caution:** [X, –] **Contra:** Severe hepatic impair, genital bleeding of unknown cause, breast CA, estrogen-dependent tumors, thromboembolic disorders, thrombosis, thrombophlebitis **Supplied:** (expressed as estrogen/medroxyprogesterone) *Prempro:* Tabs 0.625/2.5, 0.625/5 mg *Premphase:* Tabs 0.625/0 (days 1–14) & 0.625/5 mg (days 15–28) **SE:** Gallbladder Dz, thromboembolism, HA, breast tenderness

Estrogen, Conjugated + Methylprogesterone (Premarin + Methylprogesterone) Uses: *Menopausal vasomotor Sxs; osteoporosis* **Action:** Estrogen & androgen combo **Dose:** 1 tab/d **Caution:** [X, –] **Contra:** Severe hepatic impair, genital bleeding of unknown cause, breast CA, estrogen-dependent tumors, thromboembolic disorders, thrombosis, thrombophlebitis **Supplied:** Tabs 0.625 mg estrogen, conjugated & 2.5 or 5 mg of methylprogesterone **SE:** Nausea, bloating, breast enlargement/tenderness, edema, HA, hypertriglyceridemia, gallbladder Dz

Estrogen, Conjugated + Methyltestosterone (Premarin + Methyltestosterone) Uses: *Moderate–severe menopausal vasomotor Sxs*; postpartum breast engorgement **Action:** Estrogen & androgen combo **Dose:** 1 tab/d × 3 wk, then 1 wk off **Caution:** [X, –] **Contra:** Severe hepatic impair, genital bleeding of unknown cause, breast CA, estrogen-dependent tumors, thromboembolic disorders, thrombophlebitis **Supplied:** Tabs (estrogen/methyltestosterone) 0.625 mg/5 mg, 1.25 mg/10 mg **SE:** N, bloating, breast enlargement/tenderness, edema, HA, hypertriglyceridemia, gallbladder Dz

Estrogen, Conjugated Synthetic (Cenestin) **Uses:** *Rx of moderate–severe vasomotor Sxs associated with menopause* **Action:** Hormonal replacement **Dose:** 0.625–1.25 mg PO daily **Caution:** [X, –] **Contra:** See Estrogen, Conjugated **Supplied:** Tabs 0.625, 0.9, 1.25 mg **SE:** Associated with an ↑ risk of endometrial CA, gallbladder Dz, thromboembolism & possibly breast CA

Eszopiclone (Lunesta) [C-IV] **Uses:** *Insomnia* **Action:** Nonbenzodiazepine hypnotic **Dose:** 2–3 mg/d hs *Elderly:* 1–2 mg/d hs; hepatic impair/use w/ CYP3A4 inhibitor: 1 mg/d hs **Caution:** [C, ?/–] **Supplied:** Tabs 1, 2, 3 mg **SE:** HA, xerostomia, dizziness, somnolence, hallucinations, rash, Infxn, unpleasant taste **Notes:** High-fat meals slow absorption

Etanercept (Enbrel) **Uses:** *Reduces Sxs of RA when other DMARDs fail*; Crohn Dz **Action:** Binds TNF **Dose:** *Adults.* 25 mg SQ 2×/wk (separated by at least 72–96 h). *Peds 4–17 y.* 0.4 mg/kg SQ 2×/wk (max 25 mg) **Caution:** [B, ?] conditions that predispose to Infxn (eg, DM) **Contra:** Active Infxn **Supplied:** Inj 25 mg/vial **SE:** HA, rhinitis, inj site Rxn, URI, rhinitis **Notes:** Rotate inj sites

Ethambutol (Myambutol) **Uses:** *Pulmonary TB* & other mycobacterial Infxns, MAC **Action:** ↓ RNA synthesis **Dose:** *Adults & Peds > 12 y.* 15–25 mg/kg/d PO as a single dose; ↓ in renal impair, take w/food, avoid antacids **Caution:** [B, +] **Contra:** Optic neuritis **Supplied:** Tabs 100, 400 mg **SE:** HA, hyperuricemia, acute gout, abdominal pain, ↑ LFTs, optic neuritis, GI upset

Ethinyl Estradiol (Estinyl, Feminone) **Uses:** *Menopausal vasomotor Sxs; female hypogonadism* **Action:** Estrogen supl **Dose:** 0.02–1.5 mg/d ÷ daily–tid **Caution:** [X, –] **Contra:** Severe hepatic impair; genital bleeding of unknown cause, breast CA, estrogen-dependent tumors, thromboembolic disorders, thrombophlebitis **Supplied:** Tabs 0.02, 0.05, 0.5 mg **SE:** Nausea, bloating, breast enlargement/tenderness, edema, HA, hypertriglyceridemia, gallbladder Dz

Ethinyl Estradiol & Levonorgestrel (Preven) **Uses:** *Emergency contraceptive* ("morning-after pill"); prevent PRG (contraceptive failure, unprotected intercourse) **Actions:** Estrogen & progestin; interferes with implantation **Dose:** 4 tabs, take 2 tabs q12h × 2 (w/in 72 h of intercourse) **Caution:** [X, M] **Contra:** Known/suspected PRG, abnormal uterine bleeding **Supplied:** Kit: ethinyl estradiol (0.05), levonorgestrel (0.25) blister pack with 4 pills & urine PRG test **SE:** Peripheral edema, N/V/D, bloating, abdominal pain, fatigue, HA & menstrual changes **Notes:** Will not induce abortion; may ↑ risk of ectopic PRG

Ethinyl Estradiol & Norelgestromin (Ortho Evra) **Uses:** *Contraceptive patch* **Action:** Estrogen & progestin **Dose:** Apply patch to abdomen, buttocks, upper torso (not breasts) or upper outer arm at beginning of menstrual cycle; apply new patch weekly for 3 wk; week 4 is patch-free **Caution:** [X, M] **Contra:** Thrombophlebitis, undiagnosed vaginal bleeding, PRG, carcinoma of breast, estrogen-dependent tumor **Supplied:** 20 cm^2 patch (6 mg norelgestromin (active metabolite norgestimate) & 0.75 mg of ethinyl estradiol) **SE:** Breast discomfort, HA, site Rxns, nausea, menstrual cramps; thrombosis risks similar to OCP **Notes:** Less effective in women > 90 kg

Ethosuximide (Zarontin) **Uses:** *Absence (petit mal) Szs* **Action:** Anticonvulsant; ↑ Sz threshold **Dose:** *Adults.* Initial, 250 mg PO ÷ bid; ↑ by

22

250 mg/d q4–7d PRN (max 1500 mg/d). *Peds 3–6 y.* Initial: 15 mg/kg/d PO ÷ bid. *Maint:* 15–40 mg/kg/d ÷ bid, max 1500 mg/d **Caution:** [C, +] in renal/hepatic impair **Contra:** Component sensitivity **Supplied:** Caps 250 mg; syrup 250 mg/5 mL **SE:** Blood dyscrasias, GI upset, drowsiness, dizziness, irritability

Etidronate Disodium (Didronel) Uses: *↑ Ca^{2+} of malignancy, Paget Dz & heterotopic ossification* **Action:** ↓ Nl & abnormal bone resorption **Dose:** *Paget Dz:* 5–10 mg/kg/d PO ÷ doses (for 3–6 mo). ↑ Ca^{2+}: 7.5 mg/kg/d IV inf over 2 h × 3 d, then 20 mg/kg/d PO on last day of inf × 1–3 mo **Caution:** [B PO (C parenteral), ?] **Contra:** SCr > 5 mg/dL **Supplied:** Tabs 200, 400 mg; inj 50 mg/mL **SE:** GI intolerance (↓ by ÷ daily doses); hypophosphatemia, hypomagnesemia, bone pain, abnormal taste, fever, convulsions, nephrotox **Notes:** Take PO on empty stomach 2 h before any meal

Etodolac (Lodine) WARNING: May ↑ risk of CV events & GI bleeding **Uses:** *Osteoarthritis & pain,* RA **Action:** NSAID **Dose:** 200–400 mg PO bid–qid (max 1200 mg/d) **Caution:** [C (D 3rd tri), ?] ↑ bleeding risk w/aspirin, warfarin; ↑ nephrotox w/cyclosporine; Hx CHF, HTN, renal/hepatic impair, PUD **Contra:** Active GI ulcer **Supplied:** Tabs 400, 500 mg; ER tabs 400, 500, 600 mg; caps 200, 300 mg **SE:** N/V/D, gastritis, abdominal cramps, dizziness, HA, depression, edema, renal impair **Notes:** Do not crush tabs

Etonogestrel/Ethinyl Estradiol (NuvaRing) Uses: *Contraceptive* **Action:** Estrogen & progestin combo **Dose:** Rule out PRG first; insert ring vaginally for 3 wk, remove for 1 wk; insert new ring 7 d after last removed (even if bleeding) at same time of day ring removed. First day of menses is day 1, insert before day 5 even if still bleeding. Use other contraception for first 7 d of starting therapy. See insert if converting from other contraceptive; after delivery or 2nd tri abortion, insert 4 wk post partum (if not breast feeding) **Caution:** [X, ?/–] HTN, gallbladder Dz, ↑ lipids, migraines, sudden HA **Contra:** PRG, heavy smokers > 35 y, DVT, PE, cerebro-/CV Dz, estrogen-dependent neoplasm, undiagnosed abnormal genital bleeding, hepatic tumors, cholestatic jaundice **Supplied:** Intravaginal ring: ethinyl estradiol 0.015 mg/d & etonogestrel 0.12 mg/d **Notes:** If ring accidentally removed, rinse with cool/lukewarm H_2O (not hot) & reinsert ASAP; if not reinserted w/in 3 h, effectiveness ↓; do not use with diaphragm

Etoposide, VP-16 (VePesid, Toposar) Uses: *Testicular CA, NSCLC, Hodgkin Dz & NHL, ped ALL & allogeneic/autologous BMT in high doses* **Action:** Topoisomerase II inhibitor **Dose:** 50 mg/m^2/d IV for 3–5 d; 50 mg/m^2/d PO for 21 d (PO bioavailability = 50% of IV form); 2–6 g/m^2 or 25–70 mg/kg used in BMT (per protocols); ↓ in renal/hepatic impair **Caution:** [D, –] **Contra:** IT administration **Supplied:** Caps 50 mg; inj 20 mg/mL **SE:** N/V (emesis in 10–30%), myelosuppression, alopecia, ↓ BP if infused rapidly, anorexia, anemia, leukopenia, ↑ risk secondary leukemia

Exemestane (Aromasin) Uses: *Advanced breast CA in postmenopausal women w/progression after tamoxifen* **Action:** Irreversible, steroidal aromatase inhibitor; ↓ estrogens **Dose:** 25 mg PO QD after a meal **Caution:** [D, ?/–] **Contra:** Component sensitivity **Supplied:** Tabs 25 mg **SE:** Hot flashes, nausea, fatigue

22 **Exenatide (Byetta)** Uses: Type 2 DM combined w/metformin &/or sulfonylurea **Action:** Incretin mimetic: ↑ insulin release, ↓ glucagon secretion, ↓ gastric emptying, promotes satiety **Dose:** 5 mcg SQ bid w/in 60 min before AM & PM meals; ↑ to 10 mcg SQ bid after 1 mo PRN; do not give pc **Caution:** [C, ?/–] may ↓ absorption of other drugs (take antibiotics/contraceptives 1 h before) **Contra:** CrCl < 30 mL/min **Supplied:** Soln 5, 10 mcg/dose (prefilled pen) **SE:** Hypoglycemia, N/V/D, dizziness, HA, dyspepsia, ↓ appetite, jittery **Notes:** Consider ↓ sulfonylurea to ↓ risk of hypoglycemia; discard pen 30 d after 1st use

Ezetimibe (Zetia) **Uses:** *Hypercholesterolemia alone or w/HMG-CoA reductase inhibitor* **Action:** ↓ cholesterol & phytosterol absorption **Dose:** *Adults & Peds > 10 y.* 10 mg/d PO **Caution:** [C, +/–] Bile acid sequestrants ↓ bioavailability **Contra:** Hepatic impair **Supplied:** Tabs 10 mg **SE:** HA, D, abdominal pain, ↑ transaminases w/HMG-CoA reductase inhibitor

Ezetimibe/Simvastatin (Vytorin) **Uses:** *Hypercholesterolemia* **Action:** ↓ Absorption of cholesterol & phytosterols w/HMG-CoA-reductase inhibitor **Dose:** 10/10–10/80 mg/d PO; w/cyclosporine or danazol: 10/10 mg/d max; w/amiodarone or verapamil: 10/20 mg/d max; ↓ in severe renal insuff **Caution:** [X, –]; w/CYP3A4 inhibitors, gemfibrozil, niacin > 1 g/d, danazol, amiodarone, verapamil **Contra:** PRG/lactation; liver disease or ↑ LFTs **Supplied:** Tabs (ezetimibe/simvastatin) 10/10, 10/20, 10/40, 10/80 mg **SE:** HA, GI upset, myalgia, myopathy manifested as muscle pain, weakness or tenderness w/creatine kinase 10 × ULN, rhabdomyolysis, hepatitis, Infxn **Notes:** Monitor LFTs

Famciclovir (Famvir) **Uses:** *Acute herpes zoster (shingles) & genital herpes* **Action:** ↓ viral DNA synthesis **Dose:** *Zoster:* 500 mg PO q8h × 7 d. *Simplex:* 125–250 mg PO bid; ↓ in renal impair **Caution:** [B, –] **Contra:** Component sensitivity **Supplied:** Tabs 125, 250, 500 mg **SE:** Fatigue, dizziness, HA, pruritus, N/D **Notes:** Best w/in 72 h of initial lesion

Famotidine (Pepcid) **Uses:** *Short-term Rx of duodenal ulcer & benign gastric ulcer; maint for duodenal ulcer, hypersecretory conditions, GERD & heartburn* **Action:** H_2 antagonist; ↓ gastric acid secretion **Dose:** *Adults. Ulcer:* 20 mg IV q12h or 20–40 mg PO qhs × 4–8 wk. *Hypersecretion:* 20–160 mg PO q6h. *GERD:* 20 mg PO bid × 6 wk; maint: 20 mg PO hs. *Heartburn:* 10 mg PO PRN q12h. *Peds.* 0.5–1 mg/kg/d; ↓ in severe renal insuff **Caution:** [B, M] **Contra:** Component sensitivity **Supplied:** Tabs 10, 20, 40 mg; chew tabs 10 mg; susp 40 mg/5 mL; inj 10 mg/2 mL **SE:** Dizziness, HA, constipation, D, thrombocytopenia **Notes:** Chew tabs contain phenylalanine

Felodipine (Plendil) **Uses:** *HTN & CHF* **Action:** CCB **Dose:** 2.5–10 mg PO daily; ↓ in hepatic impair **Caution:** [C, ?] ↑ effect with azole antifungals, erythromycin, grapefruit juice **Contra:** Component sensitivity **Supplied:** ER tabs 2.5, 5, 10 mg **SE:** Peripheral edema, flushing, tachycardia, HA, gingival hyperplasia **Notes:** Follow BP in elderly & in impaired hepatic Fxn; swallow whole

Fenofibrate (Tricor) **Uses:** *Hypertriglyceridemia* **Action:** ↓ Triglyceride synthesis **Dose:** 48–145 mg daily; ↓ in renal impair, w/meals **Caution:** [C, ?] **Contra:** Hepatic/severe renal insuff, 1st-deg biliary cirrhosis, unexplained persistent ↑ LFTs, gallbladder Dz **Supplied:** Tabs 48, 145 mg **SE:** GI disturbances, cholecystitis, arthralgia, myalgia, dizziness **Notes:** Monitor LFTs

Fenoldopam (Corlopam) **Uses:** *Hypertensive emergency* **Action:** Rapid vasodilator **Dose:** Initial 0.03–0.1 mcg/kg/min IV inf, titrate q15 min by 0.05–0.1 mcg/kg/min **Caution:** [B, ?] ↓ BP w/β-blockers **Contra:** Allergy to sulfites

22

Supplied: Inj 10 mg/mL **SE:** ↓ BP, edema, facial flushing, N/V/D, atrial flutter/fibrillation, ↑ intraocular pressure **Notes:** Avoid concurrent β-blockers

Fenoprofen (Nalfon) WARNING: May ↑ risk of cardiovascular events and GI bleeding **Uses:** *Arthritis & pain* **Action:** NSAID **Dose:** 200–600 mg q4–8h, to 3200 mg/d max; w/food **Caution:** [B (D 3rd tri), +/–] CHF, HTN, renal/hepatic impair, Hx PUD **Contra:** NSAID sensitivity **Supplied:** Caps 200, 300 mg **SE:** GI disturbance, dizziness, HA, rash, edema, renal impair, hepatitis **Notes:** Swallow whole

Fentanyl (Sublimaze) [C-II] **Uses:** *Short-acting analgesic* in anesthesia & PCA **Action:** Narcotic analgesic **Dose:** *Adults.* 25–100 mcg/kg/dose IV/IM titrated. *Peds.* 1–2 mcg/kg IV/IM q1–4h titrated; ↓ in renal impair **Caution:** [B, +] **Contra:** ↑ ICP, resp depression, severe renal/hepatic impair **Supplied:** Inj 0.05 mg/mL **SE:** Sedation, ↓ BP, bradycardia, constipation, nausea, resp depression, miosis **Notes:** 0.1 mg fentanyl = 10 mg morphine IM

Fentanyl, Transdermal (Duragesic) [C-II] **Uses:** *Chronic pain* **Action:** Narcotic **Dose:** Apply patch to upper torso q72h; dose based on narcotic requirements in previous 24 h; ↓ in renal impair **Caution:** [B, +] **Contra:** ↑ ICP, resp depression, severe renal/hepatic impair **Supplied:** TD patches 25, 50, 75, 100 mcg/h **SE:** Sedation, ↓ BP, bradycardia, constipation, N, resp depression, miosis **Notes:** 0.1 mg fentanyl = 10 mg morphine IM

Fentanyl, Transmucosal System (Actiq) [C-II] **Uses:** *Induction of anesthesia; breakthrough CA pain* **Action:** Narcotic analgesic **Dose:** *Adults.* Anesthesia: 5–15 mcg/kg. *Pain:* 200 mcg over 15 min, titrate to effect; ↓ in renal impair **Caution:** [B, +] **Contra:** ↑ ICP, resp depression, severe renal/hepatic impair **Supplied:** Lozenges on stick 200, 400, 600, 800, 1200, 1600 mcg **SE:** Sedation, ↓ BP, bradycardia, constipation, nausea, resp depression, miosis **Notes:** 0.1 mg of fentanyl = 10 mg of morphine IM

Ferrous Gluconate (Fergon) **Uses:** *Iron deficiency anemia* & Fe supl **Action:** Dietary supl **Dose:** *Adults.* 100–200 mg of elemental Fe/d ÷ doses. *Peds.* 4–6 mg/kg/d ÷ doses; on empty stomach (OK w/meals if GI upset occurs); avoid antacids **Caution:** [A, ?] **Contra:** Hemochromatosis, hemolytic anemia **Supplied:** Tabs 300 (34 mg Fe), 325 mg (36 mg Fe) **SE:** GI upset, constipation, dark stools, discoloration of urine, may stain teeth **Notes:** 12% elemental Fe; false(+) stool guaiac

Ferrous Gluconate Complex (Ferrlecit) **Uses:** *Iron deficiency anemia or supl to erythropoietin therapy* **Action:** Fe Supl **Dose:** Test dose: 2 mL (25 mg Fe) inf over 1 h; if OK, 125 mg (10 mL) IV over 1 h. Usual cumulative dose 1 g Fe over 8 sessions (until favorable Hct) **Caution:** [B, ?] **Contra:** Anemia not due to Fe deficiency; CHF; Fe overload **Supplied:** Inj 12.5 mg/mL Fe **SE:** ↓ BP, serious allergic Rxns, GI disturbance, inj site Rxn **Notes:** Dose expressed as mg Fe; may inf during dialysis

Ferrous Sulfate **Uses:** *Fe deficiency anemia & Fe supl* **Action:** Dietary supl **Dose:** *Adults.* 100–200 mg elemental Fe/d in ÷ doses. *Peds.* 1–6 mg/kg/d ÷ daily–tid; on empty stomach (OK w/meals if GI upset occurs); avoid antacids **Caution:** [A, ?] ↑ absorption w/vitamin C; ↓ absorption w/tetracycline, fluoroquinolones, antacids, H₂-blockers, proton pump inhibitors **Contra:** Hemochromatosis, hemolytic anemia **Supplied:** Tabs 187 (60 mg Fe), 200 (65 mg Fe), 324 (65 mg Fe), 325 mg (65 mg Fe); SR caplets & tabs 160 mg (50 mg Fe), 200 mg (65 mg Fe); gtt 75 mg/0.6 mL (15 mg Fe/0.6 mL); elixir 220 mg/5 mL (44 mg Fe/5 mL); syrup 90 mg/5 mL (18 mg Fe/5 mL) **SE:** GI upset, constipation, dark stools, discolored urine

Fexofenadine (Allegra, Allegra-D)   **Uses:** *Allergic rhinitis* **Action:** Antihistamine **Dose:** *Adults & Peds > 12 y.* 60 mg PO bid or 180 mg/d; ↓ in renal impair **Caution:** [C, ?] **Contra:** Component sensitivity **Supplied:** Caps 60 mg; tabs 30, 60, 180 mg; Allegra-D (60 mg fexofenadine/120 mg pseudoephedrine) **SE:** Drowsiness (rare)

Filgrastim [G-CSF] (Neupogen)   **Uses:** *↓ Incidence of Infxn in febrile neutropenic pts; Rx chronic neutropenia* **Action:** Recombinant G-CSF **Dose:** *Adults & Peds.* 5 mcg/kg/d SQ or IV single daily dose; D/C when ANC > 10,000 **Caution:** [C, ?] w/drugs that potentiate release of neutrophils (eg, lithium) **Contra:** Allergy to *E. coli*–derived proteins or G-CSF **Supplied:** Inj 300 mcg/mL **SE:** Fever, alopecia, N/V/D, splenomegaly, bone pain, HA, rash **Notes:** Monitor CBC & plts; monitor for cardiac events; no benefit w/ANC > 10,000/μL

Finasteride (Proscar, Propecia)   **Uses:** *BPH & androgenetic alopecia* **Action:** ↓ 5α-Reductase **Dose:** *BPH:* 5 mg/d PO. *Alopecia:* 1 mg/d PO; food may ↓ absorption **Caution:** [X, –] Hepatic impair **Contra:** Pregnant women should avoid handling pills **Supplied:** Tabs 1 mg (Propecia), 5 mg (Proscar) **SE:** ↓ PSA levels (≈50% @ 6 mo) ; ↓ libido, impotence (rare) **Notes:** Reestablish PSA baseline at 6 mo; 3–6 mo for effect on urinary Sxs; continue to maintain new hair

Flavoxate (Urispas)   **Uses:** *Relief of Sx of dysuria, urgency, nocturia, suprapubic pain, urinary frequency, incontinence* **Action:** Antispasmodic **Dose:** 100–200 mg PO tid–qid **Caution:** [B, ?] **Contra:** Pyloric/duodenal obstruction, GI hemorrhage, GI obstruction, ileus, achalasia, BPH **Supplied:** Tabs 100 mg **SE:** Drowsiness, blurred vision, xerostomia

Flecainide (Tambocor)   **Uses:** Prevent AF/flutter & PSVT, *prevent/suppress life-threatening ventricular arrhythmias* **Action:** Class 1C antiarrhythmic **Dose:** *Adults.* 100 mg PO q12h; ↑ by 50 mg q12h q4d to max 400 mg/d. *Peds.* 3–6 mg/kg/d in 3 ÷ doses; ↓ in renal impair, **Caution:** [C, +] monitor in hepatic impair ↑ conc with amiodarone, digoxin, quinidine, ritonavir/amprenavir, BB, verapamil **Contra:** 2nd-/3rd-degree AV block, RBBB w/bifascicular or trifascicular block, cardiogenic shock, CAD, ritonavir/amprenavir, alkalinizing agents **Supplied:** Tabs 50, 100, 150 mg **SE:** Dizziness, visual disturbances, dyspnea, palpitations, edema, tachycardia, CHF, HA, fatigue, rash, nausea **Notes:** May cause new/worsened arrhythmias; initiate Rx in hospital; dose q8h if pt is intolerant/uncontrolled at 12–h intervals

Floxuridine (FUDR)   **Uses:** *GI adenoma, liver, renal cell carcinoma*; colon & pancreatic CAs **Action:** Inhibits thymidylate synthase; ↓ DNA synthesis (S-phase specific) **Dose:** 0.1–0.6 mg/kg/d for 1–6 wk (per protocols) **Caution:** [D, –] Drug interaction w/live & rotavirus vaccine **Contra:** BM suppression, poor nutritional status, potentially serious Infxn **Supplied:** Inj 500 mg **SE:** Myelosuppression, anorexia, abdominal cramps, N/V/D, mucositis, alopecia, skin rash & hyperpigmentation; rare neurotox (blurred vision, depression, nystagmus, vertigo & lethargy); intraarterial catheter-related problems (ischemia, thrombosis, bleeding & Infxn) **Notes:** Need effective birth control; palliative Rx for inoperable/incurable pts

Fluconazole (Diflucan) Uses: *Candidiasis (esophageal, oropharyngeal, urinary tract, vaginal, prophylaxis); cryptococcal meningitis* **Action:** Antifungal; ↓ cytochrome P-450 sterol demethylation. *Spectrum:* All *Candida* sp except *C. krusei* **Dose:** *Adults.* 100–400 mg/d PO or IV. *Vaginitis:* 150 mg PO qd. *Crypto:* 400 mg/d 1, then 200 mg × 10–12 wk after CSF (–). *Peds.* 3–6 mg/kg/d PO or IV; ↓ in renal impair **Caution:** [C, –] **Contra:** w/terfenadine **Supplied:** Tabs 50, 100, 150, 200 mg; susp 10, 40 mg/mL; inj 2 mg/mL **SE:** HA, rash, GI upset, ↓ K+, ↑ LFTs **Notes:** PO (preferred) = IV levels

Fludarabine Phosphate (FLAMP, Fludara) Uses: *Autoimmune hemolytic anemia, CLL, cold agglutinin hemolysis,* low-grade lymphoma, mycosis fungoides **Action:** ↓ Ribonucleotide reductase; blocks DNA polymerase-induced DNA repair **Dose:** 18–30 mg/m^2/d for 5 d, as a 30-min inf (per protocols) **Caution:** [D, –] Give cytarabine before fludarabine (↓ its metabolism) **Contra:** Severe Infxns; CrCl < 30 mL/min **Supplied:** Inj 50 mg **SE:** Myelosuppression, N/V/D, ↑ LFT, edema, CHF, fever, chills, fatigue, dyspnea, nonproductive cough, pneumonitis, severe CNS tox rare in leukemia

Fludrocortisone Acetate (Florinef) Uses: *Adrenocortical insuff, Addison Dz, salt-wasting syndrome* **Action:** Mineralocorticoid **Dose:** *Adults.* 0.1–0.2 mg/d PO. *Peds.* 0.05–0.1 mg/d PO **Caution:** [C, ?] **Contra:** Systemic fungal Infxns; known allergy **Supplied:** Tabs 0.1 mg **SE:** HTN, edema, CHF, HA, dizziness, convulsions, acne, rash, bruising, hyperglycemia, HPA suppression, cataracts **Notes:** For adrenal insuff, use w/glucocorticoid; dose changes based on plasma renin activity

Flumazenil (Romazicon) Uses: *Reverse sedative effects of benzodiazepines & general anesthesia* **Action:** Benzodiazepine receptor antagonist **Dose:** *Adults.* 0.2 mg IV over 15 s; repeat PRN, to 1 mg max (3 mg max in benzodiazepine OD). *Peds.* 0.01 mg/kg (0.2 mg/dose max) IV over 15 s; repeat 0.005 mg/kg at 1-min intervals to max 1 mg total; ↓ in hepatic impair **Caution:** [C, ?] **Contra:** In TCA OD; if pts given benzodiazepines to control life-threatening conditions (ICP/status epilepticus) **Supplied:** Inj 0.1 mg/mL **SE:** N/V, palpitations, HA, anxiety, nervousness, hot flashes, tremor, blurred vision, dyspnea, hyperventilation, withdrawal syndrome **Notes:** Does not reverse narcotic Sx or amnesia

Flunisolide (AeroBid, Nasalide) Uses: *Asthma in pts requiring chronic steroid therapy; relieve seasonal/perennial allergic rhinitis* **Action:** Topical steroid **Dose:** *Adults.* Met-dose inhal: 2 inhal bid (max 8/d). *Nasal:* 2 sprays/nostril bid (max 8/d). *Peds > 6 y.* Met-dose inhal: 2 inhal bid (max 4/d). *Nasal:* 1–2 sprays/nostril bid (max 4/d) **Caution:** [C, ?] **Contra:** Status asthmaticus **Supplied:** Aerosol 250 mg/actuation; nasal spray 0.025% **SE:** Tachycardia, bitter taste, local effects, oral candidiasis **Notes:** Not for acute asthma

Fluorouracil [5-FU] (Adrucil) Uses: *Colorectal, gastric, pancreatic, breast, basal cell,* head, neck, bladder, CAs **Action:** Inhibitor of thymidylate synthetase (interferes with DNA synthesis, S-phase specific) **Dose:** 370–1000 mg/m^2/d for 1–5 d IV push to 24-h cont inf; protracted venous inf of 200–300 mg/m^2/d (per protocol) **Caution:** [D, ?] ↑ tox w/allopurinol; do not give MTX before 5-FU **Contra:** Poor nutritional status, depressed BM Fxn, thrombocytopenia, major surgery w/in past mo, G6PD enzyme deficiency, PRG, serious Infxn, bilirubin > 5 mg/dL **Supplied:** Inj 50 mg/mL **SE:** Stomatitis, esophagopharyngitis, N/V/D, anorexia, myelosuppression (leukocytopenia, thrombocytopenia & anemia), rash/dry skin/photosensitivity, tingling in hands/feet w/pain (palmar–plantar erythrodysesthesia), phlebitis/discoloration at inj sites **Notes:** ↑ Thiamine intake; sun sensitivity; daily doses > 800 mg not OK; contraception recommended

Fluorouracil, Topical [5-FU] (Efudex)
Uses: *Basal cell carcinoma; actinic/solar keratosis* **Action:** Inhibits thymidylate synthetase (↓ DNA synthesis, S-phase specific) **Dose:** 5% cream bid × 3–6 wk **Caution:** [D, ?] Irritant chemo **Contra:** Component sensitivity **Supplied:** Cream 1, 5%; soln 1, 2, 5% **SE:** Rash, dry skin, photosensitivity **Notes:** Healing may not be evident for 1–2 mo; wash hands thoroughly; avoid occlusive dressings; do not overuse

Fluoxetine (Prozac, Sarafem)
WARNING: Closely monitor for worsening depression or emergence of suicidality, particularly in ped pts **Uses:** *Depression, OCD, panic disorder, bulimia, PMDD* (Sarafem) **Action:** SSRI **Dose:** 20 mg/d PO (max 80 mg/d ÷); weekly regimen 90 mg/wk after 1–2 wk of standard dose. *Bulimia:* 60 mg q AM. *Panic disorder:* 20 mg/d. *OCD:* 20–80 mg/d. *PMDD:* 20 mg/d or 20 mg intermittently, start 14 d before menses, repeat with each cycle; ↓ in hepatic failure **Caution:** [B, ?/–] Serotonin syndrome with MAOI, SSRI, serotonin agonists, linezolid; QT prolongation w/phenothiazines **Contra:** MAOI/thioridazine (wait 5 wk after D/C before MAOI) **Supplied:** *Prozac:* Caps 10, 20, 40 mg; scored tabs 10 mg; SR cap 90 mg; soln 20 mg/5 mL. *Sarafem:* Caps 10, 20 mg **SE:** Nausea, nervousness, weight loss, HA, insomnia

Fluoxymesterone (Halotestin)
Uses: Androgen-responsive metastatic *breast CA, hypogonadism* **Action:** ↓ Secretion of LH & FSH (feedback inhibition) **Dose:** *Breast CA:* 10–40 mg/d ÷ × 1–3 mo. *Hypogonadism:* 5–20 mg/d **Caution:** [X, ?/–] ↑ effect w/anticoagulants, cyclosporine, insulin, lithium, narcotics **Contra:** Serious cardiac, liver, or kidney Dz; PRG **Supplied:** Tabs 2, 5, 10 mg **SE:** Virilization, amenorrhea & menstrual irregularities, hirsutism, alopecia, acne, nausea & cholestasis. *Hematologic tox:* Suppression of clotting factors II, V, VII & × & polycythemia; ↑ libido, HA & anxiety **Notes:** Radiographic exam of hand/wrist q6mo in prepubertal children; ↓ total T_4 levels

Fluphenazine (Prolixin, Permitil)
Uses: *Schizophrenia* **Action:** Phenothiazine antipsychotic; blocks postsynaptic mesolimbic dopaminergic brain receptors **Dose:** 0.5–10 mg/d in ÷ doses PO q6–8h, average maint 5 mg/d; or 1.25 mg IM, then 2.5–10 mg/d in ÷ doses q6–8h PRN; ↓ in elderly **Caution:** [C, ?/–] **Contra:** Severe CNS depression, coma, subcortical brain damage, blood dyscrasias, hepatic Dz, w/caffeine, tannic acid, or pectin-containing products **Supplied:** Tabs 1, 2.5, 5, 10 mg; conc 5 mg/mL; elixir 2.5 mg/5 mL; inj 2.5 mg/mL; depot inj 25 mg/mL **SE:** Drowsiness, extrapyramidal effects **Notes:** Monitor LFTs; less sedative/hypotensive than chlorpromazine

Flurazepam (Dalmane) [C-IV]
Uses: *Insomnia* **Action:** Benzodiazepine **Dose:** *Adults & Peds > 15 y.* 15–30 mg PO qhs PRN; ↓ in elderly **Caution:** [X, ?/–] Elderly, low albumin, hepatic impair **Contra:** NA glaucoma; PRG **Supplied:** Caps 15, 30 mg **SE:** "Hangover" due to accumulation of metabolites, apnea **Notes:** May cause dependency

Flurbiprofen (Ansaid)
WARNING: May ↑ risk of cardiovascular events and GI bleeding **Uses:** *Arthritis* **Action:** NSAID **Dose:** 50–300 mg/d ÷ bid–qid, max 300 mg/d w/food **Caution:** [B (D in 3rd tri), +] **Contra:** PRG (3rd tri);

22

aspirin allergy **Supplied:** Tabs 50, 100 mg **SE:** Dizziness, GI upset, peptic ulcer Dz

Flutamide (Eulexin) **WARNING:** Liver failure & death reported. Measure LFT before, monthly & periodically after; D/C immediately if ALT 2 × ULN or jaundice develops **Uses:** Advanced *CAP* (in combo with LHRH agonists, eg, leuprolide or goserelin); w/radiation & GnRH for localized CAP **Action:** Nonsteroidal antiandrogen **Dose:** 250 mg PO tid (750 mg total) **Caution:** [D, ?] **Contra:** Severe hepatic impair **Supplied:** Caps 125 mg **SE:** Hot flashes, loss of libido, impotence, N/V/D, gynecomastia

Fluticasone, Nasal (Flonase) **Uses:** *Seasonal allergic rhinitis* **Action:** Topical steroid **Dose:** *Adults & Adolescents.* Nasal: 2 sprays/nostril/d. *Peds 4–11 y.* Nasal: 1–2 sprays/nostril/d **Caution:** [C, M] **Contra:** Primary Rx of status asthmaticus **Supplied:** Nasal spray 50 mcg/actuation **SE:** HA, dysphonia, oral candidiasis

Fluticasone, Oral (Flovent, Flovent Rotadisk) **Uses:** Chronic *asthma* **Action:** Topical steroid **Dose:** *Adults & Adolescents.* 2–4 puffs bid. *Peds 4–11 y.* 50 mcg bid **Caution:** [C, M] **Contra:** Primary Rx of status asthmaticus **Supplied:** Met-dose inhal 44, 110, 220 mcg/activation; Rotadisk dry powder: 50, 100, 250 mcg/activation **SE:** HA, dysphonia, oral candidiasis **Notes:** Risk of thrush; counsel on use of device

Fluticasone Propionate & Salmeterol Xinafoate (Advair Diskus) **Uses:** *Maint therapy for asthma* **Action:** Corticosteroid w/long-acting bronchodilator **Dose:** *Adults & Peds > 12 y.* 1 inhal bid q12h **Caution:** [C, M] **Contra:** Not for acute attack or in conversion from PO steroids or status asthmaticus **Supplied:** Met-dose inhal powder (fluticasone/salmeterol in mcg) 100/50, 250/50, 500/50 **SE:** URI, pharyngitis, HA **Notes:** Combo of Flovent & Serevent; do not use with spacer, do not wash mouthpiece, do not exhale into device

Fluvastatin (Lescol) **Uses:** *Atherosclerosis, primary hypercholesterolemia, hypertriglyceridemia* **Action:** HMG-CoA reductase inhibitor **Dose:** 20–80 mg PO qhs; ↓ w/hepatic impair **Caution:** [X, –] **Contra:** Active liver Dz, ↑ LFTs, PRG, breast feeding **Supplied:** Caps 20, 40 mg; XL 80 mg **SE:** HA, dyspepsia, N/D, abdominal pain

Fluvoxamine (Luvox) **WARNING:** Closely monitor for worsening depression or emergence of suicidality, particularly in ped pts **Uses:** *OCD* **Action:** SSRI **Dose:** Initial 50 mg single qhs dose, ↑ to 300 mg/d in ÷ doses; ↓ in elderly/hepatic impair, titrate slowly **Caution:** [C, ?/–] **Interactions** (MAOIs, phenothiazines, SSRIs, serotonin agonists, others) **Contra:** MAOI w/in 14 d **Supplied:** Tabs 25, 50, 100 mg **SE:** HA, N/D, somnolence, insomnia **Notes:** ÷ doses > 100 mg

Folic Acid **Uses:** *Megaloblastic anemia; folate deficiency* **Action:** Dietary supl **Dose:** *Adults.* Supl: 0.4 mg/d PO. *PRG:* 0.8 mg/d PO. *Folate deficiency:* 1 mg PO qd–tid. *Peds.* Supl: 0.04–0.4 mg/24 h PO, IM, IV, or SQ. *Folate deficiency:* 0.5–1 mg/24 h PO, IM, IV, or SQ **Caution:** [A, +] **Contra:** Pernicious, aplastic, normocytic anemias **Supplied:** Tabs 0.4, 0.8, 1 mg; inj 5 mg/mL **SE:** Well tolerated **Notes:** OK for all women of childbearing age; ↓ fetal neural tube defects by 50%; no effect on normocytic anemias

22 **Fondaparinux (Arixtra)** **WARNING:** When epidural/spinal anesthesia or spinal puncture is used, pts anticoagulated or scheduled to be anticoagulated with LMWH, heparinoids, or fondaparinux for prevention of thromboembolic complications are at risk of epidural or spinal hematoma, which can result in long-term or permanent paralysis **Uses:** *DVT prophylaxis* in hip fracture or replacement or knee replacement **Action:** Synthetic, specific inhibitor of activated factor X; a LMWH **Dose:** 2.5 mg SQ qd, up to 5–9 d; start at least 6 h postop **Caution:** [B, ?] ↑ bleeding risk w/anticoagulants, antiplatelets, drotrecogin alfa, NSAIDs **Contra:** Wt < 50 kg, CrCl < 30 mL/min, active bleeding, bacterial endocarditis, thrombocytopenia associated w/antiplatelet Ab **Supplied:** Prefilled syringes 2.5 mg/0.5 mL **SE:** Thrombocytopenia, anemia, fever, N **Notes:** D/C if plts < 100,000 μL; only give SQ; may monitor anti–factor Xa levels

Formoterol (Foradil Aerolizer) **Uses:** Maint Rx of *asthma & prevention of bronchospasm* with reversible obstructive airway Dz; exercise-induced bronchospasm **Action:** Long-acting β_2-adrenergic agonist, bronchodilator **Dose:** *Adults & Peds > 5 y.* Asthma: Inhale one 12-mcg cap q12h w/Aerolizer, 24 mcg/d max. *Adults & Peds > 12 y.* Exercise-induced bronchospasm: 1 inhal 12–mcg cap 15 min before exercise **Caution:** [C, ?] **Contra:** Need for acute bronchodilation; use w/in 2 wk of MAOI **Supplied:** 12-mcg blister pack for use in Aerolizer **SE:** Paradoxical bronchospasm; URI, pharyngitis, back pain **Notes:** Do not swallow caps; for use only with inhaler; do not start with significantly worsening or acutely deteriorating asthma

Fosamprenavir (Lexiva) **WARNING:** Do **not** use with severe liver dysfunction, reduce dose with mild–moderate liver impair (fosamprenavir 700 mg bid **w/o** ritonavir) **Uses:** HIV Infxn **Action:** Protease inhibitor **Dose:** 1400 mg bid w/o ritonavir; if w/ritonavir, fosamprenavir 1400 mg + ritonavir 200 mg qd or fosamprenavir 700 mg + ritonavir 100 mg bid. If w/efavirenz & ritonavir: fosamprenavir 1400 mg + ritonavir 300 mg qd **Caution:** [C, ?/–]; **Contra:** w/ ergot alkaloids, midazolam, triazolam, or pimozide; avoid if sulfa allergy **Supplied:** Tabs 700 mg **SE:** N/V/D, HA, fatigue, rash **Notes:** Numerous drug interactions because of hepatic metabolism

Foscarnet (Foscavir) **Uses:** *CMV retinitis*; acyclovir-resistant *herpes Infxns* **Action:** ↓ Viral DNA polymerase & RT **Dose:** *CMV retinitis: Induction:* 60 mg/kg IV q8h or 100 mg/kg q12h × 14–21 d. *Maint:* 90–120 mg/kg/d IV (Mon–Fri). *Acyclovir-resistant HSV induction:* 40 mg/kg IV q8–12h × 14–21 d; ↓ with renal impair **Caution:** [C, –] ↑ Sz potential w/fluoroquinolones; avoid nephrotoxic Rx (cyclosporine, aminoglycosides, ampho B, protease inhibitors) **Contra:** Significant renal impair (CrCl < 0.4 mL/min/kg) **Supplied:** Inj 24 mg/mL **SE:** Nephrotox, electrolyte abnormalities **Notes:** Sodium loading (500 mL 0.9% NaCl) before & after helps minimize nephrotox; monitor ionized calcium; administer through central line

Fosfomycin (Monurol) **Uses:** *Uncomplicated UTI* **Action:** ↓ bacterial cell wall synthesis. *Spectrum:* Gram(+) (staph, pneumococci); gram(−) (*E. coli, Enterococcus, Salmonella, Shigella, H. influenzae, Neisseria,* indole-negative *Proteus, Providencia*); *B. fragilis* & anaerobic gram(−) cocci are resistant **Dose:** 3 g PO dissolved in 90–120 mL of H_2O single dose; ↓ in renal impair **Caution:** [B, ?] ↓ absorption w/antacids/Ca salts **Contra:** Component sensitivity **Supplied:** Granule packets 3 g **SE:** HA, GI upset **Notes:** May take 2–3 d for Sxs to improve

Fosinopril (Monopril) **Uses:** *HTN, CHF,* DN **Action:** ACE inhibitor **Dose:** 10 mg/d PO initial; max 40 mg/d PO; ↓ in elderly; ↓ in renal impair **Cau-**

tion: [D, +] ↑ K+ w/K+ supls, ARBs, K+-sparing diuretics; ↑ renal angioedema w/NSAIDs, diuretics, hypovolemia **Contra:** Angioedema, w/ACE inhibitor, bilateral renal artery stenosis **Supplied:** Tabs 10, 20, 40 mg **SE:** Cough, dizziness, angioedema, ↑ K+

Fosphenytoin (Cerebyx) Uses: *Status epilepticus* **Action:** ↓ Sz spread in motor cortex **Dose:** As phenytoin equivalents (PE). *Load:* 15–20 mg PE/kg. *Maint:* 4–6 mg PE/kg/d; ↓ dosage, monitor levels in hepatic impair **Caution:** [D, +] May ↑ phenobarbital **Contra:** Sinus bradycardia, SA block, 2nd-/3rd-degree AV block, Adams–Stokes syndrome, rash during Rx **Supplied:** Inj 75 mg/mL **SE:** ↓ BP, dizziness, ataxia, pruritus, nystagmus **Notes:** 15 min to convert fosphenytoin to phenytoin; admin < 150 mg PE/min to prevent ↓ BP; administer with BP monitoring

Frovatriptan (Frova) See Table 22–11, page 645

Fulvestrant (Faslodex) Uses: Hormone receptor(+) metastatic *breast CA* in postmenopausal women with Dz progression following antiestrogen therapy **Action:** Estrogen receptor antagonist **Dose:** 250 mg IM monthly, either a single 5-mL inj or two concurrent 2.5-mL IM inj into buttocks **Caution:** [X, ?/–] ↑ effects w/CYP3A4 inhibitors w/hepatic impair **Contra:** PRG **Supplied:** Pre-filled syringes 50 mg/mL (single 5 mL, dual 2.5 mL) **SE:** N/V/D, constipation, abdominal pain, HA, back pain, hot flushes, pharyngitis, inj site Rxns **Notes:** Only use IM

Furosemide (Lasix) Uses: *CHF, HTN, edema,* ascites **Action:** Loop diuretic; ↓ Na & Cl reabsorption in ascending loop of Henle & distal tubule **Dose:** *Adults.* 20–80 mg PO or IV bid. *Peds.* 1 mg/kg/dose IV q6–12h; 2 mg/kg/dose PO q12–24h (max 6 mg/kg/dose) **Caution:** [C, +] ↓ K+, ↑ risk of digoxin tox; ↑ risk of ototox w/aminoglycosides, *cis*-platinum (esp in renal dysfunction) **Contra:** Allergy to sulfonylureas; anuria; hepatic coma/severe electrolyte depletion **Supplied:** Tabs 20, 40, 80 mg; soln 10 mg/mL, 40 mg/5 mL; inj 10 mg/mL **SE:** ↓ BP, hyperglycemia, ↓ K+ **Notes:** Monitor electrolytes, renal Fxn; high doses IV may cause ototox

Gabapentin (Neurontin) Uses: Adjunct in the Rx of *partial Szs;* post-herpetic neuralgia (PHN)*; chronic pain syndromes **Action:** Anticonvulsant **Dose:** *Anticonvulsant:* 300–1200 mg PO tid (max 3600 mg/d). *PHN:* 300 mg d 1, 300 mg bid d 2, 300 mg tid d 3, titrate (1800–3600 mg/d); ↓ in renal impair **Caution:** [C, ?] **Contra:** Component sensitivity **Supplied:** Caps 100, 300, 400 mg; soln 250 mg/5 mL; tab 600, 800 mg **SE:** Somnolence, dizziness, ataxia, fatigue **Notes:** Not necessary to monitor levels

Galantamine (Razadyne) Uses: *Alzheimer Dz* **Action:** Acetylcholinesterase inhibitor **Dose:** 4 mg PO bid, ↑ to 8 mg bid after 4 wk; may ↑ to 12 mg bid in 4 wk **Caution:** [B, ?] ↑ effect w/succinylcholine, amiodarone, diltiazem, verapamil, NSAIDs, digoxin; ↓ effect w/anticholinergics **Contra:** Severe renal/hepatic impair **Supplied:** Tabs 4, 8, 12 mg; soln 4 mg/mL (note old brand name: Reminyl) **SE:** GI disturbances, weight loss, sleep disturbances, dizziness, HA **Notes:** Caution w/urinary outflow obstruction, Parkinson Dz, severe asthma/COPD, severe heart Dz or ↓ BP

Gallium Nitrate (Ganite) Uses: *↑ Ca2+ of malignancy*; bladder CA **Action:** ↓ bone resorption of Ca2+ **Dose:** ↑ Ca2+: 200 mg/m²/d × 5 d. *CA:* 350 mg/m² cont inf × 5 d to 700 mg/m² rapid IV inf q2wk in antineoplastic settings (per protocols) **Caution:** [C, ?] Do not give with live vaccines or rotavirus vaccine **Contra:** SCr > 2.5 mg/dL **Supplied:** Inj 25 mg/mL **SE:** Renal insuff, ↓ Ca^{2+}, hypophosphatemia, ↓ bicarbonate, < 1% acute optic neuritis **Notes:** Bladder CA: use w/ vinblastine & ifosfamide

Ganciclovir (Cytovene, Vitrasert) Uses: *Rx & prevent CMV retinitis, prevent CMV Dz* in transplant recipients **Action:** ↓ viral DNA synthesis **Dose:** *Adults & Peds.* IV: 5 mg/kg IV q12h for 14–21 d, then maint 5 mg/kg/d IV × 7 d/ wk or 6 mg/kg/d IV × 5 d/wk. *Ocular implant:* One implant q5–8 mo. *Adults.* PO: After induction, 1000 mg PO tid. *Prevention:* 1000 mg PO tid; with food; ↓ in renal impair **Caution:** [C, –] ↑ effect w/immunosuppressives, imipenem/cilastatin, zidovudine, didanosine, other nephrotoxic Rx **Contra:** ANC < 500, plts < 25,000, intravitreal implant **Supplied:** Caps 250, 500 mg; inj 500 mg; ocular implant 4.5 mg **SE:** Granulocytopenia & thrombocytopenia, fever, rash, GI upset **Notes:** Not a cure for CMV; handle inj w/cytotox cautions; no systemic benefit w/implant

Gatifloxacin (Tequin, Zymar Ophthalmic) Uses: *Bronchitis, sinusitis, community-acquired pneumonia, UTI, uncomplicated skin/soft tissue Infxns* **Action:** Quinolone antibiotic, ↓ DNA-gyrase. *Spectrum:* Gram(+) (except MRSA, Listeria), gram(–) (not *Pseudomonas*), atypicals, some anaerobes (*Clostridium*, not *C. difficile*) **Dose:** 400 mg/d PO or IV. *Ophth:* Day 1 & 2 one gt q2h in eye while awake (8×d max) d 3–7, one gt 4×d while awake; (↓ in renal impair) **Caution:** [C, M] **Contra:** Prolonged QT interval, w/other Rx that prolong QT interval (Class Ia & III antiarrhythmics, erythromycin, antipsychotics, TCA); uncorrected ↓ K^+, children < 18 y or in PRG/lactating women **Supplied:** Tabs 200, 400 mg; inj 10 mg/mL; premixed inf D_5W 200 mg, 400 mg; ophth soln 0.3% **SE:** Prolonged QT interval, HA, N/D, tendon rupture, photosensitivity **Notes:** Reliable activity against *S. pneumoniae;* take 4 h after antacids containing Mg, Al, Fe, or Zn; drink plenty of fluids; avoid sunlight

Gefitinib (Iressa) Uses: *Rx locally advanced or metastatic NSCLC after failure of platinum-based & docetaxel chemotherapy* **Action:** ↓ intracellular phosphorylation of tyrosine kinases **Dose:** 250 mg/d PO **Caution:** [D, –] **Supplied:** Tabs 250 mg **SE:** D, rash, acne, dry skin, N/V, interstitial lung Dz, ↑ transaminases **Notes:** Follow LFTs

Gemcitabine (Gemzar) Uses: *Pancreatic CA, brain mets, NSCLC,* gastric CA **Action:** Antimetabolite; ↓ ribonucleotide reductase; produces false nucleotide base-inhibiting DNA synthesis **Dose:** 1000 mg/m² over 30 min–1 h IV inf/wk × 3–4 wk or 6–8 wk; modify dose based on hematologic Fxn (per protocol) **Caution:** [D, ?/–] **Contra:** PRG **Supplied:** Inj 200 mg, 1 g **SE:** Myelosuppression, N/V/D, drug fever, skin rash **Notes:** Reconstituted soln concn 38 mg/mL (not 40 mg/mL as earlier labeling); monitor hepatic/renal Fxn

Gemfibrozil (Lopid) Uses: *Hypertriglyceridemia, coronary heart Dz* **Action:** Fibric acid **Dose:** 1200 mg/d PO ÷ bid 30 min ac AM & PM **Caution:** [C, ?] ↑ warfarin effect, sulfonylureas; ↑ risk of myopathy w/HMG-CoA reductase inhibitors; ↓ effects w/cyclosporine **Contra:** Renal/hepatic impair (SCr > 2.0 mg/dL), gallbladder Dz, primary biliary cirrhosis **Supplied:** Tabs 600 mg **SE:** Cholelithiasis, GI upset **Notes:** Avoid use w/HMG-CoA reductase inhibitors; monitor LFTs & serum lipids

Gemifloxacin (Factive) Uses: Community-acquired pneumonia, acute exacerbation of chronic bronchitis **Action:** ↓ DNA gyrase & topoisomerase IV;

22

Spectrum: S. pneumoniae (including multidrug-resistant strains), *H. influenzae, H. parainfluenzae, M. catarrhalis, M. pneumoniae, C. pneumoniae, K. pneumoniae* **Dose:** 320 mg PO qd; CrCl < 40 mL/min: 160 mg PO qd **Caution:** [C, ?/–]; children < 18 y; Hx of ↑ QTc interval, electrolyte disorders, w/Class IA/III antiarrhythmics, erythromycin, TCAs, antipsychotics **Contra:** Fluoroquinolone allergy **Supplied:** Tab 320 mg **SE:** Rash, N/V/D, abdominal pain, dizziness, xerostomia, arthralgia, allergy/anaphylactic reactions, peripheral neuropathy, tendon rupture **Notes:** Take 3 h before or 2 h after: antacids, Fe, Zn, or other metal cations

Gemtuzumab Ozogamicin (Mylotarg) WARNING: Can cause severe allergic Rxns & other inf-related reactions including severe pulmonary events; hepatotox, including severe hepatic venoocclusive Dz reported Uses: *Relapsed CD33⁺ AML in pts > 60 y who are poor chemo candidates for chemo* Action: MoAb linked to calicheamicin; selective for myeloid cells **Dose:** Per protocol **Caution:** [D,?/–] **Contra:** Component sensitivity **Supplied:** 5 mg/20 mL vial **SE:** Myelosuppression, allergy (including anaphylaxis), inf Rxns (chills, fever, N/V, HA), pulmonary events, hepatotox **Notes:** Single agent use only, not in combo; premedicate (diphenhydramine & acetaminophen)

Gentamicin (Garamycin, G-Mycitin, others) Uses: *Serious Infxns* caused by *Pseudomonas, Proteus, E. coli, Klebsiella, Enterobacter* & *Serratia* & initial Rx of gram(–) sepsis **Action:** Bactericidal; ↓ protein synthesis. *Spectrum:* Synergy w/PCNs; gram(–) (not *Neisseria, Legionella, Acinetobacter*) **Dose:** *Adults.* 3–7 mg/kg/24h IV ÷ q8–24h. *Peds.* Infants < 7 d < 1200 g: 2.5 mg/kg/dose q18–24h. *Infants > 1200 g:* 2.5 mg/kg/dose q12–18h. *Infants > 7 d:* 2.5 mg/kg/dose IV q8–12h. *Children:* 2.5 mg/kg/d IV q8h; ↓ w/renal insuff **Caution:** [C, +/–] Avoid other nephrotoxic Rxs **Contra:** Aminoglycoside sensitivity **Supplied:** Premixed inf 40, 60, 70, 80, 90, 100, 120 mg; ADD-Vantage inj vials 10 mg/mL; inj 40 mg/mL; IT preservative-free 2 mg/mL **SE:** Nephrotox/ototox/neurotox **Notes:** Follow CrCl, SCr & serum conc for dose adjustments (Table 22–2, page 628); once daily dosing popular; follow; use IBW to dose (use adjusted if obese > 30% IBW)

Gentamicin & Prednisolone, Ophthalmic (Pred-G Ophthalmic) **Uses:** *Steroid-responsive ocular & conjunctival Infxns* sensitive to gentamicin **Action:** Bactericidal; ↓ protein synthesis w/antiinflammatory. *Spectrum: Staph, E. coli, H. influenzae, Klebsiella, Neisseria, Pseudomonas, Proteus* & *Serratia* sp **Dose:** *Oint:* 1/2 in. in conjunctival sac daily–tid. *Susp:* 1 gt bid–qid, up to 1 gt/h for severe Infxns **Contra:** Aminoglycoside sensitivity **Caution:** [C, ?] **Supplied:** *Oint, ophth:* Prednisolone acetate 0.6% & gentamicin sulfate 0.3% (3.5 g). *Susp, ophth:* Prednisolone acetate 1% & gentamicin sulfate 0.3% (2, 5, 10 mL) **SE:** Local irritation

Gentamicin, Ophthalmic (Garamycin, Genoptic, Gentacidin, Gentak, others) Uses: *Conjunctival Infxns* Action: Bactericidal; ↓ protein synthesis **Dose:** *Oint:* Apply 1/2 in bid–tid. *Soln:* 1–2 gtt q2–4h, up to 2 gtt/h for severe Infxn **Caution:** [C, ?] **Contra:** Aminoglycoside sensitivity **Supplied:** Soln & oint 0.3% **SE:** Local irritation **Notes:** Do not use other eye drops w/in 5–10 min; do not touch dropper to eye

Gentamicin, Topical (Garamycin, G-Mycitin) Uses: *Skin Infxns* caused by susceptible organisms **Action:** Bactericidal; ↓ protein synthesis **Dose:** *Adults & Peds > 1 y.* Apply tid–qid **Caution:** [C, ?] **Contra:** Aminoglycoside sensitivity **Supplied:** Cream & oint 0.1% **SE:** Irritation

Glimepiride (Amaryl) Uses: *Type 2 DM* **Action:** Sulfonylurea; ↑ pancreatic insulin release; ↑ peripheral insulin sensitivity; ↓ hepatic glucose output/production **Dose:** 1–4 mg/d, max 8 mg **Caution:** [C, –] **Contra:** DKA **Supplied:** Tabs 1, 2, 4 mg **SE:** HA, nausea, hypoglycemia **Notes:** Give w/1st meal of day

Glipizide (Glucotrol, Glucotrol XL) Uses: *Type 2 DM* **Action:** Sulfonylurea; ↑ pancreatic insulin release; ↑ peripheral insulin sensitivity; ↓ hepatic glucose output/production; ↓ intestinal glucose absorption **Dose:** 5 mg initial, ↑ by 2.5–5 mg/d, max 40 mg/d; XL max 20 mg; 30 min ac; hold if pt NPO **Caution:** [C, ?/–] Severe liver Dz **Contra:** DKA, Type 1 DM, sulfonamide sensitivity **Supplied:** Tabs 5, 10 mg; XL tabs 2.5, 5, 10 mg **SE:** HA, anorexia, N/V/D, constipation, fullness, rash, urticaria, photosensitivity **Notes:** Counsel about DM management; wait several days before adjusting dose; monitor glucose

Glucagon Uses: Severe *hypoglycemic* Rxns in DM with sufficient liver glycogen stores or β-blocker OD **Action:** Accelerates liver gluconeogenesis **Dose:** *Adults.* 0.5–1 mg SQ, IM, or IV; repeat in 20 min PRN. *Beta-blocker OD:* 3–10 mg IV; repeat in 10 min PRN; may give cont inf 1–5 mg/h. *Peds.* Neonates: 0.3 mg/kg/dose SQ, IM, or IV q4h PRN. *Children:* 0.025–0.1 mg/kg/dose SQ, IM, or IV; repeat in 20 min PRN **Caution:** [B, M] **Contra:** Pheochromocytoma **Supplied:** Inj 1 mg **SE:** N/V, ↓ BP **Notes:** Administration of glucose IV necessary; ineffective in starvation, adrenal insuff, or chronic hypoglycemia

Glyburide (DiaBeta, Micronase, Glynase) Uses: *Type 2 DM* **Action:** Sulfonylurea; ↑ pancreatic insulin release; ↑ peripheral insulin sensitivity; ↓ hepatic glucose output/production; ↓ intestinal glucose absorption **Dose:** 1.25–10 mg qd–bid, max 20 mg/d. *Micronized:* 0.75–6 mg qd–bid, max 12 mg/d **Caution:** [C, ?] Renal impair **Contra:** DKA, Type 1 DM **Supplied:** Tabs 1.25, 2.5, 5 mg; micronized tabs 1.5, 3, 6 mg **SE:** HA, hypoglycemia **Notes:** Not OK for CrCl < 50 mL/min; hold dose if NPO

Glyburide/Metformin (Glucovance) Uses: *Type 2 DM* **Action:** *Sulfonylurea:* ↑ Pancreatic insulin release. *Metformin:* ↑ Peripheral insulin sensitivity; ↓ hepatic glucose output/production; ↓ intestinal glucose absorption **Dose:** 1st line (naive pts), 1.25/250 mg PO daily–bid; 2nd line, 2.5/500 mg or 5/500 mg bid (max 20/2000 mg); take w/meals, slowly ↑ dose; hold before & 48 h after ionic contrast media **Caution:** [C, –] **Contra:** SCr > 1.4 in women or > 1.5 in men; hypoxemic conditions (CHF, sepsis, recent MI); alcoholism; metabolic acidosis; liver Dz; **Supplied:** Tabs 1.25/250 mg, 2.5/500 mg, 5/500 mg **SE:** HA, hypoglycemia, lactic acidosis, anorexia, N/V, rash **Notes:** Avoid EtOH; hold dose if NPO; monitor folate levels (megaloblastic anemia)

Glycerin Suppository Uses: *Constipation* **Action:** Hyperosmolar laxative **Dose:** *Adults.* 1 adult supp PR PRN. *Peds.* 1 infant supp PR daily–bid PRN **Caution:** [C, ?] **Supplied:** Supp (adult, infant); liq 4 mL/applicatorful **SE:** D

Gonadorelin (Lutrepulse) Uses: *Primary hypothalamic amenorrhea* **Action:** Stimulates pituitary release of LH & FSH **Dose:** 5 mcg IV q 90 min × 21 d using Lutrepulse pump kit **Caution:** [B, M] ↑ levels w/androgens, estrogens, progestins, glucocorticoids, spironolactone, levodopa; ↓ levels with OCP, digoxin, dopamine antagonists **Contra:** Condition exacerbated by PRG or reproductive hormones, ovarian cysts, causes of anovulation other than hypothalamic, hormonally dependent tumor **Supplied:** Inj 100 mcg **SE:** Multiple pregnancy risk; inj site pain **Notes:** Monitor LH, FSH

22

Goserelin (Zoladex)   Uses: Advanced *CAP* & w/radiation for localized high-risk CAP, *endometriosis, breast CA* Action: LHRH agonist, transient ↑ the ↓ in LH, w/↓ testosterone Dose: 3.6 mg SQ (implant) q 28d or 10.8 mg SQ q3mo; usually lower abdominal wall Caution: [X, –] Contra: PRG, breast feeding, 10.8-mg implant not for women Supplied: SQ implant 3.6 (1 mo), 10.8 mg (3 mo) SE: Hot flashes, ↓ libido, gynecomastia & transient exacerbation of CA-related bone pain (flare reaction 7–10 d after 1st dose) Notes: Inject SQ into fat in abdominal wall; do not aspirate; women must use contraception

Granisetron (Kytril)   Uses: *Prevention of N/V* Action: Serotonin receptor antagonist Dose: *Adults & Peds.* 10 mcg/kg/dose IV 30 min before chemo *Adults.* 2 mg PO 1 h before chemo, then 12 h later. *Postop N/V:* 1 mg IV before end of OR case Caution: [B, +/–] St. John's wort ↓ levels Contra: Liver Dz, children < 2 y Supplied: Tabs 1 mg; inj 1 mg/mL; soln 2 mg/10 mL SE: HA, constipation

Guaifenesin (Robitussin, others)   Uses: *Relief of dry, nonproductive cough* Action: Expectorant Dose: *Adults.* 200–400 mg (10–20 mL) PO q4h (max 2.4 g/d). *Peds.* < 2 y: 12 mg/kg/d in 6 ÷ doses. *2–5 y:* 50–100 mg (2.5–5 mL) PO q4h (max 600 mg/d). *6–11 y:* 100–200 mg (5–10 mL) PO q4h (max 1.2 g/d) Caution: [C, ?] Supplied: Tabs 100, 200; SR tabs 600, 1200 mg; caps 200 mg; SR caps 300 mg; liq 100 mg/5 mL SE: GI upset Notes: Give w/large amount of H_2O; some dosage forms contain EtOH

Guaifenesin & Codeine (Robitussin AC, Brontex, others) [C-V]   Uses: *Relief of dry cough* Action: Antitussive w/expectorant Dose: *Adults.* 5–10 mL or 1 tab PO q6–8h (max 60 mL/24 h). *Peds.* 2–6 y: 1–1.5 mg/kg codeine/d ÷ dose q4–6h (max 30 mg/24 h). *6–12 y:* 5 mL q4h (max 30 mL/24 h) Caution: [C, +] Supplied: Brontex tab 10 mg codeine/300 mg guaifenesin; liq 2.5 mg codeine/75 mg guaifenesin/5 mL; others 10 mg codeine/100 mg guaifenesin/5 mL SE: Somnolence

Guaifenesin & Dextromethorphan (many OTC brands)   Uses: *Cough* due to upper resp tract irritation Action: Antitussive w/expectorant Dose: *Adults & Peds > 12 y.* 10 mL PO q6–8h (max 40 mL/24 h). *Peds.* 2–6 y: Dextromethorphan 1–2 mg/kg/24 h ÷ 3–4 × d (max 10 mL/d). *6–12 y:* 5 mL q6–8h (max 20 mL/d) Caution: [C, +] Contra: Administration w/MAOI Supplied: Many OTC formulations SE: Somnolence Notes: Give with plenty of fluids

Haemophilus B Conjugate Vaccine (ActHIB, HibTITER, Pedvax-HIB, Prohibit, others)   Uses: Routine *immunization* of children against *H. influenzae* type B Dzs Action: Active immunization against *Haemophilus* B Dose: *Peds.* 0.5 mL (25 mg) IM in deltoid or vastus lateralis Caution: [C, +] Contra: Febrile illness, immunosuppression, allergy to thimerosal Supplied: Inj 7.5, 10, 15, 25 mcg/0.5 mL SE: Observe for anaphylaxis; edema, ↑ risk of *Haemophilus* B Infxn the week after vaccination Notes: Booster not required; report SAE to VAERS: 1-800-822-7967

Haloperidol (Haldol)   Uses: *Psychotic disorders, agitation, Tourette disorders, hyperactivity in children* Action: Antipsychotic, neuroleptic Dose: *Adults.* Moderate Sxs: 0.5–2 mg PO bid–tid. *Severe Sxs/agitation:* 3–5 mg PO bid–tid or 1–5 mg IM q4h PRN (max 100 mg/d). *Peds.* 3–6 y: 0.01–0.03 mg/kg/24 h PO qd. *6–12 y:* Initial, 0.5–1.5 mg/24 h PO; ↑ by 0.5 mg/24 h to maintenance of 2–4 mg/24 h (0.05–0.1 mg/kg/24 h) or 1–3 mg/dose IM q4–8h to 0.1 mg/kg/24 h max; Tourette Dz may require up to 15 mg/24 h PO; ↓ in elderly Caution: [C, ?] ↑ effects w/

22

SSRIs, CNS depressants, TCA, indomethacin, metoclopramide; avoid levodopa (↓ antiparkinsonian effects) **Contra:** NA glaucoma, severe CNS depression, coma, Parkinson Dz, BM suppression, severe cardiac/hepatic Dz **Supplied:** Tabs 0.5, 1, 2, 5, 10, 20 mg; conc liq 2 mg/mL; inj 5 mg/mL; decanoate inj 50, 100 mg/mL **SE:** Extrapyramidal Sxs (EPS), ↓ BP, anxiety, dystonias **Notes:** Do not give decanoate IV; dilute PO conc liq w/H$_2$O/juice; monitor for EPS

Haloprogin (Halotex) **Uses:** *Topical Rx of tinea pedis, tinea cruris, tinea corporis, tinea manus* **Action:** Topical antifungal **Dose:** *Adults.* Apply bid for ≤ 2 wk; intertriginous may require ≤ 4 wk **Caution:** [B, ?] **Contra:** Component sensitivity **Supplied:** 1% cream; soln **SE:** Local irritation **Notes:** Avoid contact w/eyes; improvement w/in 4 wk

Heparin **Uses:** *Rx & prevention of DVT & PE,* unstable angina, AF w/ emboli & acute arterial occlusion **Action:** Acts w/antithrombin III to inactivate thrombin & ↓ thromboplastin formation **Dose:** *Adults. Prophylaxis:* 3000–5000 units SQ q8–12h. *Thrombosis Rx:* Load 50–80 units/kg IV, then 10–20 units/kg IV qh (adjust based on PTT). *Peds.* Infants: Load 50 units/kg IV bolus, then 20 units/kg/ h IV by cont inf. *Children:* Load 50 units/kg IV, then 15–25 units/kg cont inf or 100 units/kg/dose q4h IV intermittent bolus (adjust based on PTT) **Caution:** [B, +] ↑ risk of hemorrhage w/anticoagulants, aspirin, antiplatelets, cephalosporins w/MTT side chain **Contra:** Uncontrolled bleeding, severe thrombocytopenia, suspected ICH **Supplied:** Inj 10, 100, 1000, 2000, 2500, 5000, 7500, 10,000, 20,000, 40,000 units/ mL **SE:** Bruising, bleeding, thrombocytopenia **Notes:** Follow PTT, thrombin time, or activated clotting time; little PT effect; therapeutic PTT 1.5–2 × control for most conditions; monitor for HIT w/plt counts

Hepatitis A Vaccine (Havrix, Vaqta) **Uses:** *Prevent hepatitis A* in high-risk individuals (eg, travelers, certain professions, or high-risk behaviors) **Action:** Active immunity **Dose:** (Expressed as ELISA units [EL.U.]) *Havrix: Adults.* 1440 EL.U. single IM dose. *Peds > 2 y.* 720 EL.U. single IM dose. *Vaqta: Adults.* 50 units single IM dose. *Peds.* 25 units single IM dose **Caution:** [C, +] **Contra:** Component allergy **Supplied:** Inj 720 EL.U./0.5 mL, 1440 EL.U./1 mL; 50 units/mL **SE:** Fever, fatigue, HA, inj site pain **Notes:** Booster OK 6–12 mo after primary; report SAE to VAERS: 1-800-822–7967

Hepatitis A (Inactivated) & Hepatitis B (Recombinant) Vaccine (Twinrix) **Uses:** *Active immunization against hepatitis A/B* **Action:** Active immunity **Dose:** 1 mL IM at 0, 1 & 6 mo **Caution:** [C, +] **Contra:** Component sensitivity **Supplied:** Single-dose vials, syringes **SE:** Fever, fatigue, pain at site, HA **Notes:** Booster OK 6–12 mo after vaccination; report SAE to VAERS: 1-800-822–7967

Hepatitis B Immune Globulin (HyperHep, H-BIG) **Uses:** *Exposure to HBsAg(+) material* (eg, blood, plasma, or serum [accidental needlestick, mucous membrane contact, PO]) **Action:** Passive immunization **Dose:** *Adults & Peds.* 0.06 mL/kg IM 5 mL max; w/in 24 h of exposure; w/in 14 d of sexual contact; repeat 1 & 6 mo after exposure **Caution:** [C, ?] **Contra:** Allergies to γ-globulin or antiimmunoglobulin Ab; allergies to thimerosal; IgA deficiency **Supplied:** Inj **SE:** Inj site pain, dizziness **Notes:** IM in gluteal or deltoid; w/continued exposure, give hepatitis B vaccine

Hepatitis B Vaccine (Engerix-B, Recombivax HB) **Uses:** *Prevent hepatitis B* **Action:** Active immunization; recombinant DNA **Dose:** *Adults.* 3 IM

22

doses 1 mL each; 1st 2 doses 1 mo apart; the 3rd 6 mo after the 1st. **Peds.** 0.5 mL IM adult schedule **Caution:** [C, +] ↓ effect w/immunosuppressives **Contra:** Yeast allergy **Supplied:** *Engerix-B:* Inj 20 mcg/mL; peds inj 10 mcg/0.5 mL. *Recombivax HB:* Inj 10 & 40 mcg/mL; peds inj 5 mcg/0.5 mL **SE:** Fever, inj site pain **Notes:** Deltoid IM inj adults/older peds; younger peds, use anterolateral thigh

Hetastarch (Hespan) **Uses:** *Plasma volume expansion* adjunct in shock & leukapheresis **Action:** Synthetic colloid; acts like albumin **Dose:** *Volume expansion:* 500–1000 mL (1500 mL/d max) IV (20 mL/kg/h max rate). *Leukapheresis:* 250–700 mL; ↓ in renal failure **Caution:** [C, +] **Contra:** Severe bleeding disorders, CHF, oliguric/anuric renal failure **Supplied:** Inj 6 g/100 mL **SE:** Bleeding (↑ prolongs PT, PTT, bleed time) **Notes:** Not blood or plasma substitute

Hydralazine (Apresoline, others) **Uses:** *Moderate–severe HTN; CHF* (w/Isordil) **Action:** Peripheral vasodilator **Dose:** *Adults.* Initial 10 mg PO qid, ↑ to 25 mg qid 300 mg/d max. **Peds.** 0.75–3 mg/kg/24 h PO ÷ q6–12h; ↓ in renal impair; check CBC & ANA before **Caution:** [C, +] ↓ hepatic Fxn & CAD; ↑ tox w/MAOI, indomethacin, β-blockers **Contra:** Dissecting aortic aneurysm, mitral valve/rheumatic heart Dz **Supplied:** Tabs 10, 25, 50, 100 mg; inj 20 mg/mL **SE:** SLE-like syndrome w/chronic high doses; SVT after IM inj, peripheral neuropathy **Notes:** Compensatory sinus tachycardia eliminated w/β-blocker

Hydrochlorothiazide (HydroDIURIL, Esidrix, others) **Uses:** *Edema, HTN* **Action:** Thiazide diuretic; ↓ distal tubule Na reabsorption **Dose:** *Adults.* 25–100 mg/d PO single or ÷ doses. **Peds.** < 6 mo: 2–3 mg/kg/d in 2 ÷ doses. > 6 *mo:* 2 mg/kg/d in 2 ÷ doses **Caution:** [D, +] **Contra:** Anuria, sulfonamide allergy, renal insuff **Supplied:** Tabs 25, 50, 100 mg; caps 12.5 mg; PO soln 50 mg/5 mL **SE:** ↓ K+, hyperglycemia, hyperuricemia, ↓ Na+ **Notes:** May cause sun sensitivity

Hydrochlorothiazide & Amiloride (Moduretic) **Uses:** *HTN* **Action:** Combined thiazide & a K+-sparing diuretic **Dose:** 1–2 tabs/d PO **Caution:** [D, ?] **Contra:** renal failure, sulfonamide allergy **Supplied:** Tabs (amiloride/HCTZ) 5 mg/50 mg **SE:** ↓ BP, photosensitivity, ↑ K+/↓ K+, hyperglycemia, ↓ Na+, hyperlipidemia, hyperuricemia

Hydrochlorothiazide & Spironolactone (Aldactazide) **Uses:** *Edema, HTN* **Action:** Thiazide & K+-sparing diuretic **Dose:** 25–200 mg each component/d, ÷ doses **Caution:** [D, +] **Contra:** Sulfonamide allergy **Supplied:** Tabs (HCTZ/spironolactone) 25 mg/25 mg, 50 mg/50 mg **SE:** Photosensitivity, ↓ BP, ↑ or ↓ K+, ↓ Na+, hyperglycemia, hyperlipidemia, hyperuricemia

Hydrochlorothiazide & Triamterene (Dyazide, Maxzide) **Uses:** *Edema & HTN* **Action:** Combined thiazide & K+-sparing diuretic **Dose:** *Dyazide:* 1–2 caps PO qd–bid. *Maxzide:* 1 tab/d PO **Caution:** [D, +/–] **Contra:** Sulfonamide allergy **Supplied:** (Triamterene/HCTZ) 37.5 mg/25 mg, 50 mg/25 mg, 75 mg/50 mg **SE:** Photosensitivity, ↓ BP, ↑ or ↓ K+, ↓ Na+, hyperglycemia, hyperlipidemia, hyperuricemia **Notes:** HCTZ component in Maxzide more bioavailable than in Dyazide

Hydrocodone & Acetaminophen (Lorcet, Vicodin, others) [C-III] **Uses:** *Moderate–severe pain* **Action:** Narcotic analgesic w/nonnarcotic analgesic; hydrocodone is antitussive **Dose:** 1–2 caps or tabs PO q4–6h PRN **Caution:** [C, M] **Contra:** CNS depression, severe resp depression **Supplied:** Many formulations; specify hydrocodone/APAP dose; caps 5/500; tabs 2.5/500, 5/400,

22

5/500, 7.5/400, 10/400, 7.5/500, 7.5/650, 7.5/750, 10/325, 10/400, 10/500, 10/650; elixir & soln (fruit punch) 2.5 mg hydrocodone/167 mg APAP/5 mL **SE:** GI upset, sedation, fatigue **Notes:** Do not exceed > 4 g acetaminophen/d

Hydrocodone & Aspirin (Lortab ASA, others) [C-III]
Uses: *Moderate–severe pain* **Action:** Narcotic analgesic with NSAID **Dose:** 1–2 PO q4–6h PRN, w/food/milk **Caution:** [C, M] ↓ renal Fxn, gastritis/PUD, **Contra:** Component sensitivity; children w/chickenpox (Reye syndrome) **Supplied:** 5 mg hydrocodone/500 mg ASA/tab **SE:** GI upset, sedation, fatigue **Notes:** Monitor for GI bleed

Hydrocodone & Guaifenesin (Hycotuss Expectorant, others) [C-III]
Uses: *Nonproductive cough* associated with resp Infxn **Action:** Expectorant w/cough suppressant **Dose:** *Adults & Peds > 12 y.* 5 mL q4h pc & hs. *Peds.* < 2 y: 0.3 mg/kg/d ÷ qid. *2–12 y:* 2.5 mL q4h pc & hs **Caution:** [C, M] **Contra:** Component sensitivity **Supplied:** Hydrocodone 5 mg/guaifenesin 100 mg/5 mL **SE:** GI upset, sedation, fatigue

Hydrocodone & Homatropine (Hycodan, Hydromet, others) [C-III]
Uses: *Relief of cough* **Action:** Combo antitussive **Dose:** (Based on hydrocodone) *Adults.* 5–10 mg q4–6h. *Peds.* 0.6 mg/kg/d ÷ tid–qid **Caution:** [C, M] **Contra:** NA glaucoma, ↑ ICP, depressed ventilation **Supplied:** Syrup 5 mg hydrocodone/5 mL; tabs 5 mg hydrocodone **SE:** Sedation, fatigue, GI upset **Notes:** Do not give > q4h; see individual Rx monographs

Hydrocodone & Ibuprofen (Vicoprofen) [C-III]
Uses: *Moderate–severe pain (< 10 d)* **Action:** Narcotic w/NSAID **Dose:** 1–2 tabs q4–6h PRN **Caution:** [C, M] Renal insuff; ↓ effect w/ACE inhibitors & diuretics; ↑ effect w/CNS depressants, EtOH, MAOI, aspirin, TCA, anticoagulants **Contra:** Component sensitivity **Supplied:** Tabs 7.5 mg hydrocodone/200 mg ibuprofen **SE:** Sedation, fatigue, GI upset

Hydrocodone & Pseudoephedrine (Detussin, Histussin-D, others) [C-III]
Uses: *Cough & nasal congestion* **Action:** Narcotic cough suppressant with decongestant **Dose:** 5 mL qid, PRN **Caution:** [C, M] **Contra:** MAOIs **Supplied:** 5 mg hydrocodone/60 mg pseudoephedrine/5 mL **SE:** ↑ BP, GI upset, sedation, fatigue

Hydrocodolne, Chlorpheniramine, Phenylephrine, Acetaminophen & Caffeine (Hycomine Compound) [C-III]
Uses: *Cough & Sxs of URI* **Action:** Narcotic cough suppressant w/decongestants & analgesic **Dose:** 1 tab PO q4h PRN **Caution:** [C, M] **Contra:** NAG **Supplied:** Hydrocodone 5 mg/chlorpheniramine 2 mg/phenylephrine 10 mg/APAP 250 mg/caffeine 30 mg/tab **SE:** ↑BP, GI upset, sedation, fatigue

Hydrocortisone, Rectal (Anusol-HC Suppository, Cortifoam Rectal, Proctocort, others)
Uses: *Painful anorectal conditions,* radiation proctitis, ulcerative colitis **Action:** Antiinflammatory steroid **Dose:** *Adults. Ulcerative colitis:* 10–100 mg PR qd–bid for 2–3 wk **Caution:** [B, ?/–] **Contra:** Component sensitivity **Supplied:** *Hydrocortisone acetate:* Rectal aerosol 90 mg/applicator; supp 25 mg. *Hydrocortisone base:* Rectal 1%; rectal susp 100 mg/60 mL **SE:** Minimal systemic effect

Hydrocortisone, Topical & Systemic (Cortef, Solu-Cortef)
See Steroids, page 603 & Tables 22–4 & 22–5, pages 633 & 634 **Caution:** [B, –] **Contra:**

22

Viral, fungal, or tubercular skin lesions; serious Infxns (except septic shock or tuberculous meningitis) **SE:** Systemic forms: ↑ appetite, insomnia, hyperglycemia, bruising **Notes:** May cause HPA axis suppression

Hydromorphone (Dilaudid) [C–II] Uses: *Moderate/severe pain* **Action:** Narcotic analgesic **Dose:** 1–4 mg PO, IM, IV, or PR q4–6h PRN; 3 mg PR q6–8h PRN; ↓ w/hepatic failure **Caution:** [B (D if prolonged use or high doses near term), ?] ↑ effects w/CNS depressants, phenothiazines, TCA **Contra:** Component sensitivity **Supplied:** Tabs 1, 2, 3, 4, 8 mg; liq 5 mg/mL; inj 1, 2, 4, 10 mg/mL; supp 3 mg **SE:** Sedation, dizziness, GI upset **Notes:** Morphine 10 mg IM = hydromorphone 1.5 mg IM

Hydroxyurea (Hydrea, Droxia) Uses: *CML, head & neck, ovarian & colon CA, melanoma, acute leukemia, sickle cell anemia, polycythemia vera, HIV* **Action:** ↓ ribonucleotide reductase system **Dose:** (per protocol) 50–75 mg/kg for WBC > 100,000 cells/μL; 20–30 mg/kg in refractory CML. *HIV:* 1000–1500 mg/d in single or ÷ doses; ↓ in renal insuff **Caution:** [D, –] ↑ effects w/zidovudine, zalcitabine, didanosine, stavudine, fluorouracil **Contra:** Severe anemia, BM suppression, WBC < 2500 or plt < 100,000, PRG **Supplied:** Caps 200, 300, 400, 500 mg, tabs 1000 mg **SE:** Myelosuppression (primarily leukopenia), N/V, rashes, facial erythema, radiation recall Rxns & renal dysfunction **Notes:** Open and empty capsules into H_2O

Hydroxyzine (Atarax, Vistaril) Uses: *Anxiety, sedation, itching* **Action:** Antihistamine, antianxiety **Dose:** *Adults. Anxiety or sedation:* 50–100 mg PO or IM qid or PRN (max 600 mg/d). *Itching:* 25–50 mg PO or IM tid–qid. *Peds.* 0.5–1.0 mg/kg/24 h PO or IM q6h; ↓ in hepatic failure **Caution:** [C, +/–] ↑ effects w/CNS depressants, anticholinergics, EtOH **Contra:** Component sensitivity **Supplied:** Tabs 10, 25, 50, 100 mg; caps 25, 50, 100 mg; syrup 10 mg/5 mL; susp 25 mg/5 mL; inj 25, 50 mg/mL **SE:** Drowsiness & anticholinergic effects **Notes:** Useful to potentiate narcotics effects; not for IV/SQ (thrombosis & digital gangrene)

Hyoscyamine (Anaspaz, Cystospaz, Levsin, others) Uses: *Spasm w/GI & bladder disorders* **Action:** Anticholinergic **Dose:** *Adults.* 0.125–0.25 mg (1–2 tabs) SL/PO tid–qid, ac & hs; 1 SR cap q12h **Caution:** [C, +] ↑ effects w/amantadine, antihistamines, antimuscarinics, haloperidol, phenothiazines, TCA, MAOI **Contra:** BOO, GI obstruction, glaucoma, MyG, paralytic ileus, ulcerative colitis, MI **Supplied:** (Cystospaz-M, Levsinex): Time release caps 0.375 mg; elixir (EtOH); soln 0.125 mg/5 mL; inj 0.5 mg/mL; tab 0.125 mg; tab (Cystospaz) 0.15 mg; XR tab (Levbid): 0.375 mg; SL (Levsin SL) 0.125 mg **SE:** Dry skin, xerostomia, constipation, anticholinergic SE, heat prostration w/hot weather **Notes:** Administer tabs before meals/food

Hyoscyamine, Atropine, Scopolamine & Phenobarbital (Donnatal, others) Uses: *Irritable bowel, spastic colitis, peptic ulcer, spastic bladder* **Action:** Anticholinergic, antispasmodic **Dose:** 0.125–0.25 mg (1–2 tabs) tid–qid, 1 cap q12h (SR), 5–10 mL elixir tid–qid or q8h **Caution:** [D, M] **Contra:** NAG **Supplied:** Many combos/manufacturers; *Cap* (Donnatal, others): Hyosc 0.1037 mg/atropine 0.0194 mg/scop 0.0065 mg/phenobarbital 16.2 mg. *Tabs* (Donnatal, others): Hyosc 0.1037 mg/atropine 0.0194 mg/scop 0.0065 mg/phenobarbital 16.2 mg. *Long-acting* (Donnatal): Hyosc 0.311 mg/atropine 0.0582 mg/scop 0.0195 mg/phenobarbital 48.6 mg. *Elixirs* (Donnatal, others): Hyosc 0.1037 mg/atropine 0.0194 mg/scop 0.0065 mg/phenobarbital 16.2 mg/5 mL **SE:** Sedation, xerostomia, constipation

Ibandronate (Boniva) **Uses:** Rx & prevent osteoporosis in postmenopausal women **Action:** Bisphosphonate, ↓ osteoclast-mediated bone resorption **Dose:** 2.5 mg PO qd or 150 mg once/mo on same day (do not lie down for 60 min after) **Caution:** [C, ?/–] avoid w/CrCl < 30 mL/min **Contra:** Uncorrected ↓ Ca^{2+}; inability to stand/sit upright for 60 min **Supplied:** Tabs 2.5, 150 mg **SE:** N/D, HA, dizziness, asthenia, HTN, Infxn, dysphagia, esophagitis, esophageal/gastric ulcer, musculoskeletal pain, jaw osteonecrosis (avoid extensive dental procedures) **Notes:** Take 1st thing in AM w/H_2O (6–8 oz) > 60 min before 1st food/beverage & any meds containing multivalent cations; adequate Ca^{2+} & vit D supls necessary

Ibuprofen (Motrin, Rufen, Advil, others) [OTC] **Warning:** May ↑ risk of cardiovascular events & GI bleeding **Uses:** *Arthritis, pain, fever* **Action:** NSAID **Dose:** *Adults.* 200–800 mg PO bid–qid (max 2.4 g/d) *Peds.* 30–40 mg/kg/d in 3–4 ÷ doses (max 40 mg/kg/d); w/food **Caution:** [B, +] **Contra:** 3rd tri PRG, severe hepatic impair, allergy & use w/other NSAIDs, UGI bleed, ulcers **Supplied:** Tabs 100, 200, 400, 600, 800 mg; chew tabs 50, 100 mg; caps 200 mg; susp 100 mg/2.5 mL, 100 mg/5 mL, 40 mg/mL (200 mg is OTC preparation) **SE:** Dizziness, peptic ulcer, plt inhibition, worsening of renal insuff

Ibutilide (Corvert) **Uses:** *Rapid conversion of AF/flutter* **Action:** Class III antiarrhythmic **Dose:** 0.01 mg/kg (max 1 mg) IV inf over 10 min; may repeat once; w/ECG monitoring **Caution:** [C, –] Do not use w/class I or III antiarrhythmics or w/in 4 h of ibutilide **Contra:** QTc > 440 ms **Supplied:** Inj 0.1 mg/mL **SE:** Arrhythmias, HA

Idarubicin (Idamycin) **Uses:** *Acute leukemia* (AML, ALL, ANLL), *CML in blast crisis, breast CA* **Action:** DNA intercalating agent; ↓ DNA topoisomerases I & II **Dose:** (per protocol) 10–12 mg/m²/d for 3–4 d; ↓ in renal/hepatic impairment **Caution:** [D, –] **Contra:** Bilirubin > 5 mg/dL, PRG **Supplied:** Inj 1 mg/mL (5-, 10-, 20-mg vials) **SE:** Myelosuppression, cardiotox, N/V, mucositis, alopecia & IV site Rxns, rare changes in renal/hepatic Fxn **Notes:** Avoid extravasation, potent vesicant; only given IV

Ifosfamide (Ifex, Holoxan) **Uses:** Lung, breast, pancreatic & gastric CA, HL/NHL, soft-tissue sarcoma **Action:** Alkylating agent **Dose:** (per protocol) 1.2 g/m²/d for 5 d bolus or cont inf; 2.4 g/m²/d for 3 d; w/mesna uroprotection; ↓ in renal/hepatic impair **Caution:** [D, M] ↑ effect w/phenobarbital, carbamazepine, phenytoin; St. John's wort may ↓ levels **Contra:** ↓ BM Fxn, PRG **Supplied:** Inj 1, 3 g **SE:** Hemorrhagic cystitis, nephrotox, N/V, mild–moderate leukopenia, lethargy & confusion, alopecia & ↑ hepatic enzyme **Notes:** Administer w/mesna to prevent hemorrhagic cystitis

Iloprost (Ventavis) **WARNING:** Associated with syncope; may require dosage adjustment **Uses:** *NYHA Class III/IV pulmonary arterial HTN* **Action:** Prostaglandin analogue **Dose:** Initial 2.5 mcg; if tolerated, ↑ to 5 mcg inhal 6–9 ×/d (at least 2 h apart) while awake **Caution:** [C, ?/–] Antiplatelet effects, ↑ bleeding risk w/anticoagulants; additive hypotensive effects **Contra:** SBP < 85 mm Hg **Supplied:** Inhal soln 10 mcg/mL **SE:** Syncope, ↓ BP, vasodilation, cough, HA, trismus **Notes:** Requires Pro-Dose AAD nebulizer; counsel on syncope risk

Imatinib (Gleevec) **Uses:** *Rx of CML, blast crisis, GI stromal tumors (GIST)* **Action:** ↓ Bcl-Abl tyrosine kinase (signal transduction) **Dose:** *Chronic*

22

phase CML: 400–600 mg PO qd. *Accelerated/blast crisis:* 600–800 mg PO qd. *GIST:* 400–600 mg PO qd **Caution:** [D, ?/–] w/CYP3A4 meds, (page 647), warfarin **Contra:** Component sensitivity **Supplied:** Caps 100 mg **SE:** GI upset, fluid retention, muscle cramps, musculoskeletal pain, arthralgia, rash, HA, neutropenia, thrombocytopenia **Notes:** Follow CBCs & LFTs baseline & monthly; w/large glass of H_2O & food to ↓ GI irritation

Imipenem–Cilastatin (Primaxin) Uses: *Serious Infxns* due to susceptible bacteria **Action:** Bactericidal; ↓ cell wall synthesis. *Spectrum:* Gram(+) (not *S. aureus,* group A & B streptococci), gram(–) (not *Legionella*), anaerobes **Dose:** *Adults.* 250–1000 mg (imipenem) IV q6–8h *Peds.* 60–100 mg/kg/24 h IV ÷ q6h; ↓ if CrCl is < 70 mL/min **Caution:** [C, +/–] Probenecid ↑ tox **Contra:** Ped pts w/CNS Infxn (↑ Sz risk) & < 30 kg w/renal impair **Supplied:** Inj (imipenem/cilastatin) 250/250 mg, 500/500 mg **SE:** Szs if drug accumulates, GI upset, thrombocytopenia

Imipramine (Tofranil) Uses: *Depression, enuresis,* panic attack, chronic pain **Action:** TCA; ↑ CNS synaptic serotonin or norepinephrine **Dose:** *Adults.* Hospitalized: Initial 100 mg/24 h PO in ÷ doses; ↑ over several wk 300 mg/d max. *Outpatient:* Maint 50–150 mg PO hs, 300 mg/24 h max. *Peds. Antidepressant:* 1.5–5 mg/kg/24 h ÷ qd–qid. *Enuresis:* > 6 y: 10–25 mg PO qhs; ↑ by 10–25 mg at 1–2–wk intervals (max 50 mg for 6–12 y, 75 mg for > 12 y); treat for 2–3 mo, then taper **Caution:** [D, ?/–] **Contra:** Use with MAOIs, NAG, acute recovery from MI, PRG, CHF, angina, CVD, arrhythmias **Supplied:** Tabs 10, 25, 50 mg; caps 75, 100, 125, 150 mg **SE:** CV Sxs, dizziness, xerostomia, discolored urine **Notes:** Less sedation than amitriptyline

Imiquimod Cream, 5% (Aldara) Uses: *Anogenital warts, HPV, condylomata acuminata* **Action:** Unknown; ? cytokine induction **Dose:** Apply 3×/wk, leave on 6–10 h & wash off w/soap & water, continue 16 wk max **Caution:** [B, ?] **Contra:** Component sensitivity **Supplied:** Single-dose packets 5% (250 mg cream) **SE:** Local skin reactions **Notes:** Not a cure; may weaken condoms/vaginal diaphragms, wash hands before & after use

Immune Globulin, IV (Gamimune N, Sandoglobulin, Gammar IV) Uses: *IgG Ab deficiency Dz states, (eg, congenital agammaglobulinemia, CVH & BMT), HIV, hepatitis A prophylaxis, ITP* **Action:** IgG supl **Dose:** *Adults & Peds. Immunodeficiency:* 100–200 mg/kg/mo IV at 0.01–0.04 mL/kg/min to 400 mg/kg/dose max. *ITP:* 400 mg/kg/dose IV qd × 5 d. *BMT:* 500 mg/kg/wk; ↓ in renal insuff **Caution:** [C, ?] Separate administration of live vaccines by 3 mo **Contra:** IgA deficiency w/Abs to IgA, severe thrombocytopenia or coagulation disorders **Supplied:** Inj **SE:** Associated mostly w/inf rate; GI upset

Inamrinone [Amrinone] (Inocor) Uses: *Acute CHF, ischemic cardiomyopathy* **Action:** Inotrope w/vasodilator **Dose:** IV bolus 0.75 mg/kg over 2–3 min; maint 5–10 mcg/kg/min, 10 mg/kg/d max; ↓ if ClCr < 10 mL/min **Caution:** [C, ?] **Contra:** Bisulfite allergy **Supplied:** Inj 5 mg/mL **SE:** Monitor fluid, electrolyte & renal changes **Notes:** Incompatible w/dextrose solns

Indapamide (Lozol) Uses: *HTN, edema, CHF* **Action:** Thiazide diuretic; ↑ Na, Cl & H_2O excretion in proximal segment of distal tubule **Dose:** 1.25–5 mg/d PO **Caution:** [D, ?] ↑ effect w/loop diuretics, ACE inhibitors, cyclosporine, digoxin, Li **Contra:** Anuria, thiazide/sulfonamide allergy, renal insuff, PRG **Supplied:** Tabs 1.25, 2.5 mg **SE:** ↓ BP, dizziness, photosensitivity

Notes: No additional effects w/doses > 5 mg; take early to avoid nocturia; use sunscreen; OK w/food/milk

Indinavir (Crixivan) **Uses:** *HIV Infxn* **Action:** Protease inhibitor; ↓ maturation of immature noninfectious virions to mature infectious virus **Dose:** 800 mg PO q8h; in combo w/other antiretrovirals; on empty stomach; ↓ in hepatic impair **Caution:** [C, ?] Numerous drug interactions **Contra:** w/triazolam, midazolam, pimozide, ergot alkaloids, simvastatin, lovastatin, sildenafil, St. John's wort **Supplied:** Caps 100, 200, 333, 400 mg **SE:** Nephrolithiasis, dyslipidemia, lipodystrophy, GI effects **Notes:** Drink six 8-oz glasses of H_2O/d

Indomethacin (Indocin) WARNING: May ↑ risk of cardiovascular events & GI bleeding **Uses:** *Arthritis; close ductus arteriosus; ankylosing spondylitis* **Action:** ↓ prostaglandins **Dose:** *Adults.* 25–50 mg PO bid–tid, max 200 mg/d. *Infants:* 0.2–0.25 mg/kg/dose IV; may repeat in 12–24 h up to 3 doses; w/food **Caution:** [B, +] **Contra:** ASA/NSAID sensitivity, peptic ulcer/ active GI bleed, precipitation of asthma/urticaria/rhinitis by NSAIDs/aspirin, premature neonates w/NEC, ↓ renal Fxn, active bleeding, thrombocytopenia, 3rd tri PRG **Supplied:** Inj 1 mg/vial; caps 25, 50 mg; SR caps 75 mg; susp 25 mg/5 mL **SE:** GI bleeding or upset, dizziness, edema **Notes:** Monitor renal Fxn

Infliximab (Remicade) WARNING: TB, invasive fungal Infxns & other opportunistic Infxns reported, some fatal; perform TB skin testing before therapy **Uses:** *Moderate–severe Crohn Dz; fistulizing Crohn Dz; ulcerative colitis; RA (w/MTX)* **Action:** IgG1K neutralizes TNFα **Dose:** *Crohn Dz: Induction:* 5 mg/kg IV inf, w/doses 2 & 6 wk after. *Maint:* 5 mg/kg IV inf q8wk. *RA:* 3 mg/ kg IV inf at 0, 2, 6 wk, then q8wk **Caution:** [B, ?/–] Active Infxn, hepatic impairment **Contra:** Murine allergy, moderate–severe CHF **Supplied:** Inj **SE:** Allergic Rxns; pts predisposed to Infxn (especially TB); HA, fatigue, GI upset, inf Rxns; hepatotoxicity; reactivation hepatitis B, pneumonia, BM suppression, systemic vasculitis, pericardial effusion **Notes:** monitor LFTs

Influenza Vaccine (Fluzone, FluShield, Fluvirin) **Uses:** *Prevent influenza* in all adults > 50 y, children 6–23 mo, pregnant women (2nd/3rd tri during flu season), nursing home residents, chronic Dzs, health care workers, household contacts of high-risk pts, children < 9 y receiving vaccine for the first time **Action:** Active immunization **Dose:** *Adults.* 0.5 mL/dose IM. *Peds.* ≥ 3 y: 0.5 mL IM; 6–35 mo 0.25 mL IM. *6 mo to < 9 y* (first-time vaccination): 2 doses > 4 wk apart, 2nd dose before Dec if possible **Caution:** [C, +] **Contra:** Egg, gentamicin, or thimerosal allergy, Infxn at site, high risk of influenza complications, Hx of Guillain–Barré, asthma, children 5–17 y on aspirin **Supplied:** Based on specific manufacturer, 0.25- & 0.5-mL prefilled syringes **SE:** Inj site soreness, fever, myalgia, malaise, Guillain–Barré syndrome (controversial) **Notes:** Optimal in US: Oct–Nov, protection begins 1–2 wk after, lasts up to 6 mo; each year, vaccines based on predictions of flu active in flu season (Dec–Spring in US); whole or split virus for adults; Peds < 13 y split virus or purified surface antigen to ↓ febrile Rxns

Influenza Virus Vaccine Live, Intranasal (FluMist) **Uses:** *Prevent influenza* **Action:** Live-attenuated vaccine **Dose:** *Adults 9–49 y.* 1 dose (0.5 mL)/season **Caution:** [C,?/–] **Contra:** Egg allergy, PRG, Hx Guillain–Barré syndrome, known/suspected immune deficiency, asthma or reactive airway Dz **Supplied:** Prefilled, single-use, intranasal sprayer **SE:** Runny nose, nasal congestion, HA, cough **Notes:** 0.25 mL into each nostril; do not administer concur-

22

rently w/other vaccines; avoid contact w/immunocompromised individuals for 21 d

Insulin Uses: *Type 1 or type 2 DM refractory to diet or PO hypoglycemic agents; acute life-threatening ↑ K⁺* Action: Insulin supl **Dose:** Based on serum glucose; usually SQ; can give IV (only regular)/IM; type 1 typical start dose 0.5–1 Units/kg/d; type 2 0.3–0.4 Units/kg/d; renal failure may ↓ insulin needs **Caution:** [B, +] **Contra:** Hypoglycemia **Supplied:** Table 22–6 (page 637) **SE:** Highly purified insulins ↑ free insulin; monitor for several wk when changing doses/agents

Interferon Alfa (Roferon-A, Intron A) Uses: *Hairy cell leukemia, Kaposi sarcoma, melanoma, CML, chronic hepatitis C, follicular NHL, condylomata acuminata,* multiple myeloma, kidney & bladder CA **Action:** Antiproliferative; modulates host immune response **Dose:** Per protocols. *Adults. Hairy cell leukemia:* Alfa-2a (Roferon-A): 3 M units/d for 16–24 wk SQ/IM. Alfa-2b (Intron A): 2 M units/m² IM/ SQ 3×/wk for 2–6 mo *Peds. CML:* Alfa-2a (Roferon-A): 2.5–5 M units/m² IM qd. *Chronic hepatitis B:* Alfa-2b (Intron A): 3–10 M units/m² SQ 3 ×/wk **Contra:** Benzyl alcohol sensitivity, decompensated liver Dz, autoimmune Dz, rapidly progressing AIDS-related Kaposi sarcoma **Supplied:** Injectable forms **SE:** Flu-like Sxs; fatigue; anorexia in 20–30%; neurotox at high doses; neutralizing Ab (up to 40%) if on prolonged systemic therapy

Interferon Alfa-2b & Ribavirin Combo (Rebetron) WARNING: Contraindicated for PRG women & their male partners Uses: *Chronic hepatitis C in pts w/compensated liver Dz who relapse after α-interferon therapy* **Action:** Combo antiviral agents **Dose:** 3 M units Intron A SQ 3 × wk w/1000–1200 mg of Rebetron PO ÷ bid dose for 24 wk. *Pts < 75 kg:* 1000 mg of Rebetron/d **Caution:** [X, ?] **Contra:** PRG, men w/PRG partner, autoimmune hepatitis, creatinine clearance < 50 mL/min **Supplied:** *Pts < 75 kg:* Combo packs: 6 vials Intron A (3 M Units/0.5 mL) w/6 syringes & EtOH swabs, 70 Rebetron caps; one 18 M Unit multidose vial of Intron A inj (22.8 M units/3.8 mL; 3 M units/0.5 mL) & 6 syringes & swabs, 70 Rebetron caps; one 18 M units Intron A inj multidose pen (22.5 M units/1.5 mL; 3 M units/0.2 mL) w/6 needles & swabs, 70 Rebetron caps. *Pts < 75 kg:* Identical except 84 Rebetron caps/pack **SE:** Flu-like syndrome, HA, anemia **Notes:** Monthly PRG test; instruct in self-administration of SQ Intron A

Interferon Alfacon-1 (Infergen) Uses: *Chronic hepatitis C* **Action:** Biologic response modifier **Dose:** 9 mcg SQ 3×/wk × 24 wk **Caution:** [C, M] **Contra:** *E. coli* product allergy **Supplied:** Inj 9, 15 mcg **SE:** Flu-like syndrome, depression, blood dyscrasias **Notes:** Allow > 48 h between inj

Interferon β-1b (Betaseron) Uses: *MS, relapsing-remitting & secondary progressive* **Action:** Biologic response modifier **Dose:** 0.25 mg SQ qod **Caution:** [C, ?] **Contra:** Human albumin allergy **Supplied:** Powder for inj 0.3 mg **SE:** Flu-like syndrome, depression, blood dyscrasias **Notes:** Monitor LFTs

Interferon γ-1b (Actimmune) Uses: *↓ Incidence of serious Infxns in chronic granulomatous Dz (CGD), osteopetrosis* **Action:** Biologic response modifier **Dose:** *Adults.* CGD: 50 mcg/m² SQ (1.5 million units/m²) BSA > 0.5 m²; if BSA < 0.5 m², give 1.5 mcg/kg/dose; given 3×/wk. *Peds.* BSA ≤ 0.5 m²: 1.5 mcg/kg/ SQ tid; BSA > 0.5 m²: 50 mcg/m² SQ tid **Caution:** [C, ?] **Contra:** Allergy to *E. coli*–derived products **Supplied:** Inj 100 mcg (2 million units) **SE:** Flu-like syndrome, depression, blood dyscrasias

22

Ipecac Syrup [OTC] Uses: *Drug OD, certain cases of poisoning* **Action:** Irritation of the GI mucosa; stimulation of the chemoreceptor trigger zone **Dose:** *Adults.* 15–30 mL PO, followed by 200–300 mL of H_2O; if no emesis in 20 min, repeat once. *Peds.* 6–12 y: 5–10 mL PO, followed by 10–20 mL/kg of H_2O; if no emesis in 20 min, repeat once. *1–12 y:* 15 mL PO followed by 10–20 mL/kg of H_2O; if no emesis in 20 min, repeat once **Caution:** [C, ?] **Contra:** Ingestion of petroleum distillates, strong acid, base, or other caustic agents; comatose/unconscious **Supplied:** Syrup 15, 30 mL (OTC) **SE:** Lethargy, D, cardiotox, protracted vomiting **Notes:** Usage is falling out of favor & is no longer recommended by some groups. Caution in CNS depressant OD; activated charcoal more effective (www.clintox.org/Pos_Statements/Ipecac.html)

Ipratropium (Atrovent) Uses: *Bronchospasm w/COPD, rhinitis, rhinorrhea* **Action:** Synthetic anticholinergic similar to atropine **Dose:** *Adults & Peds > 12 y.* 2–4 puffs qid. *Nasal:* 2 sprays/nostril bid–tid **Caution:** [B, +/–] **Contra:** Allergy to soya lecithin/related foods **Supplied:** Met-dose inhaler 18 mcg/dose; inhal soln 0.02%; nasal spray 0.03%, 0.06%; nasal inhaler 20 mcg/dose **SE:** Nervousness, dizziness, HA, cough, bitter taste, nasal dryness **Notes:** Not for acute bronchospasm

Irbesartan (Avapro) Uses: *HTN*, DN, CHF **Action:** Angiotensin II receptor antagonist **Dose:** 150 mg/d PO, may ↑ to 300 mg/d **Caution:** [C (1st tri; D 2nd/3rd), ?/–] **Supplied:** Tabs 75, 150, 300 mg **SE:** Fatigue, ↓ BP

Irinotecan (Camptosar) Uses: *Colorectal* & lung CA **Action:** Topoisomerase I inhibitor; ↓ DNA synthesis **Dose:** Per protocol; 125–350 mg/m^2 qwk–q3wk (↓ hepatic dysfunction, as tolerated per tox) **Caution:** [D, –] **Contra:** Allergy to component **Supplied:** Inj 20 mg/mL **SE:** Myelosuppression, N/V/D, abdominal cramping, alopecia; D is dose-limiting; Rx acute D w/atropine; Rx subacute D w/loperamide **Notes:** D correlated to levels of metabolite SN-38

Iron Dextran (Dexferrum, INFeD) Uses: *Fe deficiency when cannot supplement PO* **Action:** Fe supl **Dose:** Estimate Fe deficiency, give IM/IV. A 0.5-mL test dose; total replacement dose (mL) = 0.0476 × weight (kg) × [desired Hgb (g/dL) – measured Hgb (g/dL)] + 1 mL/5 kg weight (max 14 mL). *Adults.* Max daily dose: 100 mg Fe. *Peds.* Max daily dose: < *5 kg:* 25 mg Fe. *5–10 kg:* 50 mg Fe. *10–50 kg:* 100 mg Fe **Caution:** [C, M] **Contra:** Anemia w/o Fe deficiency. **Supplied:** Inj 50 mg (Fe)/mL **SE:** Anaphylaxis, flushing, dizziness, inj site & inf Rxns, metallic taste **Notes:** Give deep IM using "Z-track" technique; IV preferred

Iron Sucrose (Venofer) Uses: *Fe deficiency anemia w/chronic HD in those receiving erythropoietin* **Action:** Fe replacement. **Dose:** 5 mL (100 mg) IV on dialysis, 1 mL (20 mg)/min max **Caution:** [C, M] **Contra:** Anemia w/o Fe deficiency **Supplied:** 20 mg elemental Fe/mL, 5-mL vials. **SE:** Anaphylaxis, ↓ BP, cramps, N/V/D, HA **Notes:** Most pts require cumulative doses of 1000 mg; must give at slow rate

Isoniazid (INH) Uses: *Rx & prophylaxis of TB* **Action:** Bactericidal; interferes w/mycolic acid synthesis, disrupts cell wall **Dose:** *Adults.* Active TB: 5 mg/kg/24 h PO or IM (usually 300 mg/d). *Prophylaxis:* 300 mg/d PO for 6–12 mo. *Peds.* Active TB: 10–20 mg/kg/24 h PO or IM 300 mg/d max. *Prophylaxis:* 10 mg/kg/24 h PO; ↓ in hepatic/renal dysfunction **Caution:** [C, +] Liver Dz, dialysis; avoid EtOH **Contra:** Acute liver Dz, Hx INH hepatitis **Supplied:** Tabs 100, 300 mg; syrup 50 mg/5 mL; inj 100 mg/mL **SE:** Hepatitis, peripheral neuropathy, GI upset, anorexia,

22

dizziness, skin Rxn **Notes:** Use w/2–3 other drugs for active TB, based on INH resistance patterns when TB acquired & sensitivity results; prophylaxis usually w/ INH alone. IM rarely used. ↓ peripheral neuropathy w/pyridoxine 50–100 mg/d. Check CDC guidelines (MMWR) for most current recommendations

Isoproterenol (Isuprel) **Uses:** *Shock, bronchospasm, cardiac arrest, AV nodal block* **Action:** β_1- & β_2-receptor stimulant **Dose:** *Adults.* 2–10 mcg/min IV inf; titrate. *Inhal:* 1–2 inhal 4–6 × /d. *Peds.* 0.2–2 mcg/kg/min IV inf; titrate. *Inhal:* 1–2 inhal 4–6×/d **Caution:** [C, ?] **Contra:** Angina, tachyarrhythmias (digitalis-induced or others) **Supplied:** Met-inhaler; soln for neb 0.5%, 1%; inj 0.02 mg/mL, 0.2 mg/mL **SE:** Insomnia, arrhythmias, HA, trembling, dizziness **Notes:** Pulse > 130 beats/min may induce arrhythmias

Isosorbide Dinitrate (Isordil, Sorbitrate, Dilatrate-SR) **Uses:** *Rx & prevent angina,* CHF (w/hydralazine) **Action:** Relaxes vascular smooth muscle **Dose:** *Acute angina:* 5–10 mg PO (chew tabs) q2–3h or 2.5–10 mg SL PRN q5–10 min; do not give > 3 doses in a 15–30-min period. *Angina prophylaxis:* 5–40 mg PO q6h; do not give nitrates on a chronic q6h or qid basis > 7–10 d; tolerance may develop; provide 10–12–h drug-free intervals **Caution:** [C, ?] **Contra:** Severe anemia, closed-angle glaucoma, postural ↓ BP, cerebral hemorrhage, head trauma (can ↑ ICP), w/sildenafil, tadalafil, vardenafil **Supplied:** Tabs 5, 10, 20, 30, 40 mg; SR tabs 40 mg; SL tabs 2.5, 5, 10 mg; chew tabs 5, 10 mg; SR caps 40 mg **SE:** HA, ↓ BP, flushing, tachycardia, dizziness **Notes:** Higher PO dose needed for same results as SL forms

Isosorbide Mononitrate (Ismo, Imdur) **Uses:** *Prevention/Rx of angina pectoris* **Action:** Relaxes vascular smooth muscle **Dose:** 20 mg PO bid, w/the 2 doses 7 h apart or XR (Imdur) 30–120 mg/d PO **Caution:** [C, ?] **Contra:** Head trauma/cerebral hemorrhage (can ↑ ICP), w/sildenafil, tadalafil, vardenafil **Supplied:** Tabs 10, 20 mg; XR 30, 60, 120 mg **SE:** HA, dizziness, ↓ BP

Isotretinoin, 13-*cis*-Retinoic Acid (Accutane, Amnesteem, Claravis, Sotret) **WARNING:** Must not be used by PRG women; can induce severe birth defects; pt must be capable of complying w/mandatory contraceptive measures; prescribed according to product-specific risk management system. Because of teratogenicity, Accutane is approved for marketing only under a special restricted distribution FDA program called iPLEDGE **Uses:** *Refractory severe acne* **Action:** Retinoic acid derivative **Dose:** 0.5–2 mg/kg/d PO ÷ bid (↓ in hepatic Dz, take w/food) **Caution:** [X, –] Avoid tetracyclines **Contra:** Retinoid sensitivity, PRG **Supplied:** Caps 10, 20, 40 mg **SE:** Rare: Depression, psychosis, suicidal thoughts; dermatologic sensitivity, xerostomia, photosensitivity, ↑ LFTs, ↑ triglycerides **Notes:** Risk management program requires 2 (–) PRG tests before Rx & use of 2 forms of contraception 1 mo before, during & 1 mo after therapy; to prescribe isotretinoin, the prescriber must access the iPLEDGE system (www.ipledgeprogram.com); monitor LFTs & lipids

Isradipine (DynaCirc) **Uses:** *HTN* **Action:** CCB **Dose:** *Adults.* 2.5–10 mg PO bid. *Peds.* 0.05–0.15 mg/kg PO tid–qid, up to 20 mg/d (do not crush or chew) **Caution:** [C, ?] **Contra:** Severe heart block, sinus bradycardia, CHF, dosing w/in several hours of IV β-blockers **Supplied:** Caps 2.5, 5 mg; tabs CR 5, 10 mg **SE:** HA, edema, flushing, fatigue, dizziness, palpitations

22

Itraconazole (Sporanox) **WARNING:** Potential for negative inotropic effects on the heart; if signs or Sxs of CHF occur during administration, continued use should be assessed **Uses:** *Fungal Infxns (aspergillosis, blastomycosis, histoplasmosis, candidiasis)* **Action:** ↓ ergosterol synthesis **Dose:** 200 mg PO or IV qd–bid (capsule w/meals or cola/grapefruit juice); PO soln on empty stomach; avoid antacids **Caution:** [C, ?] Numerous interactions **Contra:** CrCl < 30 mL/min, Hx of CHF or ventricular dysfunction, w/H$_2$–antagonist, omeprazole **Supplied:** Caps 100 mg; soln 10 mg/mL; inj 10 mg/mL **SE:** N, rash, hepatitis, ↓ K$^+$, CHF (mostly w/IV use) **Notes:** PO soln & caps not interchangeable; useful in pts who cannot take amphotericin B

Kaolin-Pectin (Kaodene, Kao-Spen, Kapectolin) [OTC]

Uses: *Diarrhea* **Action:** Absorbent demulcent **Dose:** *Adults.* 60–120 mL PO after each loose stool or q3–4h PRN. *Peds.* 3–6 y: 15–30 mL/dose PO PRN. *6–12 y:* 30–60 mL/dose PO PRN **Caution:** [C, +] **Contra:** D secondary to pseudomembranous colitis **Supplied:** Multiple OTC forms; also available w/opium (Parepectolin [C-II]) **SE:** Constipation, dehydration

Ketoconazole (Nizoral, Nizoral AD Shampoo) [Shampoo OTC]

Uses: *Systemic fungal Infxns; topical for local fungal Infxns due to dermatophytes & yeast; shampoo for dandruff,* CAP when rapid ↓ testosterone needed (eg, cord compression) **Action:** ↓ fungal cell wall synthesis **Dose:** *Adults.* PO: 200 mg PO qd; ↑ to 400 mg PO qd for serious Infxn; CAP 400 mg PO tid (short-term). *Topical:* Apply qd (cream/shampoo). *Peds > 2 y.* 5–10 mg/kg/24 h PO ÷ q12–24h (↓ in hepatic Dz) **Caution:** [C, +/–] Any agent that ↑ gastric pH prevents absorption; may enhance anticoagulants; w/EtOH (disulfiram-like Rxn) numerous interactions **Contra:** CNS fungal Infxns (poor CNS penetration), w/ astemizole, cisapride, triazolam **Supplied:** Tabs 200 mg; topical cream 2%; shampoo 2% **SE:** N **Notes:** Monitor LFTs w/systemic use

Ketoprofen (Orudis, Oruvail)

WARNING: May ↑ risk of CV events & GI bleeding **Uses:** *Arthritis, pain* **Action:** NSAID; ↓ prostaglandins **Dose:** 25–75 mg PO tid–qid, 300 mg/d/max; w/food **Caution:** [B (D 3rd tri), ?] **Contra:** NSAID/ASA sensitivity **Supplied:** Tabs 12.5 mg; caps 25, 50, 75 mg; caps, SR 100, 150, 200 mg **SE:** GI upset, peptic ulcers, dizziness, edema, rash

Ketorolac (Toradol)

WARNING: Indicated for short-term (≥ 5 d) Rx of moderate–severe acute pain that requires opioid analgesia levels **Uses:** *Pain* **Action:** NSAID; ↓ prostaglandins **Dose:** 15–30 mg IV/IM q6h or 10 mg PO qid; max IV/IM 120 mg/d, max PO 40 mg/d; do not use for > 5 d; ↓ for age & renal dysfunction **Caution:** [B (D 3rd tri), –] **Contra:** Peptic ulcer Dz, NSAID sensitivity, advanced renal Dz, CNS bleeding, anticipated major surgery, labor & delivery, nursing mothers **Supplied:** Tabs 10 mg; inj 15 mg/mL, 30 mg/mL **SE:** Bleeding, peptic ulcer Dz, renal failure, edema, dizziness, allergy **Notes:** PO only as continuation of IM/IV therapy

Ketorolac Ophthalmic (Acular)

Uses: *Ocular itching w/seasonal allergies* **Action:** NSAID **Dose:** 1 gt qid **Caution:** [C, +] **Supplied:** Soln 0.5% **SE:** Local irritation

Ketotifen (Zaditor)

Uses: *Allergic conjunctivitis* **Action:** H$_1$–receptor antagonist, mast cell stabilizer **Dose:** *Adults & Peds.* 1 gt in eye(s) q8–12h **Caution:** [C,?/–] **Supplied:** Soln 0.025%/5 mL **SE:** Local irritation, HA, rhinitis

Labetalol (Trandate, Normodyne)

Uses: *HTN* & hypertensive emergencies **Action:** α- & β-Adrenergic blocking agent **Dose:** *Adults. HTN:* Initial, 100 mg PO bid, then 200–400 mg PO bid. *Hypertensive emergency:* 20–80 mg IV bolus, then 2 mg/min IV inf, titrate. *Peds.* PO: 3–20 mg/kg/d in ÷ doses. *Hypertensive emergency:* 0.4–1.5 mg/kg/h IV cont inf **Caution:** [C (D in 2nd or 3rd tri), +] **Contra:** Asthma/COPD, cardiogenic shock, uncompensated CHF, heart block **Supplied:** Tabs 100, 200, 300 mg; inj 5 mg/mL **SE:** Dizziness, nausea, ↓ BP, fatigue, CV effects

Lactic Acid & Ammonium Hydroxide, Ammonium Lactate (Lac-Hydrin)   Uses: *Severe xerosis & ichthyosis* Action: Emollient moisturizer Dose: Apply bid Caution: [B, ?] Supplied: Lactic acid 12% w/ammonium hydroxide SE: Local irritation

Lactobacillus (Lactinex Granules) [OTC]   Uses: Control of D, especially after antibiotic therapy **Action:** Replaces nl intestinal flora **Dose:** *Adults & Peds > 3 y.* 1 packet, 2 caps, or 4 tabs PO tid–qid (w/meals or liq) **Caution:** [A, +] **Contra:** Milk/lactose allergy **Supplied:** Tabs; caps; EC caps; powder in packets (all OTC) **SE:** Flatulence

Lactulose (Chronulac, Cephulac, Enulose)   Uses: *Hepatic encephalopathy; constipation* **Action:** Acidifies the colon, allows ammonia to diffuse into colon **Dose:** *Acute hepatic encephalopathy:* 30–45 mL PO q1h until soft stools, then tid–qid. *Chronic laxative therapy:* 30–45 mL PO tid–qid; adjust q1–2d to produce 2–3 soft stools/d. *Rectally:* 200 g in 700 mL of H_2O PR. *Peds.* Infants: 2.5–10 mL/24 h ÷ tid–qid. *Children:* 40–90 mL/24 h ÷ tid–qid **Caution:** [B, ?] **Contra:** Galactosemia **Supplied:** Syrup 10 g/15 mL, soln 10 g/15 mL, 10 g/packet **SE:** Severe D, flatulence; life-threatening electrolyte disturbances

Lamivudine (Epivir, Epivir-HBV)   WARNING: Lactic acidosis & severe hepatomegaly w/steatosis reported w/nucleoside analogues **Uses:** *HIV Infxn, chronic hepatitis B* **Action:** ↓ HIV RT & hepatitis B viral polymerase, resulting in viral DNA chain termination **Dose:** *HIV: Adults & Peds > 12 y.* 150 mg PO bid. *Peds < 12 y.* 4 mg/kg PO bid. *HBV: Adults.* 100 mg/d PO. *Peds 2–17 y.* 3 mg/kg/d PO, 100 mg max; ↓ in renal impair **Caution:** [C, ?] **Contra:** Component hypersensitivity **Supplied:** Tabs 100, 150 mg (HBV); soln 5 mg/mL, 10 mg/mL **SE:** HA, pancreatitis, anemia, GI upset, lactic acidosis

Lamotrigine (Lamictal)   WARNING: Serious rashes requiring hospitalization & D/C of Rx reported; rash less frequent in adults **Uses:** *Partial Szs, bipolar disorder, Lennox–Gastaut syndrome* **Action:** Phenyltriazine antiepileptic **Dose:** *Adults.* Szs: Initial 50 mg/d PO, then 50 mg PO bid for 2 wk, maint 300–500 mg/d in 2 ÷ doses. *Bipolar:* Initial 25 mg/d PO, 50 mg PO qd for 2 wk, 100 mg PO qd for 1 wk, maint 200 mg/d. *Peds.* 0.15 mg/kg in 1–2 ÷ doses for wk 1 & 2, then 0.3 mg/kg for wk 3 & 4, maint 1 mg/kg/d in 1–2 ÷ (↓ in hepatic Dz or if w/enzyme inducers or valproic acid) **Caution:** [C, –] Interactions w/ other antiepileptics **Supplied:** Tabs 25, 100, 150, 200 mg; chew tabs 5, 25 mg **SE:** Photosensitivity, HA, GI upset, dizziness, ataxia, rash (potentially life-threatening in children > adults) **Notes:** ? value of therapeutic monitoring

Lansoprazole (Prevacid, Prevacid IV)   Uses: *Duodenal ulcers, prevent & Rx NSAID gastric ulcers, IV alternative for ≤ 7 d/w erosive esophagitis.* H. pylori Infxn, erosive esophagitis & hypersecretory conditions **Action:** Proton pump inhibitor **Dose:** 15–30 mg/d PO; NSAID ulcer prevention 15 mg/d PO ≤ 12 wk, NSAID ulcers 30 mg/d PO, × 8 wk; 30 mg IV qd ≤ 7 d change to PO for 6–8 wk; ↓ in severe hepatic impair **Caution:** [B, ?/–] **Supplied:** Caps 15,

30 mg; inj set w/filter **SE:** HA, fatigue **Notes:** For IV provided in-line filter must be used

Lanthanum Carbonate (Fosrenol) **Uses:** *Hyperphosphatemia in renal disease* **Action:** Phosphate binder **Dose:** 750–1500 mg PO qd ÷ doses, w/or immed after meal; titrate every 2–3 wk based on PO_4^{2-} levels **Caution:** [C, ?/–], no data in GI disease **Supplied:** Chew tabs 250, 500 mg **SE:** N/V, graft occlusion **Notes:** Chew tabs before swallowing; separate from meds that interact with antacids by 2 h

Latanoprost (Xalatan) **Uses:** *Refractory glaucoma* **Action:** Prostaglandin **Dose:** 1 gt eye(s) hs **Caution:** [C, ?] **Supplied:** 0.005% soln **SE:** May darken light irises; blurred vision, ocular stinging & itching

Leflunomide (Arava) **WARNING:** PRG must be excluded before start of Rx **Uses:** *Active RA* **Action:** ↓ Pyrimidine synthesis **Dose:** Initial 100 mg/d PO for 3 d, then 10–20 mg/d **Caution:** [X, –] **Contra:** PRG **Supplied:** Tabs 10, 20, 100 mg **SE:** D, Infxn, HTN, alopecia, rash, nausea, joint pain, hepatitis **Notes:** Monitor LFTs during initial therapy

Lepirudin (Refludan) **Uses:** *HIT* **Action:** Direct thrombin inhibitor **Dose:** Bolus 0.4 mg/kg IV, then 0.15 mg/kg inf (↓ dose & inf rate if CrCl < 60 mL/min) **Caution:** [B, ?/–] Hemorrhagic event or severe HTN **Contra:** Active bleeding **Supplied:** Inj 50 mg **SE:** Bleeding, anemia, hematoma **Notes:** Adjust according to aPTT ratio, maintain aPTT 1.5–2.0

Letrozole (Femara) **Uses:** *Advanced breast CA* **Action:** Nonsteroidal aromatase inhibitor **Dose:** 2.5 mg/d PO **Caution:** [D, ?] **Contra:** PRG **Supplied:** Tabs 2.5 mg **SE:** Anemia, nausea, hot flashes, arthralgia **Notes:** CBC, thyroid Fxn, electrolyte, LFT & renal monitoring

Leucovorin (Wellcovorin) **Uses:** *OD of folic acid antagonist; augment 5-FU impaired MTX elimination* **Action:** Reduced folate source; circumvents action of folate reductase inhibitors (eg, MTX) **Dose:** *Adults & Peds.* MTX rescue: 10 mg/m²/dose IV or PO q6h for 72 h until MTX level < 10–8. *5-FU:* 200 mg/m²/d IV 1–5 d during daily 5-FU Rx or 500 mg/m²/wk w/wkly 5-FU therapy. *Adjunct to antimicrobials:* 5–15 mg/d PO **Caution:** [C, ?/–] **Contra:** Pernicious anemia **Supplied:** Tabs 5, 15, 25 mg; inj **SE:** Allergic Rxn, N/V/D, fatigue **Notes:** Many dosing schedules for leucovorin rescue following MTX therapy; do not administer IT or into ventricle

Leuprolide (Lupron, Lupron Depot, Lupron Depot-Ped, Viadur, Eligard) **Uses:** *Advanced CAP (all products), endometriosis (Lupron), uterine fibroids (Lupron) & CPP (Lupron-Ped)* **Action:** LHRH agonist; paradoxically ↓ release of gonadotropin, resulting in ↓ pituitary gonadotropins (↓ LH); in men ↓ testosterone **Dose:** *Adults.* CAP: Lupron Depot: 7.5 mg IM q28d or 22.5 mg IM q3mo or 30 mg IM q4mo; Eligard: 7.5 mg IM q28d or 22.5 mg IM q3mo or 30 mg IM q4mo 45 mg SQ 6 mo; Viadur implant (CAP only); insert in inner upper arm w/local anesthesia, replace q12mo. *Endometriosis (Lupron Depot):* 3.75 mg IM qmo X6. *Fibroids:* 3.75 mg IM qmo ×3. *Peds.* CPP (Lupron-Ped): 50 mcg/kg/d SQ inj; ↑ by 10 mcg/kg/d until total down-regulation achieved. *Depot:* < 25 kg: 7.5 mg IM q4wk. > 25–37.5 kg: 11.25 mg IM q4wk. > 37.5 kg: 15 mg IM q4wk **Caution:** [X, ?] **Contra:** Undiagnosed vaginal bleeding, implant dosage form in women & peds; PRG **Supplied:** Inj 5 mg/mL; Lupron Depot 3.75 (1 mo for fibroids, endometriosis); Lupron Depot for

22

CAP: 7.5 mg (1 mo), 22.5 (3 mo), 30 mg (4 mo); Eligard depot for CAP: 7.5 mg (1 mo); 45 mg (6 mo); Viadur 12–mo SQ implant, Lupron-Ped 7.5, 11.25, 15 mg **SE:** Hot flashes, gynecomastia, N/V, alopecia, anorexia, dizziness, HA, insomnia, paresthesias, depression exacerbation, peripheral edema & bone pain (transient "flare Rxn" 7–14 d after 1st dose [LH/testosterone surge before suppression]) **Notes:** Nonsteroidal antiandrogen (eg, bicalutamide) can block flare

Levalbuterol (Xopenex) Uses: *Asthma (Rx & prevention of bronchospasm)* **Action:** Sympathomimetic bronchodilator **Dose:** 0.63 mg neb q6–8h **Caution:** [C, ?] **Supplied:** Soln for inhal 0.63, 1.25 mg/3 mL **SE:** Tachycardia, nervousness, trembling, flu syndrome **Notes:** *R*-isomer of albuterol; may ↓ CV SEs compared with albuterol

Levamisole (Ergamisol) Uses: *Adjuvant Rx of Dukes C colon CA (in combo w/5-FU)* **Action:** Immunostimulatory **Dose:** 50 mg PO q8h for 3 d q14d during 5-FU; ↓ in hepatic impair **Caution:** [C, ?/–] **Supplied:** Tabs 50 mg **SE:** N/V/D, abdominal pain, taste disturbance, anorexia, hyperbilirubinemia, disulfiram-like Rxn on EtOH ingestion, minimal BM suppression, fatigue, fever, conjunctivitis

Levetiracetam (Keppra) Uses: *Partial onset Szs* **Action:** Unknown **Dose:** *Adults.* 500 mg PO bid, may ↑ 3000 mg/d max; *Peds. 4–16 y:* 10–20 mg/ kg/d ÷ in 2 doses, 60 mg/kg/d max (↓ in renal insuff) **Caution:** [C, ?/–] **Contra:** Component allergy **Supplied:** Tabs 250, 500, 750 mg **SE:** Dizziness & somnolence; impaired coordination

Levobunolol (A-K Beta, Betagan) Uses: *Glaucoma* **Action:** β-Adrenergic blocker **Dose:** 1–2 gtt/d 0.5% or 1–2 gtt 0.25% bid **Caution:** [C, ?] **Supplied:** Soln 0.25, 0.5% **SE:** Ocular stinging or burning **Notes:** Possible systemic effects if absorbed

Levocabastine (Livostin) Uses: *Allergic seasonal conjunctivitis* **Action:** Antihistamine **Dose:** 1 gt in eye(s) qid ≤ 4 wk **Caution:** [C, +/–] **Supplied:** 0.05% gtt **SE:** Ocular discomfort

Levofloxacin (Levaquin, Quixin & Iquix Ophthalmic) Uses: *Lower resp tract Infxns, sinusitis, UTI; topical for bacterial conjunctivitis, skin Infxns* **Action:** Quinolone antibiotic, ↓ DNA gyrase. *Spectrum:* Excellent gram(+) except MRSA & *E. faecium;* excellent gram(–) except *S. maltophilia* & *Acinetobacter* sp; poor anaerobic **Dose:** 250–500 mg/d PO or IV; community-acquired pneumonia 750 mg/d for 5 d; ophth 1–2 gtt in eye(s) q2h while awake for 2 d, then q4h while awake for 5 d; ↓ in renal impair, avoid antacids if PO **Caution:** [C, –] Interactions w/cation-containing products (eg, antacids) **Contra:** Quinolone sensitivity **Supplied:** Tabs 250, 500 mg; premixed IV 250, 500 mg; Leva-Pak 750 mg × 5 d; ophth soln 0.5% (Quixin), 1.5% (Iquix) **SE:** N/D, dizziness, rash, GI upset, photosensitivity

Levonorgestrel (Plan B) Uses: *Emergency contraceptive ("morning-after pill")*; prevents PRG if taken < 72 h after unprotected sex/contraceptive fails **Action:** Progestin **Dose:** 1 pill q12h × 2 **Caution:** [X, M] **Contra:** Known/suspected PRG, abnormal uterine bleeding **Supplied:** Tab, 0.75 mg, 2 blister pack **SE:** N/V, abdominal pain, fatigue, HA, menstrual changes. **Notes:** Will not induce abortion; ↑ risk of ectopic PRG

Levonorgestrel Implant (Norplant) Uses: *Contraceptive* **Action:** Progestin **Dose:** Implant 6 caps in midforearm **Caution:** [X, +/–] **Contra:** Undiagnosed abnormal uterine bleeding, Hepatic Dz, thromboembolism, Hx of intracranial HTN, breast CA, renal impair **Supplied:** Kits containing 6 implant-able caps, (36 mg each) **SE:** Uterine bleeding, HA, acne, nausea **Notes:** Prevents PRG for up to 5 y; remove if PRG desired

Levorphanol (Levo-Dromoran) [C-II] Uses: *Moderate–severe pain; chronic pain* **Action:** Narcotic analgesic **Dose:** 2 mg PO or SQ PRN q6–8h (↓ in hepatic failure) **Caution:** [B/D (prolonged use/high doses at term), ?] **Contra:** Component allergy **Supplied:** Tabs 2 mg; inj 2 mg/mL **SE:** Tachycardia, ↓ BP, drowsiness, GI upset, constipation, resp depression, pruritus

Levothyroxine (Synthroid, Levoxyl, others) Uses: *Hypothyroidism, myxedema coma* **Action:** Supplement L-thyroxine **Dose:** *Adults.* Initial, 25–50 mcg/d PO or IV; ↑ by 25–50 mcg/d every mo; usual 100–200 mcg/d. *Peds.* 0–1 y: 8–10 mcg/kg/24 h PO or IV. *1–5 y:* 4–6 mcg/kg/24 h PO or IV. *> 5 y:* 3–4 mcg/kg/24 h PO or IV; titrate based on response & thyroid tests; dose can ↑ rapidly in young/middle-aged **Caution:** [A, +] **Contra:** Recent MI, uncorrected adrenal insuff **Supplied:** Tabs 25, 50, 75, 88, 100, 112, 125, 137, 150, 175, 200, 300 mcg; inj 200, 500 mcg **SE:** Insomnia, weight loss, alopecia, arrhythmia **Notes:** Take w/full glass of water (prevents choking)

Lidocaine (Anestacon Topical, Xylocaine, others) Uses: *Local anesthetic; Rx cardiac arrhythmias* **Action:** Anesthetic; class IB antiarrhythmic **Dose:** *Adults.* Antiarrhythmic, ET: 5 mg/kg; follow w/0.5 mg/kg in 10 min if effective. *IV load:* 1 mg/kg/dose bolus over 2–3 min; repeat in 5–10 min; 200–300 mg/h max; cont inf 20–50 mcg/kg/min or 1–4 mg/min. *Peds.* Antiarrhythmic, ET, load: 1 mg/kg; repeat in 10–15 min 5 mg/kg max total, then IV inf 20–50 mcg/kg/min. *Topical:* Apply max 3 mg/kg/dose. *Local inj anesthetic:* Max 4.5 mg/kg (Table 22–3, page 632) **Caution:** [C, +] **Contra:** Do not use lidocaine w/epi on digits, ears, or nose (risk of vasoconstriction & necrosis); heart block **Supplied:** *Inj local:* 0.5, 1, 1.5, 2, 4, 10, 20%. *Inj IV:* 1% (10 mg/mL), 2% (20 mg/mL); admixture 4, 10, 20%. *IV inf:* 0.2%, 0.4%; cream 2%; gel 2, 2.5%; oint 2.5, 5%; liq 2.5%; soln 2, 4%; viscous 2% **SE:** Dizziness, paresthesias & convulsions associated w/tox **Notes:** 2nd line to amiodarone in ECC; dilute ET dose 1–2 mL w/NS; epi may be added for local anesthesia to ↑ effect & ↓ bleeding; for IV forms, ↓ w/liver Dz or CHF; see Table 22–2 (page 628) for levels

Lidocaine/Prilocaine (EMLA, LMX) Uses: *Topical anesthetic*; adjunct to phlebotomy or dermal procedures **Action:** Topical anesthetic **Dose:** *Adults.* EMLA cream, anesthetic disk (1 g/10 cm²): Thick layer 2–2.5 g to intact skin, cover w/occlusive dressing (eg, Tegaderm) for at least 1 h. *Anesthetic disk:* 1 g/10 cm² for at least 1 h. *Peds.* Max dose: < 3 mo or < 5 kg: 1 g/10 cm² for 1 h. *3–12 mo & > 5 kg:* 2 g/20 cm² for 4 h. *1–6 y & > 10 kg:* 10 g/100 cm² for 4 h. *7–12 y & > 20 kg:* 20 g/200 cm² for 4 h **Caution:** [B, +] Methemoglobinemia **Contra:** Do not use on mucous membranes, broken skin, eyes; allergy to amide-type anesthetics **Supplied:** Cream 2.5% lidocaine/2.5% prilocaine; anesthetic disk (1 g) **SE:** Burning, stinging, methemoglobinemia **Notes:** Longer contact time ↑ effect

Lindane (Kwell) [OTC] Uses: *Head lice, crab lice, scabies* **Action:** Ectoparasiticide & ovicide **Dose:** *Adults & Peds. Cream or lotion:* Thin layer after bathing, leave for 8–12 h, pour on laundry. *Shampoo:* Apply 30 mL, develop a lather w/warm water for 4 min, comb out nits **Caution:** [C, +/–] **Contra:** Open wounds, Sz disorder **Supplied:** Lotion 1%; shampoo 1% **SE:**

22

Arrhythmias, Szs, local irritation, GI upset **Notes:** Caution w/overuse (may be absorbed); may repeat Rx in 7 d

Linezolid (Zyvox) **Uses:** *Infxns caused by gram(+) bacteria (including vancomycin-resistant enterococcus [VRE]), pneumonia, skin Infxns* **Action:** Unique, binds ribosomal bacterial RNA; bactericidal for strep, bacteriostatic for enterococci & staph. *Spectrum:* Excellent gram(+) activity including VRE & MRSA **Dose:** *Adults.* 400–600 mg IV or PO q12h. *Peds.* 10 mg/kg IV or PO q8h (q12h in preterm neonates) **Caution:** [C, ?/–] W/ reversible MAOI, avoid foods w/tyramine & cough/cold products w/pseudoephedrine; w/myelosuppression **Supplied:** Inj 2 mg/mL; tabs 400, 600 mg; susp 100 mg/5 mL **SE:** HTN, N/D, HA, insomnia, GI upset, myelosuppression, tongue discoloration **Notes:** Follow weekly CBC

Liothyronine (Cytomel) **Uses:** *Hypothyroidism, goiter, myxedema coma, thyroid suppression therapy* **Action:** T_3 replacement **Dose:** *Adults.* Initial 25 mcg/24 h, titrate q1–2wk to response & TFT; maint of 25–100 mcg/d PO. *Myxedema coma:* 25–50 mcg IV. *Peds.* Initial 5 mcg/24 h, titrate by 5-mcg/24 h increments q1–2–wk; Maint 25–75 mcg/24 h PO qd; ↓ in elderly **Caution:** [A, +] **Contra:** Recent MI, uncorrected adrenal insuff, uncontrolled HTN **Supplied:** Tabs 5, 12.5, 25, 50 mcg; inj 10 mcg/mL **SE:** Alopecia, arrhythmias, CP, HA, sweating **Notes:** Monitor TFT

Lisinopril (Prinivil, Zestril) **Uses:** *HTN, CHF, prevent DN & AMI* **Action:** ACE inhibitor **Dose:** 5–40 mg/24 h PO qd–bid. *AMI:* 5 mg w/in 24 h of MI, then 5 mg after 24 h, 10 mg after 48 h, then 10 mg/d; ↓ in renal insuff **Caution:** [D, –] **Contra:** ACE inhibitor sensitivity **Supplied:** Tabs 2.5, 5, 10, 20, 30, 40 mg **SE:** Dizziness, HA, cough, ↓ BP, angioedema, ↑ K⁺ **Notes:** To prevent DN, start when urinary microalbuminemia begins

Lithium Carbonate (Eskalith, Lithobid, others) **Uses:** *Manic episodes of bipolar Dz* **Action:** Effects shift toward intraneuronal metabolism of catecholamines **Dose:** *Adults. Acute mania:* 600 mg PO tid or 900 mg SR bid. *Maint:* 300 mg PO tid–qid *Peds 6–12 y.* 15–60 mg/kg/d in 3–4 ÷ doses; must titrate; follow serum levels; ↓ in renal insuff, elderly **Caution:** [D, –] Many drug interactions **Contra:** Severe renal impair or CV Dz, lactation **Supplied:** Caps 150, 300, 600 mg; tabs 300 mg; SR tabs 300, 450 mg; syrup 300 mg/5 mL **SE:** Polyuria, polydipsia, nephrogenic DI, tremor; Na retention or diuretic use may ↑ tox; arrhythmias, dizziness **Notes:** See Table 22–2 (page 628) for levels

Lodoxamide (Alomide) **Uses:** *Seasonal allergic conjunctivitis* **Action:** Stabilizes mast cells **Dose:** *Adults & Peds > 2 y.* 1–2 gtt in eye(s) qid ≤ 3 mo **Caution:** [B, ?] **Supplied:** Soln 0.1% **SE:** Ocular burning, stinging, HA

Lomefloxacin (Maxaquin) **Uses:** *UTI, acute exacerbation of chronic bronchitis; prophylaxis in transurethral procedures* **Action:** Quinolone antibiotic; ↓ DNA gyrase. *Spectrum:* Good gram(–) activity including *H. influenzae* except *S. maltophilia, Acinetobacter* sp & some *P. aeruginosa* **Dose:** 400 mg/d PO; ↓ in renal insuff, avoid antacids **Caution:** [C, –] Interactions w/cation-containing products **Contra:** Allergy to other quinolones, peds < 18 y **Supplied:** Tabs 400 mg **SE:** Photosensitivity, Szs, HA, dizziness

Loperamide (Imodium) [OTC] **Uses:** *Diarrhea* **Action:** Slows intestinal motility **Dose:** *Adults.* Initial 4 mg PO, then 2 mg after each loose stool, up to 16 mg/d. *Peds.* 2–5 y, 13–20 kg: 1 mg PO tid. *6–8 y, 20–30 kg:* 2 mg PO bid.

8–12 y, > 30 kg: 2 mg PO tid **Caution:** [B, +] Not for acute diarrhea caused by *Salmonella, Shigella,* or *C. difficile* **Contra:** Pseudomembranous colitis, bloody diarrhea **Supplied:** Caps 2 mg; tabs 2 mg; liq 1 mg/5 mL (OTC) **SE:** Constipation, sedation, dizziness

Lopinavir/Ritonavir (Kaletra) Uses: *HIV Infxn* **Action:** Protease inhibitor **Dose:** *Adults.* 3 caps or 5 mL PO bid. *Peds.* 7–15 kg: 12/3 mg/kg PO bid. *15–40 kg:* 10/2.5 mg/kg PO bid. *> 40 kg:* Adult dose (w/food) **Caution:** [C, ?/–] Numerous interactions **Contra:** W/drugs dependent on CYP3A or CYP2D6 **Supplied:** Caps 133.3 mg/33.3 mg (lopinavir/ritonavir), soln 400 mg/100 mg/5 mL **SE:** Soln has EtOH, avoid disulfiram, metronidazole; GI upset, asthenia, ↑ cholesterol/triglycerides, pancreatitis; protease metabolic syndrome

Loracarbef (Lorabid) Uses: *Upper & lower resp tract, skin, bone, urinary tract, abdomen & gynecologic system bacterial Infxns* **Action:** 2nd-gen cephalosporin; ↓ cell wall synthesis. *Spectrum:* Weaker than 1st-gen against gram(+), enhanced gram(–) **Dose:** *Adults.* 200–400 mg PO bid. *Peds.* 7.5–15 mg/kg/d PO ÷ bid; on empty stomach; ↓ in severe renal insuff **Caution:** [B, +] **Supplied:** Caps 200, 400 mg; susp 125, 250 mg/5 mL **SE:** D

Loratadine (Claritin, Alavert) Uses: *Allergic rhinitis, chronic idiopathic urticaria* **Action:** Nonsedating antihistamine **Dose:** *Adults.* 10 mg/d PO *Peds.* 2–5 y: 5 mg PO qd. *> 6 y:* Adult dose; on empty stomach; ↓ in hepatic insuff **Caution:** [B, +/–] **Contra:** Component allergy **Supplied:** Tabs 10 mg (OTC); rapidly disintegrating Reditabs 10 mg; syrup 1 mg/mL **SE:** HA, somnolence, xerostomia

Lorazepam (Ativan, others) [C-IV] Uses: *Anxiety & anxiety w/depression; preop sedation; control status epilepticus*; EtOH withdrawal; antiemetic **Action:** Benzodiazepine; antianxiety agent **Dose:** *Adults. Anxiety:* 1–10 mg/d PO in 2–3 ÷ doses. *Preop:* 0.05 mg/kg to 4 mg max IM 2 h before surgery. *Insomnia:* 2–4 mg PO hs. *Status epilepticus: 4 mg/dose IV PRN q10–15 min; usual total dose 8 mg. Antiemetic:* 0.5–2 mg IV or PO q4–6h PRN. *EtOH withdrawal:* 2–5 mg IV or 1–2 mg PO initial depending on severity; titrate *Peds. Status epilepticus:* 0.05 mg/kg/dose IV, repeat at 1–20 min intervals × 2 PRN. *Antiemetic, 2–15 y:* 0.05 mg/kg (to 2 mg/dose) pre chemo; ↓ in elderly; do not administer IV > 2 mg/min or 0.05 mg/kg/min **Caution:** [D, ?/–] **Contra:** Severe pain, severe ↓ BP, sleep apnea, NAG, allergy to propylene glycol or benzyl alcohol **Supplied:** Tabs 0.5, 1, 2 mg; soln, PO conc 2 mg/mL; inj 2, 4 mg/mL **SE:** Sedation, ataxia, tachycardia, constipation, resp depression **Notes:** ≤10 min for effect if IV

Losartan (Cozaar) Uses: *HTN,* CHF, DN **Action:** Angiotensin II antagonist **Dose:** 25–50 mg PO qd–bid; ↓ in elderly/hepatic impair **Caution:** [C (1st tri, D 2nd & 3rd tri), ?/–] **Supplied:** Tabs 25, 50, 100 mg **SE:** ↓ BP in pts on diuretics; GI upset, angioedema

Lovastatin (Mevacor, Altocor) Uses: *Hypercholesterolemia* **Action:** HMG-CoA reductase inhibitor **Dose:** 20 mg/d PO w/PM meal; may ↑ at 4-wk intervals to 80 mg/d max; take w/meals **Caution:** [X, –] Avoid w/grapefruit juice, gemfibrozil. **Contra:** Active liver Dz **Supplied:** Tabs 10, 20, 40 mg **SE:** HA & GI intolerance common; promptly report any unexplained muscle pain, tenderness, or weakness (myopathy) **Notes:** Maintain cholesterol-lowering diet; monitor LFT q12wk × 1 y, then q6mo

22

Lutropin Alfa (Luveris) Uses: *Infertility* Action: Recombinant LH Dose: 75 units SC w/75–150 units FSH, 2 separate injs Caution: [X, ?/M] Contra: Primary ovarian failure, uncontrolled thyroid/adrenal dysfunction, intracranial lesion, abnormal uterine bleeding, hormone-dependent GU tumor, ovarian cyst, PRG Supplied: Inj 75 units SE: HA, N, ovarian hyperstimulation syndrome, breast pain, ovarian cysts;↑ risk of multiple births Notes: Rotate inj sites; do not exceed 14 d duration unless signs of imminent follicular development

Lymphocyte Immune Globulin, Antithymocyte Globulin, ATG (Atgam) Uses: *Allograft rejection in transplant pts; aplastic anemia if not candidate for BMT* Action: ↓ circulating T lymphocytes Dose: *Adults.* Prevent rejection: 15 mg/kg/d IV × 14 d, then qod × 7; initial w/in 24 h before/after transplant. *Rx rejection:* Same except use 10–15 mg/kg/d. *Peds.* 5–25 mg/kg/d IV. Caution: [C, ?] Contra: Hx Rxn to other equine γ-globulin preparation, leukopenia, thrombocytopenia Supplied: Inj 50 mg/mL SE: D/C w/severe thrombocytopenia/leukopenia; rash, fever, chills, ↓ BP, HA, ↑ K⁺ Notes: *Test dose:* 0.1 mL 1:1000 dilution in NS

Magaldrate (Riopan, Lowsium) [OTC] Uses: *Hyperacidity associated w/peptic ulcer, gastritis & hiatal hernia* Action: Low-Na antacid Dose: 5–10 mL PO between meals & hs Caution: [B, ?] Contra: Ulcerative colitis, diverticulitis, ileostomy/colostomy, renal insuff (Mg content) Supplied: Susp (OTC) SE: GI upset Notes: < 0.3 mg Na/tab or tsp

Magnesium Citrate (various) [OTC] Uses: *Vigorous bowel preparation*; constipation Action: Cathartic laxative Dose: *Adults.* 120–240 mL PO PRN. *Peds.* 0.5 mL/kg/dose, to 200 mL PO max; w/beverage Caution: [B, +] Contra: Severe renal Dz, heart block, N/V, rectal bleeding Supplied: Effervescent soln (OTC) SE: Abdominal cramps, gas

Magnesium Hydroxide (Milk of Magnesia) [OTC] Uses: *Constipation* Action: NS laxative Dose: *Adults.* 15–30 mL PO PRN. *Peds.* 0.5 mL/kg/dose PO PRN (follow dose w/8 oz of H₂O) Caution: [B, +] Contra: Renal insuff, intestinal obstruction, ileostomy/colostomy Supplied: Tabs 311 mg; liq 400, 800 mg/5 mL (OTC) SE: D, abdominal cramps

Magnesium Oxide (Mag-Ox 400, others) [OTC] Uses: *Replace low Mg levels* Action: Mg supl Dose: 400–800 mg/d ÷ qd–qid w/full glass of H₂O Caution: [B, +] Contra: Ulcerative colitis, diverticulitis, ileostomy/colostomy, heart block, renal insuff Supplied: Caps 140 mg; tabs 400 mg (OTC) SE: D, N

Magnesium Sulfate (various) Uses: *Replacement for low Mg levels; preeclampsia & premature labor*; refractory ↓ K⁺ & ↓ Ca²⁺ Action: Mg supl Dose: *Adults. Supl:* 1–2 g IM or IV; repeat PRN. *Preeclampsia/premature labor:* 4 g load then 1–4 g/h IV inf. *Peds.* 25–50 mg/kg/dose IM or IV q4–6h for 3–4 doses; repeat PRN; ↓ dose w/low urine output or renal insuff Caution: [B, +] Contra: Heart block, renal failure Supplied: Inj 100, 125, 250, 500 mg/mL; PO soln 500 mg/mL; granules 40 mEq/5 g SE: CNS depression, D, flushing, heart block

Mannitol (various) Uses: *Cerebral edema, ↑ intraocular pressure, renal impair, poisonings* Action: Osmotic diuretic Dose: *Diuresis: Adults.* 0.2 g/kg/dose IV over 3–5 min; if no diuresis w/in 2 h, D/C. *Peds.* 0.75 g/kg/dose IV over 3–5 min; if no diuresis w/in 2 h, D/C. *Adults & Peds.* 0.25 g/kg/dose IV push, repeated at 5-min intervals PRN; ↑ slowly to 1 g/kg/dose PRN for ↑ ICP Caution: [C, ?] w/CHF or volume overload **Contra:** Anuria, dehydration, heart failure, PE **Supplied:** Inj 5, 10, 15, 20, 25% **SE:** May exacerbate CHF, N/V/D **Notes:** Monitor for volume depletion

Measles, Mumps, Rubella and Varicella Virus Vaccine Live (Proquad) Uses:
*Simultaneous vaccination against measles, mumps, rubella & varicella in peds 12 mo–12 y or for second dose of MMR * **Action:** Active immunization, live attenuated virus **Dose:** 1 vial IM inj **Caution:** [N/A] Hx of cerebral injury or Szs (febrile reaction) **Contra:** Hx anaphylaxis to neomycin, blood dyscrasia, lymphoma, leukemia, immunosuppressive steroids, febrile illness, untreated TB **Supplied:** Inj **SE:** Fever, inj site Rxn, rash **Notes:** Allow 1 mo between inj & any other measles-containing vaccine

Mechlorethamine (Mustargen)
WARNING: Highly toxic, handle w/ care **Uses:** *Hodgkin Dz & NHL, cutaneous T-cell lymphoma (mycosis fungoides), lung CA, CML, malignant pleural effusions,* & CLL **Action:** Alkylating agent (bifunctional) **Dose:** 0.4 mg/kg single dose or 0.1 mg/kg/d for 4 d; 6 mg/m^2 1–2 ×/mo **Caution:** [D, ?] **Contra:** Known infectious Dz **Supplied:** Inj 10 mg **SE:** Myelosuppression, thrombosis, thrombophlebitis at site; tissue damage w/extravasation (Na thiosulfate used topically to treat); N/V, skin rash, amenorrhea, sterility (especially in men), secondary leukemia if treated for Hodgkin Dz **Notes:** Highly volatile; administer w/in 30–60 min of prep

Meclizine (Antivert) Uses:
Motion sickness; vertigo **Action:** Antiemetic, anticholinergic & antihistaminic properties **Dose:** *Adults & Peds > 12 y.* 25 mg PO tid–qid PRN **Caution:** [B, ?] **Supplied:** Tabs 12.5, 25, 50 mg; chew tabs 25 mg; caps 25, 30 mg (OTC) **SE:** Drowsiness, xerostomia & blurred vision

Medroxyprogesterone (Provera, Depo-Provera)
WARNING: May cause loss of bone density; associated w/duration of use **Uses:** *Contraception; secondary amenorrhea, abnormal uterine bleeding (AUB) caused by hormonal imbalance; endometrial CA* **Action:** Progestin supl **Dose:** *Contraception:* 150 mg IM q3mo or 450 mg IM q6mo. *Secondary amenorrhea: 5–10 mg/d PO for 5–10 d. AUB:* 5–10 mg/d PO for 5–10 d beginning on the 16th or 21st d of menstrual cycle. *Endometrial CA:* 400–1000 mg/wk IM; ↓ in hepatic insuff **Caution:** [X, +] **Contra:** Hx of thromboembolic disorders, hepatic Dz, PRG **Supplied:** Tabs 2.5, 5, 10 mg; depot inj 100, 150, 400 mg/mL **SE:** Breakthrough bleeding, spotting, altered menstrual flow, anorexia, edema, thromboembolic complications, depression, weight gain **Notes:** Perform breast exam & Pap smear before contraceptive therapy; obtain PRG test if last inj > 3 mo

Megestrol Acetate (Megace) Uses:
Breast/endometrial CAs; appetite stimulant in cachexia (CA & HIV) **Action:** Hormone; progesterone analogue **Dose:** *CA:* 40–320 mg/d PO in ÷ doses. *Appetite:* 800 mg/d PO ÷ **Caution:** [X, –] Thromboembolism **Contra:** PRG **Supplied:** Tabs 20, 40 mg; soln 40 mg/mL **SE:** May induce DVT; do not D/C abruptly; edema, menstrual bleeding; photosensitivity, insomnia, rash, myelosuppression

Meloxicam (Mobic)
WARNING: May ↑ risk of CV events & GI bleeding **Uses:** *Osteoarthritis* **Action:** NSAID w/↑ COX-2 activity **Dose:** 7.5–15 mg/d PO; ↓ in renal insuff; take w/food **Caution:** [C, ?/–] Peptic ulcer, NSAID, or ASA sensitivity **Supplied:** Tabs 7.5 mg **SE:** HA, dizziness, GI upset, GI bleeding, edema

22

Melphalan [l-PAM] (Alkeran) WARNING: Severe BM depression, leukemogenic & mutagenic **Uses:** *Multiple myeloma, ovarian CAs,* breast CA, testicular CA, melanoma; allogenic & ABMT (high dose) **Action:** Alkylating agent (bifunctional) **Dose:** (Per protocol) 6 mg/d or 0.25 mg/kg/d for 4–7 d, repeat 4–6-wk intervals, or 1-mg/kg × 1 q4–6wk; 0.15 mg/kg/d for 5 d q6wk. *High-dose high-risk multiple myeloma:* Single dose 140 mg/m². *ABMT:* 140–240 mg/m² IV; ↓ in renal insuff **Caution:** [D, ?] **Contra:** Allergy or resistance **Supplied:** Tabs 2 mg; inj 50, 100 mg **SE:** ↓ BM, secondary leukemia, alopecia, dermatitis, stomatitis & pulmonary fibrosis; rare allergic Rxns **Notes:** Take PO on empty stomach

Memantine (Namenda) **Uses:** Moderate/severe Alzheimer Dz **Action:** *N*-methyl-D-aspartate receptor antagonist **Dose:** Target 20 mg/d, start 5 mg/d, ↑ 5 mg/d to 20 mg/d, wait > 1 wk before ↑ dose; use ÷ doses > 5 mg/d **Caution:** [B, ?/–] Hepatic/mild–moderate renal impair **Supplied:** Tabs 5, 10 mg **SE:** Dizziness **Notes:** Renal clearance ↓ by alkaline urine (↓ 80% @ pH 8)

Meningococcal Polysaccharide Vaccine (Menomune) **Uses:** *Immunize against *N. meningitidis* (meningococcus)*; OK in some complement deficiency, asplenia, lab workers w/exposure; college students by some professional groups **Action:** Live vaccine, active immunization **Dose:** *Adults & Peds > 2 y.* 0.5 mL SQ (not intradermally or IV); keep epi (1:1000) available for anaphylactic/allergic Rxns **Caution:** [C, ?/–] **Contra:** Thimerosal sensitivity **Supplied:** Inj **SE:** Local inj site Rxns, HA **Notes:** Active against meningococcal serotypes A, C, Y & W-135; not group B

Meperidine (Demerol) [C–II] **Uses:** *Moderate–severe pain* **Action:** Narcotic analgesic **Dose:** *Adults.* 50–150 mg PO or IM q3–4h PRN. *Peds.* 1–1.5 mg/kg/dose PO or IM q3–4h PRN, up to 100 mg/dose; ↓ in elderly/renal impair **Caution:** [C/D (prolonged use or high dose at term), +] ↓ Sz threshold **Contra:** Recent/concomitant MAOIs, renal failure **Supplied:** Tabs 50, 100 mg; syrup 50 mg/mL; inj 10, 25, 50, 75, 100 mg/mL **SE:** Resp depression, Szs, sedation, constipation **Notes:** Analgesic effects potentiated w/hydroxyzine; 75 mg IM = 10 mg morphine IM

Meprobamate (Equinil, Miltown) [C–IV] **Uses:** *Short-term relief of anxiety* **Action:** Mild tranquilizer; antianxiety **Dose:** *Adults.* 400 mg PO tid–qid up to 2400 mg/d; SR 400–800 mg PO bid. *Peds 6–12 y.* 100–200 mg bid–tid; SR 200 mg bid; ↓ in renal/liver impair **Caution:** [D, +/–] **Contra:** NAG, porphyria, PRG **Supplied:** Tabs 200, 400, 600 mg; SR caps 200, 400 mg **SE:** May cause drowsiness, syncope, tachycardia, edema

Mercaptopurine, 6-MP (Purinethol) **Uses:** *Acute leukemia,* 2nd-line Rx of CML & NHL, maint ALL in children, immunosuppressant w/autoimmune Dzs (Crohn Dz) **Action:** Antimetabolite, mimics hypoxanthine **Dose:** 80–100 mg/m²/d or 2.5–5 mg/kg/d; maint 1.5–2.5 mg/kg/d; w/allopurinol requires a 67–75% ↓ dose of 6-MP (interference w/xanthine oxidase metabolism); ↓ in renal/hepatic insuff; take on empty stomach **Caution:** [D, ?] **Contra:** Severe hepatic Dz, BM suppression, PRG **Supplied:** Tabs 50 mg **SE:** Mild hematotox; uncommon GI tox, except mucositis, stomatitis & D; rash, fever, eosinophilia, jaundice, hepatitis **Notes:** Handle properly; ensure adequate hydration

22 **Meropenem (Merrem)** **Uses:** *Intraabdominal Infxns, bacterial meningitis* **Action:** Carbapenem; ↓ cell wall synthesis, a β-lactam. *Spectrum:* Excellent gram(+) (except MRSA & *E. faecium*); excellent gram(–) including extended-spectrum β-lactamase producers; good anaerobic **Dose:** *Adults.* 1 g IV q8h. *Peds.* 20–40 mg/kg IV q 8h; ↓ in renal insuff **Caution:** [B, ?] **Contra:** β-Lactam sensitivity **Supplied:** Inj 1 g/30 mL, 500 mg/20 mL **SE:** Less Sz potential than imipenem; D, thrombocytopenia **Notes:** Overuse can ↑ bacterial resistance

Mesalamine (Rowasa, Asacol, Pentasa) **Uses:** *Mild–moderate distal ulcerative colitis, proctosigmoiditis, proctitis* **Action:** Unknown; may inhibit prostaglandins **Dose:** *Retention enema:* qd hs or 1 supp bid. *PO:* 800–1000 mg PO tid–qid; ↓ initial dose in elderly **Caution:** [B, M] **Contra:** Salicylate sensitivity **Supplied:** Tabs 400 mg; caps 250 mg; supp 500 mg; rectal susp 4 g/60 mL **SE:** May discolor urine yellow-brown, HA, malaise, abdominal pain, flatulence, rash, pancreatitis, pericarditis

Mesna (Mesnex) **Uses:** *↓ ifosfamide- & cyclophosphamide-induced hemorrhagic cystitis* **Action:** Antidote **Dose:** 20% of ifosfamide dose (±) or cyclophosphamide dose IV 15 min before & 4 & 8 h after chemo **Caution:** [B; ?/–] **Contra:** Thiol sensitivity **Supplied:** Inj 100 mg/mL; tablets 400 mg **SE:** ↓ BP, allergic Rxns, HA, GI upset, taste perversion **Notes:** Hydration helps ↓ hemorrhagic cystitis

Mesoridazine (Serentil) WARNING: Can prolong QT interval in dose-related manner; torsade de pointes reported **Uses:** *Schizophrenia,* acute & chronic alcoholism, chronic brain syndrome **Action:** Phenothiazine antipsychotic **Dose:** Initial, 25–50 mg PO or IV tid; ↑ to 300–400 mg/d max **Caution:** [C, ?/–] **Contra:** Phenothiazine sensitivity, coadministration w/drugs that cause QTc prolongation, CNS depression **Supplied:** Tabs 10, 25, 50, 100 mg; PO conc 25 mg/mL; inj 25 mg/mL **SE:** Low incidence of EPS; ↓ BP, xerostomia, constipation, skin discoloration, tachycardia, lowered Sz threshold, blood dyscrasias, pigmentary retinopathy at high doses

Metaproterenol (Alupent, Metaprel) **Uses:** *Asthma & reversible bronchospasm* **Action:** Sympathomimetic bronchodilator **Dose:** *Adults.* Inhal: 1–3 inhal q3–4h, 12 inhal max/24 h; wait 2 min between inhal. *PO:* 20 mg q6–8h. *Peds.* Inhal: 0.5 mg/kg/dose, 15 mg/dose max inhaled q4–6h by neb or 1–2 puffs q4-6h. *PO:* 0.3–0.5 mg/kg/dose q6–8h **Caution:** [C, ?/–] **Contra:** Tachycardia, other arrhythmias **Supplied:** Aerosol 0.65 mg/inhal; soln for inhal 0.4, 0.6, 5%; tabs 10, 20 mg; syrup 10 mg/5 mL **SE:** Fewer β_1 effects than isoproterenol & longer acting; nervousness, tremor, tachycardia, HTN

Metaxalone (Skelaxin) **Uses:** *Painful musculoskeletal conditions* **Action:** Centrally acting skeletal muscle relaxant **Dose:** 800 mg PO tid–qid **Caution:** [C, ?/–] anemia **Contra:** Severe hepatic/renal impair **Supplied:** Tabs 400 mg **SE:** N/V, HA, drowsiness, hepatitis

Metformin (Glucophage, Glucophage XR) WARNING: Associated w/lactic acidosis **Uses:** *Type 2 DM* **Action:** ↓ Hepatic glucose production & intestinal absorption of glucose; ↑ insulin sensitivity **Dose:** *Adults.* Initial: 500 mg PO bid; may ↑ to 2550 mg/d max (w/AM & PM meals; can convert total daily dose to qd dose of XR form). *Peds 10–16 y.* 500 mg PO bid, ↑ 500 mg/wk to 2000 mg/d max in ÷ doses; do not use XR formulation in peds **Caution:** [B, +/–] **Contra:** SCr > 1.4 in females or > 1.5 in males; contra in hypoxemic conditions, including acute CHF/sepsis; avoid EtOH; hold dose before & 48 h after ionic contrast **Supplied:** Tabs 500, 850, 1000 mg; XR tabs 500 mg **SE:** Anorexia, N/V, rash, lactic acidosis (rare, but serious)

Methadone (Dolophine) [C-II] Uses: *Severe pain; detox, maint of narcotic addiction* **Action:** Narcotic analgesic **Dose:** *Adults.* 2.5–10 mg IM q3–8h or 5–15 mg PO q8h; titrate as needed *Peds.* 0.7 mg/kg/24 h PO or IM ÷ q8h; ↑ slowly to avoid resp depression; ↓ in renal impair **Caution:** [B/D (prolonged use/high doses at term) + (w/doses = 20 mg/24 h)], severe liver Dz **Supplied:** Tabs 5, 10, 40 mg; PO soln 5, 10 mg/5 mL; PO conc 10 mg/mL; inj 10 mg/mL **SE:** Resp depression, sedation, constipation, urinary retention, ventricular arrhythmias **Notes:** Equianalgesic w/parenteral morphine; longer half-life; prolongs QT interval

Methenamine (Hiprex, Urex, others) Uses: *Suppress/eliminate bacteriuria associated w/chronic/recurrent UTI* **Action:** Converted to formaldehyde & ammonia in acidic urine; nonspecific bactericidal action **Dose:** *Adults.* *Hippurate:* 1 g bid. *Mandelate:* 1 g qid PO pc & hs *Peds 6–12 y. Hippurate:* 25–50 mg/kg/d PO ÷ bid. *Mandelate:* 50–75 mg/kg/d PO ÷ qid (take w/food, ascorbic acid w/adequate hydration) **Caution:** [C, +] **Contra:** Renal insuff, severe hepatic Dz & severe dehydration; sulfonamide allergy **Supplied:** *Methenamine hippurate* (Hiprex, Urex): Tabs 1 g. *Methenamine mandelate:* 500 mg, 1g EC tabs **SE:** Rash, GI upset, dysuria, ↑ LFTs

Methimazole (Tapazole) Uses: *Hyperthyroidism, thyrotoxicosis,* prep for thyroid surgery or radiation **Action:** Blocks T_3 & T_4 formation **Dose:** *Adults. Initial:* 15–60 mg/d PO ÷ tid. *Maint:* 5–15 mg PO qd. *Peds.* Initial: 0.4–0.7 mg/kg/24 h PO ÷ tid. *Maint:* $^1/_3$–$^2/_3$ of initial dose PO qd; w/food **Caution:** [D, +/–] **Contra:** Breast-feeding **Supplied:** Tabs 5, 10 mg **SE:** GI upset, dizziness, blood dyscrasias **Notes:** Follow clinically & w/TFT

Methocarbamol (Robaxin) Uses: *Relief of discomfort associated w/ painful musculoskeletal conditions* **Action:** Centrally acting skeletal muscle relaxant **Dose:** *Adults.* 1.5 g PO qid for 2–3 d, then 1-g PO qid maint therapy; IV form rarely indicated. *Peds.* 15 mg/kg/dose, may repeat PRN (OK for tetanus only) **Caution:** Sz disorders [C, +] **Contra:** MyG, renal impair **Supplied:** Tabs 325, 500, 750 mg; inj 100 mg/mL **SE:** Can discolor urine; drowsiness, GI upset

Methotrexate (Folex, Rheumatrex) Uses: *ALL & AML (including leukemic meningitis), trophoblastic tumors (chorioepithelioma, choriocarcinoma, chorioadenoma destruens, hydatidiform mole), breast, lung, head & neck CAs, Burkitt lymphoma, mycosis fungoides, osteosarcoma, Hodgkin Dz & NHL, psoriasis; RA* **Action:** ↓ Dihydrofolate reductase-mediated gen of tetrahydrofolate **Dose:** *CA:* Per protocol. *RA:* 7.5 mg/wk PO × 1 or 2.5 mg q12h PO for 3 doses/wk; high dose Rx requires leucovorin rescue (↓ hematologic/ mucosal tox); ↓ in renal/hepatic impair **Caution:** [D, –] **Contra:** Severe renal/ hepatic impair, PRG/lactation **Supplied:** Tabs 2.5, 5, 7.5, 10, 15 mg; inj 2.5, 25 mg/mL; preservative-free inj 25 mg/mL **SE:** Myelosuppression, N/V/D, anorexia, mucositis, hepatotox (transient & reversible; may progress to atrophy, necrosis, fibrosis, cirrhosis), rashes, dizziness, malaise, blurred vision, alopecia, photosensitivity, renal failure, pneumonitis; rarely, pulmonary fibrosis; chemical arachnoiditis & HA w/IT delivery **Notes:** Monitor CBC, LFTs, Cr, MTX levels & CXR

Methyldopa (Aldomet) Uses: *HTN* **Action:** Centrally acting antihypertensive **Dose:** *Adults.* 250–500 mg PO bid–tid (max 2–3 g/d) or 250 mg–1 g IV q6–8h. *Peds.* 10 mg/kg/24 h PO in 2–3 ÷ doses (max 40 mg/kg/24 h ÷ q6–12h) or 5–10 mg/kg/dose IV q6–8h to total dose of 20–40 mg/kg/24 h; ↓ in renal

22

insuff/elderly **Caution:** [B (PO), C (IV), +] **Contra:** Liver Dz; MAOIs **Supplied:** Tabs 125, 250, 500 mg; PO susp 50 mg/mL; inj 50 mg/mL **SE:** Discolors urine; initial transient sedation or drowsiness frequent, edema, hemolytic anemia, hepatic disorders

Methylergonovine (Methergine) Uses: *Postpartum bleeding (uterine subinvolution)* **Action:** Ergotamine derivative **Dose:** 0.2 mg IM after placental delivery, may repeat 2–4-h intervals or 0.2–0.4 mg PO q6–12h for 2–7 d **Caution:** [C, ?] **Contra:** HTN, PRG **Supplied:** Injectable forms; tabs 0.2 mg **SE:** HTN, N/V **Notes:** Give IV doses over a period of > 1 min w/BP monitoring

Methylprednisolone (Solu-Medrol) (See Steroids, Table 22–4, page 633)

Metoclopramide (Reglan, Clopra, Octamide) Uses: *Relief of diabetic gastroparesis, symptomatic GERD; chemo-induced N/V, facilitate small-bowel intubation & radiologic evaluation of the upper GI tract,* stimulate gut in prolonged postop ileus **Action:** Stimulates upper GI tract motility; blocks dopamine in chemoreceptor trigger zone **Dose:** *Adults. Diabetic gastroparesis:* 10 mg PO 30 min ac & hs for 2–8 wk PRN, or same dose given IV for 10 d, then PO. *Reflux:* 10–15 mg PO 30 min ac & hs. *Antiemetic:* 1–3 mg/kg/dose IV 30 min before chemo, then q2h × 2 doses, then q3h × 3 doses. *Peds. Reflux:* 0.1 mg/kg/ dose PO qid. *Antiemetic:* 1–2 mg/kg/dose IV as adults **Caution:** [B, –] Drugs w/ extrapyramidal ADRs **Contra:** Sz disorders, GI obstruction **Supplied:** Tabs 5, 10 mg; syrup 5 mg/5 mL; soln 10 mg/mL; inj 5 mg/mL **SE:** Dystonic Rxns common w/high doses, (Rx w/IV diphenhydramine); restlessness, D, drowsiness,

Metolazone (Mykrox, Zaroxolyn) Uses: *Mild–moderate essential HTN & edema of renal Dz or cardiac failure* **Action:** Thiazide-like diuretic; ↓ distal tubule Na reabsorption **Dose:** *HTN:* 2.5–5 mg/d PO. *Edema:* 5–20 mg/d PO. *Peds.* 0.2–0.4 mg/kg/d PO ÷ q12h–qd **Caution:** [D, +] **Contra:** Thiazide/sulfonamide sensitivity, anuria **Supplied:** *Tabs:* Mykrox (rapid acting) 0.5 mg, Zaroxolyn 2.5, 5, 10 mg **SE:** Monitor fluid/electrolytes; dizziness, ↓ BP, tachycardia, CP, photosensitivity **Notes:** Mykrox & Zaroxolyn not bioequivalent

Metoprolol (Lopressor, Toprol XL) WARNING: Do not acutely stop therapy as marked worsening of angina can result Uses: *HTN, angina, AMI, CHF* **Action:** β-Adrenergic receptor blocker **Dose:** *Angina:* 50–100 mg PO bid. *HTN:* 100–450 mg/d PO. *AMI:* 5 mg IV X3 doses, then 50 mg PO q6h × 48 h, then 100 mg PO bid. *CHF:* 12–25 mg/d PO × 2 wk, ↑ at 2–wk intervals to 200 mg/max, use low dose in pts w/greatest severity; ↓ in hepatic failure **Caution:** [C, +] Uncompensated CHF, bradycardia, heart block **Contra:** Arrhythmia w/tachycardia **Supplied:** Tabs 50, 100 mg; ER tabs 50, 100, 200 mg; inj 1 mg/ mL **SE:** Drowsiness, insomnia, ED, bradycardia, bronchospasm

Metronidazole (Flagyl, MetroGel) Uses: *Bone/joint, endocarditis, intra-abdominal, meningitis & skin Infxns; amebiasis; trichomoniasis; bacterial vaginosis* **Action:** Interferes w/DNA synthesis *Spectrum:* Excellent anaerobic *C. difficile,* also *H. pylori* in combo therapy **Dose:** *Adults. Anaerobic Infxns:* 500 mg IV q6–8h. *Amebic dysentery:* 750 mg/d PO for 5–10 d. *Trichomoniasis:* 250 mg PO tid for 7 d or 2 g PO × 1. *C. difficile Infxn:* 500 mg PO or IV q8h for 7– 10 d (PO preferred; IV only if pt NPO). *Vaginosis:* 1 applicatorful intravag bid or 500 mg PO bid for 7 d. *Acne rosacea/skin:* Apply bid. *Peds.* Anaerobic Infxns: 15 mg/kg/24 h PO or IV ÷ q6h. *Amebic dysentery:* 35–50 mg/kg/24 h

22

PO in 3 ÷ doses for 5–10 d; ↓ in hepatic impair **Caution:** [B, M] Avoid EtOH **Contra:** First tri of PRG **Supplied:** Tabs 250, 500 mg; XR tabs 750 mg; caps 375 mg; topical lotion & gel 0.75%; intravag gel 0.75% (5 g/applicator 37.5 mg in 70-g tube), cream 1% **SE:** Disulfiram-like Rxn; dizziness, HA, GI upset, anorexia, urine discoloration **Notes:** For trichomoniasis, Rx pt's partner; no aerobic bacteria activity; use in combo w/serious mixed Infxns

Mexiletine (Mexitil) Uses: *Suppression of symptomatic ventricular arrhythmias*; diabetic neuropathy **Action:** Class IB antiarrhythmic **Dose:** *Adults.* 200–300 mg PO q8h; 1200 mg/d max. *Peds.* 2.5–5 mg/kg PO q8h; drug interactions w/hepatic enzyme inducers & suppressors requiring dosage changes; w/food or antacids **Caution:** [C, +] May worsen severe arrhythmias **Contra:** Cardiogenic shock or 2nd-/3rd-degree AV block w/o pacemaker **Supplied:** Caps 150, 200, 250 mg **SE:** Monitor LFTs; light-headedness, dizziness, anxiety, incoordination, GI upset, ataxia, hepatic damage, blood dyscrasias

Mezlocillin (Mezlin) Uses: *Infxns caused by susceptible gram(–) bacteria (skin, bone, resp tract, urinary tract, abdomen, septicemia) * **Action:** Bactericidal; ↓ cell wall synthesis. *Spectrum:* Gram(–) *Klebsiella, Proteus, E. coli, Enterobacter, P. aeruginosa* & *Serratia* **Dose:** *Adults.* 3 g IV q4–6h. *Peds.* 200–300 mg/kg/d ÷ q4–6h; ↓ in renal/hepatic insuff **Caution:** [B, M] **Contra:** PCN sensitivity **Supplied:** Inj **SE:** GI upset, agranulocytosis, thrombocytopenia **Notes:** Often used w/aminoglycoside

Miconazole (Monistat, others) Uses: *Candidal Infxns, dermatomycoses (various tinea forms)* **Action:** Fungicide; alters fungal membrane permeability **Dose:** Apply to area bid for 2–4 wk. *Intravag:* 1 applicatorful or supp hs for 3 (4% or 200 mg) or 7 d (2% or 100 mg) **Caution:** [C, ?] Azole sensitivity **Supplied:** Topical cream 2%; lotion 2%; powder 2%; spray 2%; vaginal supp 100, 200 mg; vaginal cream 2%, 4% [OTC] **SE:** Vaginal burning, may ↑ warfarin **Notes:** Antagonistic to amphotericin B in vivo

Midazolam (Versed) [C-IV] Uses: *Preop sedation, conscious sedation for short procedures & mechanically ventilated pts, induction of general anesthesia* **Action:** Short-acting benzodiazepine **Dose:** *Adults.* 1–5 mg IV or IM; titrate to effect. *Peds. Preop:* 0.25–1 mg/kg, 20 mg max PO. *Conscious sedation:* 0.08 mg/kg IM × 1. *General anesthesia:* 0.15 mg/kg IV, then 0.05 mg/kg/dose q2min for 1–3 doses PRN to induce anesthesia (↓ in elderly, w/narcotics or CNS depressants) **Caution:** [D, +/–] CYP3A4 substrate, several drug interactions **Contra:** NAG; use of amprenavir, nelfinavir, ritonavir **Supplied:** Inj 1, 5 mg/mL; syrup 2 mg/mL **SE:** Monitor for resp depression; ↓ BP in conscious sedation, nausea **Notes:** Reversal w/flumazenil

Mifepristone, RU 486 (Mifeprex) WARNING: Pt counseling & information required; associated w/fatal infections & bleeding Uses: *Termination of intrauterine PRG of < 49 d* **Action:** Antiprogestin; ↑ prostaglandins, results in uterine contraction **Dose:** Administered w/3 office visits: d 1, three 200-mg tabs PO; d 3 if no abortion, two 200-mg misoprostol PO; on or about d 14, verify termination of PRG **Caution:** [X, –] **Contra:** Anticoagulation therapy, bleeding disorders **Supplied:** Tabs 200 mg **SE:** Abdominal pain & 1–2 wk of uterine bleeding **Notes:** Give under physician's supervision

22 **Miglitol (Glyset)** Uses: *Type 2 DM* **Action:** α-Glucosidase inhibitor; delays digestion of ingested carbohydrates **Dose:** Initial 25 mg PO tid; maint

50–100 mg tid (w/1st bite of each meal) **Caution:** [B, –] **Contra:** Obstructive or inflammatory GI disorders; SCr > 2 **Supplied:** Tabs 25, 50, 100 mg **SE:** Flatulence, D, abdominal pain **Notes:** Use alone or w/sulfonylureas

Milrinone (Primacor) **Uses:** *CHF* **Action:** Positive inotrope & vasodilator; little chronotropic activity **Dose:** 50 mcg/kg, then 0.375–0.75 mcg/kg/min inf; ↓ in renal impair **Caution:** [C, ?] **Contra:** Allergy to drug or amrinone **Supplied:** Inj 1 mcg/mL **SE:** Arrhythmias, ↓ BP, HA **Notes:** Monitor fluid/electrolyte status & BP/HR

Mineral Oil [OTC] **Uses:** *Constipation* **Action:** Emollient laxative **Dose:** *Adults.* 5–45 mL PO PRN. *Peds > 6 y.* 5–20 mL PO bid **Caution:** [C, ?] N/V, difficulty swallowing, bedridden pts **Contra:** Appendicitis, diverticulitis, ulcerative colitis **Supplied:** Liq [OTC] **SE:** Lipid pneumonia, anal incontinence, impaired vitamin absorption

Minoxidil (Loniten, Rogaine) **Uses:** *Severe HTN; male & female pattern baldness* **Action:** Peripheral vasodilator; stimulates vertex hair growth **Dose:** *Adults. PO:* 2.5–10 mg PO bid–qid. *Topical:* Apply bid to affected area. *Peds.* 0.2–1 mg/kg/24 h ÷ PO q12–24h; ↓ PO dose in elderly **Caution:** [C, +] **Contra:** Pheochromocytoma, allergy to components **Supplied:** Tabs 2.5, 5, 10 mg; topical soln (Rogaine) 2% **SE:** Pericardial effusion & volume overload w/ PO use; hypertrichosis w/chronic use, edema, ECG changes, weight gain

Mirtazapine (Remeron) **WARNING:** Closely monitor for worsening depression or emergence of suicidality, particularly in ped pts **Uses:** *Depression* **Action:** Tetracyclic antidepressant **Dose:** 15 mg PO hs, up to 45 mg/d hs **Caution:** [C, ?] **Contra:** MAOIs w/in 14 d **Supplied:** Tabs 15, 30, 45 mg **SE:** Somnolence, ↑ cholesterol, constipation, xerostomia, weight gain, agranulocytosis **Notes:** Do not ↑ dose at intervals of less than 1–2 wk

Misoprostol (Cytotec) **Uses:** *Prevent NSAID-induced gastric ulcers*; induction of labor, incomplete & therapeutic abortion **Action:** Prostaglandin w/ both antisecretory & mucosal protective properties **Dose:** *Ulcer prevention:* 200 mcg PO qid w/meals; in women, start on 2nd or 3rd d of next nl menstrual period; 25–50 mcg for induction of labor (term); 400 mcg on d 3 of mifepristone for PRG termination (take w/food) **Caution:** [X, –] **Contra:** PRG, component allergy **Supplied:** Tabs 100, 200 mcg **SE:** Can cause miscarriage w/potentially dangerous bleeding; HA, GI Sxs common (D, abdominal pain, constipation)

Mitomycin (Mutamycin) **Uses:** *Stomach, pancreas,* breast, colon CA; squamous cell CA of anus; non-small-cell lung, head & neck, cervical; bladder CA (intravesically) **Action:** Alkylating agent; may generate oxygen free radicals w/DNA strand breaks **Dose:** 20 mg/m^2 q6–8wk or 10 mg/m^2 in combo w/other myelosuppressive drugs; bladder CA 20–40 mg in 40 mL NS via a urethral catheter once/wk × 8 wk, followed by monthly treatments for 1 y; ↓ in renal/hepatic impair **Caution:** [D, –] **Contra:** Thrombocytopenia, leukopenia, coagulation disorders, SCr > 1.7 mg/dL **Supplied:** Inj **SE:** Myelosuppression (may persist up to 3–8 wk after dose, may be cumulative; minimize by a lifetime dose < 50–60 mg/m^2), N/V, anorexia, stomatitis & renal tox; microangiopathic hemolytic anemia (similar to HUS) w/progressive renal failure; venoocclusive Dz of the liver, interstitial pneumonia, alopecia (rare); extravasation Rxns; contact dermatitis

Mitoxantrone (Novantrone) **Uses:** *AML (w/cytarabine), ALL, CML, CAP, MS,* breast CA & NHL **Action:** DNA-intercalating agent; ↓ DNA topo-

22

isomerase II **Dose:** Per protocol; ↓ in hepatic impair, leukopenia, thrombocytopenia; maintain hydration **Caution:** [D, –] reports of secondary AML (monitor CBC) **Contra:** PRG **Supplied:** Inj 2 mg/mL **SE:** Myelosuppression, N/V, stomatitis, alopecia (infrequent), cardiotox, urine discoloration; **Notes:** cardiac monitoring before each dose

Modafinil (Provigil) **Uses:** *Improve wakefulness in pts w/narcolepsy & excessive daytime sleepiness* **Action:** May alter dopamine & norepinephrine release, ↓ GABA-mediated neurotransmission **Dose:** 200 mg PO q morning **Caution:** [C, ?/–] in pts w/CV Dz; ↑ effects of warfarin, diazepam, phenytoin; ↓ OCP effects, cyclosporine & theophylline **Contra:** Component allergy **Supplied:** Tablets 100 mg, 200 mg **SE:** HA, N, D, paresthesias, rhinitis, agitation **Notes:** ↓ dose in elderly/hepatic impair by 50%

Moexipril (Univasc) **Uses:** *HTN, post-MI,* DN **Action:** ACE inhibitor **Dose:** 7.5–30 mg in 1–2 ÷ doses 1 h ac **Caution:** [C (1st tri, D 2nd & 3rd tri), ?] **Contra:** ACE inhibitor sensitivity **Supplied:** Tabs 7.5, 15 mg; ↓ in renal impair **SE:** ↓ BP, edema, angioedema, HA, dizziness, cough

Molindone (Moban) **Uses:** *Psychotic disorders* **Action:** Piperazine phenothiazine **Dose:** *Adults.* 50–75 mg/d, ↑ to 225 mg/d if necessary. *Peds.* 3–5 y: 1–2.5 mg/d in 4 ÷ doses. *5–12 y:* 0.5–1.0 mg/kg/d in 4 ÷ doses **Caution:** [C, ?] NAG **Contra:** Drug or EtOH-induced CNS depression **Supplied:** Tabs 5, 10, 25, 50, 100 mg; conc 20 mg/mL **SE:** ↓ BP, tachycardia, arrhythmias, EPS, Szs, constipation, xerostomia, blurred vision

Montelukast (Singulair) **Uses:** *Prophylaxis & Rx of chronic asthma, seasonal allergic rhinitis* **Action:** Leukotriene receptor antagonist **Dose:** *Asthma: Adults & Peds > 15 y.* 10 mg/d PO taken in PM. *Peds.* 2–5 y: 4 mg/d PO taken in PM. *6–14 y:* 5 mg/d PO in PM. *Rhinitis: Adults & Peds > 15 y.* 10 mg qd *Peds.* 2–5 y: 4 mg qd. *6–14 y:* 5 mg qd **Caution:** [B, M] **Contra:** Component allergy **Supplied:** Tabs 10 mg; chew tabs 4, 5 mg **SE:** HA, dizziness, fatigue, rash, GI upset, Churg–Strauss syndrome **Notes:** Not for acute asthma

Morphine (Avinza XR, Duramorph, Infumorph, MS Contin, Kadian SR, Oramorph SR, Palladone, Roxanol) [C-II] **Uses:** *Relief of severe pain* **Action:** Narcotic analgesic **Dose:** *Adults.* PO: 5–30 mg q4h PRN; SR tabs 30–60 mg q8–12h (do not chew/crush). IV/IM: 2.5–15 mg q2–6h; supp 10–30 mg q4h. *IT:* (Duramorph, Infumorph): Per protocol *Peds.* 0.1–0.2 mg/kg/dose IM/IV q2–4h PRN to 15 mg/dose max **Caution:** [B (D if prolonged use or high doses at term), +/–] **Contra:** Severe asthma, resp depression, GI obstruction **Supplied:** Immediate-release tabs 10, 14, 20 mg; MS Contin CR tabs 15, 30, 60, 100, 200 mg; Oramorph SR CR tabs 15, 30, 60, 100 mg; Kadian SR caps 20, 30 50, 60, 100 mg; Palladone ER caps 12, 16, 24, 32 mg; Avinza XR caps 30, 60, 90, 120 mg; soln 10, 20, 100 mg; supp 5, 10, 20 mg; inj 2, 4, 5, 8, 10, 15 mg/mL; Duramorph/Infumorph inj 0.5, 1 mg/mL; supp 5, 10, 20, 30 mg **SE:** Narcotic SE (resp depression, sedation, constipation, N/V, pruritus), granulomas w/IT **Notes:** May require scheduled dosing to relieve severe chronic pain; do not crush/chew SR/ER forms

Morphine Liposomal (DepoDur) **Uses:** *Long-lasting epidural analgesia* **Action:** ER morphine analgesia **Dose:** 10–20 mg lumbar epidural inj (c-section 10 mg after cord clamped) **Caution:** [C, +/–] elderly, biliary Dz (sphincter of Oddi spasm) **Contra:** paralytic ileus, resp depression, asthma, obstructed airway, suspected/known head injury ↑ ICP, allergy to morphine. **Supplied:** Inj

10 mg/mL **SE:** Hypoxia, resp depression, ↓ BP, retention, N/V, constipation, flatulence, pruritus, pyrexia, anemia, HA, dizziness, tachycardia, insomnia, ileus **Notes:** Effect ≤ 48 h; not for IT/IV/IM use

Moxifloxacin (Avelox, Vigamox Ophthalmic) **Uses:** *Acute sinusitis, acute bronchitis, skin/soft tissue Infxns, conjunctivitis & community-acquired pneumonia* **Action:** 4th-gen quinolone; ↓ DNA gyrase. *Spectrum:* Excellent gram(+) coverage except MRSA & *E. faecium;* good gram(–) coverage except *P. aeruginosa, S. maltophilia* & *Acinetobacter* sp; good anaerobic coverage **Dose:** 400 mg/d PO (avoid cation products, antacids) /IV qd. *Ophth:* 1 gt tid × 7d **Caution:** [C, ?/–] Quinolone sensitivity; interactions w/Mg-, Ca-, Al- & Fe-containing products & class IA & III antiarrhythmic agents **Contra:** Quinolone or component sensitivity **Supplied:** Tabs 400 mg, inj, ophth 0.5% **SE:** Dizziness, nausea, QT prolongation, Szs, photosensitivity, tendon rupture **Notes:** Take PO 4h before or 8h after antacids

Mupirocin (Bactroban) **Uses:** *Impetigo; eradication of MRSA in nasal carriers* **Action:** ↓ Bacterial protein synthesis **Dose:** *Topical:* Apply small amount to area. *Nasal:* Apply bid in nostrils **Caution:** [B, ?] **Contra:** Do not use w/other nasal products **Supplied:** Oint 2%; cream 2% **SE:** Local irritation, rash

Muromonab-CD3 (Orthoclone OKT3) **WARNING:** Can cause anaphylaxis; monitor fluid status **Uses:** *Acute rejection after organ transplantation* **Action:** Blocks T-cell Fxn **Dose:** *Adults.* 5 mg/d IV for 10–14 d. *Peds.* 0.1 mg/kg/d for 10–14 d **Caution:** [C, ?/–] Murine sensitivity, fluid overload **Contra:** Heart failure/fluid overload, Hx of Szs, PRG, uncontrolled HTN **Supplied:** Inj 5 mg/5 mL **SE:** Murine Ab; fever & chills after the 1st dose (premedicate w/ steroid/APAP/antihistamine); monitor for anaphylaxis or pulmonary edema **Notes:** 0.22–μm filter for administration

Mycophenolate Mofetil (CellCept) **WARNING:** ↑ Risk of Infxns, possible development of lymphoma **Uses:** *Prevent organ rejection after transplant* **Action:** ↓ immunologically mediated inflammatory responses **Dose:** *Adults.* 1 g PO bid; *Peds.* BSA 1.2–1.5 m^2: 750 mg PO bid; *BSA > 1.5 m^2*: 1 g PO bid; may taper up to 600 mg/m^2 PO bid; used w/steroids & cyclosporine; ↓ in renal insuff or neutropenia. *IV:* Infuse over > 2 h. *PO:* Take on empty stomach; do not open capsules **Caution:** [C, ?/–] **Contra:** Component allergy; IV use in polysorbate 80 allergy **Supplied:** Caps 250, 500 mg; inj 500 mg **SE:** N/V/D, pain, fever, HA, Infxn, HTN, anemia, leukopenia, edema

Mycophenolic Acid (Myfortic) **WARNING:** ↑ Risk of Infxns, possible development of lymphoma **Uses:** *Prevent rejection after renal transplant* **Action:** Cytostatic to lymphocytes **Dose:** *Adults.* 720 mg PO bid; *Peds.* BSA 400–720 mg/m^2: 750 mg PO bid; ↓ in renal insuff/neutropenia (on empty stomach) **Caution:** [C, ?/–] **Contra:** Component allergy **Supplied:** DR tabs 180, 360 mg **SE:** N/V/D, pain, fever, HA, Infxn, HTN, anemia, leukopenia, edema

Nabumetone (Relafen) **WARNING:** May ↑ risk of CV events & GI bleeding **Uses:** *Arthritis & pain* **Action:** NSAID; ↓ prostaglandins **Dose:** 1000–2000 mg/d ÷ qd–bid w/food **Caution:** [C (D 3rd tri), +] **Contra:** Peptic ulcer, NSAID sensitivity, severe hepatic Dz **Supplied:** Tabs 500, 750 mg **SE:** Dizziness, rash, GI upset, edema, peptic ulcer

Nadolol (Corgard) **Uses:** *HTN & angina* **Action:** Competitively blocks β-adrenergic receptors, $β_1$, $β_2$ **Dose:** 40–80 mg/d; ↑ to 240 mg/d (angina) or 320 mg/d (HTN) may be needed; ↓ in renal insuff & elderly **Caution:** [C (1st tri; D

22

if 2nd or 3rd tri), +] **Contra:** Uncompensated CHF, shock, heart block, asthma **Supplied:** Tabs 20, 40, 80, 120, 160 mg **SE:** Nightmares, paresthesias, ↓ BP, bradycardia, fatigue

Nafcillin (Nallpen) **Uses:** *Infxns due to susceptible strains of *Staphylococcus* & *Streptococcus** **Action:** Bactericidal; ↓ cell wall synthesis. *Spectrum:* Good gram(+) **Dose:** *Adults.* 1–2 g IV q4–6h. *Peds.* 50–200 mg/kg/d ÷ q4–6h **Caution:** [B, ?] PCN allergy **Supplied:** Inj **SE:** Interstitial nephritis, D, fever, nausea **Notes:** No adjustments for renal Fxn

Naftifine (Naftin) **Uses:** *Tinea pedis, cruris & corporis* **Action:** Antifungal antibiotic **Dose:** Apply bid **Caution:** [B, ?] **Contra:** Component sensitivity **Supplied:** 1% cream; gel **SE:** Local irritation

Nalbuphine (Nubain) **Uses:** *Moderate–severe pain; preop & obstetric analgesia* **Action:** Narcotic agonist–antagonist; ↓ ascending pain pathways **Dose:** *Adults.* 10–20 mg IM or IV q4–6h PRN; max of 160 mg/d; single max dose, 20 mg. *Peds.* 0.2 mg/kg IV or IM to a max dose of 20 mg; ↓ in hepatic insuff **Caution:** [B (D if prolonged or high doses at term), ?] **Contra:** Sulfite sensitivity **Supplied:** Inj 10, 20 mg/mL **SE:** CNS depression, drowsiness; caution in pts receiving opiates

Naloxone (Narcan) **Uses:** *Opioid addiction (diagnosis) & OD* **Action:** Competitive narcotic antagonist **Dose:** *Adults.* 0.4–2.0 mg IV, IM, or SQ q5min; max total dose, 10 mg. *Peds.* 0.01–1 mg/kg/dose IV, IM, or SQ; repeat IV q3min × 3 doses PRN **Caution:** [B, ?] May precipitate acute withdrawal in addicts **Supplied:** Inj 0.4, 1.0 mg/mL; neonatal inj 0.02 mg/mL **SE:** ↓ BP, tachycardia, irritability, GI upset, pulmonary edema **Notes:** If no response after 10 mg, suspect nonnarcotic cause

Naltrexone (ReVia) **Uses:** *EtOH & narcotic addiction* **Action:** Competitively binds to opioid receptors **Dose:** 50 mg/d PO; do not give until opioid-free for 7–10 d **Caution:** [C, M] **Contra:** Acute hepatitis, liver failure; opioid use **Supplied:** Tabs 50 mg **SE:** May cause hepatotox; insomnia, GI upset, joint pain, HA, fatigue

Naphazoline & Antazoline (Albalon-A Ophthalmic, others), Naphazoline & Pheniramine Acetate (Naphcon A) **Uses:** *Relieve ocular redness & itching caused by allergy* **Action:** Vasoconstrictor & antihistamine **Dose:** 1–2 gtt up to qid **Caution:** [C, +] **Contra:** Glaucoma, children < 6 y & w/contact lenses **Supplied:** Soln 15 mL **SE:** CV stimulation, dizziness, local irritation

Naproxen (Aleve [OTC], Naprosyn, Anaprox) **WARNING:** May ↑ risk of CV events & GI bleeding **Uses:** *Arthritis & pain* **Action:** NSAID; ↓ prostaglandins **Dose:** *Adults & Peds > 12 y.* 200–500 mg bid–tid to 1500 mg/d max; ↓ in hepatic impair **Caution:** [B (D 3rd tri), +] **Contra:** NSAID sensitivity, peptic ulcer **Supplied:** Tabs 200, 220, 250, 375, 500 mg; DR (EC) tabs 375, 500 mg; susp 125 mg/5 mL **SE:** Dizziness, pruritus, GI upset, peptic ulcer, edema

Naratriptan (Amerge) [OTC] **Uses:** *Acute migraine attacks* **Action:** Serotonin 5-HT$_1$ receptor antagonist **Dose:** 1–2.5 mg PO once; repeat PRN in 4 h; ↓ in mild renal/hepatic insuff, take w/fluids **Caution:** [C, M] **Contra:** Severe renal/hepatic impair, avoid in angina, ischemic heart Dz, uncontrolled HTN, cerebrovascular syndromes & ergot use **Supplied:** Tabs 1, 2.5 mg **SE:** Dizziness, sedation, GI upset, paresthesias, ECG changes, coronary vasospasm, arrhythmias

Natalizumab (Tysabri) Uses: *Relapsing MS* Withdrawn due to safety concerns

Nateglinide (Starlix) Uses: *Type 2 DM* **Action:** ↑ Pancreatic release of insulin **Dose:** 120 mg PO tid 1–30 min pc; ↓ to 60 mg tid if near target HbA_{1c}, (take 1–30 min ac) **Caution:** [C, –]. Caution w/drugs metabolized by CYP2C9/3A4 **Contra:** Diabetic ketoacidosis, type 1 DM **Supplied:** Tabs 60, 120 mg **SE:** Hypoglycemia, URI; salicylates, nonselective β-blockers may enhance hypoglycemia

Nedocromil (Tilade) Uses: *Mild–moderate asthma* **Action:** Antiinflammatory agent **Dose:** *Inhal:* 2 inhal qid **Caution:** [B, ?/–] **Contra:** Component allergy **Supplied:** Met-dose inhaler **SE:** Chest pain, dizziness, dysphonia, rash, GI upset, Infxn **Notes:** Not for acute asthma attacks

Nefazodone (Serzone) WARNING: Fatal hepatitis & liver failure possible, D/C if LFT > 3 × ULN, do not re-treat; closely monitor for worsening depression or emergence of suicidality, particularly in ped pts Uses: *Depression* **Action:** ↓ Neuronal uptake of serotonin & norepinephrine **Dose:** Initial 100 mg PO bid; usual 300–600 mg/d in 2 ÷ doses **Caution:** [C, ?] **Contra:** MAOIs, pimozide, cisapride, carbamazepine **Supplied:** Tabs 100, 150, 200, 250 mg **SE:** Postural ↓ BP & allergic Rxns; HA, drowsiness, xerostomia, constipation, GI upset, liver failure **Notes:** Monitor LFTs, HR/BP

Nelfinavir (Viracept) Uses: *HIV Infxn* **Action:** Protease inhibitor; results in formation of immature, noninfectious virion **Dose:** *Adults.* 750 mg PO tid or 1250 mg PO bid. *Peds.* 20–30 mg/kg PO tid; take w/food **Caution:** [B, ?] Many drug interactions **Contra:** Phenylketonuria, triazolam/midazolam use or drug dependent on CYP3A4 (page 647) **Supplied:** Tabs 250 mg; PO powder **SE:** Food ↑ absorption; interacts w/St. John's wort; dyslipidemia, lipodystrophy, D, rash

Neomycin, Bacitracin & Polymyxin B (Neosporin Ointment) (See Neomycin & Polymyxin B, below)

Neomycin, Colistin & Hydrocortisone (Cortisporin-TC Otic Drops); Neomycin, Colistin, Hydrocortisone & Thonzonium (Cortisporin-TC Otic Suspension) Uses: *External otitis,* Infxns of mastoid/fenestration cavities **Action:** Antibiotic w/antiinflammatory **Dose:** *Adults.* 4–5 gtt in ear(s) tid–qid. *Peds.* 3–4 gtt in ear(s) tid–qid **Caution:** [C, ?] **Supplied:** Otic gtt & susp **SE:** Local irritation

Neomycin & Dexamethasone (AK-Neo-Dex Ophthalmic, Neo-Decadron Ophthalmic) Uses: *Steroid-responsive inflammatory conditions of the cornea, conjunctiva, lid & anterior segment* **Action:** Antibiotic w/ antiinflammatory corticosteroid **Dose:** 1–2 gtt in eye(s) q3–4h or thin coat tid–qid until response, then ↓ to qd **Caution:** [C, ?] **Supplied:** Cream neomycin 0.5%/dexamethasone 0.1%; oint neomycin 0.35%/dexamethasone 0.05%; soln neomycin 0.35%/dexamethasone 0.1% **SE:** Local irritation **Notes:** Use under supervision of ophthalmologist

Neomycin & Polymyxin B (Neosporin Cream) [OTC] Uses: *Infxn in minor cuts, scrapes & burns* **Action:** Bactericidal **Dose:** Apply bid–qid **Caution:** [C, ?] **Contra:** Component allergy **Supplied:** Cream neomycin 3.5 mg/polymyxin B 10,000 Units/g **SE:** Local irritation **Notes:** Different from Neosporin oint

22

Neomycin, Polymyxin B & Dexamethasone (Maxitrol) Uses:
Steroid-responsive ocular conditions w/bacterial Infxn **Action:** Antibiotic w/ antiinflammatory corticosteroid **Dose:** 1–2 gtt in eye(s) q4–6h; apply oint in eye(s) tid–qid **Caution:** [C, ?] **Supplied:** Oint neomycin sulfate 3.5 mg/polymyxin B sulfate 10,000 units/dexamethasone 0.1%/g; susp identical/5 mL **SE:** Local irritation **Notes:** Use under supervision of ophthalmologist

Neomycin, Polymyxin & Hydrocortisone (Cortisporin Ophthalmic & Otic) Uses:
Ocular & otic bacterial Infxns **Action:** Antibiotic & antiinflammatory **Dose:** *Otic:* 3–4 gtt in the ear(s) tid–qid. *Ophth:* Apply a thin layer to the eye(s) or 1 gt qd–qid **Caution:** [C, ?] **Supplied:** Otic susp; ophth soln; ophth oint **SE:** Local irritation

Neomycin, Polymyxin B & Prednisolone (Poly-Pred Ophthalmic)
Uses: *Steroid-responsive ocular conditions w/bacterial Infxn* **Action:** Antibiotic & antiinflammatory **Dose:** 1–2 gtt in eye(s) q4–6h; apply oint in eye(s) tid–qid **Caution:** [C, ?] **Supplied:** Susp neomycin 0.35%/polymyxin B 10,000 Units/prednisolone 0.5%/mL **SE:** Irritation **Notes:** Use under supervision of ophthalmologist

Neomycin–Polymyxin Bladder Irrigant (Neosporin GU Irrigant)
Uses: *Continuous irrigant for prophylaxis against bacteriuria & gram(−) bacteremia associated w/indwelling catheter use* **Action:** Bactericide **Dose:** 1 mL irrigant in 1 L of 0.9% NaCl; cont bladder irrigation w/1 L of soln/24 h **Caution:** [D] **Contra:** Component allergy **Supplied:** Soln neomycin sulfate 40 mg & polymyxin B 200,000 Units/mL; amp 1, 20 mL **SE:** Neomycin-induced ototox or nephrotox (rare) **Notes:** Potential for bacterial/fungal super Infxn; not for inj

Neomycin Sulfate (Myciguent) [OTC] Uses:
Hepatic coma, bowel prep **Action:** Aminoglycoside, poorly absorbed PO; ↓ GI bacterial flora **Dose:** *Adults.* 3–12 g/24 h PO in 3–4 ÷ doses. *Peds.* 50–100 mg/kg/24 h PO in 3–4 ÷ doses **Caution:** [C, ?/–] Renal failure, neuromuscular disorders, hearing impair **Contra:** Intestinal obstruction **Supplied:** Tabs 500 mg; PO soln 125 mg/5 mL **SE:** Hearing loss w/long-term use; rash, N/V **Notes:** Do not use parenterally (↑ tox); part of the Condon bowel prep

Nesiritide (Natrecor) Uses:
Acutely decompensated CHF **Action:** Human B-type natriuretic peptide **Dose:** 2 mcg/kg IV bolus, then 0.01 mcg/kg/min IV **Caution:** [C, ?/–] When vasodilators are not appropriate **Contra:** SBP < 90, cardiogenic shock **Supplied:** Vials 1.5 mg **SE:** ↓ BP, HA, GI upset, arrhythmias, ↑ Cr **Notes:** Requires continuous BP monitoring; some studies indicate ↑ in mortality

Nevirapine (Viramune) WARNING:
Reports of fatal hepatotox even after short-term use; severe life-threatening skin reactions (Stevens–Johnson, toxic epidermal necrolysis & allergic Rxns); monitor closely during 1st 8 wk of Rx **Uses:** *HIV Infxn* **Action:** Nonnucleoside RT inhibitor **Dose:** *Adults.* Initial 200 mg/d PO × 14 d, then 200 mg bid. *Peds.* < 8 y: 4 mg/kg/d × 14 d, then 7 mg/kg bid. > *8 y:* 4 mg/kg/d × 14 d, then 4 mg/kg bid (w/o regard to food) **Caution:** [C, +/–] OCP **Supplied:** Tabs 200 mg; susp 50 mg/5 mL **SE:** Life-threatening rash; HA, fever, D, neutropenia, hepatitis. **Notes:** Give w/out regard to food; not recommended in women if CD4 > 250 or men > 400 unless benefit > risk of hepatotoxicity

Niacin (Niaspan) Uses: *Adjunct in significant hyperlipidemia* **Action:** ↓ Lipolysis; ↓ esterification of triglycerides; ↑ lipoprotein lipase **Dose:** 1–6 g ÷ doses PO tid; 9 g/d max (w/food) **Caution:** [A (C if doses > RDA), +] **Contra:** Liver Dz, peptic ulcer, arterial hemorrhage **Supplied:** SR caps 125, 250, 300, 400, 500 mg; tabs 25, 50, 100, 250, 500 mg; SR tabs 150, 250, 500, 750 mg; elixir 50 mg/5 mL **SE:** Upper body/facial flushing & warmth; GI upset, flatulence, exacerbate peptic ulcer; HA, paresthesias, liver damage, gout, or altered glucose control in DM. **Notes:** Flushing ↓ by taking aspirin or NSAID 30–60 min before dose

Nicardipine (Cardene) Uses: *Chronic stable angina & HTN*; prophylaxis of migraine **Action:** CCB **Dose:** *Adults. PO:* 20–40 mg PO tid. *SR:* 30–60 mg PO bid. *IV:* 5 mg/h IV cont inf; ↑ by 2.5 mg/h q15min to max 15 mg/h. *Peds. PO:* 20–30 mg PO q 8h. *IV:* 0.5–5 mcg/kg/min; ↓ in renal/hepatic impair **Caution:** [C, ?/–] Heart block, CAD **Contra:** Cardiogenic shock **Supplied:** Caps 20, 30 mg; SR caps 30, 45, 60 mg; inj 2.5 mg/mL **SE:** Flushing, tachycardia, ↓ BP, edema, HA **Notes:** PO-to-IV conversion: 20 mg tid = 0.5 mg/h, 30 mg tid = 1.2 mg/h, 40 mg tid = 2.2 mg/h; take w/food (not high fat)

Nicotine Gum (Nicorette) [OTC] Uses: *Aid to smoking cessation for relief of nicotine withdrawal* **Action:** Systemic delivery of nicotine **Dose:** Chew 9–12 pieces/d PRN; max 30 pieces/d **Caution:** [C, ?] **Contra:** Life-threatening arrhythmias, unstable angina **Supplied:** 2 mg, 4 mg/piece; mint, orange, original flavors **SE:** Tachycardia, HA, GI upset, hiccups **Notes:** Must stop smoking & perform behavior modification for max effect

Nicotine Nasal Spray (Nicotrol NS) Uses: *Aid to smoking cessation for relief of nicotine withdrawal* **Action:** Systemic delivery of nicotine **Dose:** 0.5 mg/actuation; 1–2 sprays/h, 10 sprays/h max **Caution:** [D, M] **Contra:** Life-threatening arrhythmias, unstable angina **Supplied:** Nasal inhaler 10 mg/mL **SE:** Local irritation, tachycardia, HA, taste perversion **Notes:** Must stop smoking & perform behavior modification for max effect

Nicotine Transdermal (Habitrol, Nicoderm CQ [OTC], Nicotrol [OTC]) Uses: *Aid to smoking cessation; relief of nicotine withdrawal* **Action:** Systemic delivery of nicotine **Dose:** Individualized; 1 patch (14–22 mg/d) & taper over 6 wk **Caution:** [D, M] **Contra:** Life-threatening arrhythmias, unstable angina **Supplied:** Habitrol & Nicoderm CQ 7, 14, 21 mg of nicotine/24 h; Nicotrol 5, 10, 15 mg/24 h **SE:** Insomnia, pruritus, erythema, local site Rxn, tachycardia **Notes:** Nicotrol worn for 16 h to mimic smoking patterns; others worn for 24 h; must stop smoking & perform behavior modification for max effect

Nifedipine (Procardia, Procardia XL, Adalat, Adalat CC) Uses: *Vasospastic or chronic stable angina & HTN*; tocolytic **Action:** CCB **Dose:** *Adults. SR* tabs 30–90 mg/d. *Tocolysis:* 10–20 mg PO q4–6h. *Peds.* 0.6–0.9 mg/kg/24 h ÷ tid–qid **Caution:** [C, +] Heart block, aortic stenosis **Contra:** Immediate-release preparation for urgent or emergency HTN; acute MI **Supplied:** Caps 10, 20 mg; SR tabs 30, 60, 90 mg **SE:** HA common on initial Rx; reflex tachycardia may occur w/regular release dosage forms; peripheral edema, ↓ BP, flushing, dizziness **Notes:** Adalat CC & Procardia XL not interchangeable; SL administration not OK

Nilutamide (Nilandron) **WARNING:** Interstitial pneumonitis possible; most cases in 1st 3 mo; follow CXR before Rx Uses: *Combo w/surgical castra-

22

tion for metastatic CAP* **Action:** Nonsteroidal antiandrogen **Dose:** 300 mg/d PO in ÷ doses for 30 d, then 150 mg/d **Caution:** [N/A] **Contra:** Severe hepatic impair or resp insuff **Supplied:** Tabs 150 mg **SE:** Hot flashes, loss of libido, impotence, N/V/D, gynecomastia, hepatic dysfunction (follow LFTs), interstitial pneumonitis **Notes:** May cause Rxn when taken w/EtOH

Nimodipine (Nimotop) **Uses:** *Prevent vasospasm following subarachnoid hemorrhage* **Action:** CCB **Dose:** 60 mg PO q4h for 21 d; ↓ in hepatic failure **Caution:** [C, ?] **Contra:** Component allergy **Supplied:** Caps 30 mg **SE:** ↓ BP, HA, constipation **Notes:** Administered via NG tube if caps cannot be swallowed whole

Nisoldipine (Sular) **Uses:** *HTN* **Action:** CCB **Dose:** 10–60 mg/d PO; do not take w/grapefruit juice or high-fat meal; ↓ starting doses in elderly or hepatic impair **Caution:** [C, ?] **Supplied:** ER tabs 10, 20, 30, 40 mg **SE:** Edema, HA, flushing

Nitazoxanide (Alinia) **Uses:** *Cryptosporidium-* or *Giardia*-induced diarrhea in pts 1–11 y* **Action:** Antiprotozoal. *Spectrum: Cryptosporidium* and *Giardia* **Dose:** *Peds.* 12–47 mo. 5 mL (100 mg) PO q 12h × 3 d. *4–11 y:* 10 mL (200 mg) PO q 12h × 3 d; take w/food **Caution:** [B, ?] **Contra:** N/A **Supplied:** 100 mg/5 mL PO susp **SE:** Abdominal pain **Notes:** Susp contains sucrose, interacts w/highly protein-bound drugs

Nitrofurantoin (Macrodantin, Furadantin, Macrobid) WARNING: Pulmonary reactions possible **Uses:** *Prevention & Rx UTI* **Action:** Bacteriostatic; interferes w/carbohydrate metabolism. *Spectrum:* Susceptible gram(−) & some gram(+) bacteria; *Pseudomonas, Serratia* & most sp *Proteus*-resistant **Dose:** *Adults. Suppression:* 50–100 mg/d PO. *Rx:* 50–100 mg PO qid. *Peds.* 4–7 mg/kg/24 h in 4 ÷ doses (w/food/milk/antacid) **Caution:** [B, +] Avoid if CrCl < 50 mL/min, PRG at term **Contra:** Renal failure, infants < 1 mo **Supplied:** Caps/tabs 50, 100 mg; SR caps 100 mg; susp 25 mg/5 mL **SE:** GI SEs; dyspnea & a variety of acute/chronic pulmonary reactions, peripheral neuropathy **Notes:** Macrocrystals (Macrodantin) cause < N than other forms

Nitroglycerin (Nitrostat, Nitrolingual, Nitro-Bid Ointment, Nitro-Bid IV, Nitrodisc, Transderm-Nitro, others) **Uses:** *Angina pectoris, acute & prophylactic therapy, CHF, BP control* **Action:** Relaxation of vascular smooth muscle, dilates coronary arteries **Dose:** *Adults.* SL: 1 tab q5min SL PRN for 3 doses. *Translingual:* 1–2 met-doses sprayed onto PO mucosa q3–5min, max 3 doses. *PO:* 2.5–9 mg tid. IV: 5–20 mcg/min, titrated to effect. *Topical:* Apply ½ in of oint to chest wall tid, wipe off at night. *TD:* 0.2–0.4 mg/h/ patch qd. *Peds.* 1 mcg/kg/min IV, titrate **Caution:** [B, ?] Restrictive cardiomyopathy **Contra:** *IV:* Pericardial tamponade, constrictive pericarditis. *PO:* Use w/ sildenafil, tadalafil, vardenafil, head trauma, closed-angle glaucoma **Supplied:** SL tabs 0.3, 0.4, 0.6 mg; translingual spray 0.4 mg/dose; SR caps 2.5, 6.5, 9, 13 mg; SR tabs 2.6, 6.5, 9.0 mg; inj 0.5, 5, 10 mg/mL; oint 2%; TD patches 0.1, 0.2, 0.4, 0.6 mg/h; buccal CR 2, 3 mg **SE:** HA, ↓ BP, light-headedness, GI upset **Notes:** Nitrate tolerance w/chronic use after 1–2 wk; minimize by providing nitrate-free period qd, using shorter-acting nitrates tid & removing long-acting patches & oint before sleep to ↓ tolerance

Nitroprusside (Nipride, Nitropress) **Uses:** *Hypertensive crisis, CHF, controlled ↓ BP periop (↓ bleeding),* aortic dissection, pulmonary edema

22

Action: ↓ Systemic vascular resistance **Dose:** *Adult & Peds.* 0.5–10 mcg/kg/min IV inf, titrate; usual dose 3 mcg/kg/min **Caution:** [C, ?] ↓ cerebral perfusion **Contra:** High output failure, compensatory HTN **Supplied:** Inj 25 mg/mL **SE:** Excessive hypotensive effects, palpitations, HA **Notes:** Thiocyanate (metabolite w/renal excretion) w/tox at 5–10 mg/dL, more likely if used for > 2–3 d; to Rx aortic dissection, use β-blocker concomitantly

Nizatidine (Axid, Axid AR) [OTC] Uses: *Duodenal ulcers, GERD, heartburn* **Action:** H₂-receptor antagonist **Dose:** *Adults. Active ulcer:* 150 mg PO bid or 300 mg PO hs; maint 150 mg PO hs. *GERD:* 300 mg PO bid; maint PO bid. *Heartburn:* 75 mg PO bid. *Peds.* GERD: 10 mg/kg PO bid in ÷ doses, 150 mg bid max; ↓ in renal impair **Caution:** [B, +] **Contra:** H₂-receptor antagonist sensitivity **Supplied:** Caps 75 [OTC], 150, 300 mg **SE:** Dizziness, HA, constipation, D

Norepinephrine (Levophed) Uses: *Acute ↓ BP, cardiac arrest (adjunct)* **Action:** Peripheral vasoconstrictor acts on arterial/venous beds **Dose:** *Adults.* 8–12 mcg/min IV, titrate. *Peds.* 0.05–0.1 mg/kg/min IV, titrate **Caution:** [C, ?] **Contra:** ↓ BP due to hypovolemia **Supplied:** Inj 1 mg/mL **SE:** Bradycardia, arrhythmia **Notes:** Correct volume depletion as much as possible before vasopressors; interaction w/ TCAs leads to severe HTN; infuse into large vein to avoid extravasation; phentolamine 5–10 mg/10 mL NS injected locally for extravasation

Norethindrone Acetate/Ethinyl Estradiol (FemHRT) WARNING: Estrogens & progestins should not be used for the prevention of CV Dz; the WHI study reported ↑ risks of MI, breast CA & DVT in postmenopausal women during 5 y of treatment with estrogens combined with medroxyprogesterone acetate relative to placebo Uses: *Rx of moderate–severe vasomotor Sxs associated w/ menopause; prevent osteoporosis* **Action:** Hormone replacement **Dose:** 1 tablet qd **Caution:** [X, –] **Contra:** PRG; Hx breast CA; estrogen-dependent neoplasia; abnormal genital bleeding; Hx DVT, PE, or related disorders; recent (w/in past year) arterial thromboembolic Dz (CVA, MI) **Supplied:** 1 mg norethindrone/5 mcg ethinyl estradiol tablets **SE:** Thrombosis, dizziness, HA, libido changes **Notes:** Use in women w/intact uterus

Norfloxacin (Noroxin, Chibroxin ophthal) Uses: *Complicated & uncomplicated UTI due to gram(–) bacteria, prostatitis, gonorrhea,* & infectious D **Action:** Quinolone, ↓ DNA gyrase. *Spectrum:* Susceptible *E. faecalis, E. coli, K. pneumoniae, P. mirabilis, P. aeruginosa, S. epidermidis, S. saprophyticus* **Dose:** 400 mg PO bid (↓ in renal impair). *Gonorrhea:* 800 mg single dose. *Prostatitis:* 400 mg PO bid *Adults, Peds > 1 y:* 1 gt each eye qid for 7 d **Caution:** [C, –] Tendinitis/tendon rupture, quinolone sensitivity, **Contra:** Hx of allergy or tendinitis w/fluoroquinolones **Supplied:** Tabs 400 mg; ophth 3 mg/mL **SE:** Photosensitivity, HA, GI; ocular burning w/ophth **Notes:** Interactions w/antacids, theophylline, caffeine; good concn in the kidney & urine, poor blood levels; not for urosepsis

Norgestrel (Ovrette) Uses: *PO Contraceptive* **Action:** Prevent follicular maturation & ovulation **Dose:** 1 tab/d; begin d 1 of menses **Caution:** [X, ?] **Contra:** Thromboembolic disorders, breast CA, PRG, severe hepatic Dz **Supplied:** Tabs 0.075 mg **SE:** Edema, breakthrough bleeding, thromboembolism **Notes:** Progestin-only products have ↑ risk of failure in prevention of PRG

Nortriptyline (Aventyl, Pamelor) Uses: *Endogenous depression* **Action:** TCA; ↑ synaptic CNS levels of serotonin &/or norepinephrine **Dose:** *Adults.* 25

22

mg PO tid–qid; > 150 mg/d not OK. *Elderly:* 10–25 mg hs. ***Peds.*** 6–7 y: 10 mg/d. *8–11 y:* 10–20 mg/d. > *11 y:* 25–35 mg/d, ↓ w/hepatic insuff **Caution:** [D, +/–] NAG, CV Dz **Contra:** TCA allergy, use w/MAOI **Supplied:** Caps 10, 25, 50, 75 mg; soln 10 mg/5 mL **SE:** Anticholinergic (blurred vision, retention, xerostomia) **Notes:** Max effect seen after 2 wk

Nystatin (Mycostatin) Uses: *Mucocutaneous *Candida* Infxns (oral, skin, vaginal)* **Action:** Alters membrane permeability. *Spectrum:* Susceptible *Candida* sp **Dose:** ***Adults & Peds.*** PO: 400,000–600,000 units PO "swish & swallow" qid. *Vaginal:* 1 tab vaginally hs × 2 wk. *Topical:* Apply bid–tid to area. ***Peds.*** Infants: 200,000 Units PO q6h. **Caution:** [B (C PO), +] **Supplied:** PO susp 100,000 units/mL; PO tabs 500,000 units; troches 200,000 units; vaginal tabs 100,000 units; topical cream/oint 100,000 units/g **SE:** GI upset, Stevens–Johnson syndrome **Notes:** Not absorbed PO; not for systemic Infxns

Octreotide (Sandostatin, Sandostatin LAR) Uses: *↓ Severe diarrhea associated w/carcinoid & neuroendocrine GI tumors (eg, VIPoma, ZE syndrome)*; bleeding esophageal varices **Action:** Long-acting peptide; mimics natural hormone somatostatin **Dose:** *Adults.* 100–600 mcg/d SQ/IV in 2–4 ÷ doses; start 50 mcg qd–bid. *Sandostatin LAR (depot):* 10–30 mg IM q4wk ***Peds.*** 1–10 mcg/kg/24 h SQ in 2–4 ÷ doses. **Caution:** [B, +] Hepatic/renal impair **Supplied:** Inj 0.05, 0.1, 0.2, 0.5, 1 mg/mL; 10, 20, 30 mg/5 mL depot **SE:** N/V, abdominal discomfort, flushing, edema, fatigue, cholelithiasis, hyper/hypoglycemia, hepatitis

Ofloxacin (Floxin, Ocuflox Ophthalmic) Uses: *Lower resp tract, skin & skin structure & UTI, prostatitis, uncomplicated gonorrhea & *Chlamydia* Infxns; topical (bacterial conjunctivitis; otitis externa; perforated ear drum > 12 y)* **Action:** Bactericide; ↓ DNA gyrase. *Spectrum: S. pneumoniae, S. aureus, S. pyogenes, H. influenzae, P. mirabilis, N. gonorrhoeae, C. trachomatis, E. coli* **Dose:** *PO: Adults.* 200–400 mg PO bid or IV q12h. ***Ophth: Adults & Peds > 1 y.*** 1–2 gtt in eye(s) q2–4h for 2 d, then qid × 5 more d. ***Otic: Adults & Peds > 12 y.*** 10 gtt in ear(s) bid for 10 d. ***Peds 1–12 y.*** 5 gtt in ear(s) bid for 10 d. ↓ in renal impair; on empty stomach **Caution:** [C, –] Interacts w/antacids, sucralfate, Al-, Ca-, Mg-, Fe-, and Zn-containing drugs (↓ absorption) **Contra:** Quinolone allergy **Supplied:** Tabs 200, 300, 400 mg; inj 20, 40 mg/mL; ophth & otic 0.3% **SE:** N/V/D, photosensitivity, insomnia, HA **Notes:** Use ophth form in ears

Olanzapine (Zyprexa, Zyprexa, Zydis) WARNING: Mortality in elderly w/dementia-related psychosis **Uses:** *Bipolar mania, schizophrenia,* psychotic disorders, acute agitation in schizophrenia **Action:** Dopamine & serotonin antagonist **Dose:** *Bipolar/schizophrenia:* 5–10 mg/d, ↑ wkly PRN, 20 mg/d max *Agitation:* 10–20 mg IMq2–4h PRN, 40 mg d/max **Caution:** [C, –] **Supplied:** Tabs 2.5, 5, 7.5, 10, 15, 20 mg; PO disintegrating tabs 5, 10, 15, 20 mg **SE:** HA, somnolence, orthostatic ↓ BP, tachycardia, dystonia, xerostomia, constipation **Notes:** Takes weeks to titrate dose; smoking ↓ levels; may be confused w/Zyrtec

Olopatadine (Patanol) Uses: *Allergic conjunctivitis* **Action:** H_1-receptor antagonist **Dose:** 1–2 gtt in eye(s) bid q6–8h **Caution:** [C, ?] **Supplied:** Soln 0.1% 5 mL **SE:** Local irritation, HA, rhinitis **Notes:** Do not instill w/contacts in

Olsalazine (Dipentum) Uses: *Maint remission in ulcerative colitis* **Action:** Topical antiinflammatory **Dose:** 500 mg PO bid (w/food) **Caution:** [C, M] Salicylate sensitivity **Supplied:** Caps 250 mg **SE:** D, HA, blood dyscrasias, hepatitis

Omalizumab (Xolair) Uses: *Moderate–severe asthma in ≥12 y w/reactivity to an allergen & when Sxs inadequately controlled w/inhaled steroids* **Action:** Anti-IgE Ab **Dose:** 150–375 mg SQ q2–4wk (dose/frequency based on serum IgE level & BW, see package insert) **Caution:** [B,?/–] **Contra:** Component allergy **Supplied:** 150 mg single-use 5-mL vial **SE:** Site Rxn, sinusitis, HA, anaphylaxis reported in 3 pts **Notes:** Continue other asthma medications as indicated

Omeprazole (Prilosec, Zegerid) Uses: *Duodenal/gastric ulcers, ZE syndrome, GERD,* *H. pylori* Infxns **Action:** Proton-pump inhibitor **Dose:** 20–40 mg PO qd–bid Zegerid powder 1 h ac; in small cup w/2 tbsp H_2O (not food or other liquids); refill and drink **Caution:** [C, –] **Supplied:** Caps 10, 20, 40 mg; powder packets 20 mg; Zegerid PO powder 20, 40 mg **SE:** HA, D **Notes:** Combo (ie, antibiotic) Rx for *H. pylori*

Ondansetron (Zofran) Uses: *Prevent chemo-associated & postop N/V* **Action:** Serotonin receptor antagonist **Dose:** *Adults & Peds.* 0.15 mg/kg/dose IV before chemo, then 4 & 8 h after 1st dose or 4–8 mg PO tid; 1st dose 30 min before chemo & give on a schedule, not PRN. *Postop: Adults.* 4 mg IV immediately before anesthesia or postop. *Peds.* < 40 kg: 0.1 mg/kg. *> 40 kg:* 4 mg IV ↓ dose w/hepatic impair **Caution:** [B, +/–] **Supplied:** Tabs 4, 8 mg; inj 2 mg/mL **SE:** D, HA, constipation, dizziness

Oprelvekin (Neumega) Uses: *Prevent severe thrombocytopenia w/ chemo* **Action:** ↑ Proliferation & maturation of megakaryocytes (IL-11) **Dose:** *Adults.* 50 mcg/kg/d SQ for 10–21 d. *Peds.* > 12 y: 75–100 mcg/kg/d SQ for 10–21 d. *< 12 y:* Use only in clinical trials. **Caution:** [C, ?/–] **Supplied:** 5 mg powder for inj **SE:** Tachycardia, palpitations, arrhythmias, edema, HA, dizziness, insomnia, fatigue, fever, nausea, anemia, dyspnea

Oral Contraceptives, Biphasic, Monophasic, Triphasic, Progestin Only (Table 22–7, page 638)
Uses: *Birth control & regulation of anovulatory bleeding* **Action:** *Birth control:* Suppresses LH surge, prevents ovulation; progestins thicken cervical mucus; ↓ fallopian tubule cilia, ↓ endometrial thickness to ↓ chances of fertilization. *Anovulatory bleeding:* Cyclic hormones mimic body's natural cycle & regulate endometrial lining, results in regular bleeding q28d; may also ↓ uterine bleeding & dysmenorrhea **Dose:** 28-d cycle pills take qd; 21-d cycle pills take qd, no pills during last 7 d of cycle (during menses); some available as TD patch **Caution:** [X, +] Migraine, HTN, DM, sickle cell Dz, gallbladder Dz **Contra:** Undiagnosed vaginal bleeding, PRG, estrogen-dependent malignancy, hypercoagulation disorders, liver Dz, hemiplegic migraine, smokers > 35 y **Supplied:** 28-d cycle pills (21 active pills + 7 placebo/Fe supl); 21-d cycle pills (21 active pills) **SE:** Intramenstrual bleeding, oligomenorrhea, amenorrhea, ↑ appetite/weight gain, ↓ libido, fatigue, depression, mood swings, mastalgia, HA, melasma, ↑ vaginal discharge, acne/greasy skin, corneal edema, nausea **Notes:** Taken correctly, 99.9% effective for preventing PRG; no STD prevention, use additional barrier contraceptive; long term, can ↓ risk of ectopic PRG, benign breast Dz, ovarian & uterine CA. *Rx of menstrual cycle control:* Start w/monophasic; take for 3 mo before switching to another brand; if bleeding continues, change to pill w/higher estrogen dose. *Rx for birth control:* Choose pill w/lowest SE profile for particular pt; SEs numerous, due to Sxs of estrogen excess and progesterone deficiency; each pill's side effect profile is unique (see insert)

22

Orlistat (Xenical) Uses: *Manage obesity w/BMI 30 or 27 w/other risk factors; type 2 DM, dyslipidemia* Action: Reversible inhibitor of gastric & pancreatic lipases. Dose: 120 mg PO tid w/fat-containing meal Caution: [B, ?] May ↓ cyclosporine & warfarin dose requirements Contra: Cholestasis, malabsorption Supplied: Capsules 120 mg SE: Abdominal pain/discomfort, fatty/oily stools, fecal urgency Notes: Do not use if meal contains no fat; GI effects ↑ w/ higher-fat meals; supplement w/fat-soluble vitamins

Orphenadrine (Norflex) Uses: *Muscle spasms* Action: Central atropine-like effects cause indirect skeletal muscle relaxation, euphoria, analgesia Dose: 100 mg PO bid, 60 mg IM/IV q12h Caution: [C, +] Contra: Glaucoma, GI obstruction, cardiospasm, MyG Supplied: Tabs 100 mg; SR tabs 100 mg; inj 30 mg/mL SE: Drowsiness, dizziness, blurred vision, flushing, tachycardia, constipation

Oseltamivir (Tamiflu) Uses: * Prevention & Rx influenza A & B* Action: ↓ viral neuraminidase Dose: *Adults.* 75 mg PO bid for 5 d. *Peds.* PO bid dosing: < 14 kg: 30 mg. *16–23 kg:* 45 mg. *24–40 kg:* 60 mg; > *40 kg:* As adults; ↓ in renal impair Caution: [C, ?/–] Contra: Component allergy Supplied: Caps 75 mg, powder 12 mg/mL SE: N/V, insomnia Notes: Initiate w/in 48 h of Sx onset or exposure

Oxacillin (Bactocill, Prostaphlin) Uses: *Infxns due to susceptible *S. aureus* & *Streptococcus** Action: Bactericidal; ↓ cell wall synthesis. *Spectrum:* Excellent gram(+), poor gram(–) Dose: *Adults.* 250–500 mg (1 g severe) IM/IV q4–6h. *Peds.* 150–200 mg/kg/d IV ÷ q4–6h; ↓ in significant renal Dz Caution: [B, M] Contra: PCN sensitivity Supplied: Inj; caps 250, 500 mg; soln 250 mg/ 5 mL SE: GI upset, interstitial nephritis, blood dyscrasias

Oxaliplatin (Eloxatin) WARNING: Administer w/supervision of physician experienced in chemo. Appropriate management is possible only w/adequate diagnostic & Rx facilities. Anaphylactic-like Rxns reported. Uses: *Adjuvant Rx stage-III colon CA (primary resected) & metastatic colon CA w/ 5-FU* Action: Metabolized to platinum derivatives, crosslinks DNA Dose: Per protocol; see insert. *Premedicate:* Antiemetics w/or w/o dexamethasone Caution: [D, –] see Warning Contra: Allergy to components or platinum Supplied: Inj forms SE: Anaphylaxis, granulocytopenia, paresthesia, N/V/D, stomatitis, fatigue, neuropathy (common) hepatotox Notes: 5-FU & leucovorin are given in combo; epi, corticosteroids & antihistamines alleviate severe Rxns

Oxaprozin (Daypro) WARNING: May ↑ risk of CV events & GI bleeding Uses: *Arthritis & pain* Action: NSAID; ↓ prostaglandins synthesis Dose: 600–1200 mg/d; ↓ in renal/hepatic impair Caution: [C (D in 3rd tri or near term), ?] ASA/NSAID sensitivity, peptic ulcer, bleeding disorders Supplied: Caps 600 mg SE: CNS inhibition, sleep disturbance, rash, GI upset, peptic ulcer, edema, renal failure

Oxazepam (Serax) [C-IV] Uses: *Anxiety, acute EtOH withdrawal,* anxiety w/depressive Sxs Action: Benzodiazepine Dose: *Adults.* 10–15 mg PO tid–qid; severe anxiety & EtOH withdrawal may require up to 30 mg qid. *Peds.* 1 mg/kg/d in ÷ doses Caution: [D, ?] Supplied: Caps 10, 15, 30 mg; tabs 15 mg SE: Sedation, ataxia, dizziness, rash, blood dyscrasias, dependence Notes: Avoid abrupt D/C; metabolite of diazepam (Valium)

22

Oxcarbazepine (Trileptal) Uses: *Partial Szs,* bipolar disorders Action: Blocks voltage-sensitive Na⁺ channels, stabilization of hyperexcited neural membranes **Dose: *Adults.*** 300 mg PO bid, ↑ wkly to target maint 1200–2400 mg/d. ***Peds.*** 8–10 mg/kg bid, 500 mg/d max, ↑ wkly to target maint dose; ↓ in renal insuff **Caution:** [C, –] Cross-sensitivity to carbamazepine; reports of fatal skin and multiorgan hypersensitivity Rxns **Contra:** Components sensitivity **Supplied:** Tabs 150, 300, 600 mg **SE:** ↓ Na⁺, HA, dizziness, fatigue, somnolence, GI upset, diplopia, mental concentration difficulties **Notes:** Do not abruptly D/C, check Na⁺ if fatigue reported; advise about symptoms of Stevens–Johnson syndrome and topic epidermal necrolysis

Oxiconazole (Oxistat) Uses: *Tinea pedis, cruris & corporis* **Action:** Antifungal antibiotic. *Spectrum:* Most strains of *E. floccosum, T. mentagrophytes, T. rubrum, M. furfur* **Dose:** Apply bid **Caution:** [B, M] **Contra:** Component allergy **Supplied:** Cream 1%; lotion **SE:** Local irritation

Oxybutynin (Ditropan, Ditropan XL) Uses: *Symptomatic relief of urgency, nocturia & incontinence w/neurogenic or reflex neurogenic bladder* **Action:** Direct smooth muscle antispasmodic; ↑ bladder capacity **Dose: *Adults & Peds > 5 y.*** 5 mg PO tid–qid; XL 5 mg PO qd; ↑ to 30 mg/d PO (5 & 10 mg/tab). ***Peds 1–5 y.*** 0.2 mg/kg/dose bid–qid (syrup 5 mg/5 mL); ↓ in elderly; periodic drug holiday OK **Caution:** [B, ? (use w/caution)] **Contra:** Glaucoma, MyG, GI or GU obstruction, ulcerative colitis, megacolon **Supplied:** Tabs 5 mg; XL tabs 5, 10, 15 mg; syrup 5 mg/5 mL **SE:** Anticholinergic (drowsiness, xerostomia, constipation, tachycardia)

Oxybutynin Transdermal System (Oxytrol) Uses: *Rx OAB* **Action:** Smooth muscle antispasmodic; ↑ bladder capacity **Dose:** One 3.9 mg/d system apply 2×/wk to abdomen, hip, or buttock **Caution:** [B, ?/–] **Contra:** Urinary or gastric retention, uncontrolled narrow-angle glaucoma **Supplied:** 3.9 mg/d TD system **SE:** Anticholinergic effects, itching/redness at site **Notes:** Avoid reapplication to the same site w/in 7 d

Oxycodone [Dihydrohydroxycodeinone] (OxyContin, OxyIR, Roxicodone) [C-II] WARNING: Swallow whole, do not crush; high abuse potential Uses: *Moderate/severe pain, usually in combo w/nonnarcotic analgesics* **Action:** Narcotic analgesic **Dose: *Adults.*** 5 mg PO q6h PRN. ***Peds.*** 6–12 y: 1.25 mg PO q6h PRN. *> 12 y:* 2.5 mg q6h PRN. ↓ In severe liver Dz **Caution:** [B (D if prolonged use or near term), M] **Contra:** Allergy, resp depression **Supplied:** Immediate-release caps (OxyIR) 5 mg; tabs (Percolone) 5 mg; CR (OxyContin) 10, 20, 40, 80 mg; liq 5 mg/5 mL; soln conc 20 mg/mL **SE:** ↓ BP, sedation, dizziness, GI upset, constipation, risk of abuse **Notes:** OxyContin for chronic CA pain; sought after as drug of abuse

Oxycodone & Acetaminophen (Percocet, Tylox) [C-II] Uses: *Moderate–severe pain* **Action:** Narcotic analgesic **Dose: *Adults.*** 1–2 tabs/caps PO q4–6h PRN (acetaminophen max dose 4 g/d). ***Peds.*** Oxycodone 0.05–0.15 mg/kg/dose q4–6h PRN, up to 5 mg/dose **Caution:** [B (D prolonged use or near term), M] **Contra:** Allergy, resp depression **Supplied:** Percocet tabs, mg oxycodone/mg APAP: 2.5/325, 5/325, 7.5/325, 10/325, 7.5/500, 10/650; Tylox caps 5 mg oxycodone, 500 mg APAP; soln 5 mg oxycodone & 325 mg APAP/5 mL **SE:** ↓ BP, sedation, dizziness, GI upset, constipation

Oxycodone & Aspirin (Percodan, Percodan-Demi) [C-II] Uses: *Moderate–moderately severe pain* **Action:** Narcotic analgesic w/NSAID **Dose: *Adults.*** 1–2 tabs/caps PO q4–6h PRN. ***Peds.*** Oxycodone 0.05–0.15 mg/kg/dose q4–

22

6h PRN, up to 5 mg/dose; ↓ in severe hepatic failure **Caution:** [B (D prolonged use or near term), M] Peptic ulcer **Contra:** Component allergy **Supplied:** Percodan 4.5 mg oxycodone hydrochloride, 0.38 mg oxycodone terephthalate, 325 mg ASA; Percodan-Demi 2.25 mg oxycodone hydrochloride, 0.19 mg oxycodone terephthalate, 325 mg ASA **SE:** Sedation, dizziness, GI upset, constipation

Oxycodone/Ibuprofen (Combunox) [C-II] Uses: *Short term (not > 7 d) management of acute moderate–severe pain* **Action:** Narcotic w/NSAID **Dose:** Initial **Caution:** [C, –] w/impaired renal/hepatic Fxn; COPD, CNS depression **Contra:** Paralytic ileus, 3rd tri PRG, allergy to ASA or NSAIDs, when opioids are contraindicated, PRG **Supplied:** Tabs 5 mg oxycodone/400 mg ibuprofen **SE:** N/V, somnolence, dizziness, sweating, flatulence, ↑ LFTs **Notes:** Monitor renal Fxn; abuse potential w/oxycodone

Oxymorphone (Numorphan) [C-II] Uses: *Moderate–severe pain, sedative* **Action:** Narcotic analgesic **Dose:** 0.5 mg IM, SQ, IV initial, 1–1.5 mg q4–6h PRN. *PR:* 5 mg q4–6h PRN **Caution:** [B, ?] **Contra:** ↑ ICP, severe resp depression **Supplied:** Inj 1, 1.5 mg/mL; supp 5 mg **SE:** ↓ BP, sedation, GI upset, constipation, histamine release **Notes:** Chemically related to hydromorphone

Oxytocin (Pitocin) Uses: *Induce labor, control postpartum hemorrhage*; promote milk letdown in lactating women **Action:** Stimulate muscular contractions of the uterus & milk flow during nursing **Dose:** 0.001–0.002 units/min IV inf; titrate 0.02 units/min max. *Breast feeding:* 1 spray in both nostrils 2–3 min before feeding **Caution:** [Uncategorized, no anomalies expected, +/–] **Contra:** When vaginal delivery not favorable, fetal distress **Supplied:** Inj 10 units/mL; nasal soln 40 units/mL **SE:** Uterine rupture, fetal death; arrhythmias, anaphylaxis, H_2O intox **Notes:** Monitor vital signs; nasal form for breast feeding only

Paclitaxel (Taxol, Abraxane) Uses: *Ovarian & breast CA* CAP **Action:** Mitotic spindle poison promotes microtubule assembly & stabilization against depolymerization **Dose:** Per protocols; use glass or polyolefin containers (eg, nitroglycerin tubing set); PVC sets result in plasticizer leaching; ↓ in hepatic failure; maintain hydration **Caution:** [D, –] **Contra:** Neutropenia < 1500 WBC/μL; solid tumors **Supplied:** Inj 6 mg/mL, 5 mg/mL albumin bound (Abraxane) **SE:** Myelosuppression, peripheral neuropathy, transient ileus, myalgia, bradycardia, ↓ BP, mucositis, N/V/D, fever, rash, HA & phlebitis; hematologic tox schedule-dependent; leukopenia dose-limiting by 24-h inf; neurotox dose-limiting by short (1–3 h) inf **Notes:** Allergic Rxns (dyspnea, ↓ BP, urticaria, rash) usually w/in 10 min of inf; minimize w/corticosteroid, antihistamine pretreatment.

Palifermin (Kepivance) Uses: *Oral mucositis w/BMT* **Action:** Synthetic keratinocyte GF **Dose:** *Phase 1:* 60 mcg/kg IV qd × 3, 3rd dose 24–48 h before chemo *Phase 2:* 60 mcg/kg IV qd × 3, immediately after stem cell infusion **Caution:** [C, ?/–] **Contra:** N/A **Supplied:** Inj 6.25 mg **SE:** Unusual mouth sensations, tongue thickening, rash, ↑ amylase & lipase **Notes:** *E. coli*–derived; separate phases by 4 d; safety unknown w/nonhematologic malignancies

Palivizumab (Synagis) Uses: *Prevent RSV Infxn* **Action:** MoAb **Dose:** *Peds.* 15 mg/kg IM monthly, typically Nov–Apr **Caution:** [C, ?] Renal/hepatic dysfunction **Contra:** Component allergy **Supplied:** Vials 50, 100 mg **SE:** URI, rhinitis, cough, ↑ LFT, local irritation

22

Palonosetron (Aloxi) **WARNING:** May ↑ QTc interval Uses: *Prevention acute & delayed N/V w/emetogenic chemo* **Action:** $5HT_3$-receptor antagonist **Dose:** 0.25 mg IV 30 min before chemo; do not repeat w/in 7 d **Caution:** [B, ?] **Contra:** Component allergy **Supplied:** 0.25 mg/5 mL vial **SE:** HA, constipation, dizziness, abdominal pain, anxiety

Pamidronate (Aredia) **Uses:** *↑ Ca^{2+} of malignancy, Paget Dz, palliate symptomatic bone metastases* **Action:** ↓ Nl & abnormal bone resorption **Dose:** ↑ Ca^{2+}: 60 mg IV over 4 h or 90 mg IV over 24 h. *Paget Dz:* 30 mg/d IV slow inf for 3 d **Caution:** [C, ?/–] Avoid invasive dental procedures in CA patients **Contra:** PRG **Supplied:** Powder for inj 30, 60, 90 mg **SE:** Fever, inj site Rxn, uveitis, fluid overload, HTN, abdominal pain, N/V, constipation, UTI, bone pain,↓ K^+, ↓ Ca^{2+},↓ Mg^{2+}, hypophosphatemia; jaw osteonecrosis in CA patients, dental exam pretherapy

Pancrelipase (Pancrease, Cotazym, Creon, Ultrase) **Uses:** *Exocrine pancreatic secretion deficiency (eg, CF, chronic pancreatitis, pancreatic insuff), steatorrhea of malabsorption* **Action:** Pancreatic enzyme supl **Dose:** 1–3 caps (tabs) w/meals & snacks; ↑ to 8 caps (tabs); do not crush or chew EC products; dose-dependent on digestive requirements of pt; avoid antacids **Caution:** [C, ?/–] **Contra:** Pork product allergy **Supplied:** Caps, tabs **SE:** N/V, abdominal cramps **Notes:** Individualize therapy

Pancuronium (Pavulon) **Uses:** *Paralysis w/mechanical ventilation* **Action:** Nondepolarizing neuromuscular blocker **Dose:** *Adults.* 2–4 mg IV q2–4h PRN. *Peds.* 0.02–0.1 mg/kg/dose q2–4h PRN; ↓ in renal/hepatic impair; intubate pt & keep on controlled ventilation; use adequate sedation or analgesia **Caution:** [C, ?/–] **Contra:** Component or bromide sensitivity **Supplied:** Inj 1, 2 mg/mL **SE:** Tachycardia, HTN, pruritus, other histamine reactions

Pantoprazole (Protonix) **Uses:** *GERD, erosive gastritis,* ZE syndrome, PUD **Action:** Proton-pump inhibitor **Dose:** 40 mg/d PO; do not crush/ chew tabs; 40 mg IV/d (not > 3 mg/min, use Protonix filter) **Caution:** [B, ?/–] **Supplied:** Tabs 40 mg; inj **SE:** Chest pain, anxiety, GI upset, ↑ LFTs

Paregoric, Camphorated Tincture of Opium [C-III] **Uses:** *Diarrhea,* pain & neonatal opiate withdrawal syndrome **Action:** Narcotic **Dose:** *Adults.* 5–10 mL PO qd–qid PRN. *Peds.* 0.25–0.5 mL/kg qd–qid. *Neonatal withdrawal syndrome:* 3–6 gtt PO q3–6 h PRN to relieve Sxs for 3–5 d, then taper over 2–4 wk **Caution:** [B (D w/prolonged use/high dose near term, +] **Contra:** Tincture (children); convulsive disorder **Supplied:** Liq 2 mg morphine = 20 mg opium/5 mL **SE:** ↓ BP, sedation, constipation **Notes:** Contains anhydrous morphine from opium; short-term use only

Paroxetine (Paxil, Paxil CR) **WARNING:** Closely monitor for worsening depression or emergence of suicidality, particularly in ped pts **Uses:** *Depression, OCD, panic disorder, social anxiety disorder,* PMDD **Action:** SSRI **Dose:** 10–60 mg PO single daily dose in AM; CR 25 mg/d PO; ↑ 12.5 mg/ wk (max range 26–62.5 mg/d) **Caution:** [B, ?/] **Contra:** MAOI **Supplied:** Tabs 10, 20, 30, 40 mg; susp 10 mg/5 mL; CR 12.5, 25 mg **SE:** Sexual dysfunction, HA, somnolence, dizziness, GI upset, D, xerostomia, tachycardia

Pegfilgrastim (Neulasta) **Uses:** *↓ Frequency of Infxn in pts w/nonmyeloid malignancies receiving myelosuppressive anti-CA drugs that cause febrile neutropenia* **Action:** Colony-stimulating factor **Dose:** *Adults.* 6 mg SQ × 1/ chemo cycle. *Peds.* 100 mcg/kg SQ × 1/chemo cycle **Caution:** [C, M] in sickle cell **Contra:** Allergy to *E. coli*–derived proteins or filgrastim **Supplied:**

22

Syringes: 6 mg/0.6 mL **SE:** Splenic rupture HA, fever, weakness, fatigue, dizziness, insomnia, edema, N/V/D, stomatitis, anorexia, constipation, taste perversion, dyspepsia, abdominal pain, granulocytopenia, neutropenic fever, ↑ LFT & uric acid, arthralgia, myalgia, bone pain, ARDS, alopecia, aggravation of sickle cell Dz **Notes:** Never give between 14 d before & 24 h after dose of cytotoxic chemo

Peg Interferon Alfa-2a (Pegasys)   **Uses:** *Chronic hepatitis C w/compensated liver Dz* **Action:** Biologic response modifier **Dose:** 180 mcg (1 mL) SQ qwk × 48 wk; ↓ in renal impair **Caution:** [C, /?–] **Contra:** Autoimmune hepatitis, decompensated liver Dz **Supplied:** 180 mcg/mL inj **SE:** Depression, insomnia, suicidal behavior, GI upset, neutropenia & thrombocytopenia, alopecia, pruritus **Notes:** May aggravate neuropsychiatric, autoimmune, ischemic & infectious disorders

Peg Interferon Alfa-2b (PEG-Intron)   **Uses:** *Rx hepatitis C* **Action:** Immune modulation **Dose:** 1 mcg/kg/wk SQ; 1.5 mcg/kg/wk combined w/ribavirin **Caution:** [C, ?/–] w/psychiatric Hx **Contra:** Autoimmune hepatitis, decompensated liver Dz, hemoglobinopathy **Supplied:** Vials 50, 80, 120, 150 mcg/0.5 mL **SE:** Depression, insomnia, suicidal behavior, GI upset, neutropenia, thrombocytopenia, alopecia, pruritus **Notes:** Give hs or w/APAP to ↓ flulike Sxs; monitor CBC/platelets

Pemetrexed (Alimta)   **Uses:** *W/cisplatin in nonresectable mesothelioma* NSCLC **Action:** Antifolate antineoplastic **Dose:** 500 mg/m² IV over 10 min every 3 wk; hold if CrCl < 45 mL/min; give w/vitamin B₁₂ (1000 mcg IM every 9 wk) & folic acid (350–1000 mcg PO qd); start 1 wk before; dexamethasone 4 mg PO bid × 3 start 1 d before each Rx **Caution:** [D, –] Renal/hepatic/BM impair **Contra:** Component sensitivity **Supplied:** 500-mg vial **SE:** Neutropenia, thrombocytopenia, N/V/D, anorexia, stomatitis, renal failure, neuropathy, fever, fatigue, mood changes, dyspnea, anaphylactic reactions **Notes:** Avoid NSAIDs, follow CBC/platelets

Pemirolast (Alamast)   **Uses:** *Allergic conjunctivitis* **Action:** Mast cell stabilizer **Dose:** 1–2 gtt in each eye qid **Caution:** [C, ?/–] **Supplied:** 1 mg/mL **SE:** HA, rhinitis, cold/flu symptoms, local irritation **Notes:** Wait 10 min before inserting contacts

Penbutolol (Levatol)   **Uses:** *HTN* **Action:** β-adrenergic receptor blocker, β₁, β₂ **Dose:** 20–40 mg/d; ↓ in hepatic insuff **Caution:** [C (1st tri; D if 2nd/3rd tri), M] **Contra:** Asthma, cardiogenic shock, cardiac failure, heart block, bradycardia **Supplied:** Tabs 20 mg **SE:** Flushing, ↓ BP, fatigue, hyperglycemia, GI upset, sexual dysfunction, bronchospasm

Penciclovir (Denavir)   **Uses:** *Herpes simplex (herpes labialis/cold sores)* **Action:** Competitive inhibitor of DNA polymerase **Dose:** Apply at 1st sign of lesions, then q2h × 4 d **Caution:** [B, ?/–] **Contra:** Allergy **Supplied:** Cream 1% [OTC] **SE:** Erythema, HA **Notes:** Do not apply to mucous membranes

Penicillin G, Aqueous (Potassium or Sodium) (Pfizerpen, Pentids)   **Uses:** *Bacteremia, endocarditis, pericarditis, resp tract Infxns, meningitis, neurosyphilis, skin/skin structure Infxns* **Action:** Bactericide; ↓ cell wall synthesis. *Spectrum:* Most gram(+) (not staphylococci), streptococci, *N. meningitidis,* syphilis, clostridia & anaerobes (not *Bacteroides*) **Dose:** *Adults.* 400,000–800,000 units PO qid; IV doses vary depending on indications; range

0.6–24 MU/d in ÷ doses q4h. **Peds.** *Newborns* < 1 wk: 25,000–50,000 units/kg/dose IV q12h. *Infants 1 wk–< 1 mo:* 25,000–50,000 units/kg/dose IV q8h. *Children:* 100,000–300,000 units/kg/24h IV ÷ q4h; ↓ in renal impair **Caution:** [B, M] **Contra:** Allergy **Supplied:** Tabs 200,000, 250,000, 400,000, 800,000 units; susp 200,000, 400,000 units/5 mL; powder for inj **SE:** Allergic Rxns; interstitial nephritis, D, Szs **Notes:** Contains 1.7 mEq of K^+/MU

Penicillin G Benzathine (Bicillin) Uses: *Single-dose regimen for streptococcal pharyngitis, rheumatic fever, glomerulonephritis prophylaxis & syphilis* **Action:** Bactericidal; ↓ cell wall synthesis. *Spectrum:* See Penicillin G **Dose:** *Adults.* 1.2–2.4 million units deep IM inj q2–4wk. **Peds.** 50,000 units/kg/dose, 2.4 million units/dose max; deep IM inj q2–4 wk **Caution:** [B, M] **Contra:** Allergy **Supplied:** Inj 300,000, 600,000 units/mL; Bicillin L-A benzathine salt only; Bicillin C-R combo of benzathine & procaine (300,000 units procaine w/300,000 units benzathine/mL or 900,000 units benzathine w/300,000 units procaine/2 mL) **SE:** Inj site pain, acute interstitial nephritis, anaphylaxis **Notes:** Sustained action, detectable levels up to 4 wk; drug of choice for noncongenital syphilis

Penicillin G Procaine (Wycillin, others) Uses: *Infxns of respir tract, skin/soft tissue, scarlet fever, syphilis* **Action:** Bactericidal; ↓ cell wall synthesis. *Spectrum:* PCN G-sensitive organisms that respond to low, persistent serum levels **Dose:** *Adults.* 0.6–4.8 million units/d in ÷ doses q12–24h; give probenecid at least 30 min before PCN to prolong action. **Peds.** 25,000–50,000 units/kg/d IM ÷ qd–bid **Caution:** [B, M] **Contra:** Allergy **Supplied:** Inj 300,000, 500,000, 600,000 units/mL **SE:** Pain at inj site, interstitial nephritis, anaphylaxis **Notes:** Long-acting parenteral PCN; levels up to 15 h

Penicillin V (Pen-Vee K, Veetids, others) Uses: Susceptible streptococci Infxns, otitis media, URIs, skin/soft tissue Infxns (PCN-sensitive staph) **Action:** Bactericidal; ↓ cell wall synthesis. *Spectrum:* Most gram(+), including strep **Dose:** *Adults.* 250–500 mg PO q6h, q8h, q12h. **Peds.** 25–50 mg/kg/25h PO in 4 doses; ↓ in renal impair; on empty stomach **Caution:** [B, M] **Contra:** Allergy **Supplied:** Tabs 125, 250, 500 mg; susp 125, 250 mg/5 mL **SE:** GI upset, interstitial nephritis, anaphylaxis, convulsions **Notes:** Well-tolerated PO PCN; 250 mg = 400,000 units of PCN G

Pentamidine (Pentam 300, NebuPent) Uses: *Rx & prevention of PCP* **Action:** ↓ DNA, RNA, phospholipid & protein synthesis **Dose:** *Adults & Peds.* 4 mg/kg/24 h IV qd for 14–21 d. *Prevention: Adults & Peds > 5 y.* 300 mg once q4wk, give via Respigard II neb; IV requires ↓ in renal impair **Caution:** [C, ?] **Contra:** Component allergy **Supplied:** Inj 300 mg/vial; aerosol 300 mg **SE:** Associated w/pancreatic cell necrosis w/hyperglycemia; pancreatitis, CP, fatigue, dizziness, rash, GI upset, renal impair, blood dyscrasias (leukopenia & thrombocytopenia) **Notes:** Follow CBC, glucose, pancreatic Fxn monthly for 1st 3 mo; monitor for ↓ BP following IV administration

Pentazocine (Talwin) [C-IV] Uses: *Moderate–severe pain* **Action:** Partial narcotic agonist–antagonist **Dose:** *Adults.* 30 mg IM or IV; 50–100 mg PO q3–4h PRN. **Peds.** 5–8 y: 15 mg IM q4h PRN. *8–14 y:* 30 mg IM q4h PRN; ↓ in renal/hepatic impair **Caution:** [C (1st tri, D w/prolonged use/high dose near term), +/–] **Contra:** Allergy **Supplied:** Tabs 50 mg (+ naloxone 0.5 mg); inj 30 mg/mL **SE:** Considerable dysphoria; drowsiness, GI upset, xerostomia, Szs **Notes:** 30–60 mg IM = 10 mg of morphine IM

22

Pentobarbital (Nembutal, others) [C-II] **Uses:** *Insomnia, convulsions,* induced coma after severe head injury **Action:** Barbiturate **Dose:** *Adults.* Sedative: 20–40 mg PO or PR q6–12h. *Hypnotic:* 100–200 mg PO or PR hs PRN. *Induced coma:* Load 5–10 mg/kg IV, then maint 1–3 mg/kg/h IV inf (keep serum level 20–50 mg/mL). *Peds.* Hypnotic: 2–6 mg/kg/dose PO hs PRN. *Induced coma:* As adult **Caution:** [D, +/–] Severe hepatic impair **Contra:** Allergy **Supplied:** Caps 50, 100 mg; elixir 18.2 mg/5 mL (= 20 mg pentobarbital); supp 30, 60, 120, 200 mg; inj 50 mg/mL **SE:** Resp depression, ↓ BP w/ aggressive IV use for cerebral edema; bradycardia, ↓ BP, sedation, lethargy, resp depression, hangover, rash, Stevens–Johnson syndrome, blood dyscrasias **Notes:** Tolerance to sedative–hypnotic effect w/in 1–2 wk

Pentosan Polysulfate Sodium (Elmiron) **Uses:** *Relief of pain/discomfort associated w/interstitial cystitis* **Action:** Bladder wall buffer **Dose:** 100 mg PO tid on empty stomach w/H_2O 1 h ac or 2 h pc **Caution:** [B, ?/–] **Contra:** Allergy **Supplied:** Caps 100 mg **SE:** Alopecia, N/D, HA, ↑ LFTs, anticoagulant effects, thrombocytopenia **Notes:** Reassess after 3 mo

Pentoxifylline (Trental) **Uses:** *Symptomatic management of peripheral vascular Dz* **Action:** ↓ Blood cell viscosity by restoring erythrocyte flexibility **Dose:** *Adults.* 400 mg PO tid pc; Rx for at least 8 wk for full effect; ↓ to bid w/ GI/CNS SEs **Caution:** [C, +/–] **Contra:** Cerebral/retinal hemorrhage **Supplied:** Tabs 400 mg **SE:** Dizziness, HA, GI upset

Pergolide (Permax) **Uses:** *Parkinson Dz* **Action:** Centrally active dopamine receptor agonist **Dose:** Initial, 0.05 mg PO tid, titrated q2–3d to effect; maint 2–3 mg/d in ÷ doses **Caution:** [B, ?/–] **Contra:** Ergot sensitivity **Supplied:** Tabs 0.05, 0.25, 1.0 mg **SE:** Dizziness, somnolence, confusion, nausea, constipation, dyskinesia, rhinitis, MI **Notes:** May ↓ BP during start of therapy

Perindopril Erbumine (Aceon) **Uses:** *HTN,* CHF, DN, post-MI **Action:** ACE inhibitor **Dose:** 4–8 mg/d; avoid w/food; ↓ in elderly/renal impair **Caution:** [C (1st tri, D 2nd & 3rd tri), ?/–] ACE-inhibitor-induced angioedema **Contra:** Bilateral renal artery stenosis, primary hyperaldosteronism **Supplied:** Tabs 2, 4, 8 mg **SE:** HA, ↓ BP, dizziness, GI upset, cough **Notes:** OK w/diuretics

Permethrin (Nix, Elimite) [OTC] **Uses:** *Eradication of lice/scabies* **Action:** Pediculicide **Dose:** *Adults & Peds.* Saturate hair & scalp; allow 10 min before rinsing **Caution:** [B, ?/–] **Contra:** Allergy **Supplied:** Topical liq 1%; cream 5% **SE:** Local irritation **Notes:** Disinfect clothing, bedding, combs & brushes

Perphenazine (Trilafon) **Uses:** *Psychotic disorders, severe nausea,* intractable hiccups **Action:** Phenothiazine; blocks brain dopaminergic receptors **Dose:** *Antipsychotic:* 4–16 mg PO tid; max 64 mg/d. *Hiccups:* 5 mg IM q6h PRN or 1 mg IV at intervals not < 1–2 mg/min, 5 mg max. *Peds.* 1–6 y: 4–6 mg/ d PO in ÷ doses. *6–12 y:* 6 mg/d PO in ÷ doses. *> 12 y:* 4–16 mg PO bid–qid; ↓ in hepatic insuff **Caution:** [C, ?/–] narrow-angle glaucoma, severe HTN/↓ BP **Contra:** Phenothiazine sensitivity, BM depression, severe liver or cardiac Dz **Supplied:** Tabs 2, 4, 8, 16 mg; PO conc 16 mg/5 mL; inj 5 mg/mL **SE:** ↓ BP, tachycardia, bradycardia, EPS, drowsiness, Szs, photosensitivity, skin discoloration, blood dyscrasias, constipation

22

Phenazopyridine (Pyridium, others) **Uses:** *Lower urinary tract irritation* **Action:** Local anesthetic on urinary tract mucosa **Dose:** *Adults.* 100–200

mg PO tid. **Peds.** **6–12 y.** 12 mg/kg/24 h PO in 3 ÷ doses; ↓ in renal insuff **Caution:** [B, ?] Hepatic Dz **Contra:** Renal failure **Supplied:** Tabs 100, 200 mg; some available OTC **SE:** GI disturbances; red-orange urine color (can stain clothing); HA, dizziness, acute renal failure, methemoglobinemia

Phenelzine (Nardil) Uses: *Depression* **Action:** MAOI **Dose:** 15 mg PO tid. *Elderly:* 15–60 mg/d ÷ doses **Caution:** [C, –] Interacts w/SSRI, ergots, triptans **Contra:** CHF, Hx liver Dz **Supplied:** Tabs 15 mg **SE:** Postural ↓ BP; edema, dizziness, sedation, rash, sexual dysfunction, xerostomia, constipation, urinary retention **Notes:** May take 2–4 wk for effect; avoid tyramine-containing foods (eg, cheeses)

Phenobarbital [C-IV] Uses: *Sz disorders,* insomnia, anxiety **Action:** Barbiturate **Dose:** **Adults.** Sedative–hypnotic: 30–120 mg/d PO or IM PRN. *Anticonvulsant:* Load 10–12 mg/kg in 3 ÷ doses, then 1–3 mg/kg/24 h PO, IM, or IV. **Peds.** Sedative–hypnotic: 2–3 mg/kg/24 h PO or IM hs PRN. *Anticonvulsant:* Load 15–20 mg/kg ÷ in 2 equal doses 4 h apart, then 3–5 mg/kg/24h PO ÷ in 2–3 doses. **Caution:** [D, M] **Contra:** Porphyria, liver dysfunction **Supplied:** Tabs 8, 15, 16, 30, 32, 60, 65, 100 mg; elixir 15, 20 mg/5 mL; inj 30, 60, 65, 130 mg/mL **SE:** Bradycardia, ↓ BP, hangover, Stevens–Johnson syndrome, blood dyscrasias, resp depression **Notes:** Tolerance develops to sedation; paradoxic hyperactivity seen in ped pts; long half-life allows single daily dosing (Table 22–2, page 628)

Phenylephrine (Neo-Synephrine) Uses: *Vascular failure in shock, allergy, or drug-induced ↓ BP; nasal congestion*; mydriatic **Action:** α-Adrenergic agonist **Dose:** **Adults.** Mild–moderate ↓ BP: 2–5 mg IM or SQ ↑ BP for 2 h; 0.1–0.5 mg IV elevates BP for 15 min. *Severe ↓ BP/shock:* Cont inf at 100–180 mg/min; after BP stabilized, maint 40–60 mg/min. *Nasal congestion:* 1–2 sprays/nostril PRN. *Ophth:* 1 gtt 15–30 min before exam. **Peds.** ↓ BP: 5–20 mcg/kg/dose IV q10–15 min or 0.1–0.5 mg/kg/min IV inf, titrate to effect. *Nasal congestion:* 1 spray/nostril q3–4h PRN **Caution:** [C, +/–] HTN, acute pancreatitis, hepatitis, coronary Dz, narrow-angle glaucoma, hyperthyroidism **Contra:** Bradycardia, arrhythmias **Supplied:** Inj 10 mg/mL; nasal soln 0.125, 0.16, 0.25, 0.5, 1%; ophth soln 0.12, 2.5, 10% **SE:** Arrhythmias, HTN, peripheral vasoconstriction activity potentiated by oxytocin, MAOIs & TCAs; HA, weakness, necrosis, ↓ renal perfusion **Notes:** Promptly restore blood volume if loss has occurred; use large veins to avoid extravasation; phentolamine 10 mg in 10–15 mL of NS for local inj to Rx extravasation

Phenytoin (Dilantin) Uses: *Sz disorders* **Action:** ↓ Sz spread in the motor cortex **Dose:** **Load: Adults & Peds.** 15–20 mg/kg IV, 25 mg/min max or PO in 400-mg doses at 4-h intervals. *Maint:* **Adults.** Initial, 200 mg PO or IV bid or 300 mg hs; then follow levels. **Peds.** 4–7 mg/kg/24h PO or IV ÷ qd–bid; avoid PO susp (erratic absorption) **Caution:** [D, +] **Contra:** Heart block, sinus bradycardia **Supplied:** Caps 30, 100 mg; chew tabs 50 mg; PO susp 30, 125 mg/5 mL; inj 50 mg/mL **SE:** Nystagmus/ataxia early signs of tox; gum hyperplasia w/long-term use. *IV:* ↓ BP, bradycardia, arrhythmias, phlebitis; peripheral neuropathy, rash, blood dyscrasias, Stevens–Johnson syndrome **Notes:** Follow levels (Table 22–2, page 628); phenytoin albumin bound & levels reflect bound & free phenytoin; w/↓ albumin & azotemia, low levels may be therapeutic (nl free levels); do not change dosage at intervals < 7–10 d

Physostigmine (Antilirium) Uses: *Antidote for TCA, atropine & scopolamine OD; glaucoma* **Action:** Reversible cholinesterase inhibitor **Dose:**

22

Adults. 2 mg IV or IM q 20 min. *Peds.* 0.01–0.03 mg/kg/dose IV q15–30 min up to 2 mg total if needed **Caution:** [C, ?] **Contra:** GI/GU obstruction, CV Dz **Supplied:** Inj 1 mg/mL; ophth oint 0.25% **SE:** Rapid IV admin associated w/ Szs; cholinergic side effects; sweating, salivation, lacrimation, GI upset, asystole, changes in heart rate **Notes:** Excessive readministration can result in cholinergic crisis; crisis reversed w/atropine

Phytonadione, Vitamin K (AquaMEPHYTON, others) Uses: *Coagulation disorders due to faulty production of factors II, VII, IX, X*; hyperalimentation **Action:** Cofactor for production of factors II, VII, IX & X **Dose:** *Adults & Peds. Anticoagulant-induced prothrombin deficiency:* 1–10 mg PO or IV slowly. *Hyperalimentation:* 10 mg IM or IV qwk. *Infants.* 0.5–1 mg/dose IM, SQ, or PO **Caution:** [C, +] **Contra:** Allergy **Supplied:** Tabs 5 mg; inj 2, 10 mg/mL **SE:** Anaphylaxis from IV dosage; give IV slowly; GI upset (PO), inj site Rxns **Notes:** W/parenteral Rx, 1st change in PT usually seen in 12–24 h; use makes re-Coumadinization more difficult

Pimecrolimus (Elidel) Uses: *Atopic dermatitis* refractory, severe perianal itching **Action:** Inhibits T-lymphocytes **Dose:** Apply bid; use at least 1 wk after resolution **Caution:** [C, ?/–] w/local Infxn, lymphadenopathy; immunocompromise; avoid age < 2 y **Contra:** Allergy **Supplied:** Oint 0.03%, 0.1%; 30-g, 60-g tubes **SE:** Phototox, local irritation/burning, flu-like Sxs, may ↑ malignancy **Notes:** Apply to dry skin only; wash hands after use; ? ↑ cancer risk; second-line/short-term use only

Pindolol (Visken) Uses: *HTN* **Action:** β-Adrenergic receptor blocker, β_1, β_2, ISA **Dose:** 5–10 mg bid, 60 mg/d max; ↓ in hepatic/renal failure **Caution:** [B (1st tri; D if 2nd or 3rd tri), +/–] **Contra:** Uncompensated CHF, cardiogenic shock, bradycardia, heart block, asthma, COPD **Supplied:** Tabs 5, 10 mg **SE:** Insomnia, dizziness, fatigue, edema, GI upset, dyspnea; fluid retention may exacerbate CHF

Pioglitazone (Actos) Uses: *Type 2 DM* **Action:** ↑ Insulin sensitivity **Dose:** 15–45 mg/d PO **Caution:** [C, –] **Contra:** Hepatic impair **Supplied:** Tabs 15, 30, 45 mg **SE:** Weight gain, URI, HA, hypoglycemia, edema

Pioglitazone/Metformin (ActoPlus Met) WARNING: Can cause lactic acidosis which is fatal in 50% of cases Uses: *Type 2 DM as adjunct to diet and exercise* **Action:** Combined ↑ insulin sensitivity w/↓ hepatic glucose release **Dose:** Initial 1 tab PO qd or bid, titrate; max daily pioglitazone 45 mg & metformin 2550 mg **Caution:** [C, –] stop w/radiologic contrast agents **Contra:** Renal impair, acidosis **Supplied:** Tabs pioglitazone mg/metformin mg: 15/500, 15/850 **SE:** Lactic acidosis, hypoglycemia, edema, weight gain, URI, HA, GI upset, liver damage **Notes:** Follow LFTs

Piperacillin (Pipracil) Uses: *Infxns of skin, bone, resp & urinary tract, abdomen, sepsis* **Action:** 4th-gen PCN; bactericidal; ↓ cell wall synthesis. *Spectrum:* Primarily gram(+), better *Enterococcus, H. influenza,* not staph; gram(–) *E. coli, Proteus, Shigella, Pseudomonas,* not β-lactamase-producing **Dose:** *Adults.* 3 g IV q4–6h. *Peds.* 200–300 mg/kg/d IV ÷ q4–6h; ↓ in renal failure **Caution:** [B, M] PCN sensitivity **Supplied:** Inj **SE:** ↓ Plt aggregation, interstitial nephritis, renal failure, anaphylaxis, hemolytic anemia **Notes:** Often used w/aminoglycoside

Piperacillin–Tazobactam (Zosyn) Uses: *Infxns of skin, bone, resp & urinary tract, abdomen, sepsis* **Action:** PCN plus β-lactamase inhibitor; bactericidal; ↓ cell wall synthesis. *Spectrum:* Good gram(+), excellent gram(−); covers β-lactamase producers **Dose:** *Adults.* 3.375–4.5 g IV q6h; ↓ in renal failure **Caution:** [B, M] PCN or β-lactam sensitivity **Supplied:** Inj **SE:** D, HA, insomnia, GI upset, serum sickness–like reaction, pseudomembranous colitis **Notes:** Often used in combo w/aminoglycoside

Pirbuterol (Maxair) **Uses:** *Prevention & Rx reversible bronchospasm* **Action:** β$_2$-Adrenergic agonist **Dose:** 2 inhal q4–6h; max 12 inhal/d **Caution:** [C, ?/–] **Supplied:** Aerosol 0.2 mg/actuation; Autohaler dry powder 0.2 mg/actuation **SE:** Nervousness, restlessness, trembling, HA, taste changes, tachycardia

Piroxicam (Feldene) WARNING: May ↑ risk of CV events & GI bleeding **Uses:** *Arthritis & pain* **Action:** NSAID; ↓ prostaglandins **Dose:** 10–20 mg/d **Caution:** [B (1st tri; D if 3rd tri or near term), +] GI bleeding **Contra:** ASA or NSAID sensitivity; use after CABG **Supplied:** Caps 10, 20 mg **SE:** Dizziness, rash, GI upset, edema, acute renal failure, peptic ulcer

Plasma Protein Fraction (Plasmanate, others) **Uses:** *Shock & ↓ BP* **Action:** Plasma volume expander **Dose:** Initial, 250–500 mL IV (not > 10 mL/min); subsequent inf based on response. *Peds.* 10–15 mL/kg/dose IV; subsequent inf based on response **Caution:** [C, +] **Contra:** Renal insuff, CHF **Supplied:** Inj 5% **SE:** ↓ BP w/rapid inf; hypocoagulability, metabolic acidosis, PE **Notes:** 130–160 mEq Na/L; not substitute for RBC

Pneumococcal 7-Valent Conjugate Vaccine (Prevnar) **Uses:** *Immunization against pneumococcal Infxns in infants & children* **Action:** Active immunization **Dose:** 0.5 mL IM/dose; series of 3 doses; 1st dose age 2 mo w/subsequent doses q2mo **Caution:** [C, +] Thrombocytopenia **Contra:** Diphtheria toxoid sensitivity, febrile illness **Supplied:** Inj **SE:** Local reactions, arthralgia, fever, myalgia

Pneumococcal Vaccine, Polyvalent (Pneumovax-23) **Uses:** *Immunization against pneumococcal Infxns in pts at high risk (eg, all age ≥ 65 y)* **Action:** Active immunization **Dose:** 0.5 mL IM. **Caution:** [C, ?] **Contra:** *Do not vaccinate during immunosuppressive therapy* **Supplied:** Inj 25 mg each of polysaccharide isolates per 0.5-mL dose **SE:** Fever, inj site Rxn, hemolytic anemia, thrombocytopenia, anaphylaxis

Podophyllin (Podocon-25, Condylox Gel 0.5%, Condylox) **Uses:** *Topical therapy for benign growths (genital & perianal warts [condylomata acuminata],* papillomas, fibromas) **Action:** Direct antimitotic effect; exact mechanism unknown **Dose:** *Condylox gel & Condylox:* Apply 3 consecutive d/ wk for 4 wk. *Podocon-25:* Use sparingly on the lesion, leave on for 1–4 h, thoroughly wash off **Caution:** [C, ?] Immunosuppression **Contra:** DM, bleeding lesions **Supplied:** Podocon-25 (w/benzoin) 15-mL bottles; Condylox gel 0.5% 35 g clear gel; Condylox soln 0.5% 35 g clear **SE:** Local reactions, significant absorption; anemia, tachycardia, paresthesias, GI upset, renal/hepatic damage **Notes:** Podocon-25 applied only by clinician; do not dispense directly to patient

Polyethylene Glycol, PEG 3350 (MiraLax) **Uses:** *Occasional constipation* **Action:** Osmotic laxative **Dose:** 17 g powder (1 heaping tbsp) in 8 oz (1 cup) of H$_2$O & drink; max 14 d **Caution:** [C, ?] R/O bowel obstruction before use **Contra:** GI obstruction, allergy to PEG **Supplied:** Powder for reconstitution; bottle cap holds 17 g **SE:** Upset stomach, bloating, cramping, gas, severe D, hives **Notes:** Can add to H$_2$O, juice, soda, coffee, or tea

22

Polyethylene Glycol, PEG Electrolyte Solution (GoLYTELY, CoLyte) **Uses:** *Bowel prep before examination or surgery* **Action:** Osmotic cathartic **Dose:** *Adults.* Following 3–4-h fast, drink 240 mL of soln q10min until 4 L consumed. *Peds.* 25–40 mL/kg/h for 4–10 h **Caution:** [C, ?] **Contra:** GI obstruction, bowel perforation, megacolon, ulcerative colitis **Supplied:** Powder for reconstitution to 4 L **SE:** Cramping or nausea, bloating **Notes:** 1st BM should occur in approximately 1 h

Polymyxin B & Hydrocortisone (Otobiotic Otic) **Uses:** *Superficial bacterial Infxns of external ear canal* **Action:** Antibiotic/antiinflammatory combo **Dose:** 4 gtt in ear(s) tid–qid **Caution:** [B, ?] **Supplied:** Soln polymyxin B 10,000 units/hydrocortisone 0.5%/mL **SE:** Local irritation **Notes:** Useful in neomycin allergy

Potassium Citrate (Urocit-K) **Uses:** *Alkalinize urine, prevent urinary stones (uric acid, calcium stones if hypocitraturic)* **Action:** Urinary alkalinization **Dose:** 10–20 mEq PO tid w/meals, max 100 mEq/d **Caution:** [A, +] **Contra:** Severe renal impair, dehydration, $\uparrow$ K^+, peptic ulcer; use of K^+-sparing diuretics or salt substitutes **Supplied:** 540-, 1080-mg tabs **SE:** GI upset, $\downarrow$ Ca^{2+}, $\uparrow$ K^+, metabolic alkalosis **Notes:** Tabs 540 mg = 5 mEq, 1080 mg = 10 mEq

Potassium Citrate & Citric Acid (Polycitra-K) **Uses:** *Alkalinize urine, prevent urinary stones (uric acid, Ca stones if hypocitraturic)* **Action:** Urinary alkalinization **Dose:** 10–20 mEq PO tid w/meals, max 100 mEq/d **Caution:** [A, +] **Contra:** Severe renal impair, dehydration, $\uparrow$ K^+, peptic ulcer; use of K^+-sparing diuretics or salt substitutes **Supplied:** Soln 10 mEq/5 mL; powder 30 mEq/ packet **SE:** GI upset, $\downarrow$ Ca^{2+}, $\uparrow$ K^+, metabolic alkalosis

Potassium Iodide [Lugol Solution] (SSKI, Thyro-Block) **Uses:** *Thyroid storm,* $\downarrow$ vascularity before thyroid surgery, block thyroid uptake of radioactive iodine, thin bronchial secretions **Action:** Iodine supl **Dose:** *Adults & Peds > 2 y.* Preop thyroidectomy: 50–250 mg PO tid (2–6 gtt strong iodine soln); give 10 d preop. *Peds 1 y.* Thyroid crisis: 300 mg (6 gtt SSKI q8h). *Peds < 1 y:* 1/2 adult dose **Caution:** [D, +] $\uparrow$ K^+, TB, PE, bronchitis, renal impair **Contra:** Iodine sensitivity **Supplied:** Tabs 130 mg; soln (SSKI) 1 g/mL; Lugol soln, strong iodine 100 mg/mL; syrup 325 mg/5 mL **SE:** Fever, HA, urticaria, angioedema, goiter, GI upset, eosinophilia

Potassium Supplements (Kaon, Kaochlor, K-Lor, Slow-K, Micro-K, Klorvess, others) **Uses:** *Prevention or Rx of $\downarrow$ K^+* (eg, diuretic use) **Action:** K^+ supl **Dose:** *Adults.* 20–100 mEq/d PO ÷ qd–bid; IV 10–20 mEq/h, max 40 mEq/h & 150 mEq/d (monitor K^+ levels frequently w/high-dose IV). *Peds.* Calculate K^+ deficit; 1–3 mEq/kg/d PO ÷ qd–qid; IV max dose 0.5–1 mEq/kg/h **Caution:** [A, +] Renal insuff, use w/NSAIDs & ACE inhibitors **Contra:** $\uparrow$ K^+ **Supplied:** PO forms (Table 22–8, page 642); injectable forms **SE:** Can cause GI irritation; bradycardia, $\uparrow$ K^+, heart block **Notes:** Mix powder & liq w/beverage (unsalted tomato juice, etc); follow K^+; Cl– salt OK w/alkalosis; w/ acidosis use acetate, bicarbonate, citrate, or gluconate salt

Pramipexole (Mirapex) **Uses:** *Parkinson Dz* **Action:** Dopamine agonist **Dose:** 1.5–4.5 mg/d PO, initial 0.375 mg/d in 3 ÷ doses; titrate slowly **Caution:** [C, ?/–] **Contra:** Component allergy **Supplied:** Tabs 0.125, 0.25, 1, 1.5 mg **SE:** Postural $\downarrow$ BP, asthenia, somnolence, abnormal dreams, GI upset, EPS

22

Pramoxine (Anusol Ointment, Proctofoam-NS, others) **Uses:** *Relief of pain & itching from hemorrhoids, anorectal surgery*; topical for burns & dermatosis **Action:** Topical anesthetic **Dose:** Apply freely to anal area q3h **Caution:** [C, ?] **Supplied:** [OTC] All 1%; foam (Proctofoam-NS), cream, oint, lotion, gel, pads, spray **SE:** Contact dermatitis, mucosal thinning w/chronic use

Pramoxine + Hydrocortisone (Enzone, Proctofoam-HC) Uses: *Relief of pain & itching from hemorrhoids* **Action:** Topical anesthetic, antiinflammatory **Dose:** Apply freely to anal area tid–qid **Caution:** [C, ?/–] **Supplied:** Cream pramoxine 1% acetate 0.5/1%; foam pramoxine 1% hydrocortisone 1%; lotion pramoxine 1% hydrocortisone 0.25%/2.5%, pramoxine 2.5% & hydrocortisone 1% **SE:** Contact dermatitis, mucosal thinning with chronic use

Pravastatin (Pravachol) Uses: ↓ Cholesterol **Action:** HMG-CoA reductase inhibitor **Dose:** 10–40 mg PO hs; ↓ in significant renal/hepatic impair **Caution:** [X, –] **Contra:** Liver Dz or persistent LFT ↑ **Supplied:** Tabs 10, 20, 40 mg **SE:** Use caution w/concurrent gemfibrozil; HA, GI upset, hepatitis, myopathy, renal failure

Prazosin (Minipress) Uses: *HTN* **Action:** Peripherally acting α-adrenergic blocker **Dose:** *Adults.* 1 mg PO tid; can ↑ to 20 mg/d max. *Peds.* 5–25 mcg/kg/dose q6h, to 25 mcg/kg/dose max **Caution:** [C, ?] **Contra:** Component allergy **Supplied:** Caps 1, 2, 5 mg **SE:** Dizziness, edema, palpitations, fatigue, GI upset **Notes:** Can cause orthostatic ↓ BP, take the 1st dose hs; tolerance develops to this effect; tachyphylaxis may result

Prednisolone (See Table 22–4, page 633)

Prednisone (See Table 22–4, page 633)

Pregabalin (Lyrica) Uses: *DM peripheral neuropathy pain; postherpetic neuralgia; adjunct Rx adult partial onset seizures* **Action:** Nerve transmission modulator **Dose:** *Neuropathic pain:* 50 mg PO tid, ↑ to 300 mg/d w/in 1 wk based on response (300 mg/d max) *Postherpetic neuralgia:* 75–150 mg bid, or 50–100 mg tid; start 75 mg bid or 50 mg tid; ↑ to 300 mg/d w/in 1 wk based on response; if pain persists after 2–4 wk,↑ to 600 mg/d; *Epilepsy:* Start 150 mg/d (75 mg bid or 50 mg tid) may ↑ to max 600 mg/d; ↓ w/renal insuff; w/or w/o food **Caution:** [X, –] with significant renal impair, see insert for dosing **Contra:** PRG **Supplied:** Tabs 25, 50, 75, 100, 150, 200, 225, 300 mg **SE:** Dizziness, drowsiness, xerostomia, peripheral edema, blurred vision, weight gain, difficulty concentrating **Notes:** Related to gabapentin; w/D/C, taper over at least 1 wk

Probenecid (Benemid, others) Uses: *Prevent gout & hyperuricemia; prolongs levels of PCNs & cephalosporins* **Action:** Renal tubular blocking agent **Dose:** *Adults.* Gout: 250 mg bid × 1 wk, then 0.5 g PO bid; can ↑ by 500 mg/mo up to 2–3 g/d. *Antibiotic effect:* 1–2 g PO 30 min before dose. *Peds > 2 y.* 25 mg/kg, then 40 mg/kg/d PO ÷ qid **Caution:** [B, ?] **Contra:** High-dose ASA, moderate–severe renal impair, age < 2 y **Supplied:** Tabs 500 mg **SE:** HA, GI upset, rash, pruritus, dizziness, blood dyscrasias **Notes:** Do not use during acute gout attack

Procainamide (Pronestyl, Procan) Uses: *Supraventricular/ventricular arrhythmias* **Action:** Class 1A antiarrhythmic **Dose:** *Adults. Recurrent VF/VT:* 20 mg/min IV (total 17 mg/kg max). *Maint:* 1–4 mg/min. *Stable wide-complex tachycardia of unknown origin, AF w/rapid rate in WPW:* 20 mg/min IV until arrhythmia suppression, ↓ BP, QRS widens > 50%, then 1–4 mg/min. *Chronic dosing:* 50 mg/kg/d PO in ÷ doses q4–6h. *Peds. Chronic maint:* 15–50 mg/kg/24 h PO ÷ q3–6h; ↓ in renal/hepatic impair **Caution:** [C, +] **Contra:**

22

Complete heart block, 2nd- or 3rd-degree heart block w/o pacemaker, torsade de pointes, SLE **Supplied:** Tabs & caps 250, 375, 500 mg; SR tabs 250, 500, 750, 1000 mg; inj 100, 500 mg/mL **SE:** ↓ BP, lupus-like syndrome, GI upset, taste perversion, arrhythmias, tachycardia, heart block, angioneurotic edema **Notes:** Follow levels (Table 22–2, page 628)

Procarbazine (Matulane) WARNING: Highly toxic; handle w/care **Uses:** *Hodgkin Dz,* NHL, brain tumors **Action:** Alkylating agent; ↓ DNA & RNA synthesis **Dose:** Per protocol **Caution:** [D, ?] W/EtOH ingestion **Contra:** Inadequate BM reserve **Supplied:** Caps 50 mg **SE:** Myelosuppression, hemolytic reactions (w/G6PD deficiency), N/V/D; disulfiram-like Rxn; cutaneous & constitutional Sxs, myalgia, arthralgia, CNS effects, azoospermia, cessation of menses

Prochlorperazine (Compazine) **Uses:** *N/V, agitation & psychotic disorders* **Action:** Phenothiazine; blocks postsynaptic dopaminergic CNS receptors **Dose:** *Adults. Antiemetic:* 5–10 mg PO tid–qid or 25 mg PR bid or 5–10 mg deep IM q4–6h. *Antipsychotic:* 10–20 mg IM acutely or 5–10 mg PO tid–qid for maint; ↑ doses may be required for antipsychotic effect. *Peds.* 0.1–0.15 mg/kg/dose IM q4–6h or 0.4 mg/kg/24 h PO ÷ tid–qid **Caution:** [C, +/–] narrow-angle glaucoma, severe liver/cardiac Dz **Contra:** Phenothiazine sensitivity, BM suppression **Supplied:** Tabs 5, 10, 25 mg; SR caps 10, 15, 30 mg; syrup 5 mg/5 mL; supp 2.5, 5, 25 mg; inj 5 mg/mL **SE:** EPS common; Rx w/diphenhydramine

Promethazine (Phenergan) **Uses:** *N/V, motion sickness* **Action:** Phenothiazine; blocks CNS postsynaptic mesolimbic dopaminergic receptors **Dose:** *Adults.* 12.5–50 mg PO, PR, or IM bid–qid PRN. *Peds.* 0.1–0.5 mg/kg/dose PO or IM q2–6h PRN **Caution:** [C, +/–] use w/agents w/resp depressant effects **Contra:** Component allergy, narrow-angle glaucoma, age < 2 y **Supplied:** Tabs 12.5, 25, 50 mg; syrup 6.25 mg/5 mL, 25 mg/5 mL; supp 12.5, 25, 50 mg; inj 25, 50 mg/mL **SE:** Drowsiness, tardive dyskinesia, EPS, lowered Sz threshold, ↓ BP, GI upset, blood dyscrasias, photosensitivity, resp depression in children

Propafenone (Rythmol) **Uses:** *Life-threatening ventricular arrhythmias, AF* **Action:** Class IC antiarrhythmic; **Dose:** *Adults.* 150–300 mg PO q8h. *Peds.* 8–10 mg/kg/d ÷ in 3–4 doses; may ↑ 2 mg/kg/d, to max of 20 mg/kg/d **Caution:** [C, ?] w/amprenavir, ritonavir **Contra:** Uncontrolled CHF, bronchospasm, cardiogenic shock, conduction disorders **Supplied:** Tabs 150, 225, 300 mg **SE:** Dizziness, unusual taste, 1st-degree heart block, arrhythmias, prolongs QRS & QT intervals; fatigue, GI upset, blood dyscrasias

Propantheline (Pro-Banthine) **Uses:** *PUD,* symptomatic Rx of small-intestinal hypermotility, spastic colon, ureteral spasm, bladder spasm, pylorospasm **Action:** Antimuscarinic **Dose:** *Adults.* 15 mg PO ac & 30 mg PO hs; ↓ in elderly. *Peds.* 2–3 mg/kg/24h PO ÷ tid–qid **Caution:** [C, ?] **Contra:** narrow-angle glaucoma, ulcerative colitis, toxic megacolon, GI/GU obstruction **Supplied:** Tabs 7.5, 15 mg **SE:** Anticholinergic (eg, xerostomia, blurred vision)

Propofol (Diprivan) **Uses:** *Induction & maint of anesthesia; sedation in intubated pts* **Action:** Sedative–hypnotic; mechanism unknown **Dose:** *Adults. Anesthesia:* 2–2.5 mg/kg induction, then 0.1–0.2 mg/kg/min inf *ICU sedation:* 5–50 mcg/kg/min cont inf; ↓ in elderly, debilitated, ASA II/IV pts *Peds. Anesthesia:* 2.5–3.5 mg/kg induction; then 125–300 mcg/kg/min **Caution:** [B, +] **Contra:** If general anesthesia contraindicated **Supplied:** Inj 10 mg/mL **SE:** May

↑ triglycerides w/extended dosing; ↓ BP, pain at site, apnea, anaphylaxis **Note:** 1 mL of propofol has 0.1 g fat

Propoxyphene (Darvon), Propoxyphene & Acetaminophen (Darvocet) & Propoxyphene & Aspirin (Darvon Compound-65, Darvon-N + Aspirin) [C-IV]

Uses: *Mild–moderate pain* **Action:** Narcotic analgesic **Dose:** 1–2 PO q4h PRN; ↓ in hepatic impair, elderly **Caution:** [C (D if prolonged use), M] Hepatic impair (APAP), peptic ulcer (ASA); severe renal impair **Contra:** Allergy **Supplied:** *Darvon:* Propoxyphene HCl caps 65 mg. *Darvon-N:* Propoxyphene napsylate 100-mg tabs. *Darvocet-N:* Propoxyphene napsylate 50 mg/APAP 325 mg. *Darvocet-N 100:* Propoxyphene napsylate 100 mg/APAP 650 mg. *Darvon Compound-65:* Propoxyphene HCl caps 65-mg/ASA 389 mg/caffeine 32 mg. *Darvon-N w/ASA:* Propoxyphene napsylate 100 mg/ASA 325 mg **SE:** OD can be lethal; ↓ BP, dizziness, sedation, GI upset, ↑ levels on LFTs

Propranolol (Inderal)

Uses: *HTN, angina, MI, hyperthyroidism, essential tremor, hypertrophic subaortic stenosis, pheochromocytoma; prevents migraines & atrial arrhythmias* **Action:** β-Adrenergic receptor blocker, β_1, β_2; only β-blocker to block conversion of T_4 to T_3 **Dose:** *Adults. Angina:* 80–320 mg/d PO ÷ bid–qid or 80–160 mg/d SR. *Arrhythmia:* 10–80 mg PO tid–qid or 1 mg IV slowly, repeat q5min, 5 mg max. *HTN:* 40 mg PO bid or 60–80 mg/d SR, ↑ wkly to max 640 mg/d. *Hypertrophic subaortic stenosis: 20–40 mg PO tid–qid. MI:* 180–240 mg PO ÷ tid–qid. *Migraine prophylaxis:* 80 mg/d ÷ qid–tid, ↑ wkly 160–240 mg/d ÷ tid–qid max; wean if no response in 6 wk. *Pheochromocytoma:* 30–60 mg/d ÷ tid–qid. *Thyrotoxicosis:* 1–3 mg IV × 1; 10–40 mg PO q6h. *Tremor:* 40 mg PO bid, ↑ PRN 320 mg/d max. *Peds. Arrhythmia:* 0.5–1.0 mg/kg/d ÷ tid–qid, ↑ PRN q3–7d to 60 mg/d max; 0.01–0.1 mg/kg IV over 10 min, 1 mg max. *HTN:* 0.5–1.0 mg/kg ÷ bid–qid, ↑ PRN q3–7d to 2 mg/kg/d max; ↓ in renal impair **Caution:** [C (1st tri, D if 2nd or 3rd tri), +] **Contra:** Uncompensated CHF, cardiogenic shock, bradycardia, heart block, PE, severe resp Dz **Supplied:** Tabs 10, 20, 40, 60, 80 mg; SR caps 60, 80, 120, 160 mg; oral soln 4, 8, 80 mg/mL; inj 1 mg/mL **SE:** Bradycardia, ↓ BP, fatigue, GI upset, ED

Propylthiouracil, PTU

Uses: *Hyperthyroidism* **Action:** ↓ Production of T_3 & T_4 & conversion of T_4 to T_3 **Dose:** *Adults.* Initial: 100 mg PO q8h (may need up to 1200 mg/d); after pt euthyroid (6–8 wk), taper dose by $^1/_2$ q4–6wk to maint, 50–150 mg/24 h; can usually D/C in 2–3 y; ↓ in elderly *Peds.* Initial: 5–7 mg/kg/24 h PO ÷ q8h. *Maint:* $^1/_3$–$^2/_3$ of initial dose **Caution:** [D, –] **Contra:** Allergy **Supplied:** Tabs 50 mg **SE:** Fever, rash, leukopenia, dizziness, GI upset, taste perversion, SLE-like syndrome **Notes:** Monitor pt clinically, check TFT

Protamine (generic)

Uses: *Reverse heparin effect* **Action:** Neutralize heparin by forming a stable complex **Dose:** Based on degree of heparin reversal; give IV slowly; 1 mg reverses approx 100 units of heparin given in the preceding 3–4 h, 50 mg max **Caution:** [C, ?] **Contra:** Allergy **Supplied:** Inj 10 mg/mL **SE:** Follow coags; anticoag effect if given w/o heparin; ↓ BP, bradycardia, dyspnea, hemorrhage

Pseudoephedrine (Sudafed, Novafed, Afrinol, others) [OTC]

Uses: *Decongestant* **Action:** Stimulates α-adrenergic receptors w/vasoconstriction **Dose:** *Adults.* 30–60 mg PO q6–8h; SR caps 120 mg PO q12h. *Peds.* 4 mg/kg/24 h PO ÷ qid; ↓ in renal insuff **Caution:** [C, +] **Contra:** Poorly con-

_AD, w/MAOIs **Supplied:** Tabs 30, 60 mg; caps 60 mg; SR
g; SR caps 120 mg; liq 7.5 mg/0.8 mL, 15, 30 mg/5 mL **SE:**
a, tachycardia, arrhythmias, nervousness, tremor *Notes:* Found in
ough/cold preparations; OTC restricted in most states

n (Metamucil, Serutan, Effer-Syllium) Uses: *Constipation
ic diverticular Dz* **Action:** Bulk laxative **Dose:** 1 tsp (7 g) in glass of H_2O
d–tid **Caution:** [B, ?] Effer-syllium (effervescent psyllium) usually contains
caution w/renal failure; phenylketonuria (in products w/aspartame) **Contra:**
suspected bowel obstruction **Supplied:** Granules 4, 25 g/tsp; powder 3.5 g/packet
SE: D, abdominal cramps, bowel obstruction, constipation, bronchospasm

Pyrazinamide (generic) Uses: *Active TB in combo w/other agents*
Action: Bacteriostatic; unknown mechanism **Dose:** *Adults.* 15–30 mg/kg/24 h PO
÷ tid–qid; max 2 g/d. *Peds.* 15–30 mg/kg/d PO ÷ qd–bid; ↓ w/renal/hepatic impair
Caution: [C, +/–] **Contra:** Severe hepatic damage, acute gout **Supplied:** Tabs
500 mg **SE:** Hepatotox, malaise, GI upset, arthralgia, myalgia, gout, photosensitivity **Notes:** Use in combo w/other anti-TB drugs; consult *MMWR* for latest TB
recommendations; dosage regimen differs for "directly observed" therapy

Pyridoxine, Vitamin B$_6$ Uses: *Rx & prevention of vitamin B$_6$ deficiency* **Action:** Vitamin B$_6$ supl **Dose:** *Adults.* Deficiency: 10–20 mg/d PO.
Drug-induced neuritis: 100–200 mg/d; 25–100 mg/d prophylaxis. *Peds.* 5–25 mg/
d × 3 wk **Caution:** [A (C if doses exceed RDA), +] **Contra:** Component allergy
Supplied: Tabs 25, 50, 100 mg; inj 100 mg/mL **SE:** Allergic Rxns, HA, N

Quazepam (Doral) [C-IV] Uses: *Insomnia* **Action:** Benzodiazepine
Dose: 7.5–15 mg PO hs PRN; ↓ in elderly & hepatic failure **Caution:** [X, ?/–]
narrow-angle glaucoma **Contra:** PRG, sleep apnea **Supplied:** Tabs 7.5, 15 mg
SE: Sedation, hangover, somnolence, resp depression **Notes:** Do not D/C
abruptly

Quetiapine (Seroquel) WARNING: ↑ Mortality in elderly with dementia-related psychosis **Uses:** *Acute exacerbations of schizophrenia* **Action:** Serotonin & dopamine antagonism **Dose:** 150–750 mg/d; initiate at 25–100 mg bid–
tid; slowly ↑ dose; ↓ dose for hepatic & geriatric pts **Caution:** [C, –] **Contra:**
Component allergy **Supplied:** Tabs 25, 100, 200 mg **SE:** Reports of confusion w/
nefazodone; HA, somnolence, weight gain, orthostatic ↓ BP, dizziness, cataracts,
neuroleptic malignant syndrome, tardive dyskinesia, QT prolongation

Quinapril (Accupril) WARNING: ACE inhibitors used during the 2nd &
3rd tri of PRG can cause fetal injury & death **Uses:** *HTN, CHF, DN, post-MI*
Action: ACE inhibitor **Dose:** 10–80 mg PO qd ×1; ↓ in renal impair **Caution:**
[D, +] **Contra:** ACE inhibitor sensitivity or angioedema **Supplied:** Tabs 5, 10,
20, 40 mg **SE:** Dizziness, HA, ↓ BP, impaired renal Fxn, angioedema, taste perversion, cough

Quinidine (Quinidex, Quinaglute) Uses: *Prevention of tachydys-
rhythmias, malaria* **Action:** Class 1A antiarrhythmic **Dose:** *Adults. AF/flutter
conversion:* After digitalization, 200 mg q2–3h × 8 doses; ↑ qd to 3–4 g max or
nl rhythm. *Peds.* 15–60 mg/kg/24 h PO in 4–5 ÷ doses; ↓ in renal impair **Caution:** [C, +] w/ritonavir **Contra:** Digitalis tox & AV block; conduction disorders
Supplied: *Sulfate:* Tabs 200, 300 mg; SR tabs 300 mg. *Gluconate:* SR tabs 324
mg; inj 80 mg/mL **SE:** Extreme ↓ BP w/IV use; syncope, QT prolongation, GI
upset, arrhythmias, fatigue, cinchonism (tinnitus, hearing loss, delirium, visual

changes), fever, hemolytic anemia, thrombocytopenia, rash **Notes:** Check le (Table 22–2, page 628); sulfate salt 83% quinidine; gluconate salt 62% quiⁱ dine; use w/drug that slows AV conduction (eg, digoxin, diltiazem, β-blocker)

Quinupristin–Dalfopristin (Synercid) Uses: *Vancomycin-resistan Infxns due to *E. faecium* & other gram(+)* **Action:** ↓ Ribosomal protein synthesis. *Spectrum:* Vancomycin-resistant *E. faecium,* methicillin-susceptible *S. aureus, S. pyogenes;* not active against *E. faecalis* **Dose:** *Adults & Peds.* 7.5 mg/kg IV q8–12h (use central line if possible); incompatible w/NS or heparin; flush IV w/dextrose; ↓ in hepatic failure **Caution:** [B, M] Multiple drug interactions (eg, cyclosporine) **Contra:** Component allergy **Supplied:** Inj 500 mg (150 mg quinupristin/350 mg dalfopristin) **SE:** Hyperbilirubinemia, inf site Rxns & pain, arthralgia, myalgia

Rabeprazole (Aciphex) Uses: *PUD, GERD, ZE* **Action:** Proton-pump inhibitor **Dose:** 20 mg/d; may ↑ to 60 mg/d; do not crush tabs **Caution:** [B, ?/–] **Supplied:** Tabs 60 mg **SE:** HA, fatigue, GI upset

Raloxifene (Evista) Uses: *Prevent osteoporosis* **Action:** Partial antagonist of estrogen, behaves like estrogen **Dose:** 60 mg/d **Caution:** [X, –] **Contra:** Thromboembolism, PRG **Supplied:** Tabs 60 mg **SE:** Chest pain, insomnia, rash, hot flashes, GI upset, hepatic dysfunction

Ramipril (Altace) WARNING: ACE inhibitors used during the 2nd & 3rd tri of PRG can cause fetal injury & death Uses: *HTN, CHF, DN, post-MI* **Action:** ACE inhibitor **Dose:** 2.5–20 mg/d PO ÷ qd–bid; ↓ in renal failure **Caution:** [D, +] **Contra:** ACE-inhibitor-induced angioedema **Supplied:** Caps 1.25, 2.5, 5, 10 mg **SE:** Cough, HA, dizziness, ↓ BP, renal impair, angioedema **Notes:** OK in combo w/diuretics

Ranitidine Hydrochloride (Zantac) Uses: *Duodenal ulcer, active benign ulcers, hypersecretory conditions & GERD* **Action:** H₂-receptor antagonist **Dose:** *Adults. Ulcer:* 150 mg PO bid, 300 mg PO hs, or 50 mg IV q6–8h; or 400 mg IV/d cont inf, then maint of 150 mg PO hs. *Hypersecretion:* 150 mg PO bid, up to 600 mg/d. *GERD:* 300 mg PO bid; maint 300 mg PO hs. *Dyspepsia:* 75 mg PO qd–bid *Peds.* 0.75–1.5 mg/kg/dose IV q6–8h or 1.25–2.5 mg/kg/dose PO q12h; ↓ in renal failure **Caution:** [B, +] **Contra:** Component allergy **Supplied:** Tabs 75 [OTC], 150, 300 mg; effervescent tabs 150 mg; syrup 15 mg/mL; inj 25 mg/mL **SE:** Dizziness, sedation, rash, GI upset **Notes:** PO & parenteral doses differ

Rasburicase (Elitek) Uses: *Reduce ↑ uric acid due to tumor lysis (peds)* **Action:** Catalyzes uric acid **Dose:** *Peds.* 0.15 or 0.20 mg/kg IV over 30 min, qd × 5 **Caution:** [C, ?/–] Falsely ↓ uric acid values **Contra:** Anaphylaxis, screen for G6PD deficiency to avoid hemolysis, methemoglobinemia **Supplied:** 1.5 mg inj **SE:** Fever, neutropenia, GI upset, HA, rash

Repaglinide (Prandin) Uses: *Type 2 DM* **Action:** ↑ pancreatic insulin release **Dose:** 0.5–4 mg ac, PO start 1–2 mg, ↑ to 16 mg/d max; take pc **Caution:** [C, ?/–] **Contra:** DKA, type 1 DM **Supplied:** Tabs 0.5, 1, 2 mg **SE:** HA, hyper/hypoglycemia, GI upset

Reteplase (Retavase) Uses: *Post-AMI* **Action:** Thrombolytic agent **Dose:** 10 units IV over 2 min, 2nd dose in 30 min, 10 units IV over 2 min **Caution:** [C, ?/–] **Contra:** Internal bleeding, spinal surgery/trauma, Hx CNS vascu-

.ontrolled ↓ BP, sensitivity to thrombolytics **Supplied:** Inj
. Bleeding, allergic reactions

azole) Uses: *RSV Infxn in infants; hepatitis C (in combo
.fa-2b)* **Action:** Unknown **Dose:** *RSV:* 6 g in 300 mL sterile H₂O,
.2–18 h. *Hep C:* 600 mg PO bid in combo w/interferon alfa-2b (see
Alfa-2b & Ribavirin Combo [Rebetron], page 552) **Caution:** [X, ?]
.umulate on soft contact lenses **Contra:** PRG, autoimmune hepatitis,
< 50 mL/min **Supplied:** Powder for aerosol 6 g; caps 200 mg **SE:** fatigue,
, GI upset, anemia, myalgia, alopecia, bronchospasm **Notes:** Aerosolized by
SPAG; monitor Hbg/Hct; PRG test monthly

Rifabutin (Mycobutin) Uses: *Prevent *M. avium* complex Infxn in AIDS
pts w/CD4 count < 100* **Action:** ↓ DNA-dependent RNA polymerase activity
Dose: *Adults.* 150–300 mg/d PO. *Peds.* 1 y: 15–25 mg/kg/d PO. *2–10 y:*
4.4–18.8 mg/kg/d PO. *14–16 y:* 2.8–5.4 mg/kg/d PO **Caution:** [B; ?/–] WBC
< 1000/μL or platelets < 50,000/μL; ritonavir **Contra:** Allergy **Supplied:** Caps
150 mg **SE:** Discolored urine, rash, neutropenia, leukopenia, myalgia, ↑ LFTs
Notes: SEs/interactions similar to rifampin

Rifampin (Rifadin) Uses: *TB & Rx & prophylaxis of *N. meningitidis, H.
influenzae,* or *S. aureus* carriers*; adjunct for severe *S. aureus* **Action:** ↓ DNA-
dependent RNA polymerase **Dose:** *Adults.* N. meningitidis & *H. influenzae carrier:* 600 mg/d PO for 4 d. *TB:* 600 mg PO or IV qd or 2×/wk w/combo regimen.
Peds. 10–20 mg/kg/dose PO or IV qd–bid; ↓ in hepatic failure **Caution:** [C, +]
Amprenavir, multiple drug interactions **Contra:** Allergy, presence of active *N.
meningitidis* Infxn, w/saquinavir/ritonavir **Supplied:** Caps 150, 300 mg; inj 600
mg **SE:** Orange-red discoloration of bodily fluids, ↑ LFTs, flushing, HA **Notes:**
Never use as single agent w/active TB

Rifapentine (Priftin) Uses: *Pulmonary TB* **Action:** ↓ DNA-dependent
RNA polymerase. *Spectrum: M. tuberculosis* **Dose:** *Intensive phase:* 600 mg PO
2×/wk for 2 mo; separate doses by 3 or more d. *Continuation phase:* 600 mg/wk
for 4 mo; part of 3–4 drug regimen **Caution:** [C, red-orange breast milk] ↓ protease inhibitor efficacy, antiepileptics, β-blockers, CCBs **Contra:** Allergy to rifamycin **Supplied:** 150-mg tabs **SE:** Neutropenia, hyperuricemia, HTN, HA,
dizziness, rash, GI upset, blood dyscrasias, ↑ LFTs, hematuria, discolored secretions **Notes:** Monitor LFTs

Rifaximin (Xifaxan) Uses: *Travelers' diarrhea (noninvasive strains of *E.
coli*) in patients > 12 y* **Action:** Not absorbed, derivative of rifamycin. *Spectrum: E. coli* **Dose:** 1 tab PO qd × 3 d **Caution:** [C, ?/–] Allergy (rash,
angioedema, urticaria); pseudomembranous colitis **Contra:** Allergy to rifamycin **Supplied:** Tabs 200 mg **SE:** Flatulence, HA, abdominal pain, GI distress,
fever **Notes:** D/C if Sx worsen or persist > 24–48 h, or w/fever or blood in stool

Rimantadine (Flumadine) Uses: *Prophylaxis & Rx of influenza A viral
Infxns Antiviral* **Action:Dose:** *Adults & Peds > 9 y.* 100 mg PO bid. *Peds 1–9 y.*
5 mg/kg/d PO, 150 mg/d max; qd w/severe renal/hepatic impair & elderly; initiate
w/in 48 h of Sx onset **Caution:** [C, –] w/cimetidine; avoid in PRG or breast feeding
Contra: Component & amantadine allergy **Supplied:** Tabs 100 mg; syrup 50 mg/5
mL **SE:** Orthostatic ↓ BP, edema, dizziness, GI upset, ↓ Sz threshold

22

Rimexolone (Vexol Ophthalmic) Uses: *Postop inflammation & uve-
itis* **Action:** Steroid **Dose:** *Adults & Peds > 2 y.* *Uveitis:* 1–2 gtt/h daytime &

q2h at night, taper to 1 gt q4h. *Postop:* 1–2 gtt qid < 2 wk **Caution:** [C, ?/–] Ocular Infxns **Supplied:** Susp 1%; **SE:** Blurred vision, local irritation **Notes:** Taper dose

Risedronate (Actonel) Uses: *Paget Dz; treat/prevent glucocorticoid-induced/postmenopausal osteoporosis* **Action:** Bisphosphonate; ↓ osteoclast-mediated bone resorption **Dose:** *Paget Dz:* 30 mg/d PO for 2 mo. *Osteoporosis Rx/prevention:* 5 mg qd or 35 mg qwk; 30 min before 1st food/drink of the d; stay upright for at least 30 min after **Caution:** [C, ?/–] Ca supls & antacids ↓ absorption **Contra:** Component allergy, ↓ Ca^{2+}, esophageal abnormalities, unable to stand/sit for 30 min, CrCl < 30 mL/min **Supplied:** Tabs 5, 30, 35 mg **SE:** HA, D, abdominal pain, arthralgia; flu-like Sxs, rash, esophagitis, bone pain **Notes:** Monitor LFT, Ca^{2+}, PO_4^{3-}, K^+

Risperidone (Risperdal) WARNING: ↑ Mortality in elderly with dementia-related psychosis Uses: *Psychotic disorders (schizophrenia),* dementia of the elderly, bipolar disorder, mania, Tourette disorder, autism **Action:** Benzisoxazole antipsychotic **Dose:** *Adults.* 0.5–6 mg PO bid. *Peds & Adolescents.* 0.25 mg PO bid, ↑ q5–7d; ↓ start dose w/elderly, renal/hepatic impair *Caution:* [C, –], ↑ BP w/antihypertensives, clozapine **Contra:** Component allergy **Supplied:** Tabs 0.25, 0.5, 1, 2, 3, 4 mg; soln 1 mg/mL **SE:** Orthostatic ↓ BP, EPS w/ high dose, tachycardia, arrhythmias, sedation, dystonia, neuroleptic malignant syndrome, sexual dysfunction, constipation, xerostomia, blood dyscrasias, cholestatic jaundice, weight gain **Notes:** Several weeks for effect

Ritonavir (Norvir) Uses: *HIV* **Action:** Protease inhibitor; ↓ maturation of immature noninfectious virions to mature infectious virus **Dose:** *Adults.* Initial 300 mg PO bid, titrate over 1 wk to 600 mg PO bid (titration will ↓ GI SE). *Peds* ≥2 y. 250 mg/m^2 titrate to 400 mg bid (adjust w/amprenavir, indinavir, nelfinavir & saquinavir); (w/food) **Caution:** [B, +] w/ergotamine, amiodarone, bepridil, flecainide, propafenone, quinidine, pimozide, midazolam, triazolam **Contra:** W/ergotamine, amiodarone, bepridil, flecainide, propafenone, quinidine, pimozide, midazolam, triazolam, St. John's wort **Supplied:** Caps 100 mg; soln 80 mg/mL **SE:** ↑ triglycerides, ↑ LFTs, N/V/D/cramps, abdominal pain, taste perversion, anemia, weakness, HA, fever, malaise, rash, paresthesias **Notes:** Refrigerate

Rivastigmine (Exelon) Uses: *Mild–moderate dementia in Alzheimer Dz* **Action:** Enhances cholinergic activity **Dose:** 1.5 mg bid; ↑ to 6 mg bid, w/ ↑ at 2–wk intervals (w/food) **Caution:** [B, ?] β-Blockers, CCBs, smoking, neuromuscular blockade, digoxin **Contra:** Allergy to rivastigmine or carbamates **Supplied:** Caps 1.5, 3, 4.5, 6 mg; soln 2 mg/mL **SE:** Dose-related GI effects, N/ V/D; dizziness, insomnia, fatigue, tremor, diaphoresis, HA **Notes:** Swallow capsules whole, do not break, chew, or crush; avoid EtOH

Rizatriptan (Maxalt, Maxalt MLT) (See Table 22–11, page 645)

Rocuronium (Zemuron) Uses: *Skeletal muscle relaxation during rapid-sequence intubation, surgery, or mechanical ventilation* **Action:** Nondepolarizing neuromuscular blocker **Dose:** *Rapid sequence intubation:* 0.6–1.2 mg/kg IV. *Continuous inf:* 4–16 mcg/kg/min IV; ↓ in hepatic impair **Caution:** [C, ?] Aminoglycosides, vancomycin, tetracycline, polymyxins enhance blockade **Contra:** Component or pancuronium allergy **Supplied:** 10 mg/mL 5,10 mL vials **SE:** BP changes, tachycardia

22

Ropinirole (Requip) Uses: *Rx of Parkinson Dz* Action: Dopamine agonist Dose: Initial 0.25 mg PO tid, wkly ↑ 0.25 mg/dose, to 3 mg max Caution: [C, ?/–] Severe CV, renal, or hepatic impair Contra: Component allergy Supplied: Tabs 0.25, 0.5, 1, 2, 5 mg SE: Syncope, postural ↓ BP, N/V, HA, somnolence, hallucinations, dyskinesias Notes: D/C w/7-d taper

Rosiglitazone (Avandia) Uses: *Type 2 DM* Action: ↑ insulin sensitivity Dose: 4–8 mg/d PO or in 2 ÷ doses (w/o regard to meals) Caution: [C, –] Not for DKA; w/ESRD (renal elimination) Contra: Active liver Dz Supplied: Tabs 2, 4, 8 mg SE: Weight gain, hyperlipidemia, HA, edema, fluid retention, exacerbated CHF, hyper/hypoglycemia, hepatic damage

Rosuvastatin (Crestor) Uses: *Rx primary hypercholesterolemia & mixed dyslipidemia* Action: HMG-CoA reductase inhibitor Dose: 5–40 mg PO qd; max 5 mg/d w/cyclosporine, 10 mg/d w/gemfibrozil or CrCl < 30 mL/min (avoid Al-/Mg-based antacids for 2 h after) Caution: [X,?/–] Contra: Active liver Dz or unexplained ↑ LFT Supplied: Tabs 5, 10, 20, 40 mg SE: Myalgia, constipation, asthenia, abdominal pain, nausea, myopathy, rarely rhabdomyolysis Notes: May ↑ warfarin effect; monitor LFTs at baseline, 12 wk, then q6mo; ↓ dose in Asian patients

Salmeterol (Serevent) Uses: *Asthma, exercise-induced asthma, COPD* Action: Sympathomimetic bronchodilator, β_2–agonist Dose: *Adults & Peds* ≥12 y. 1 Diskus-dose inhaled bid Caution: [C, ?/–] Contra: Acute asthma; w/in 14 d of MAOI Supplied: Dry powder disk SE: HA, pharyngitis, tachycardia, arrhythmias, nervousness, GI upset, tremors Notes: Not for acute attacks; also prescribe short-acting β-agonist

Saquinavir (Fortovase) Uses: *HIV Infxn* Action: HIV protease inhibitor Dose: 1200 mg PO tid w/in 2 h pc (dose adjust w/ritonavir, delavirdine, lopinavir & nelfinavir) Caution: [B, +] w/rifampin, ketoconazole, statins, sildenafil Contra: Allergy, sun exposure w/o sunscreen/clothing, triazolam, midazolam, ergots, rifampin Supplied: Caps 200 mg SE: Dyslipidemia, lipodystrophy, rash, hyperglycemia, GI upset, weakness, hepatic dysfunction Notes: Take 2h after meal, avoid direct sunlight

Sargramostim, GM-CSF (Prokine, Leukine) Uses: *Myeloid recovery after BMT or chemo* Action: Recombinant GF, Activates mature granulocytes & macrophages Dose: *Adults & Peds.* 250 mcg/m^2/d IV for 21 d (BMT) Caution: [C, ?/–] Lithium, corticosteroids Contra: > 10% blasts, allergy to yeast, concurrent chemo/RT Supplied: Inj 250, 500 mcg SE: Bone pain, fever, ↓ BP, tachycardia, flushing, GI upset, myalgia Notes: Rotate inj sites; use APAP PRN for pain

Scopolamine, Scopolamine Transdermal (Scopace, Transderm-Scop) Uses: *Prevent N/V associated w/motion sickness, anesthesia, opiates; mydriatic,* cycloplegic, Rx iridocyclitis Action: Anticholinergic, antiemetic Dose: 1 patch behind ear q3d; apply > 4 h before exposure; 0.4–0.8 PO, repeat PRN q4–6h; ↓ in elderly Caution: [C, +] APAP, levodopa, ketoconazole, digitalis, KCl Contra: narrow-angle glaucoma, GI or GU obstruction, thyrotoxicosis, paralytic ileus Supplied: Patch 1.5 mg, tabs 0.4 mg, ophth 0.25% SE: Xerostomia, drowsiness, blurred vision, tachycardia, constipation Notes: Do not blink excessively after dose, wait 5 min before dosing other eye; activity w/ patch requires several hours

22

Secobarbital (Seconal) [C-II] Uses: *Insomnia,* preanesthetic agent **Action:** Rapid-acting barbiturate **Dose:** *Adults.* 100–200 mg, 100–300 mg preop. *Peds.* 2–6 mg/kg/dose, 100 mg/max, ↓ in elderly **Caution:** [D, +] CYP2C9, 3A3/4, 3A5–7 inducer (page 647); ↑ tox w/other CNS depressants **Contra:** Porphyria, PRG **Supplied:** Caps 100 mg **SE:** Tolerance in 1–2 wk; resp depression, CNS depression, porphyria, photosensitivity

Selegiline (Eldepryl) Uses: Parkinson Dz **Action:** MAOI **Dose:** 5 mg PO bid; ↓ in elderly **Caution:** [C, ?] Meperidine, SSRI, TCAs **Contra:** Concurrent meperidine **Supplied:** Tabs/caps 5 mg **SE:** N, dizziness, orthostatic ↓ BP, arrhythmias, tachycardia, edema, confusion, xerostomia **Notes:** ↓ carbidopa/levodopa if used in combo

Selenium Sulfide (Exsel Shampoo, Selsun Blue Shampoo, Selsun Shampoo) Uses: *Scalp seborrheic dermatitis,* scalp itching & flaking due to *dandruff*; tinea versicolor **Action:** Antiseborrheic **Dose:** *Dandruff, seborrhea:* Massage 5–10 mL into wet scalp, leave on 2–3 min, rinse, repeat; use 2×wk, then once q1–4wk PRN. *Tinea versicolor:* Apply 2.5% qd × d on area & lather w/small amounts of water; leave on 10 min, then rinse **Caution:** [C, ?] **Contra:** Open wounds **Supplied:** Shampoo [OTC] 1, 2.5% **SE:** Dry or oily scalp, lethargy, hair discoloration, local irritation **Notes:** Do not use more than 2×/wk

Sertaconazole (Ertaczo) Uses: *Topical Rx interdigital tinea pedis* **Action:** Imidazole antifungal. *Spectrum: T. rubrum, T. mentagrophytes, E. floccosum* **Dose:** *Adults & Peds > 12.* Apply between toes & immediate surrounding healthy skin bid × 4 wk **Caution:** [C, ?] **Contra:** Component allergy **Supplied:** 2% cream **SE:** Contact dermatitis, dry/burning skin, tenderness **Notes:** Use in immunocompetent pts

Sertraline (Zoloft) **WARNING:** Closely monitor pts for worsening depression or emergence of suicidality, particularly in ped pts **Uses:** *Depression, panic disorders, OCD, posttraumatic stress disorders (PTSD),* social anxiety disorder, eating disorders, premenstrual disorders **Action:** ↓ neuronal uptake of serotonin **Dose:** *Adults. Depression:* 50–200 mg/d PO. *PTSD:* 25 mg PO qd × wk, then 50 mg PO qd, 200 mg/d max. *Peds.* 6–12 y: 25 mg PO qd. *13–17 y:* 50 mg PO qd **Caution:** [C, ?/–] w/haloperidol (serotonin syndrome); sumatriptan, linezolid, hepatic impair **Contra:** MAOI use w/in 14 d; concomitant pimozide **Supplied:** Tabs 25, 50, 100 mg **SE:** Can activate manic/hypomanic state; weight loss; insomnia, somnolence, fatigue, tremor, xerostomia, N/D, dyspepsia, ejaculatory dysfunction, ↓ libido, hepatotox

Sevelamer (Renagel) Uses: *↓ serum phosphorus in ESRD* **Action:** Binds intestinal PO_4^- **Dose:** 2–4 capsules PO tid w/meals; adjust based on PO_4^- **Caution:** [C, ?] **Contra:** Bowel obstruction **Supplied:** Capsules 403 mg **SE:** BP changes, N/V/D, dyspepsia, thrombosis **Notes:** Do not open or chew capsules; may ↓ fat-soluble vitamin absorption; 800 mg sevelamer = 667 mg Ca acetate

Sibutramine (Meridia) [C-IV] Uses: *Obesity* **Action:** Blocks uptake of norepinephrine, serotonin, dopamine **Dose:** 10 mg/d PO, may ↓ to 5 mg after 4 wk **Caution:** [C, –] SSRIs, lithium, dextromethorphan, opioids **Contra:** MAOI w/in 14 d, uncontrolled HTN, arrhythmias **Supplied:** Caps 5, 10, 15 mg **SE:** HA, insomnia, xerostomia, constipation, rhinitis, tachycardia, HTN **Notes:** Use w/low-calorie diet, monitor BP & HR

22

Sildenafil (Viagra, Revatio) Uses: *Viagra:* *Erectile dysfunction,* *Revatio:* *Pulmonary artery HTN* **Action:** ↓ Phosphodiesterase type 5 (responsible for cGMP breakdown); ↑ cGMP activity, causing smooth-muscle relaxation & ↑ flow to the corpus cavernosum and pulmonary vasculature; possible antiproliferative effect on pulmonary artery smooth muscle **Dose:** 25–100 mg PO 1 h before sexual activity, max × 1 d; ↓ if > 65 y; avoid fatty foods w/dose; Revatio 20 mg PO tid **Caution:** [B, ?] CYP3A4 inhibitors **Contra:** W/nitrates; retinitis pigmentosa; hepatic/severe renal impair **Supplied:** Tabs (Viagra) 25, 50, 100 mg, tabs (Revatio) 20 mg **SE:** HA; flushing; dizziness; blue haze visual disturbance (usually reversible) **Notes:** Cardiac events in absence of nitrates debatable

Silver Nitrate (Dey-Drop, others) Uses: *Removal of granulation tissue & warts; prophylaxis in burns* **Action:** Caustic antiseptic & astringent **Dose:** *Adults & Peds.* Apply to moist surface 2–3 × wk for several wks or until effect **Caution:** [C, ?] **Contra:** Do not use on broken skin **Supplied:** Topical impregnated applicator sticks, oint 10%, soln 10, 25, 50%; ophth 1% amp **SE:** May stain tissue black, usually resolves; local irritation, methemoglobinemia **Notes:** D/C if redness or irritation develops; no longer used in US for newborn prevention of GC conjunctivitis

Silver Sulfadiazine (Silvadene) Uses: *Prevention & Rx of Infxn in 2nd- & 3rd-degree burns* **Action:** Bactericidal **Dose:** *Adults & Peds.* Aseptically cover the area w/¹/₁₆-in coating bid **Caution:** [B unless near term, ?/–] **Contra:** Infants < 2 mo, PRG near term **Supplied:** Cream 1% **SE:** Itching, rash, skin discoloration, blood dyscrasias, hepatitis, allergy **Notes:** Systemic absorption w/extensive application

Simethicone (Mylicon) [OTC] Uses: Flatulence **Action:** Defoaming action **Dose:** *Adults & Peds.* 40–125 mg PO pc & hs PRN **Caution:** [C, ?] **Contra:** Intestinal perforation or obstruction **Supplied:** OTC Tabs 80, 125 mg; caps 125 mg; gt 40 mg/0.6 mL **SE:** N/D **Notes:** Available in combo products OTC

Simvastatin (Zocor) Uses: ↓ Cholesterol **Action:** HMG-CoA reductase inhibitor **Dose:** 5–80 mg PO; w/meals; ↓ in renal insuff **Caution:** [X, –] Avoid concurrent use of gemfibrozil **Contra:** PRG, liver Dz **Supplied:** Tabs 5, 10, 20, 40 mg **SE:** HA, GI upset, myalgia, myopathy (muscle pain, tenderness or weakness with creatine kinase 10 × ULN), hepatitis **Notes:** Follow LFTs

Sirolimus, Rapamycin (Rapamune) WARNING: Can cause immunosuppression & Infxns Uses: Prophylaxis of organ rejection **Action:** ↓ T-lymphocyte activation **Dose:** *Adults > 40 kg.* 6 mg PO on d 1, then 2 mg/d PO. *Adults < 40 kg & Peds* ≥ 13 y. 3 mg/m² load, then 1 mg/m²/d (in H_2O/orange juice; no grapefruit juice while on sirolimus); take 4 h after cyclosporine; ↓ in hepatic impair **Caution:** [C, ?/–] Grapefruit juice, ketoconazole **Contra:** Component allergy **Supplied:** Soln 1 mg/mL, tab 1 mg **SE:** HTN, edema, CP, fever, HA, insomnia, acne, rash, ↑ cholesterol, GI upset, ↑/↓ K^+, Infxns, blood dyscrasias, arthralgia, tachycardia, renal impair, hepatic artery thrombosis, graft loss & death in de novo liver transplant **Notes:** Levels not needed except in liver failure (trough 9–17 ng/mL)

Smallpox Vaccine (Dryvax) Uses: Immunization against smallpox (variola virus) **Action:** Active immunization (live attenuated vaccinia virus) **Dose:** *Adults (routine nonemergency) or all ages (emergency):* 2–3 punctures w/bifurcated needle dipped in vaccine into deltoid, posterior triceps muscle; check site for Rxn in 6–8 d; if major Rxn, site scabs & heals, leaving scar; if mild/equivocal

Rxn, repeat w/15 punctures **Caution:** [X, N/A] **Contra:** *Nonemergency use: Febrile* illness, immunosuppression, Hx eczema & their household contacts. *Emergency:* No absolute contraindications **Supplied:** Vial for reconstitution: 100 million pock-forming units/mL **SE:** Malaise, fever, regional lymphadenopathy, encephalopathy, rashes, spread of inoculation to other sites administered; Stevens–Johnson syndrome, eczema vaccinatum w/severe disability

Sodium Bicarbonate, NaHCO$_3$ Uses: *Alkalinize urine,* RTA, *metabolic acidosis, $\uparrow$ K$^+$, TCA OD* **Action:** Alkalinization **Dose:** *Adults.* Cardiac arrest: Initiate ventilation, 1 mEq/kg/dose IV; repeat 0.5 mEq/kg in 10 min once or based on acid–base status. *Metabolic acidosis:* 2–5 mEq/kg IV over 8 h & PRN according to acid–base status. *Alkalinize urine:* 4 g (48 mEq) PO, then 1–2 g q4h; adjust based on urine pH; 2 amp/1 L D$_5$W at 100–250 mL/h IV, monitor urine pH & serum bicarbonate. *Chronic renal failure:* 1–3 mEq/kg/d. *Distal RTA:* 1 mEq/ kg/d PO. *Peds > 1 y:* Cardiac arrest: See Adult dosage. *Peds < 1 y:* ECC: Initiate ventilation, 1:1 dilution 1 mEq/mL dosed 1 mEq/kg IV; can repeat w/0.5 mEq/kg in 10 min × 1 or according to acid–base status. *Chronic renal failure:* See Adult dosage. *Distal RTA:* 2–3 mEq/kg/d PO. *Proximal RTA:* 5–10 mEq/kg/d; titrate according to serum bicarbonate. *Alkalinize urine:* 84–840 mg/kg/d (1–10 mEq/kg/ d) in ÷ doses; adjust based on urine pH **Caution:** [C, ?] **Contra:** Alkalosis, $\uparrow$ Na$^+$, severe pulmonary edema, $\downarrow$ Ca^{2+} **Supplied:** Powder, tabs; 300 mg = 3.6 mEq; 325 mg = 3.8 mEq; 520 mg = 6.3 mEq; 600 mg = 7.3 mEq; 650 mg = 7.6 mEq; inj 1 mEq/1 mL vial or amp **SE:** Belching, edema, flatulence, $\uparrow$ Na$^+$, metabolic alkalosis **Notes:** 1 g neutralizes 12 mEq of acid; 50 mEq bicarb = 50 mEq Na; can make 3 amps in 1 L D$_5$W to = D$_5$NS w/150 mEq bicarb

Sodium Citrate (Bicitra) Uses: Alkalinize urine; dissolve uric acid & cysteine stones **Action:** Urinary alkalinization **Dose:** *Adults.* 2–6 tsp (10–30 mL) diluted in 1–3 oz H$_2$O pc & hs. *Peds.* 1–3 tsp (5–15 mL) diluted in 1–3 oz H$_2$O pc & hs; best after meals **Caution:** [C, +] **Contra:** Aluminum-based antacids; severe renal impair or Na-restricted diets **Supplied:** 15- or 30-mL unit dose: 16 (473 mL) or 4 (118 mL) fl oz **SE:** Tetany, metabolic alkalosis, $\uparrow$ K$^+$, GI upset; avoid use of multiple 50-mL amps; can cause $\uparrow$ Na$^+$/hyperosmolality **Notes:** 1 mL = 1 mEq Na & 1 mEq bicarb

Sodium Oxybate (Xyrem) [C-III] Uses: *Narcolepsy-associated cataplexy* **Action:** Inhibitory neurotransmitter **Dose:** *Adults & Peds* $\geq$ 16 y: 2.25 g PO qhs, second dose 2.5–4 h later; may $\uparrow$ 9 g/d max **Caution:** [B, ?/–] **Contra:** Succinic semialdehyde dehydrogenase deficiency; potentiates EtOH **Supplied:** 500 mg/mL 180-mL PO soln **SE:** Confusion, depression, diminished level of consciousness, incontinence, significant vomiting, resp depression, psychiatric Sxs **Notes:** May lead to dependence; synonym for γ-hydroxybutyrate (GHB), abused as a "date rape drug"; controlled distribution (prescriber & pt registration); must be administered when pt in bed

Sodium Phosphate (Visicol) Uses: Bowel prep before colonoscopy **Action:** Hyperosmotic laxative **Dose:** 3 tabs PO w/at least 8 oz clear liq every 15 min (20 tabs total night before procedure; 3–5 h before colonoscopy, repeat) **Caution:** [C, ?] Renal impair, electrolyte disturbances **Contra:** Megacolon, bowel obstruction, CHF, ascites, unstable angina, gastric retention, bowel perforation, colitis, hypomotility. **Supplied:** Tablets 2 g **SE:** QT prolongation, D, $\uparrow$ Na$^+$, flatulence, cramps

Sodium Polystyrene Sulfonate (Kayexalate) Uses: *$\uparrow$ K$^+$* **Action:** Na$^+$/K$^+$ ion-exchange resin **Dose:** *Adults.* 15–60 g PO or 30–60 g PR q6h based

22

on serum K⁺. **Peds.** 1 g/kg/dose PO or PR q6h based on serum K⁺ (given w/ agent, eg, sorbitol, to promote movement through the bowel) **Caution:** [C, M] **Contra:** ↑ Na⁺ **Supplied:** Powder; susp 15 g/60 mL sorbitol **SE:** ↑ Na⁺, ↓ K⁺, Na retention, GI upset, fecal impaction **Notes:** Enema acts more quickly than PO; PO most effective

Solifenacin (VESIcare) **Uses:** OAB **Action:** Antimuscarinic **Dose:** 5 mg PO qd, 10 mg max **Caution:** [C, ?/–] Bladder outflow or GI obstruction, ulcerative colitis, MyG, renal/hepatic impair, QT prolongation risk **Contra:** narrow-angle glaucoma, urinary/gastric retention **Supplied:** Tabs 5, 10 mg **SE:** Constipation, xerostomia **Notes:** Interacts w/azole antifungals; do not ↑ dose w/severe renal/moderate hepatic impair

Sorbitol (generic) **Uses:** *Constipation* **Action:** Laxative **Dose:** 30–60 mL PO of a 20–70% soln PRN **Caution:** [B, +] **Contra:** Anuria **Supplied:** Liq 70% **SE:** Edema, electrolyte losses, lactic acidosis, GI upset, xerostomia **Notes:** May be vehicle for many liq formulations (eg, zinc, Kayexalate)

Sotalol (Betapace) **WARNING:** Monitor pts for 1st 3 d of Rx to ↓ risks of arrhythmia **Uses:** *Ventricular arrhythmias, AF* **Action:** β-Adrenergic-blocking agent **Dose:** *Adults.* 80 mg PO bid; may be ↑ to 240–320 mg/d. *Peds.* Neonates: 9 mg/m² tid. *1–19 mo:* 20 mg/m² tid. *20–23 mo:* 29.1 mg/m² tid. ≥ 2 y: 30 mg/m² tid; ↓ in renal failure **Caution:** [B (1st tri) (D if 2nd or 3rd tri), +] **Contra:** Asthma, bradycardia, prolonged QT interval, 2nd- or 3rd-degree heart block w/o pacemaker, cardiogenic shock, uncontrolled CHF, CrCl < 40 mL/min **Supplied:** Tabs 80, 120, 160, 240 mg **SE:** Bradycardia, CP, palpitations, fatigue, dizziness, weakness, dyspnea **Notes:** Betapace should not be substituted for Betapace AF because of differences in labeling

Sotalol (Betapace AF) **WARNING:** To minimize risk of induced arrhythmia, pts initiated/reinitiated on Betapace AF should be placed for a minimum of 3 d (on their maint dose) in a facility that can provide cardiac resuscitation, continuous ECG monitoring & calculations of CrCl; Betapace should not be substituted for Betapace AF because of labeling differences **Uses:** *Maintain sinus rhythm for symptomatic A fib/flutter* **Action:** β-Adrenergic-blocking agent **Dose:** *Adults.* Initial CrCl > 60 mL/min: 80 mg PO q12h. *CrCl 40–60 mL/min:* 80 mg PO q2h; ↑ to 120 mg during hospitalization; monitor QT interval 2–4 h after each dose, w/ dose reduction or D/C if QT interval > 500 ms. *Peds.* Neonates: 9 mg/m² tid. *1–19 mo:* 20 mg/m² tid. *20–23 mo:* 29.1 mg/m² tid. ≥ 2 y: 30 mg/m² tid; can double all doses as max daily dose; allow ≥ 36 h between dosage titrations **Caution:** [B (1st tri; D if 2nd or 3rd tri), +] if converting from previous antiarrhythmic therapy **Contra:** Asthma, bradycardia, prolonged QT interval, 2nd- or 3rd-degree heart block w/o pacemaker, cardiogenic shock, uncontrolled CHF, CrCl < 40 mL/min **Supplied:** Tabs 80, 120, 160 mg **SE:** Bradycardia, CP, palpitations, fatigue, dizziness, weakness, dyspnea **Notes:** Follow renal Fxn & QT interval

Sparfloxacin (Zagam) **Uses:** *Community-acquired pneumonia, acute exacerbations of chronic bronchitis* **Action:** Quinolone; ↓ DNA gyrase **Dose:** 400 mg PO d 1, then 200 mg q24h × 10 d; ↓ in renal impair **Caution:** [C, ?/–] w/ theophylline, caffeine, sucralfate, warfarin & antacids **Contra:** w/QT prolongation & drugs that prolong QT interval **Supplied:** Tabs 200 mg **SE:** Phototox (even daylight through windows); restlessness, N/V/D, rash, ruptured tendons, ↑ LFTs, sleep disorders, confusion, convulsions **Notes:** Protect from sunlight up to 5 d after last dose

Spironolactone (Aldactone) Uses: *Hyperaldosteronism, ascites from CHF or cirrhosis* **Action:** Aldosterone antagonist; K^+-sparing diuretic **Dose:** *Adults.* 25–100 mg PO qid; CHF (NYHA class III–IV) 25–50 mg/d. *Peds.* 1–3.3 mg/kg/24 h PO ÷ bid–qid. *Neonates:* 0.5–1 mg/kg/dose q8h; w/food **Caution:** [D, +] **Contra:** ↑ K^+, renal failure, anuria **Supplied:** Tabs 25, 50, 100 mg **SE:** ↑ K^+ & gynecomastia, arrhythmia, sexual dysfunction, confusion, dizziness

Stavudine (Zerit) **WARNING:** Lactic acidosis & severe hepatomegaly w/ steatosis & pancreatitis reported **Uses:** *Advanced HIV* **Action:** RT inhibitor **Dose:** *Adults.* > 60 kg: 40 mg bid. *< 60 kg:* 30 mg bid. *Peds.* Birth–13 d: 0.5 mg/kg q12h. *> 14 d & < 30 kg:* 1 mg/kg q12h. ≥ 30 kg: Adult dose; ↓ in renal failure **Caution:** [C, +] **Contra:** Allergy **Supplied:** Caps 15, 20, 30, 40 mg; soln 1 mg/mL **SE:** Peripheral neuropathy, HA, chills, fever, malaise, rash, GI upset, anemia, lactic acidosis, ↑ LFTs, pancreatitis **Notes:** Take w/plenty of H_2O

Steroids, Systemic (See also Table 22–4, page 633) The following relates only to the commonly used systemic glucocorticoids **Uses:** *Endocrine disorders* (adrenal insuff), *rheumatoid disorders, collagen–vascular Dzs, dermatologic Dzs, allergic states, cerebral edema,* nephritis, nephrotic syndrome, immunosuppression for transplantation, ↑ Ca^{2+}, malignancies (breast, lymphomas), preop (in any pt who has been on steroids in the previous year, known hypoadrenalism, preop for adrenalectomy); inj into joints/tissue **Action:** Glucocorticoid **Dose:** Varies w/use & institutional protocols. *Adrenal insuff, acute: Adults.* Hydrocortisone: 100 mg IV; then 300 mg/d ÷ q6h; convert to 50 mg PO q8h × 6 doses, taper to 30–50 mg/d ÷ bid. *Peds.* Hydrocortisone: 1–2 mg/kg IV, then 150–250 mg/d ÷ tid. *Adrenal insuff, chronic (physiologic replacement):* May need mineralocorticoid supl such as Florinef. *Adults.* Hydrocortisone 20 mg PO qAM, 10 mg PO qPM; cortisone 0.5–0.75 mg/kg/d ÷ bid; cortisone 0.25–0.35 mg/kg/d IM; dexamethasone 0.03–0.15 mg/kg/d or 0.6–0.75 mg/m²/d ÷ q6–12h PO, IM, IV. *Peds.* Hydrocortisone: 0.5–0.75 mg/kg/d PO tid; hydrocortisone succinate 0.25–0.35 mg/kg/d IM. *Asthma, acute: Adults.* Methylprednisolone 60 mg PO/IV q6h or dexamethasone 12 mg IV q6h. *Peds.* Prednisolone 1–2 mg/kg/d or prednisone 1–2 mg/kg/d ÷ qd–bid for up to 5 d; methylprednisolone 2–4 mg/kg/d IV ÷ tid; dexamethasone 0.1–0.3 mg/kg/d divided q6h. *Congenital adrenal hyperplasia: Peds.* Initial hydrocortisone 30–36 mg/m²/d PO ÷ ¹/₃ dose qAM, ²/₃ dose qPM; maint 20–25 mg/m²/d ÷ bid. *Extubation/airway edema: Adults.* Dexamethasone 0.5–1 mg/kg/d IM/IV ÷ q6h (start 24 h before extubation; continue × 4 more doses). *Peds.* Dexamethasone 0.1–0.3 mg/kg/d ÷ q6h × 3–5 d (start 48–72h before extubation) *Immunosuppressive/antiinflammatory: Adults & Older Peds. Hydrocortisone:* 15–240 mg PO, IM, IV q12h. *Methylprednisolone:* 4–48 mg/d PO, taper to lowest effective dose. *Methylprednisolone Na succinate:* 10–80 mg/d IM. *Adults.* Prednisone or prednisolone: 5–60 mg/d PO ÷ qd–qid. *Infants & Younger Children.* Hydrocortisone 2.5–10 mg/kg/d PO ÷ q6–8h; 1–5 mg/kg/d IM/IV ÷ bid. *Nephrotic syndrome: Peds.* Prednisolone or prednisone 2 mg/kg/d PO tid–qid until urine is protein-free for 5 d, use up to 28 d; for persistent proteinuria, 4 mg/kg/dose PO qod max 120 mg/d for an additional 28 d; maint 2 mg/kg/d qod for 28 d; taper over 4–6 wk (max 80 mg/d). *Septic shock* (controversial): *Adults.* Hydrocortisone 500 mg–1 g IM/IV q2–6h. *Peds.* Hydrocortisone 50 mg/kg IM/IV, repeat q4–24 h PRN. *Status asthmaticus: Adults & Peds.* Hydrocortisone 1–2 mg/kg/dose IV q6h; then ↓ by 0.5–1 mg/kg q6h. *Rheumatic Dz: Adults.* Intraarticular: Hydrocortisone acetate 25–37.5 mg large joint, 10–25 mg small joint; methylprednisolone acetate 20–

22

80 mg large joint, 4–10 mg small joint. *Intrabursal:* Hydrocortisone acetate 25–37.5 mg. *Intraganglial:* Hydrocortisone acetate 25–37.5 mg. *Tendon sheath:* Hydrocortisone acetate 5–12.5 mg. *Periop steroid coverage:* Hydrocortisone 100 mg IV night before surgery, 1 h preop, intraop & 4, 8 & 12 h postop; postop day 1 100 mg IV q6h; postop day 2 100 mg IV q8h; postop day 3 100 mg IV q12h; postop day 4 50 mg IV q12h; postop day 5 25 mg IV q12h; resume prior PO dosing if chronic use or D/C if only periop coverage required. *Cerebral edema:* Dexamethasone 10 mg IV; then 4 mg IV q4–6h **Caution:** [C, ?/–] **Contra:** Active varicella Infxn, serious Infxn except TB, fungal Infxns **Supplied:** See Table 22–4, page 633. **SE:** ↑ appetite, hyperglycemia, ↓ K⁺, osteoporosis, nervousness, insomnia, "steroid psychosis," adrenal suppression **Notes:** Hydrocortisone succinate for systemic, acetate for intraarticular; never abruptly D/C steroids, taper dose

Streptokinase (Streptase, Kabikinase)   **Uses:** *Coronary artery thrombosis, acute massive PE, DVT & some occluded vascular grafts* **Action:** Activates plasminogen to plasmin that degrades fibrin **Dose:** *Adults.* PE: Load 250,000 units peripheral IV over 30 min, then 100,000 units/h IV for 24–72 h. *Coronary artery thrombosis:* 1.5 million units IV over 60 min. *DVT or arterial embolism:* Load as w/PE, then 100,000 units/h for 72 h. *Peds.* 3500–4000 units/ kg over 30 min, followed by 1000–1500 units/kg/h. *Occluded catheter* (controversial): 10,000–25,000 units in NS to final volume of catheter (leave in place for 1h, aspirate & flush catheter w/NS) **Caution:** [C, +] **Contra:** Streptococcal Infxn or streptokinase in last 6 mo, active bleeding, CVA, TIA, spinal surgery, or trauma in last month, vascular anomalies, severe hepatic or renal Dz, endocarditis, pericarditis, severe uncontrolled HTN **Supplied:** Powder for inj 250,000, 600,000, 750,000, 1,500,000 units **SE:** Bleeding, ↓ BP, fever, bruising, rash, GI upset, hemorrhage, anaphylaxis **Notes:** If maint inf inadequate to maintain thrombin clotting time 2–5 × control, see package for adjustments; antibodies remain 3–6 mo after dose

Streptomycin   **Uses:** *TB,* streptococcal or enterococcal endocarditis **Action:** Aminoglycoside; interferes w/protein synthesis **Dose:** *Adults.* Endocarditis: 1 g q12h 1–2 wk, then 500 mg q12h 1–4 wk. *TB:* 15 mg/kg/d (up to 1 g), directly observed therapy (DOT) 2 × wk 20–30 mg/kg/dose (max 1.5 g), DOT 3 × wk 25–30 mg/kg/dose (max 1g). *Peds.* 15 mg/kg/d; DOT 2 × wk 20–40 mg/ kg/dose (max 1 g); DOT 3 × wk 25–30 mg/kg/dose (max 1 g); ↓ in renal failure, either IM or IV over 30–60 min **Caution:** [D, +] **Contra:** PRG **Supplied:** Inj 400 mg/mL (1-g vial) **SE:** ↑ incidence of vestibular & auditory tox, neurotox, nephrotox **Notes:** Monitor levels: peak 20–30 mcg/mL, trough < 5 mcg/mL; toxic peak > 50, trough > 10

Streptozocin (Zanosar)   **Uses:** *Pancreatic islet cell tumors* & carcinoid tumors **Action:** DNA–DNA (interstrand) cross-linking; DNA, RNA & protein synthesis inhibitor **Dose:** Per protocol; ↓ in renal failure **Caution:** W/renal failure [D, ?/–] **Contra:** Caution, PRG **Supplied:** Inj 1 g **SE:** N/V, duodenal ulcers; myelosuppression rare (20%) & mild; nephrotox (proteinuria & azotemia often heralded by hypophosphatemia) dose-limiting; hypo/hyperglycemia; inj site Rxns **Notes:** Monitor Cr

Succimer (Chemet)   **Uses:** *Lead poisoning (levels > 45 mcg/mL)* **Action:** Heavy-metal chelating agent **Dose:** *Adults & Peds.* 10 mg/kg/dose q8h × 5 d, then 10 mg/kg/dose q12h for 14 d; ↓ in renal impair **Caution:** [C, ?] **Con-**

tra: Allergy **Supplied:** Caps 100 mg **SE:** Rash, fever, GI upset, hemorrhoids, metallic taste, drowsiness, ↑ LFTs **Notes:** Monitor lead levels, maintain hydration, may open capsules

Succinylcholine (Anectine, Quelicin, Sucostrin)
Uses: *Adjunct to general anesthesia to facilitate ET intubation & to induce skeletal muscle relaxation during surgery or mechanical ventilation* **Action:** Depolarizing neuromuscular blocking agent **Dose:** *Adults.* 1–1.5 mg/kg IV over 10–30 s, followed by 0.04–0.07 mg/kg PRN or 10–100 mcg/kg/min inf. *Peds.* 1–2 mg/kg/dose IV, followed by 0.3–0.6 mg/kg/dose q5min; ↓ in severe liver Dz **Caution:** [C, M] **Contra:** If risk for malignant hyperthermia; myopathy; recent major burn, multiple trauma, extensive skeletal muscle denervation **Supplied:** Inj 20, 50, 100 mg/mL; powder for inj 500 mg, 1 g/vial **SE:** May precipitate malignant hyperthermia, resp depression, or prolonged apnea; multiple drugs potentiate; observe for CV effects (arrhythmias, ↓ BP, brady/tachycardia); ↑ intraocular pressure, postop stiffness, salivation, myoglobinuria **Notes:** May be given IVP/inf/IM deltoid

Sucralfate (Carafate)
Uses: *Duodenal ulcers,* gastric ulcers, stomatitis, GERD, preventing stress ulcers, esophagitis **Action:** Forms ulcer-adherent complex that protects against acid, pepsin & bile acid **Dose:** *Adults.* 1 g PO qid, 1 h before meals & hs. *Peds.* 40–80 mg/kg/d ÷ q6h; continue 4–8 wk unless healing demonstrated by x-ray or endoscopy; separate from other drugs by 2 h; on empty stomach ac **Caution:** [B, +] **Contra:** Component allergy **Supplied:** Tabs 1 g; susp 1 g/10 mL **SE:** Constipation; D, dizziness, xerostomia **Notes:** Aluminum may accumulate in renal failure

Sulfacetamide (Bleph-10, Cetamide, Sodium Sulamyd)
Uses: *Conjunctival Infxns* **Action:** Sulfonamide antibiotic **Dose:** 10% oint apply qid & hs; soln for keratitis apply q2–3h based on severity **Caution:** [C, M] **Contra:** Sulfonamide sensitivity; age < 2 mo **Supplied:** Oint 10%; soln 10, 15, 30% **SE:** Irritation, burning; blurred vision, brow ache, Stevens–Johnson syndrome, photosensitivity

Sulfacetamide & Prednisolone (Blephamide, others)
Uses: *Steroid-responsive inflammatory ocular conditions w/Infxn or a risk of Infxn* **Action:** Antibiotic & antiinflammatory **Dose:** *Adults & Peds > 2 y.* Apply oint to lower conjunctival sac qd–qid; soln 1–3 gtt 2–3 h while awake **Caution:** [C, ?/–] Sulfonamide sensitivity; age < 2 mo **Supplied:** Oint sulfacetamide 10%/prednisolone 0.5%, sulfacetamide 10%/prednisolone 0.2%, sulfacetamide 10%/prednisolone 0.25%; susp sulfacetamide 10%/prednisolone 0.25%, sulfacetamide 10%/prednisolone 0.5%, sulfacetamide 10%/prednisolone 0.2% **SE:** Irritation, burning, blurred vision, brow ache, Stevens–Johnson syndrome, photosensitivity **Notes:** OK ophth susp use as otic agent

Sulfasalazine (Azulfidine, Azulfidine EN)
Uses: *Ulcerative colitis, RA, juvenile RA,* active Crohn Dz, ankylosing spondylitis, psoriasis **Action:** Sulfonamide; actions unclear **Dose:** *Adults.* Initial, 1 g PO tid–qid; ↑ to a max of 8 g/d in 3–4 ÷ doses; maint 500 mg PO qid. *Peds.* Initial, 40–60 mg/kg/24 h PO ÷ q4–6h; maint, 20–30 mg/kg/24 h PO ÷ q6h. *RA > 6 y:* 30–50 mg/kg/d in 2 doses, start w/ 1/4–1/3 maint dose, ↑ weekly until dose reached at 1 mo, 2 g/d max; ↓ in renal failure **Caution:** [B (D if near term), M] **Contra:** Sulfonamide or salicylate sensitivity, porphyria, GI or GU obstruction; avoid in hepatic impair **Supplied:** Tabs 500 mg; EC tabs 500 mg; PO susp 250 mg/5 mL **SE:** GI

22

upset; discolors urine; dizziness, HA, photosensitivity, oligospermia, anemias, Stevens–Johnson syndrome **Notes:** May cause yellow-orange skin/contact lens discoloration; avoid sunlight exposure

Sulfinpyrazone (Anturane) Uses: *Acute & chronic gout* Action: ↓
Renal tubular absorption of uric acid **Dose:** 100–200 mg PO bid for 1 wk, ↑ PRN to maint of 200–400 mg bid; max 800 mg/d; take w/food or antacids & plenty of fluids; avoid salicylates **Caution:** [C (D if near term), ?/–] **Contra:** Renal impair, avoid salicylates; peptic ulcer; blood dyscrasias, near term PRG, allergy **Supplied:** Tabs 100 mg; caps 200 mg **SE:** N/V, stomach pain, urolithiasis, leukopenia **Notes:** Take w/plenty of H_2O

Sulindac (Clinoril) WARNING: May ↑ risk of CV events & GI bleeding
Uses: *Arthritis & pain* **Action:** NSAID; ↓ prostaglandins **Dose:** 150–200 mg bid w/food **Caution:** [B (D if 3rd tri or near term), ?] **Contra:** NSAID or ASA sensitivity, ulcer, GI bleeding **Supplied:** Tabs 150, 200 mg **SE:** Dizziness, rash, GI upset, pruritus, edema, ↓ renal blood flow, renal failure (? fewer renal effects than other NSAIDs), peptic ulcer, GI bleeding

Sumatriptan (Imitrex) Uses: Rx acute migraine attacks Action: Vascular
serotonin receptor agonist **Dose:** *Adults.* SQ: 6 mg SQ as a single dose PRN; repeat PRN in 1 h to a max of 12 mg/24 h. *PO:* 25 mg, repeat in 2 h, PRN, 100 mg/d max PO dose; max 300 mg/d. *Nasal spray:* 1 spray into 1 nostril, repeat in 2 h to 40 mg/24 h max. *Peds. Nasal spray:* 6–9 y: 5–20 mg/d. *12–17 y:* 5–20 mg, up to 40 mg/d **Caution:** [C, M] **Contra:** Angina, ischemic heart Dz, uncontrolled HTN, ergot use, MAOI use w/in 14 d **Supplied:** Inj 6 mg/mL; orally disintegrating tabs 25, 50, 100 mg; nasal spray 5, 20 mg **SE:** Pain & bruising at site; dizziness, hot flashes, paresthesias, CP, weakness, numbness, coronary vasospasm, HTN

Tacrine (Cognex) Uses: *Mild–moderate Alzheimer dementia* Action:
Cholinesterase inhibitor **Dose:** 10–40 mg PO qid to 160 mg/d; separate doses from food **Caution:** [C, ?] **Contra:** Previous tacrine-induced jaundice **Supplied:** Caps 10, 20, 30, 40 mg **SE:** ↑ LFT, HA, dizziness, GI upset, flushing, confusion, ataxia, myalgia, bradycardia **Notes:** Serum conc > 20 ng/mL have more SE; monitor LFTs

Tacrolimus, FK 506 (Prograf, Protopic) Uses: *Prophylaxis against
organ rejection,* eczema **Action:** Macrolide immunosuppressant **Dose:** *Adults.* IV: 0.05–0.1 mg/kg/d cont inf. *PO:* 0.15–0.3 mg/kg/d ÷ 2 doses. *Peds.* IV: 0.03–0.05 mg/kg/d as cont inf. *PO:* 0.15–0.2 mg/kg/d PO ÷ q 12 h. *Adults & Peds.* Eczema: Apply bid, continue 1 wk after clearing; ↓ in hepatic/renal impair **Caution:** [C, –] Do not use w/cyclosporine; avoid topical if age < 2 y **Contra:** Component allergy **Supplied:** Caps 1, 5 mg; inj 5 mg/mL; oint 0.03, 0.1% **SE:** Neurotox & nephrotox, HTN, edema, HA, insomnia, fever, pruritus, ↓/↑ K^+, hyperglycemia, GI upset, anemia, leukocytosis, tremors, paresthesias, pleural effusion, Szs, lymphoma **Notes:** Monitor levels; reports of ↑ cancer risk; topical use for short term/second line

Tadalafil (Cialis) Uses: *Erectile dysfunction* Action: Phosphodiesterase
5 inhibitor **Dose:** *Adults.* 10 mg PO before sexual activity w/o regard to meals (20 mg max); ↓ 5 mg (10 mg max) in renal & hepatic insuff **Caution:** [B, –] **Contra:** Nitrates, α-blockers (except tamsulosin), severe hepatic insuff **Supplied:** 5-, 10-, 20-mg tabs **SE:** HA, flushing, dyspepsia, rhinitis, back pain, myalgia **Notes:** Longest acting of class (36 h)

Talc (Sterile Talc Powder) Uses: *↓ Recurrence of malignant pleural effusions (pleurodesis)* **Action:** Sclerosing agent **Dose:** Mix slurry: 50 mL NS w/5-g vial, mix, distribute 25 mL into two 60-mL syringes, volume to 50 mL/syringe w/NS. Infuse each into chest tube, flush w/25 mL NS. Keep tube clamped; have pt change positions q15min for 2 h; unclamp tube **Caution:** [X, –] **Contra:** Planned further surgery on site **Supplied:** 5 g powder **SE:** Pain, Infxn **Notes:** May add 10–20 mL 1% lidocaine/syringe; must have chest tube placed, monitor closely while tube clamped (tension pneumothorax), not antineoplastic

Tamoxifen (Nolvadex) Uses: *Breast CA [postmenopausal, estrogen receptor(+)], reduction of breast CA in high-risk women, metastatic male breast CA,* mastalgia, pancreatic CA, gynecomastia, ovulation induction **Action:** Nonsteroidal antiestrogen; mixed agonist–antagonist effect **Dose:** 20–40 mg/d (typically 10 mg bid or 20 mg/d) **Caution:** [D, –] **Contra:** Caution in leukopenia, thrombocytopenia, hyperlipidemia **Supplied:** Tabs 10, 20 mg **SE:** Uterine malignancy & thrombotic events noted in breast CA prevention trials; menopausal Sxs (hot flashes, N/V) in premenopausal pts; vaginal bleeding & menstrual irregularities; rash, pruritus vulvae, dizziness, HA, peripheral edema; acute flare of bone metastasis pain & ↑ Ca^{2+}; retinopathy reported (high dose) **Notes:** ↑ Risk of PRG in premenopausal women (induces ovulation)

Tamsulosin (Flomax) Uses: *BPH* **Action:** Antagonist of prostatic α-receptors **Dose:** 0.4 mg/d PO; do not crush, chew, or open caps **Caution:** [B, ?] **Contra:** Female sex **Supplied:** Caps 0.4, 0.8 mg **SE:** HA, dizziness, syncope, somnolence, ↓ libido, GI upset, retrograde ejaculation, rhinitis, rash, angioedema **Notes:** Not for use as antihypertensive

Tazarotene (Tazorac) Uses: *Facial acne vulgaris; stable plaque psoriasis up to 20% body surface area* **Action:** Keratolytic **Dose:** *Adults & Peds > 12 y.* Acne: Cleanse face, dry & apply thin film qd hs on acne lesions. *Psoriasis:* Apply hs **Caution:** [X, ?/–] **Contra:** Retinoid sensitivity **Supplied:** Gel 0.05, 0.1% **SE:** Burning, erythema, irritation, rash, photosensitivity, desquamation, bleeding, skin discoloration **Notes:** D/C w/excessive pruritus, burning, skin redness or peeling occur until Sxs resolve

Tegaserod (Zelnorm) **WARNING:** Rare reports of ischemic colitis **Uses:** *Short-term Rx of constipation-predominant IBS in women*, chronic idiopathic constipation in pts < 65 y **Action:** $5HT_4$ serotonin agonist **Dose:** 6 mg PO bid pc for 4–6 wk; may continue for 2nd course **Caution:** [B, ?/–] **Contra:** Severe renal, moderate–severe hepatic impair, Hx of bowel obstruction, gallbladder Dz, sphincter of Oddi dysfunction, abdominal adhesions **Supplied:** Tabs 2, 6 mg **SE:** Do not administer if D present, as GI motility ↑; D/C if abdominal pain worsens **Notes:** Maintain hydration

Telithromycin (Ketek) **WARNING:** May be associated with pseudomembranous colitis and hepatic failure **Uses:** *Acute bacterial exacerbations of chronic bronchitis, acute bacterial sinusitis; mild–moderate community-acquired pneumonia* **Action:** Unique macrolide, blocks protein synthesis; bacteriocidal. *Spectrum: S. aureus, S. pneumoniae, H. influenzae, M. catarrhalis, C. pneumoniae, M. pneumoniae* **Dose:** *Chronic bronchitis/sinusitis:* 800 mg (2 tabs) PO qd × 5. *Pneumonia:* 800 mg (2 tabs) PO qd × 7–10 d **Caution:** [C, M] pseudomembranous colitis, ↑QTc interval, MyG exacerbations, visual disturbances, hepatic dysfunction; dosing in renal impair unknown **Contra:** Macrolide allergy, use w/

cisapride or pimozide **Supplied:** Tabs 400 mg **SE:** N/V/D, dizziness **Notes:** CYP450 inhibitor; multiple drug interactions

Telmisartan (Micardis) Uses: *HTN, CHF,* DN **Action:** Angiotensin II receptor antagonist **Dose:** 40–80 mg/d **Caution:** [C (1st tri; D 2nd & 3rd tri), ?/–] **Contra:** Angiotensin II receptor antagonist sensitivity **Supplied:** Tabs 40, 80 mg **SE:** Edema, GI upset, HA, angioedema, renal impair, orthostatic ↓ BP

Temazepam (Restoril) [C-IV] Uses: *Insomnia,* anxiety, depression, panic attacks **Action:** Benzodiazepine **Dose:** 15–30 mg PO hs PRN; ↓ in elderly **Caution:** [X, ?/–] Potentiates CNS depressive effects of opioids, barbs, EtOH, antihistamines, MAOIs, TCAs **Contra:** Narrow-angle glaucoma **Supplied:** Caps 7.5, 15, 30 mg **SE:** Confusion, dizziness, drowsiness, hangover **Notes:** Abrupt D/C after > 10 d use may cause withdrawal

Tenecteplase (TNKase) Uses: *Restore perfusion & mortality w/AMI* **Action:** Thrombolytic; TPA **Dose:** 30–50 mg; see the following table:

Weight (kg)	TNKase (mg)	TNKase[a] Volume (mL)
<60	30	6
≥60–70	35	7
≥70–80	40	8
≥80–90	45	9
≥90	50	10

[a]From one vial of reconstituted TNKase.

Caution: [C, ?], ↑ bleeding w/NSAIDs, ticlopidine, clopidogrel, GPIIb/IIIa antagonists **Contra:** Bleeding, CVA, major surgery (intracranial, intraspinal) or trauma w/in 2 mo **Supplied:** Inj 50 mg, reconstitute w/10 mL sterile H_2O **SE:** Bleeding, allergy **Notes:** Do not shake w/reconstitution; do *not* use w/D_5W

Tenofovir (Viread) Uses: *HIV Infxn* **Action:** Nucleotide RT inhibitor **Dose:** 300 mg PO qd w/meal **Caution:** [B, ?/–] Didanosine (separate admin times), lopinavir, ritonavir w/known risk factors for liver Dz **Contra:** CrCl < 60 mL/min; **Supplied:** Tabs 300 mg **SE:** GI upset, metabolic syndrome, hepatotox; separate didanosine doses by 2 h **Notes:** Take w/fatty meal; combo product w/ emtricitabine known as Truvada

Tenofovir/Emtricitabine (Truvada) WARNING: Lactic acidosis & severe hepatomegaly with steatosis, including fatal cases, have been reported with the use of nucleoside analogs alone or in combo w/other antiretrovirals. Not OK w/chronic hepatitis; effects in patients coinfected with hepatitis B & HIV unknown Uses: *HIV Infxn* **Action:** Dual nucleotide RT inhibitor Dose: 300 mg PO qd w/or w/o meal **Caution:** W/known risk factors for liver Dz [B, ?/–] **Contra:** CrCl < 30 mL/min; **Supplied:** Tabs: 200 mg emtricitabine/300 mg tenofovir **SE:** GI upset, metabolic syndrome, hepatotox **Notes:** Take w/fatty meal

Terazosin (Hytrin) Uses: *BPH & HTN* **Action:** α_1-Blocker (blood vessel & bladder neck/prostate) **Dose:** Initial, 1 mg PO hs; ↑ 20 mg/d max **Caution:** [C, ?] w/BB, CCB, ACE inhibitor **Contra:** α-Antagonist sensitivity **Supplied:** Tabs 1, 2, 5, 10 mg; caps 1, 2, 5, 10 mg **SE:** ↓ BP & syncope following 1st dose; dizziness, weakness, nasal congestion, peripheral edema, palpitations, GI upset **Notes:** Caution w/1st dose syncope; if for HTN, combine w/thiazide diuretic

Terbinafine (Lamisil) Uses: *Onychomycosis, athlete's foot, jock itch, ringworm,* cutaneous candidiasis, pityriasis versicolor **Action:** ↓ squalene epoxidase resulting in fungal death **Dose:** *PO:* 250 mg/d PO for 6–12 wk. *Topical:* Apply to area; ↓ in renal/hepatic impair **Caution:** [B, –] ↑ effects of drug metab by CYP2D6 **Contra:** Liver Dz/kidney failure **Supplied:** Tabs 250 mg; cream 1% **SE:** HA, dizziness, rash, pruritus, alopecia, GI upset, taste perversion, neutropenia, retinal damage, Stevens–Johnson syndrome **Notes:** Effect may take months owing to need for new nail growth; do not use occlusive dressings

Terbutaline (Brethine, Bricanyl) Uses: *Reversible bronchospasm (asthma, COPD); inhibits labor* **Action:** Sympathomimetic; tocolytic **Dose:** *Adults. Bronchodilator:* 2.5–5 mg PO qid or 0.25 mg SQ; may repeat in 15 min (max 0.5 mg in 4 h). *Met-dose inhaler:* 2 inhal q4–6h. *Premature labor:* Acutely 2.5–10 mg/min/IV, gradually ↑ as tolerated q10–20min; maint 2.5–5 mg PO q4–6h until term *Peds.* PO: 0.05–0.15 mg/kg/dose PO tid; max 5 mg/24h; ↓ in renal failure **Caution:** [B, +] ↑ tox w/MAOIs, TCAs; diabetes, HTN, hyperthyroidism **Contra:** Tachycardia, component allergy **Supplied:** Tabs 2.5, 5 mg; inj 1 mg/mL; met-dose inhaler **SE:** HTN, hyperthyroidism, β$_1$-adrenergic effects w/high dose, nervousness, trembling, tachycardia, HTN, dizziness

Terconazole (Terazol 7) Uses: *Vaginal fungal Infxns* **Action:** Topical antifungal **Dose:** 1 applicatorful or 1 supp intravag hs × 3–7 d **Caution:** [C, ?] **Contra:** Component allergy **Supplied:** Vaginal cream 0.4%, vaginal supp 80 mg **SE:** Vulvar/vaginal burning **Notes:** Insert high into vagina

Teriparatide (Forteo) Uses: *Severe/refractory osteoporosis* **Action:** PTH (recombinant) **Dose:** 20 mcg SQ qd in thigh or abdomen **Caution:** [C, ?/–] **Contra:** w/Paget Dz, prior radiation, bone metastasis, ↑ Ca^{2+}; caution in urolithiasis **Supplied:** 3-mL prefilled device (discard after 28 d) **SE:** Orthostatic ↓ BP on administration, N/D, ↑ Ca, leg cramps **Notes:** 2–y max use; osteosarcoma in animals

Testosterone (AndroGel, Androderm, Striant, Testim, Testoderm) [CIII] Uses: *Male hypogonadism* **Action:** Testosterone replacement; ↑ lean body mass, libido **Dose:** All daily *AndroGel:* 5 g gel. *Androderm:* Two 2.5-mg or one 5-mg patch qd. *Striant:* 30-mg buccal tabs bid. *Testim:* one 5-g gel tube. *Testoderm:* one 4- or 6-mg scrotal patch **Caution:** [N/A, N/A] **Supplied:** *AndroGel, Testim:* 5-gm gel (50-mg test); *Androderm:* 2.5-, 5-mg patches; *Striant:* 30-mg buccal tabs; *Testoderm:* 4- or 6-mg scrotal patch **SE:** Site Rxns, acne, edema, weight gain, gynecomastia, HTN, ↑ sleep apnea, prostate enlargement **Notes:** Injectable testosterone enanthate (Delatestryl; Testro-LA) & cypionate (Depo-Testosterone) require inj every 14–28 d with highly variable serum levels; PO agents (methyltestosterone & oxandrolone) associated w/hepatitis/hepatic tumors; transdermal/mucosal forms preferred

Tetanus Immune Globulin Uses: *Passive tetanus immunization* (suspected contaminated wound w/unknown immunization status; see also Table 22–9, page 643) **Action:** Passive immunization **Dose:** *Adults & Peds.* 250–500 units IM (higher dose w/delayed Rx) **Caution:** [C, ?] **Contra:** Thimerosal sensitivity **Supplied:** Inj 250-unit vial or syringe **SE:** Pain, tenderness, erythema at inj site; fever, angioedema, muscle stiffness, anaphylaxis **Notes:** May begin active immunization series at different inj site if required

22

Tetanus Toxoid Uses: *Tetanus prophylaxis* See also Table 22–9, page 643 **Action:** Active immunization **Dose:** Based on previous immunization Table 22–9 **Caution:** [C, ?] **Contra:** Chloramphenicol use, neurologic Sxs w/previous use, active Infxn (for routine primary immunization) **Supplied:** Inj tetanus toxoid, fluid, 4–5 Lf units/0.5 mL; tetanus toxoid, adsorbed, 5, 10 Lf units/0.5 mL **SE:** Local erythema, induration, sterile abscess; chills, fever, neurologic disturbances

Tetracycline (Achromycin V, Sumycin) Uses: *Broad-spectrum antibiotic* **Action:** Bacteriostatic; ↓ protein synthesis. *Spectrum:* Gram(+): *Staph, Strep.* Gram(–): *H. pylori.* Atypicals: *Chlamydia, Rickettsia & Mycoplasma* **Dose:** *Adults.* 250–500 mg PO bid–qid. *Peds > 8 y.* 25–50 mg/kg/24 h PO q6–12h; ↓ in renal/hepatic impair **Caution:** [D, +] **Contra:** PRG, antacids, w/dairy products; children ≤ 8 y **Supplied:** Caps 100, 250, 500 mg; tabs 250, 500 mg; PO susp 250 mg/5 mL **SE:** Photosensitivity, GI upset, renal failure, pseudotumor cerebri, hepatic impair **Notes:** Can stain tooth enamel & depress bone formation in children

Thalidomide (Thalomid) Uses: *Erythema nodosum leprosum (ENL),* graft-versus-host Dz, aphthous ulceration in HIV(+) pts **Action:** ↓ Neutrophil chemotaxis, ↓ monocyte phagocytosis **Dose:** *GVHD:* 100–1600 mg PO qd. *Stomatitis:* 200 mg bid for 5 d, then 200 mg qd up to 8 wk. *ENL:* 100–300 mg PO qhs **Caution:** [X, –] May ↑ HIV viral load; Hx Szs **Contra:** PRG; sexually active men not using latex condoms and women not using 2 forms of contraception **SE:** Dizziness, drowsiness, rash, fever, orthostasis, Stevens–Johnson syndrome, peripheral neuropathy, Szs **Supplied:** 50-mg cap **Notes:** Physician must register w/STEPS risk management program; informed consent necessary; immediately D/C if rash develops

Theophylline (Theo24, TheoChron) Uses: *Asthma, bronchospasm* **Action:** Relaxes smooth muscle of the bronchi & pulmonary blood vessels **Dose:** *Adults.* 900 mg PO ÷ q6h; SR products may be ÷ q8–12h (maint). *Peds.* 16–22 mg/kg/24 h PO ÷ q6h; SR products may be ÷ q8–12h (maint); ↓ in hepatic failure **Caution:** [C, +] Multiple interactions (eg, caffeine, smoking, carbamazepine, barbiturates, β-blockers, ciprofloxacin, E-mycin, INH, loop diuretics) **Contra:** Arrhythmia, hyperthyroidism, uncontrolled Szs **Supplied:** Elixir 80, 150 mg/15 mL; liq 80, 160 mg/15 mL; caps 100, 200, 250 mg; tabs 100, 125, 200, 225, 250, 300 mg; SR caps 50, 75, 100, 125, 200, 250, 260, 300 mg; SR tabs 100, 200, 250, 300, 400, 450, 500 mg **SE:** N/V, tachycardia & Szs; nervousness, arrhythmias **Notes:** See levels, Table 22–2 (page 628)

Thiamine, Vitamin B₁ Uses: *Thiamine deficiency (beriberi), alcoholic neuritis, Wernicke encephalopathy* **Action:** Dietary supl **Dose:** *Adults.* Deficiency: 100 mg/d IM for 2 wk, then 5–10 mg/d PO for 1 mo. *Wernicke encephalopathy:* 100 mg IV single dose, then 100 mg/d IM for 2 wk. *Peds.* 10–25 mg/d IM for 2 wk, then 5–10 mg/24 h PO for 1 mo **Caution:** [A (C if doses exceed RDA), +] **Contra:** Component allergy **Supplied:** Tabs 5, 10, 25, 50, 100, 500 mg; inj 100, 200 mg/mL **SE:** Angioedema, paresthesias, rash, anaphylaxis w/ rapid IV **Notes:** IV use associated w/anaphylactic Rxn; give IV slowly

Thiethylperazine (Torecan) Uses: *N/V* **Action:** Antidopaminergic antiemetic **Dose:** 10 mg PO, PR, or IM qd–tid; ↓ in hepatic failure **Caution:** [X, ?] **Contra:** Phenothiazine & sulfite sensitivity, PRG **Supplied:** Tabs 10 mg; supp 10 mg; inj 5 mg/mL **SE:** EPS, xerostomia, drowsiness, orthostatic ↓ BP, tachycardia, confusion

22

6-Thioguanine, 6-TG (Tabloid) Uses: *AML, ALL, CML* Action: Purine-based antimetabolite (substitutes for natural purines interfering w/ nucleotide synthesis) Dose: 2–3 mg/kg/d; ↓ in severe renal/hepatic impair Caution: [D, –] Contra: Resistance to mercaptopurine Supplied: Tabs 40 mg SE: Myelosuppression (leukopenia/thrombocytopenia), N/V/D, anorexia, stomatitis, rash, hyperuricemia, rare hepatotox

Thioridazine (Mellaril) WARNING: Dose-related QT prolongation Uses: *Schizophrenia,* psychosis Action: Phenothiazine antipsychotic Dose: *Adults.* Initial, 50–100 mg PO tid; maint 200–800 mg/24 h PO in 2–4 ÷ doses. *Peds > 2 y.* 0.5–3 mg/kg/24 h PO in 2–3 ÷ doses Caution: [C, ?] Phenothiazines, QTc-prolonging agents, aluminum Contra: Phenothiazine sensitivity Supplied: Tabs 10, 15, 25, 50, 100, 150, 200 mg; PO conc 30, 100 mg/mL; PO susp 25, 100 mg/5 mL SE: Low incidence of EPS; ventricular arrhythmias; ↓ BP, dizziness, drowsiness, neuroleptic malignant syndrome, Szs, skin discoloration, photosensitivity, constipation, sexual dysfunction, blood dyscrasias, pigmentary retinopathy, hepatic impair Notes: Avoid EtOH, dilute PO conc in 2–4 oz liq

Thiothixene (Navane) Uses: *Psychotic disorders* Action: Antipsychotic Dose: *Adults & Peds > 12 y.* Mild–moderate psychosis: 2 mg PO tid, up to 20–30 mg/d. *Severe psychosis:* 5 mg PO bid; ↑ to a max of 60 mg/24 h PRN. *IM use:* 16–20 mg/24 h ÷ bid–qid; max 30 mg/d. *Peds < 12 y.* 0.25 mg/kg/24 h PO ÷ q6–12h Caution: [C, ?] Contra: Phenothiazine sensitivity Supplied: Caps 1, 2, 5, 10, 20 mg; PO conc 5 mg/mL; inj 2, 5 mg/mL SE: Drowsiness, EPS most common; ↓ BP, dizziness, drowsiness, neuroleptic malignant syndrome, Szs, skin discoloration, photosensitivity, constipation, sexual dysfunction, blood dyscrasias, pigmentary retinopathy, hepatic impair Notes: Dilute PO conc immediately before administration

Tiagabine (Gabitril) Uses: *Adjunct in Rx of partial Szs,* bipolar disorder Action: Inhibition of GABA Dose: *Adults & Peds* ≥12 y. Initial 4 mg/d PO, ↑ by 4 mg during 2nd wk; ↑ PRN by 4–8 mg/d based on response, 56 mg/d max Caution: [C, M] Contra: Component allergy Supplied: Tabs 4, 12, 16, 20 mg SE: Dizziness, HA, somnolence, memory impair, tremors Notes: Use gradual withdrawal; used in combo w/other anticonvulsants

Ticarcillin (Ticar) Uses: Infxns due to gram(–) bacteria (*Klebsiella, Proteus, E. coli, Enterobacter, P. aeruginosa* & *Serratia*) involving the skin, bone, resp & urinary tract, abdomen, sepsis Action: 4th-gen PCN, bactericidal; ↓ cell wall synthesis. *Spectrum:* Some gram(+) (strep, fair enterococcus, not MRSA), gram(–); enhanced w/aminoglycoside use, good anaerobes (bactericides) Dose: *Adults.* 3 g IV q4–6h. *Peds.* 200–300 mg/kg/d IV ÷ q4–6h; ↓ in renal failure Caution: [B, +] PCN sensitivity Supplied: Inj SE: Interstitial nephritis, anaphylaxis, bleeding, rash, hemolytic anemia Notes: Used in combo w/aminoglycosides

Ticarcillin/Potassium Clavulanate (Timentin) Uses: *Infxns of the skin, bone, resp & urinary tract, abdomen, sepsis* Action: 4th-gen PCN; bactericidal; ↓ cell wall synthesis; clavulanic acid blocks β-lactamase. *Spectrum:* Good gram(+), not MRSA; good gram(–) & anaerobes Dose: *Adults.* 3.1 g IV q4–6h. *Peds.* 200–300 mg/kg/d IV ÷ q4–6h; ↓ in renal failure Caution: [B, +/–] PCN sensitivity Supplied: Inj SE: Hemolytic anemia, false(+) proteinuria Notes: Often used in combo w/aminoglycosides; penetrates CNS with meningeal irritation

22

Ticlopidine (Ticlid) **WARNING:** Neutropenia/agranulocytosis, TTP, aplastic anemia reported **Uses:** *↓ Risk of thrombotic stroke,* protect grafts status post CABG, diabetic microangiopathy, ischemic heart Dz, DVT prophylaxis, graft prophylaxis after renal transplant **Action:** Plt aggregation inhibitor **Dose:** 250 mg PO bid w/food **Caution:** [B, ?/−], ↑ tox of ASA, anticoagulation, NSAIDs, theophylline **Contra:** Bleeding, hepatic impair, neutropenia, thrombocytopenia **Supplied:** Tabs 250 mg **SE:** Bleeding, GI upset, rash, ↑ on LFTs **Notes:** Follow CBC 1st 3 mo

Tigecycline (Tygacil) **Uses:** *Rx complicated skin & soft-tissue Infxns & complicated intraabdominal Infxns* **Action:** New class: related to tetracycline. *Spectrum:* Broad gram(+), gram(−), anaerobic, some mycobacterial; *E. coli, E. faecalis* (vanco-susceptible isolates), *S. aureus* (meth-susceptible/resistant), *Strep* (*agalactiae, anginosus* grp, *pyogenes*), *C. freundii, E. cloacae, B. fragilis* group, *C. perfringens, Peptostreptococcus* **Dose:** *Adults.* 100 mg, then 50 mg q12h IV over 30–60 min every 12 h **Caution:** [D, ?] hepatic impair, monotherapy w/intestinal perf, not OK in peds **Contra:** Component sensitivity **Supplied:** Inj **SE:** N/V, inj site Rxn

Timolol (Blocadren) **WARNING:** Exacerbation of ischemic heart Dz w/ abrupt D/C **Uses:** *HTN & MI* **Action:** β-Adrenergic receptor blocker, β_1, β_2 **Dose:** *HTN:* 10–20 mg bid, up to 60 mg/d. *MI:* 10 mg bid **Caution:** [C (1st tri; D if 2nd or 3rd tri), +] **Contra:** CHF, cardiogenic shock, bradycardia, heart block, COPD, asthma **Supplied:** Tabs 5, 10, 20 mg **SE:** Sexual dysfunction, arrhythmia, dizziness, fatigue, CHF

Timolol, Ophthalmic (Timoptic) **Uses:** *Glaucoma* **Action:** β-Blocker **Dose:** 0.25% 1 gt bid; ↓ to qd when controlled; use 0.5% if needed; 1 gt/d gel **Caution:** [C (1st tri; D 2nd or 3rd), ?/+] **Supplied:** Soln 0.25/0.5%; Timoptic XE (0.25, 0.5%) gel-forming soln **SE:** Local irritation

Tinidazole (Tindamax) **WARNING:** Off-label use discouraged (animal carcinogenicity w/other drugs in class) **Uses:** *Adults/children > 3 y.* *Trichomoniasis & giardiasis; intestinal amebiasis, amebic liver abscess* **Action:** Antiprotozoal nitroimidazole *Spectrum: T. vaginalis, G. duodenalis, E. histolytica* **Dose:** *Adults. Trichomoniasis:* 2 g PO; Rx partner; *Giardiasis:* 2 g PO. *Amebiasis:* 2 g PO qd × 3. *Amebic liver abscess:* 2 g PO qd × 3–5. *Peds.* Trichomoniasis: 50 mg/kg PO, 2 g/d max. *Giardiasis:* 50 mg/kg PO, 2 g max. *Amebiasis:* 50 mg/kg PO qd × 3, 2 g/d max. *Amebic liver abscess:* 50 mg/kg PO qd × 3–5, 2 g/ d max (w/food) **Caution:** [C, D in 1st trimester; −] May be cross-resistant with metronidazole; Sz/peripheral neuropathy may require D/C; w/CNS/hepatic impair **Contra:** Metronidazole allergy, 1st trimester PRG, w/EtOH use **Supplied:** Tabs 250, 500 **SE:** CNS disturbances; blood dyscrasias, taste disturbances, N/V, darkens urine **Notes:** D/C EtOH during & 3 d after Rx; potentiates warfarin & lithium; clearance ↓ w/other drugs; crush & disperse in cherry syrup for peds; removed by HD

Tinzaparin (Innohep) **Uses:** *Rx of DVT w/or w/o PE* **Action:** LMWH **Dose:** 175 units/kg SQ qd at least 6 d until warfarin dose stabilized **Caution:** [B, ?] Pork allergy, active bleeding, mild–moderate renal dysfunction **Contra:** Allergy to sulfites, heparin, benzyl alcohol, HIT **Supplied:** 20,000 units/mL **SE:** Bleeding, bruising, thrombocytopenia, inj site pain, ↑ LFTs **Notes:** Monitor via Anti-Xa levels; no effect on: bleeding time, plt Fxn, PT, aPTT

22

Tioconazole (Vagistat) **Uses:** *Vaginal fungal Infxns* **Action:** Topical antifungal **Dose:** 1 applicatorful intravag hs (single dose) **Caution:** [C, ?] **Con-**

tra: Component allergy **Supplied:** Vaginal oint 6.5% **SE:** Local burning, itching, soreness, polyuria **Notes:** Insert high into vagina

Tiotropium (Spiriva) **Uses:** Bronchospasm w/COPD, bronchitis, emphysema **Action:** Synthetic anticholinergic like atropine **Dose:** 1 cap/d inhaled using HandiHaler, *do not* use w/spacer **Caution:** [C, ?/–] BPH, narrow-angle glaucoma, MyG, renal impair **Contra:** Acute bronchospasm **Supplied:** Caps 18 mcg **SE:** URI, xerostomia **Notes:** Monitor FEV_1 or peak flow

Tirofiban (Aggrastat) **Uses:** *Acute coronary syndrome* **Action:** Glycoprotein IIB/IIIa inhibitor **Dose:** Initial 0.4 mcg/kg/min for 30 min, followed by 0.1 mcg/kg/min; use in combo w/heparin; ↓ in renal insuff **Caution:** [B, ?/–] **Contra:** Bleeding, intracranial neoplasm, vascular malformation, stroke/surgery/trauma w/in last 30 d, severe HTN **Supplied:** Inj 50, 250 mcg/mL **SE:** Bleeding, bradycardia, coronary dissection, pelvic pain, rash

Tobramycin (Nebcin) **Uses:** *Serious gram(–) Infxns* **Action:** Aminoglycoside; ↓ protein synthesis. *Spectrum:* Gram(–) bacteria (including *Pseudomonas*) **Dose:** *Adults.* 1–2.5 mg/kg/dose IV q8–24h. *Peds.* 2.5 mg/kg/dose IV q8h; ↓ w/renal insuff **Caution:** [C, M] **Contra:** Aminoglycoside sensitivity **Supplied:** Inj 10, 40 mg/mL **SE:** Nephrotox & ototox **Notes:** Follow CrCl & levels for dosage adjustments (Table 22–2, page 628)

Tobramycin Ophthalmic (AKTob, Tobrex) **Uses:** *Ocular bacterial Infxns* **Action:** Aminoglycoside **Dose:** 1–2 gtt q4h; oint bid–tid; if severe, use oint q3–4h, or 2 gtt q30–60min, then less frequently **Caution:** [C, M] **Contra:** Aminoglycoside sensitivity **Supplied:** Oint & soln tobramycin 0.3% **SE:** Ocular irritation

Tobramycin & Dexamethasone Ophthalmic (TobraDex) **Uses:** *Ocular bacterial Infxns associated w/significant inflammation* **Action:** Antibiotic w/antiinflammatory **Dose:** 0.3% oint apply q3–8h or soln 0.3% apply 1–2 gtt q1–4h **Caution:** [C, M] **Contra:** Aminoglycoside sensitivity **Supplied:** Oint & soln tobramycin 0.3% & dexamethasone 0.1% **SE:** Local irritation/edema **Notes:** Use under ophthalmologist's direction

Tolazamide (Tolinase) **Uses:** *Type 2 DM* **Action:** Sulfonylurea; ↑ pancreatic insulin release; ↑ peripheral insulin sensitivity; ↓ hepatic glucose output **Dose:** 100–500 mg/d (no benefit > 1 g/d) **Caution:** [C, +/–] Elderly, hepatic or renal impair **Supplied:** Tabs 100, 250, 500 mg; soln 1 mg/mL **SE:** HA, dizziness, GI upset, rash, hyperglycemia, photosensitivity, blood dyscrasias

Tolazoline (Priscoline) **Uses:** *Peripheral vasospastic disorders* **Action:** Competitively blocks α-adrenergic receptors **Dose:** *Adults.* 10–50 mg IM/IV/SQ qid. *Neonates.* 1–2 mg/kg IV over 10–15 min, then 1–2 mg/kg/h (adjust w/↓ renal Fxn) **Caution:** [C, ?] **Contra:** CAD **Supplied:** Inj 25 mg/mL **SE:** ↓ BP, peripheral vasodilation, tachycardia, arrhythmias, GI upset & bleeding, blood dyscrasias, renal failure

Tolbutamide (Orinase) **Uses:** *Type 2 DM* **Action:** Sulfonylurea; ↑ pancreatic insulin release; ↑ peripheral insulin sensitivity; ↓ hepatic glucose output **Dose:** 500–1000 mg bid; ↓ in hepatic failure **Caution:** [C, +] **Contra:** Sulfonylurea sensitivity **Supplied:** Tabs 500 mg **SE:** HA, dizziness, GI upset, rash, photosensitivity, blood dyscrasias, hypoglycemia

Tolcapone (Tasmar) **Uses:** *Adjunct to carbidopa/levodopa in Parkinson Dz* **Action:** Catechol-*O*-methyltransferase inhibitor slows levodopa metabolism **Dose:** 100 mg PO w/first daily levodopa/carbidopa dose, then dose 6 & 12 h later; ↓/w renal impair **Caution:** [C, ?] **Contra:** Hepatic impair; w/nonselective MAOI **Supplied:** Tablets 100 mg, 200 mg **SE:** Constipation, xerostomia, vivid dreams, hallucinations, anorexia, N/D, orthostasis, liver failure **Notes:** Do not abruptly D/C or ↓ dose; monitor LFTs

Tolmetin (Tolectin) WARNING: May ↑ risk of CV events & GI bleeding **Uses:** *Arthritis & pain* **Action:** NSAID; ↓ prostaglandins **Dose:** 200–600 mg PO tid; 2000 mg/d max **Caution:** [C (D in 3rd tri or near term), +] **Contra:** NSAID or ASA sensitivity **Supplied:** Tabs 200, 600 mg; caps 400 mg **SE:** Dizziness, rash, GI upset, edema, GI bleeding, renal failure

Tolnaftate (Tinactin) [OTC] **Uses:** *Tinea pedis, cruris, corporis, manus, versicolor* **Action:** Topical antifungal **Dose:** Apply to area bid for 2–4 wk **Caution:** [C, ?] **Contra:** Nail & scalp Infxns **Supplied:** OTC 1% liq; gel; powder; cream; soln **SE:** Local irritation **Notes:** Avoid ocular contact, Infxn should improve in 7–10 d

Tolterodine (Detrol, Detrol LA) **Uses:** *OAB (frequency, urgency, incontinence)* **Action:** Anticholinergic **Dose:** Detrol 1–2 mg PO bid; Detrol LA 2–4 mg/d **Caution:** [C, ?/–] w/CYP2D6 & 3A3/4 inhibitor **Contra:** Urinary retention, gastric retention, or uncontrolled narrow-angle glaucoma **Supplied:** Tabs 1, 2 mg; Detrol LA tabs 2, 4 mg **SE:** Xerostomia, blurred vision

Topiramate (Topamax) **Uses:** *Adjunctive Rx for complex partial Szs & tonic–clonic Szs,* bipolar disorder, neuropathic pain, migraine prophylaxis **Action:** Anticonvulsant **Dose:** *Adults. Seizures:* Total dose 400 mg/d; see insert for 8-wk titration schedule. *Migraine prophylaxis:* titrate 100 m/d total *Peds 2–16 y:* Initial, 1–3 mg/kg/d PO qhs; titrate per insert to 5–9 mg/kg/d; ↓ w/renal impair **Caution:** [C, ?/–] **Contra:** Component allergy **Supplied:** Tabs 25, 100, 200 mg; caps sprinkles 15, 25, 50 mg **SE:** Metabolic acidosis, kidney stones, fatigue, dizziness, psychomotor slowing, memory impair, GI upset, tremor, nystagmus, weight loss, acute secondary glaucoma requiring drug D/C **Notes:** Metabolic acidosis responsive to ↓ dose or D/C; D/C w/taper

Topotecan (Hycamtin) WARNING: Chemo precautions, BM suppression possible **Uses:** *Ovarian CA (cisplatin-refractory), small-cell lung CA,* sarcoma, ped NSCLC **Action:** Topoisomerase I inhibitor; ↓DNA synthesis **Dose:** 1.5 mg/m^2/d as a 1-h IV inf × 5 d, repeat q3wk; ↓ w/renal impair **Caution:** [D, –] **Contra:** PRG, breast feeding **Supplied:** 4-mg vials **SE:** Myelosuppression, N/V/D, drug fever, rash

Torsemide (Demadex) **Uses:** *Edema, HTN, CHF & hepatic cirrhosis* **Action:** Loop diuretic; ↓ reabsorption of Na$^+$ & Cl– in ascending loop of Henle & distal tubule **Dose:** 5–20 mg/d PO or IV **Caution:** [B, ?] **Contra:** Sulfonylurea sensitivity **Supplied:** Tabs 5, 10, 20, 100 mg; inj 10 mg/mL **SE:** Orthostatic ↓ BP, HA, dizziness, photosensitivity, electrolyte imbalance, blurred vision, renal impair **Notes:** 20 mg torsemide = 40 mg furosemide

Tramadol (Ultram) **Uses:** *Moderate–severe pain* **Action:** Centrally acting analgesic **Dose:** *Adults.* 50–100 mg PO q4–6h PRN, 400 mg/d max. *Peds.* 0.5–1 mg/kg PO q 4–6h PRN **Caution:** [C, ?/–] **Contra:** Opioid dependency; w/ MAOIs; sensitivity to codeine **Supplied:** Tabs 50 mg **SE:** Dizziness, HA, somnolence, GI upset, resp depression, anaphylaxis **Notes:** ↓ Sz threshold; tolerance or dependence may develop

Tramadol/Acetaminophen (Ultracet) Uses: *Short-term Rx acute pain (< 5 d)* Action: Centrally acting analgesic; nonnarcotic analgesic Dose: 2 tabs PO q4–6h PRN; 8 tabs/d max. *Elderly/renal impair:* Lowest possible dose; 2 tabs q12h max if CrCl < 30 Caution: [C, –] Szs, hepatic/renal impair, or Hx addictive tendencies Contra: Acute intox Supplied: Tab 37.5 mg tramadol/ 325 mg APAP SE: SSRIs, TCAs, opioids, MAOIs ↑ risk of Szs; dizziness, somnolence, tremor, HA, N/V/D, constipation, xerostomia, liver tox, rash, pruritus, ↑ sweating, physical dependence Notes: Avoid EtOH

Trandolapril (Mavik) WARNING: Use in PRG in 2nd/3rd tri can result in fetal death Uses: *HTN,* CHF, LVD, post-AMI Action: ACE inhibitor Dose: *HTN:* 2–4 mg/d. *CHF/LVD:* 4 mg/d; ↓ w/severe renal/hepatic impair Caution: [D, +] ACE inhibitor sensitivity, angioedema w/ACE inhibitors Supplied: Tabs 1, 2, 4 mg SE: ↓ BP, bradycardia, dizziness, ↑ K+, GI upset, renal impair, cough, angioedema Notes: African American pts min dose is 2 mg vs 1 mg in white pts

Trastuzumab (Herceptin) Uses: *Metastatic breast CAs that overexpress HER2/neu protein* breast CA adjuvant, w/doxorubicin, cyclophosphamide, and paclitaxel if pt HER2(+) Action: MoAb; binds human epidermal GF receptor 2 protein (HER2); mediates cellular cytotox Dose: Per protocol Caution: [B, ?] CV dysfunction, allergy/inf Rxns Contra: None known Supplied: Inj form SE: Anemia, cardiomyopathy, nephrotic syndrome, pneumonitis Notes: Inf related Rxns minimized w/APAP, diphenhydramine & meperidine

Trazodone (Desyrel) Uses: *Depression,* hypnotic, augment other antidepressants Action: Antidepressant; ↓ reuptake of serotonin & norepinephrine Dose: *Adults & Adolescents.* 50–150 mg PO qd–qid; max 600 mg/d. *Sleep:* 50 mg PO, qhs, PRN Caution: [C, ?/–] Contra: Component allergy Supplied: Tabs 50, 100, 150, 300 mg SE: Dizziness, HA, sedation, nausea, xerostomia, syncope, confusion, tremor, hepatitis, EPS Notes: Takes 1–2 wk for symptom improvement; may interact with CYP3A4 inhibitors to ↑ trazodone concentrations, carbamazepine to ↓ trazodone concentrations

Treprostinil Sodium (Remodulin) Uses: *NYHA class II–IV pulmonary arterial HTN* Action: Vasodilation, inhibits plt aggregation Dose: 0.625– 1.25 ng/kg/min cont inf Caution: [B, ?/–] Contra: Component allergy Supplied: 1, 2.5, 5, 10 mg/mL inj SE: Additive effects w/anticoagulants, antihypertensives; inf site Rxns Notes: Initiate in monitored setting; do not D/C or ↓ dose abruptly

Tretinoin, Topical Retinoic Acid (Retin-A, Avita, Renova) Uses: *Acne vulgaris, sun-damaged skin, wrinkles* (photo aging), some skin CAs Action: Exfoliant retinoic acid derivative Dose: *Adults & Peds > 12 y.* Apply qd hs (w/irritation, ↓ frequency). *Photoaging:* Start w/0.025%, ↑ to 0.1% over several months (apply only q3d if on neck area; dark skin may require bid use) Caution: [C, ?] Contra: Retinoid sensitivity Supplied: Cream 0.025, 0.05, 0.1%; gel 0.01, 0.025, 0.1%; microformulation gel 0.1%; liq 0.05% SE: Avoid sunlight; edema; skin dryness, erythema, scaling, changes in pigmentation, stinging, photosensitivity

Triamcinolone (Azmacort) Uses: *Chronic asthma* Action: Topical steroid Dose: Two inhalations tid–qid or 4 inhal bid Caution: [C, ?] SE: Cough, oral candidiasis Contra: Component allergy Supplied: Inhaler 100 mcg/met spray Notes: Instruct pts to rinse mouth after use; not for acute asthma

Triamcinolone & Nystatin (Mycolog-II) Uses: *Cutaneous candidiasis* Action: Antifungal & antiinflammatory Dose: Apply lightly to area bid; max 25 mg/d Caution: [C, ?] Contra: Varicella; systemic fungal Infxns Supplied: Cream & oint 15, 30, 60, 120 mg SE: Local irritation, hypertrichosis, pigmentation changes Notes: For short-term use (< 7 d)

Triamterene (Dyrenium) Uses: *Edema associated w/CHF, cirrhosis* Action: K⁺-sparing diuretic Dose: *Adults.* 100–300 mg/24 h PO ÷ qd–bid. *Peds.* 2–4 mg/kg/d in 1–2 ÷ doses; ↓ w/renal/hepatic impair Caution: [B (manufacturer; D ed. opinion), ?/–] Contra: ↑ K⁺, renal impair, DM; caution w/other K⁺-sparing diuretics Supplied: Caps 50, 100 mg SE: ↓ K⁺, blood dyscrasias, liver damage, other Rxns

Triazolam (Halcion) [C-IV] Uses: *Short-term management of insomnia* Action: Benzodiazepine Dose: 0.125–0.25 mg/d PO hs PRN; ↓ in elderly Caution: [X, ?/–] Contra: narrow-angle glaucoma; cirrhosis; concurrent amprenavir, ritonavir, or nelfinavir Supplied: Tabs 0.125, 0.25 mg SE: Tachycardia, CP, drowsiness, fatigue, memory impair, GI upset Notes: Additive CNS depression w/EtOH & other CNS depressants

Triethanolamine (Cerumenex) [OTC] Uses: *Cerumen (ear wax) removal* Action: Ceruminolytic agent Dose: Fill ear canal & insert cotton plug; irrigate w/H₂O after 15 min; repeat PRN Caution: [C, ?] Contra: Perforated tympanic membrane, otitis media Supplied: Soln 6, 12 mL SE: Local dermatitis, pain, erythema, pruritus

Triethylenethiophosphamide (Thio-Tepa, Tespa, TSPA) Uses: *Hodgkin Dz & NHL; leukemia; breast, ovarian, CAs,* preparative regimens for allogeneic & ABMT w/high doses Action: Polyfunctional alkylating agent Dose: 0.5 mg/kg q1–4wk, 6 mg/m² IM or IV × 4 d q2–4wk, 15–35 mg/m² by cont IV inf over 48 h; 60 mg into the bladder & retained 2 h q1–4wk; 900–125 mg/m² in ABMT regimens (highest dose w/o ABMT is 180 mg/m²); 1–10 mg/m² (typically 15 mg) IT 1 or 2 × /wk; 0.8 mg/kg in 1–2 L of soln may be instilled intraperitoneally; ↓ in renal failure Caution: [D, –] Contra: Component allergy Supplied: Inj 15 mg SE: Myelosuppression, N/V, dizziness, HA, allergy, paresthesias, alopecia Notes: Intravesical use in bladder CA infrequent today

Trifluoperazine (Stelazine) Uses: *Psychotic disorders* Action: Phenothiazine; blocks postsynaptic CNS dopaminergic receptors Dose: *Adults.* 2–10 mg PO bid. *Peds 6–12 y.* 1 mg PO qd–bid initial, gradually ↑ to 15 mg/d; ↓ in elderly/debilitated pts Caution: [C, ?/–] Contra: Hx blood dyscrasias; phenothiazine sensitivity Supplied: Tabs 1, 2, 5, 10 mg; PO conc 10 mg/mL; inj 2 mg/mL SE: Orthostatic ↓ BP, EPS, dizziness, neuroleptic malignant syndrome, skin discoloration, lowered Sz threshold, photosensitivity, blood dyscrasias Notes: PO conc must be diluted to 60 mL or more before administration; requires several weeks for onset of effects

Trifluridine (Viroptic) Uses: *Herpes simplex keratitis & conjunctivitis* Action: Antiviral Dose: 1 gt q2h (max 9 gtt/d); ↓ to 1 gt q4h after healing begins; Rx up to 14 d Caution: [C, M] Contra: Component allergy Supplied: Soln 1% SE: Local burning, stinging

22 **Trihexyphenidyl (Artane)** Uses: *Parkinson Dz* Action: Blocks excess acetylcholine at cerebral synapses Dose: 2–5 mg PO qd–qid Caution: [C, +]

Contra: Narrow-angle glaucoma, GI obstruction, MyG, bladder obstructions **Supplied:** Tabs 2, 5 mg; SR caps 5 mg; elixir 2 mg/5 mL **SE:** Dry skin, constipation, xerostomia, photosensitivity, tachycardia, arrhythmias

Trimethobenzamide (Tigan) Uses: *N/V* **Action:** ↓ Medullary chemoreceptor trigger zone **Dose:** *Adults.* 250 mg PO or 200 mg PR or IM tid–qid PRN. *Peds.* 20 mg/kg/24 h PO or 15 mg/kg/24 h PR or IM in 3–4 ÷ doses **Caution:** [C, ?] **Contra:** Benzocaine sensitivity **Supplied:** Caps 100, 250 mg; supp 100, 200 mg; inj 100 mg/mL **SE:** Drowsiness, ↓ BP, dizziness; hepatic impair, blood dyscrasias, Szs, parkinsonian-like syndrome **Notes:** In the presence of viral Infxns, may mask emesis or mimic CNS effects of Reye syndrome

Trimethoprim (Trimpex, Proloprim) Uses: *UTI due to susceptible gram(+) & gram(−) organisms;* suppression of UTI **Action:** ↓ Dihydrofolate reductase. *Spectrum:* Many gram(+) & (−) except *Bacteroides, Branhamella, Brucella, Chlamydia, Clostridium, Mycobacterium, Mycoplasma, Nocardia, Neisseria, Pseudomonas & Treponema* **Dose:** *Adults.* 100 mg/d PO bid or 200 mg/d PO. *Peds.* 4 mg/kg/d in 2 ÷ doses; ↓ w/renal failure **Caution:** [C, +] **Contra:** Megaloblastic anemia due to folate deficiency **Supplied:** Tabs 100, 200 mg; PO soln 50 mg/5 mL **SE:** Rash, pruritus, megaloblastic anemia, hepatic impair, blood dyscrasias **Notes:** Take w/plenty of H_2O

Trimethoprim (TMP)–Sulfamethoxazole (SMX), Cotrimoxazole (Bactrim, Septra) Uses: *UTI Rx & prophylaxis, otitis media, sinusitis, bronchitis* **Action:** SMX ↓ synthesis of dihydrofolic acid, TMP ↓ dihydrofolate reductase to impair protein synthesis. *Spectrum:* Includes *Shigella, P. jiroveci* (formerly *carinii*) & *Nocardia* Infxns, *Mycoplasma, Enterobacter* sp, *Staph, Strep* & more **Dose:** *Adults.* 1 DS tab PO bid or 5–20 mg/kg/24 h (based on TMP) IV in 3–4 ÷ doses. *P. jiroveci:* 15–20 mg/kg/d IV or PO (TMP) in 4 ÷ doses. *Nocardia:* 10–15 mg/kg/d IV or PO (TMP) in 4 ÷ doses. *UTI prophylaxis:* 1 PO qd. *Peds.* 8–10 mg/kg/24 h (TMP) PO ÷ into 2 doses or 3–4 doses IV; do not use in newborns; ↓ in renal failure; maintain hydration **Caution:** [B (D if near term), +] **Contra:** Sulfonamide sensitivity, porphyria, megaloblastic anemia w/folate deficiency, significant hepatic impair **Supplied:** Regular tabs 80 mg TMP/400 mg SMX; DS tabs 160 mg TMP/800 mg SMX; PO susp 40 mg TMP/200 mg SMX/5 mL; inj 80 mg TMP/ 400 mg SMX/5 mL **SE:** Allergic skin Rxns, photosensitivity, GI upset, Stevens–Johnson syndrome, blood dyscrasias, hepatitis **Notes:** Synergistic combo, interacts w/warfarin

Trimetrexate (Neutrexin) WARNING: Must be used w/leucovorin to avoid tox **Uses:** *Moderate–severe PCP* **Action:** ↓ dihydrofolate reductase **Dose:** 45 mg/m² IV q24h for 21 d; administer w/leucovorin 20 mg/m² IV q6h for 24 d; ↓ in hepatic impair **Caution:** [D, ?/–] **Contra:** MTX sensitivity **Supplied:** Inj **SE:** Sz, fever, rash, GI upset, anemias, ↑ LFTs, peripheral neuropathy, renal impair **Notes:** Use cytotoxic cautions; inf over 60 min

Triptorelin (Trelstar Depot, Trelstar LA) Uses: *Palliation of advanced CAP* **Action:** LHRH analog; ↓ GNRH w/continuous dosing; transient ↑ in LH, FSH, testosterone & estradiol 7–10 d after first dose; w/chronic/continuous use (usually 2–4 wk), sustained ↓ LH & FSH w/↓ testicular & ovarian steroidogenesis similar to surgical castration **Dose:** 3.75 mg IM monthly or 11.25 mg IM q3mo **Caution:** [X, N/A] **Contra:** Not indicated in females **Supplied:** Inj depot 3.75 mg; LA 11.25 mg **SE:** Dizziness, emotional lability, fatigue, HA, insomnia,

HTN, D, vomiting, ED, retention, UTI, pruritus, anemia, inj site pain, musculo-skeletal pain, osteoporosis, allergic Rxns

Trospium Chloride (Sanctura) Uses: *OAB* **Action:** Antimuscarinic, antispasmodic **Dose:** 20 mg PO bid, ↓ w/renal impair or > 75 y; on empty stom-ach or 1 h ac **Caution:** [C, ?/–] BOO, GI obstruction, ulcerative colitis, MyG, renal/hepatic impair **Contra:** Narrow-angle glaucoma, urinary/gastric retention **Supplied:** Tabs 20 mg **SE:** Constipation, xerostomia

Trovafloxacin (Trovan) WARNING: Trovan has been associated w/seri-ous liver injury leading to need for liver transplant &/or death. **Uses:** *Life-threatening Infxns* including pneumonia, complicated intraabdominal, gyneco-logic/pelvic, or skin Infxns **Action:** Fluoroquinolone antibiotic; ↓ DNA gyrase. *Spectrum:* Broad-spectrum gram(+) & gram(–), including anaerobes; TB typi-cally resistant **Dose:** 200 mg/d; ↓ w/hepatic impair **Caution:** [C, –] in children **Contra:** Hepatic impair **Supplied:** Inj 5 mg/mL in 40 & 60 mL; tabs 100, 200 mg **SE:** Liver failure, dizziness, HA, nausea, rash **Notes:** Use restricted to hos-pitals; hepatotox led to restricted availability

Urokinase (Abbokinase) Uses: *PE, DVT, restore patency to IV cathe-ters* **Action:** Converts plasminogen to plasmin; causes clot lysis **Dose:** *Adults & Peds.* Systemic effect: 4400 units/kg IV over 10 min, then by 4400–6000 units/kg/h for 12 h. *Restore catheter patency:* Inject 5000 units into catheter & aspirate **Caution:** [B, +] **Contra:** Do not use w/in 10 d of surgery, delivery, or organ biopsy; bleeding, CVA, vascular malformation **Supplied:** Powder for inj 5000 units/mL, 250,000-unit vial **SE:** Bleeding, ↓ BP, dyspnea, bronchospasm, anaphylaxis, cholesterol embolism

Valacyclovir (Valtrex) Uses: *Herpes zoster; genital herpes* **Action:** Prodrug of acyclovir; ↓ viral DNA replication. *Spectrum:* Herpes simplex I & II **Dose:** 1 g PO tid. *Genital herpes:* 500 mg bid × 7 d. *Herpes prophylaxis:* 500–1000 mg/d; ↓ w/renal failure **Caution:** [B, +] **Supplied:** Caplets 500 mg **SE:** HA, GI upset, dizziness, pruritus, photophobia

Valdecoxib (Bextra) Uses: *RA, osteoarthritis, primary dysmenorrhea* **Action:** COX-2 inhibition **Dose:** *Arthritis:* 10 mg PO qd. *Dysmenorrhea:* 20 mg PO bid, PRN **Caution:** [C, ?] Asthma, urticaria, allergic-type reactions after ASA or NSAIDs, sulfonamide allergy **Supplied:** Tabs 10, 20 mg **SE:** ↑ LFT, GI ulceration or bleeding; dizziness, edema, HTN, HA, peptic ulcer, renal failure; serious allergic reactions have occurred, including Stevens–Johnson syndrome

Valganciclovir (Valcyte) Uses: *CMV* **Action:** Ganciclovir prodrug; ↓ viral DNA synthesis **Dose:** Induction, 900 mg PO bid w/food × 21 d, then 900 mg PO qd; ↓ in renal dysfunction **Caution:** [C, ?/–] Use w/imipenem/cilastatin, nephrotoxic drugs **Contra:** Allergy to acyclovir, ganciclovir, valganciclovir; ANC < 500/mm^2; plt < 25 K; Hgb < 8 g/dL **Supplied:** Tabs 450 mg **SE:** BM suppression **Notes:** Monitor CBC & Cr

Valproic Acid (Depakene, Depakote) Uses: *Rx epilepsy, mania; prophylaxis of migraines,* Alzheimer behavior disorder **Action:** Anticonvul-sant; ↑ availability of GABA **Dose:** *Adults & Peds.* Szs: 30–60 mg/kg/24 h PO ÷ tid (after initiation of 10–15 mg/kg/24 h). *Mania:* 750 mg in 3 ÷ doses, ↑ 60 mg/kg/d max. *Migraines:* 250 mg bid, ↑ 1000 mg/d max; ↓ w/hepatic impair **Caution:** [D, +] **Contra:** Severe hepatic impair **Supplied:** Caps 250 mg; syrup 250 mg/5 mL **SE:** Somnolence, dizziness, GI upset, diplopia, ataxia, rash, thrombocytopenia, hepatitis, pancreatitis, prolonged bleeding times, alopecia, weight gain, hyperammonemic encephalopathy reported in pts w/urea cycle disorders **Notes:** Monitor LFTs & serum levels (Table 22–2, page 628); phenobarbital & phenytoin may alter levels

Valsartan (Diovan) WARNING: Use during 2nd/3rd tri of PRG can cause fetal harm **Uses:** HTN, CHF, DN **Action:** Angiotensin II receptor antagonist **Dose:** 80–160 mg/d **Caution:** [C (1st tri; D 2nd & 3rd tri), ?/–] W/ K$^+$-sparing diuretics or K$^+$ supls **Contra:** Severe hepatic impair, biliary cirrhosis/obstruction, primary hyperaldosteronism, bilateral renal artery stenosis **Supplied:** Caps 80, 160 mg **SE:** ↓ BP, dizziness

Vancomycin (Vancocin, Vancoled) **Uses:** *Serious MRSA Infxns; enterococcal Infxns; PO Rx of *C. difficile* pseudomembranous colitis* **Action:** ↓ Cell wall synthesis. *Spectrum:* Gram(+) bacteria & some anaerobes (includes MRSA, *Staphylococcus* sp, *Enterococcus* sp, *Streptococcus* sp, *C. difficile*) **Dose:** *Adults.* 1 g IV q12h; for colitis 125–500 mg PO q6h. *Peds.* 40–60 mg/kg/24 h IV in ÷ doses q6–12 h. *Neonates.* 10–15 mg/kg/dose q12h; ↓ in renal insuff **Caution:** [C, M] **Contra:** Component allergy; avoid in Hx hearing loss **Supplied:** Caps 125, 250 mg; powder for PO soln; powder for inj 500 mg, 1000 mg, 10 g/vial **SE:** Ototoxic & nephrotoxic; GI upset (PO), neutropenia **Notes:** See drug levels (Table 22–2, page 628); not absorbed PO, local effect in gut only; give IV dose slowly (over 1–3 h) to prevent "red-man syndrome" (red flushing of head, neck, upper torso); IV product may be given PO for colitis

Vardenafil (Levitra) WARNING: May prolong QTc interval **Uses:** *ED* **Action:** Phosphodiesterase 5 inhibitor **Dose:** 10 mg PO 60 min before sexual activity; 2.5 mg if administered w/CYP3A4 inhibitors; max × 1 ≤ 20 mg **Caution:** [B, –] w/CV, hepatic, or renal Dz **Contra:** Nitrates **Supplied:** 2.5-mg, 5-mg, 10-mg, 20-mg tabs **SE:** ↓ BP, HA, dyspepsia, priapism **Notes:** Concomitant α-blockers may cause ↓ BP

Varicella Virus Vaccine (Varivax) **Uses:** *Prevent varicella (chickenpox)* **Action:** Active immunization; live attenuated virus **Dose:** *Adults & Peds.* 0.5 mL SQ, repeat 4–8 wk **Caution:** [C, M] **Contra:** Immunocompromise; neomycin-anaphylactoid Rxn, blood dyscrasias; immunosuppressive drugs; avoid PRG for 3 mo after **Supplied:** Powder for inj **SE:** Mild varicella Infxn; fever, local Rxns, irritability, GI upset **Notes:** OK for all children & adults who have not had chickenpox

Vasopressin [Antidiuretic Hormone, ADH] (Pitressin) **Uses:** *DI; Rx postop abdominal distention*; adjunct Rx of GI bleeding & esophageal varices; pulseless VT & VF, adjunct systemic vasopressor (IV drip) **Action:** Posterior pituitary hormone, potent GI and peripheral vasoconstrictor **Dose:** *Adults & Peds.* DI: 2.5–10 units SQ or IM tid–qid. *GI hemorrhage:* 0.2–0.4 units/min; ↓ in cirrhosis; caution in vascular Dz. *VT/VF:* 40 units IVP X1. *Vasopressor:* 0.01–0.1 units/kg/min **Caution:** [B, +] **Contra:** Allergy **Supplied:** Inj 20 units/mL **SE:** HTN, arrhythmias, fever, vertigo, GI upset, tremor **Notes:** Addition of vasopressor to concurrent norepinephrine or epi inf

Vecuronium (Norcuron) **Uses:** *Skeletal muscle relaxation during surgery or mechanical ventilation* **Action:** Nondepolarizing neuromuscular blocker **Dose:** *Adults & Peds.* 0.08–0.1 mg/kg IV bolus; maint 0.010–0.015 mg/kg after 25–40 min; additional doses q12–15min PRN; ↓ in severe renal/hepatic

22

impair **Caution:** [C, ?] Drug interactions cause ↑ effect (eg, aminoglycosides, tetracycline, succinylcholine) **Supplied:** Powder for inj 10 mg **SE:** Bradycardia, ↓ BP, itching, rash, tachycardia, CV collapse **Notes:** Fewer cardiac effects than pancuronium

Venlafaxine (Effexor) WARNING: Closely monitor for worsening depression or emergence of suicidality, particularly in ped pts **Uses:** *Depression, generalized anxiety,* social anxiety disorder; obsessive–compulsive disorder, chronic fatigue syndrome, ADHD, autism **Action:** Potentiation of CNS neurotransmitter activity **Dose:** 75–375 mg/d ÷ into 2–3 equal doses; ↓ w/renal/ hepatic impair **Caution:** [C, ?/–] **Contra:** MAOIs **Supplied:** Tabs 25, 37.5, 50, 75, 100 mg; ER caps 37.5, 75, 150 mg **SE:** HTN, ↑ HR, HA, somnolence, GI upset, sexual dysfunction; actuates mania or Szs **Notes:** Avoid EtOH

Verapamil (Calan, Isoptin) Uses: *Angina, HTN, PSVT, AF, atrial flutter,* migraine prophylaxis, hypertrophic cardiomyopathy, bipolar Dz **Action:** CCB **Dose:** *Adults. Arrhythmias:* 2nd line for PSVT w/narrow QRS complex & adequate BP 2.5–5 mg IV over 1–2 min; repeat 5–10 mg in 15–30 min PRN (30 mg max). *Angina:* 80–120 mg PO tid, ↑ 480 mg/24 h max. *HTN:* 80–180 mg PO tid or SR tabs 120–240 mg PO qd to 240 mg bid. *Peds.* < 1 y: 0.1–0.2 mg/kg IV over 2 min (may repeat in 30 min). *1–16 y:* 0.1–0.3 mg/kg IV over 2 min (may repeat in 30 min); 5 mg max. *PO: 1–5 y:* 4–8 mg/kg/d in 3 ÷ doses. > *5 y:* 80 mg q6–8h; ↓ in renal/hepatic impair **Caution:** [C, +] Amiodarone/β-blockers/ flecainide can cause bradycardia; statins, midazolam, tacrolimus, theophylline levels may be ↑ **Contra:** Conduction disorders, cardiogenic shock; caution w/ elderly pts **Supplied:** Tabs 40, 80, 120 mg; SR tabs 120, 180, 240 mg; SR caps 120, 180, 240, 360 mg; inj 5 mg/2 mL **SE:** Gingival hyperplasia, constipation, ↓ BP, bronchospasm, heart rate or conduction disturbances

Vinblastine (Velban, Velbe) WARNING: Chemotherapeutic agent; handle w/caution **Uses:** *Hodgkin Dz & NHL, mycosis fungoides, CA (testis, renal cell, breast, NSCLC, AIDS-related Kaposi sarcoma,* choriocarcinoma), histiocytosis **Action:** ↓ Microtubule assembly **Dose:** 0.1–0.5 mg/kg/wk (4–20 mg/ m²); ↓ in hepatic failure **Caution:** [D, ?] **Contra:** IT use **Supplied:** Inj 1 mg/mL **SE:** Myelosuppression (especially leukopenia), N/V, constipation, neurotox, alopecia, rash, myalgia, tumor pain

Vincristine (Oncovin, Vincasar PFS) WARNING: Chemotherapeutic agent; handle w/caution; **fatal if administered IT Uses:** *ALL, breast & small-cell lung CA, sarcoma (eg, Ewing tumor, rhabdomyosarcoma), Wilms tumor, Hodgkin Dz & NHL, neuroblastoma, multiple myeloma* **Action:** Promotes disassembly of mitotic spindle, causing metaphase arrest **Dose:** 0.4–1.4 mg/m² (single doses 2 mg/ max); ↓ in hepatic failure **Caution:** [D, ?] **Contra:** IT use **Supplied:** Inj 1 mg/mL **SE:** Neurotox commonly dose limiting, jaw pain (trigeminal neuralgia), fever, fatigue, anorexia, constipation & paralytic ileus, bladder atony; no significant myelosuppression w/standard doses; tissue necrosis w/extravasation

Vinorelbine (Navelbine) WARNING: Chemotherapeutic agent; handle w/caution **Uses:** *Breast & NSCLC* (alone or w/cisplatin) **Action:** ↓ Polymerization of microtubules, impairing mitotic spindle formation; semisynthetic vinca alkaloid **Dose:** 30 mg/m²/wk; ↓ in hepatic failure **Caution:** [D, ?] **Contra:** IT use **Supplied:** Inj 10 mg **SE:** Myelosuppression (leukopenia), mild GI effects, infrequent neurotox (6–29%); constipation & paresthesias (rare); tissue damage from extravasation

Vitamin B$_1$ See Thiamine (page 610)

Vitamin B$_6$ See Pyridoxine (page 594)

Vitamin B$_{12}$ See Cyanocobalamin (page 511)

Vitamin K See Phytonadione (page 588)

Voriconazole (VFEND) Uses: *Invasive aspergillosis, serious fungal Infxns* **Action:** ↓ Ergosterol synthesis. *Spectrum:* Several types of fungus: *Aspergillus, Scedosporium* sp, *Fusarium* sp **Dose: *Adults & Peds*** ≥ 12 y. IV: 6 mg/kg q12h × 2, then 4 mg/kg bid; may ↓ to 3 mg/kg/dose. *PO:* < 40 kg: 100 mg q12h, up to 150 mg; > 40 kg: 200 mg q 12 h, up to 300 mg; ↓ w/mild–moderate hepatic impair; IV only one dose w/renal impair (PO empty stomach) **Caution:** [D, ?/–] **Contra:** Severe hepatic impair **Supplied:** Tabs 50, 200 mg; 200-mg inj **SE:** Vision changes, fever, rash, GI upset, ↑ LFTs **Notes:** Screen for multiple drug interactions (eg, ↑ dose w/phenytoin)

Warfarin (Coumadin) Uses: *Prophylaxis & Rx of PE & DVT, AF w/ embolization,* other postop indications **Action:** ↓ Vitamin K–dependent clotting factors in order: VII-IX-X-II **Dose: *Adults.*** Titrate, INR 2.0–3.0 for most; mechanical valves INR is 2.5–3.5. *ACCP guidelines:* 5 mg initial (unless rapid therapeutic INR needed), may use 7.5–10 mg; if pt elderly or has other bleeding risk factors ↓. *Alternative:* 10–15 mg PO, IM, or IV qd for 1–3 d; maint 2–10 mg/ d PO, IV, or IM; follow daily INR initial to adjust dosage (see Table 22–10, page 644). *Peds.* 0.05–0.34 mg/kg/24 h PO, IM, or IV; follow PT/INR to adjust dosage; monitor vitamin K intake; ↓ w/hepatic impair/elderly **Caution:** [X, +] **Contra:** Severe hepatic/renal Dz, bleeding, peptic ulcer, PRG **Supplied:** Tabs 1, 2, 2.5, 3, 4, 5, 6, 7.5, 10 mg; inj **SE:** Bleeding due to overanticoagulation (PT > 3 × control or INR > 5.0–6.0) or injury & INR w/in therapeutic range; bleeding, alopecia, skin necrosis, purple toe syndrome **Notes:** INR preferred test; to rapidly correct overanticoagulation, use vitamin K, FFP or both; highly teratogenic; do *not* use in PRG. Caution pt on taking w/other meds, especially ASA. *Common warfarin interactions:* Potentiated by APAP, EtOH (w/liver Dz), amiodarone, cimetidine, ciprofloxacin, cotrimoxazole, erythromycin, fluconazole, flu vaccine, isoniazid, itraconazole, metronidazole, omeprazole, phenytoin, propranolol, quinidine, tetracycline. Inhibited by barbiturates, carbamazepine, chlordiazepoxide, cholestyramine, dicloxacillin, nafcillin, rifampin, sucralfate, high-vitamin K foods

Zafirlukast (Accolate) Uses: *Adjunctive Rx of asthma* **Action:** Selective & competitive inhibitor of leukotrienes **Dose: *Adults & Peds*** ≥ 12 y. 20 mg bid. *Peds 5–11 y.* 10 mg PO bid (empty stomach) **Caution:** [B, –] Interacts w/ warfarin, ↑ INR **Contra:** Component allergy **Supplied:** Tabs 20 mg **SE:** Hepatic dysfunction, usually reversible on D/C; HA, dizziness, GI upset; Churg–Strauss syndrome **Notes:** Not for acute asthma

Zalcitabine (Hivid) **WARNING:** Use w/caution in pts w/neuropathy, pancreatitis, lactic acidosis, hepatitis Uses: *HIV* **Action:** Antiretroviral agent **Dose: *Adults.*** 0.75 mg PO tid. *Peds.* 0.015–0.04 mg/kg PO q 6h; ↓ in renal failure **Caution:** [C, +] **Contra:** Component allergy **Supplied:** Tabs 0.375, 0.75 mg **SE:** Peripheral neuropathy, pancreatitis, fever, malaise, anemia, hypo/hyperglycemia, hepatic impair **Notes:** May be used in combo w/zidovudine

Zaleplon (Sonata) [C-IV] Uses: *Insomnia* **Action:** Nonbenzodiazepine sedative/hypnotic; pyrazolopyrimidine **Dose:** 5–20 mg hs PRN; ↓ w/renal/

22

hepatic insuff, elderly **Caution:** [C, ?/–] w/mental/psychological conditions **Contra:** Component allergy **Supplied:** Caps 5, 10 mg **SE:** HA, edema, amnesia, somnolence, photosensitivity **Notes:** Take immediately before desired onset

Zanamivir (Relenza) Uses: *Influenza A & B* **Action:** ↓ Viral neuraminidase **Dose:** *Adults & Peds > 7 y.* 2 inhal (10 mg) bid for 5 d; initiate w/in 48 h of Sxs **Caution:** [C, M] **Contra:** Pulmonary Dz **Supplied:** Powder for inhal 5 mg **SE:** Bronchospasm, HA, GI upset **Notes:** Use Diskhaler for administration

Ziconotide (Prialt) WARNING: Psychiatric, cognitive, neurologic impair may develop over several weeks; monitor frequently; may necessitate D/C **Uses:** *IT Rx of severe, refractory, chronic pain* **Action:** N-type CCB in spinal cord **Dose:** 2.6 mcg/d IT at 0.1 mcg/h; may ↑ 0.8 mcg/h to total 19.2 mcg/d by d 21 **Caution:** [C, ?/–] Reversible psychiatric/neurologic impair **Contra:** Psychosis **Supplied:** Inj 25, 100 mg/mL **SE:** Dizziness, N/V, confusion, abnormal vision; may require dosage adjustment **Notes:** May D/C abruptly; uses specific pumps; do not ↑ more frequently than 2–3 ×/wk

Zidovudine (Retrovir) WARNING: Neutropenia, anemia, lactic acidosis & hepatomegaly w/steatosis **Uses:** *HIV Infxn, prevention of maternal transmission of HIV* **Action:** ↓ RT **Dose:** *Adults.* 200 mg PO tid or 300 mg PO bid or 1–2 mg/kg/dose IV q4h. *PRG:* 100 mg PO 5 ×/d until labor starts; during labor 2 mg/kg over 1 h followed by 1 mg/kg/h until clamping of the cord. *Peds.* 160 mg/m²/dose q8h; ↓ in renal failure **Caution:** [C, ?/–] **Contra:** Allergy **Supplied:** Caps 100 mg; tabs 300 mg; syrup 50 mg/5 mL; inj 10 mg/mL **SE:** Hematologic tox, HA, fever, rash, GI upset, malaise

Zidovudine & Lamivudine (Combivir) WARNING: Neutropenia, anemia, lactic acidosis & hepatomegaly w/steatosis **Uses:** *HIV Infxn* **Action:** Combo of RT inhibitors **Dose:** *Adults & Peds > 12 y.* 1 tab PO bid; ↓ in renal failure **Caution:** [C, ?/–] **Contra:** Component allergy **Supplied:** Caps zidovudine 300 mg/lamivudine 150 mg **SE:** Hematologic tox, HA, fever, rash, GI upset, malaise, pancreatitis **Notes:** Combo product ↓ daily pill burden

Zileuton (Zyflo) Uses: *Chronic Rx of asthma* **Action:** Inhibitor of 5-lipoxygenase **Dose:** *Adults & Peds ≥ 12 y.* 600 mg PO qid **Caution:** [C, ?/–] **Contra:** Hepatic impair **Supplied:** Tabs 600 mg **SE:** Hepatic damage, HA, GI upset, leukopenia **Notes:** Monitor LFTs every month × 3, then q2–3 mo; take on regular basis; not for acute asthma

Ziprasidone (Geodon) WARNING: ↑ mortality in elderly with dementia-related psychosis **Uses:** *Schizophrenia, acute agitation* **Action:** Atypical antipsychotic **Dose:** 20 mg PO bid, may ↑ in 2–d intervals up to 80 mg bid; agitation 10–20 mg IM PRN up to 40 mg/d; separate 10 mg doses by 2 h & 20 mg doses by 4h (w/food) **Caution:** [C, –] w/↓ Mg²⁺, ↓ K⁺ **Contra:** QT prolongation, recent MI, uncompensated heart failure, meds that ↑ QT interval **Supplied:** Caps 20, 40, 60, 80 mg; Inj 20 mg/mL **SE:** Bradycardia; rash, somnolence, resp disorder, EPS, weight gain, orthostatic ↓ BP **Notes:** Monitor electrolytes

Zoledronic Acid (Zometa) Uses: *↑ Ca²⁺ of malignancy (HCM),* ↓ skeletal-related events in CAP, multiple myeloma & metastatic bone lesions **Action:** Bisphosphonate; ↓ osteoclastic bone resorption **Dose:** *HCM:* 4 mg IV over at least 15 min; may re-treat in 7 d if adequate renal Fxn. *Bone lesions/myeloma:* 4 mg IV over at least 15 min, repeat q3–4wk PRN; prolonged w/Cr ↑ **Caution:** [C, ?/–] Loop

diuretics, aminoglycosides; ASA-sensitive asthmatics; avoid invasive dental procedures in CA patients; renal dysfunction **Contra:** Bisphosphonate allergy **Supplied:**
Vial 4 mg **SE:** Adverse effects ↑ w/renal dysfunction; fever, flu-like syndrome, GI
upset, insomnia, anemia; electrolyte abnormalities, osteonecrosis of jaw **Notes:**
Requires vigorous prehydration; do not exceed recommended doses/inf duration to
↓ dose-related renal dysfunction; follow Cr; avoid oral surgery; dental examination
recommended before therapy; ↓ dose w/renal dysfunction

Zolmitriptan (Zomig, Zomig XMT, Zomig Nasal) Uses: *Acute Rx
migraine* **Action:** Selective serotonin agonist; causes vasoconstriction **Dose:** Initial
2.5 mg PO, may repeat after 2 h, 10 mg max in 24 h; nasal 5 mg; HA returns, repeated
after 2 h 10 mg max 24 h **Caution:** [C, ?/–] **Contra:** Ischemic heart Dz, Prinzmetal
angina, uncontrolled HTN, accessory conduction pathway disorders, ergots, MAOIs
Supplied: Tabs 2.5, 5 mg; Rapid tabs (ZMT) 2.5 mg; nasal 5.0, 2.5, 1.0, 0.5 mg, **SE:**
Dizziness, hot flashes, paresthesias, chest tightness, myalgia, diaphoresis

Zolpidem (Ambien, Ambien CR) [C-IV] Uses: *Short-term Rx of insomnia* **Action:** Hypnotic agent **Dose:** 5–10 mg or 12.5 mg CR PO hs PRN; ↓ in
elderly (use 6.25 mg CR), hepatic insuff **Caution:** [B, –] **Contra:** Breast feeding
Supplied: Tabs 5, 10 mg; CR 6.25, 12.5 mg **SE:** HA, dizziness, drowsiness, nausea,
myalgia **Notes:** May be habit-forming; CR delivers a rapid then a longer lasting dose

Zonisamide (Zonegran) Uses: *Adjunct Rx complex partial Szs* **Action:**
Anticonvulsant **Dose:** Initial 100 mg/d PO; may ↑ to 400 mg/d **Caution:** [C, –] ↑
tox w/CYP3A4 inhibitor; ↓ levels w/concurrent carbamazepine, phenytoin, phenobarbital, valproic acid **Contra:** Allergy to sulfonamides; oligohidrosis & hypothermia in peds **Supplied:** Caps 100 mg **SE:** Dizziness, drowsiness, confusion,
ataxia, memory impair, paresthesias, psychosis, nystagmus, diplopia, tremor; anemia, leukopenia; GI upset, nephrolithiasis, Stevens–Johnson syndrome; monitor for
↓ sweating & ↑ body temperature **Notes:** Swallow capsules whole

NATURAL AND HERBAL AGENTS

The following is a guide to some common herbal products. These agents may be
sold separately or in combination with other products. According to the FDA:
"Manufacturers of dietary supplements can make claims about how their products affect the structure or function of the body, but they may not claim to prevent, treat, cure, mitigate, or diagnose a disease without prior FDA approval"*

Black Cohosh Uses: Sx of menopause (eg, hot flashes), PMS, hyperchole-
terolemia, peripheral arterial Dz; has antiinflammatory & sedative effects **Efficacy:** May have short-term benefit on menopausal Sx **Dose:** 40–160 mg PO qd.
Caution: May further ↓ lipids &/or BP w/prescription meds **Contra:** PRG (miscarriage, prematurity reports) **SE:** OD can cause N/V, dizziness, nervous system
& visual changes, bradycardia & (possibly) Szs, liver damage/failure

Chamomile Uses: Antispasmodic, sedative, antiinflammatory, astringent,
antibacterial. **Dose:** 10–15 g PO qd (3 g dried flower heads tid–qid between
meals; can steep in 250 mL hot H_2O) **Caution:** W/allergy to chrysanthemums,
ragweed, asters (family Compositae) **SE:** Contact dermatitis; allergy, anaphy-

---

*Based on data in Haist SA and Robbins JB: *Internal Medicine on Call,* 4th ed,
2005, McGraw-Hill. See also www.fda.gov.

laxis **Interactions:** W/anticoagulants, additive w/sedatives (benzodiazepines); delayed gastric absorption of meds if taken together (↓ GI motility)

Cranberry (*Vaccinium macrocarpon*) **Uses:** Prevention & Rx UTI. **Efficacy:** Possibly effective **Dose:** 150 mg/d PO **Caution:** May ↑ kidney stones in susceptible individuals **SE:** None known **Interactions:** None significant

Dong Quai (*Angelica polymorpha, sinensis*) **Uses:** Uterine stimulant; menstrual cramps, irregular menses & menopausal Sx; antiinflammatory, vasodilator, CNS stimulant, immunosuppressant, analgesic, antipyretic, antiasthmatic **Efficacy:** Possibly effective for menopausal Sx **Dose:** 9–12 g PO tab bid. **Caution:** Avoid in PRG & lactation. **SE:** D, photosensitivity, skin cancer. **Interactions:** Anticoagulants (↑ INR w/warfarin).

Echinacea (*Echinacea purpurea*) **Uses:** Immune system stimulant; prevention/Rx of colds, flu; supportive care chronic infections of the resp/lower urinary tract **Efficacy:** Not established; may ↓ severity & duration of URI **Dose:** 6–9 mL expressed juice or 2–5 g dried root PO **Caution:** Do not use w/progressive systemic or immune Dzs (eg, TB, collagen–vascular disorders, MS); may interfere with immunosuppressive therapy, not OK w/PRG; do not use > 8 consecutive wk; possible immunosuppression **SE:** N, rash **Interactions:** Anabolic steroids, amiodarone, MTX, corticosteroids, cyclosporine.

Ephedra/Ma Huang **Uses:** Stimulant, aid in weight loss, bronchial dilation. **Dose:** Not OK owing to **reported deaths** (> 100 mg/d can be life-threatening). US sales banned by FDA in 2004 **Caution:** Adverse cardiac events, stroke, death **SE:** Nervousness, HA, insomnia, palpitations, V, hyperglycemia **Interactions:** Digoxin, antihypertensives, antidepressants, diabetic medications

Evening Primrose Oil **Uses:** PMS, diabetic neuropathy, ADHD **Efficacy:** Possibly for PMS, not for menopausal Sx **Dose:** 2–4 g/d PO **SE:** Indigestion, N, soft stools, HA **Interactions:** ↑ Phenobarbital metabolism, ↓ Sz threshold

Feverfew (*Tanacetum parthenium*) **Uses:** Prevent/Rx migraine; fever; menstrual disorders; arthritis; toothache; insect bites **Efficacy:** Weak for migraine prevention **Dose:** 125 mg of dried leaf (w/at least 0.2% of parthenolide) PO **Caution:** Do not use in PRG **SE:** Oral ulcers, gastric disturbance, swollen lips, abdominal pain; long-term SE unknown. **Interactions:** ASA, warfarin

Garlic (*Allium sativum*) **Uses:** Antioxidant; hyperlipidemia, HTN; antiinfective (antibacterial, antifungal); tick repellant (oral) **Efficacy:** ↓ Cholesterol by 4–6%; soln ↓ BP; possible ↓ GI/CAP risk **Dose:** 400–1200 mg powder (2–5 mg allicin) PO **Caution:** Do not use in PRG (abortifacient); D/C 7 d preop (bleeding risk) **SE:** ↑ Insulin levels, ↑ lipid/cholesterol levels, anemia, oral burning sensation, N/V/D **Interactions:** Warfarin & ASA (↓ plt aggregation), additive w/DM agents (↑ hypoglycemia). CYP450, 3A4 inducer (may ↑ cyclosporine, HIV antivirals, OCP)

Ginger (*Zingiber officinale*) **Uses:** Prevent motion sickness; N/V due to anesthesia **Efficacy:** Benefit in ↓ N/V w/motion or PRG; weak for postop or chemo **Dose:** 1–4 g rhizome or 0.5–2 g powder PO qd **Caution:** Pt w/gallstones; excessive dose (↑ depression & may interfere w/cardiac Fxn or anticoagulants) **SE:** Heartburn **Interactions:** Excessive consumption may interfere with cardiac, DM, or anticoagulant meds (↓ plt aggregation)

Ginkgo Biloba **Uses:** Memory deficits, dementia, anxiety, improvement Sx peripheral vascular Dz, vertigo, tinnitus, asthma/bronchospasm, antioxidant, premenstrual Sx (especially breast tenderness), impotence, SSRI-induced sexual

22

dysfunction **Dose:** 60–80 mg standardized dry extract PO bid–tid **Efficacy:** Small cognition benefit w/dementia; no other demonstrated benefit in healthy adults **Caution:** ↑ Bleeding risk (antagonism of plt-activating factor), concerning w/antiplatelet agents (D/C 3 d preop); reports of ↑ Sz risk **SE:** GI upset, HA, dizziness, heart palpitations, rash **Interactions:** ASA, salicylates, warfarin

Ginseng **Uses:** "Energy booster," stress reduction, enhance brain activity & physical endurance (adaptogenic), antioxidant, aid in glucose control **Efficacy:** Not established **Dose:** 1–2 g of root or 100–300 mg of extract (7% ginsenosides) PO TID **Caution:** W/ cardiac Dz, DM, hypotension, HTN, mania, schizophrenia, w/corticosteroids; avoid in PRG; D/C 7 d preop (bleeding risk) **SE:** Controversial "ginseng abuse syndrome" w/high dose (nervousness, excitation, HA, insomnia); palpitations, vaginal bleeding, breast nodules, hypoglycemia **Interactions:** Warfarin, antidepressants & caffeine (↑ stimulant effect), DM meds (↑ hypoglycemia)

Glucosamine Sulfate (Chitosamine) and Chondroitin Sulfate
Uses: Osteoarthritis (glucosamine: rate-limiting step in glycosaminoglycan synthesis), ↑ cartilage rebuilding; chondroitin: biological polymer, flexible matrix between protein filaments in cartilage; draws fluids/nutrients into joint, "shock absorption" **Efficacy:** Controversial **Dose:** Glucosamine 500 PO tid, chondroitin 400 mg PO tid **Caution:** None known **SE:** ↑ Insulin resistance in DM; concentrated in cartilage; theoretically unlikely to cause toxic/teratogenic effects **Interactions:** *Glucosamine:* None. *Chondroitin:* Monitor anticoagulant therapy

Kava Kava (Kava Kava Root Extract, *Piper methysticum*)
Uses: Anxiety, stress, restlessness, insomnia **Efficacy:** Possible mild anxiolytic **Dose:** Standardized extract (70% kavalactones) 100 mg PO bid–tid **Caution:** Hepatotox risk, banned in Europe/Canada. Not OK in PRG, lactation. D/C 24 h preop (may ↑ sedative effect of anesthetics) **SE:** Mild GI disturbances; rare allergic skin/rash reactions, may ↑ cholesterol; ↑ LFT /jaundice; vision changes, red eyes, puffy face, muscle weakness **Interactions:** Avoid w/sedatives, alcohol, stimulants, barbiturates (may potentiate CNS effect)

Melatonin **Uses:** Insomnia, jet lag, antioxidant, immunostimulant **Efficacy:** Sedation most pronounced w/elderly patients with ↑ endogenous melatonin levels; some evidence for jet lag **Dose:** 1–3 mg 20 min before hs (w/CR 2 h before hs) **Caution:** Use synthetic rather than animal pineal gland, "heavy head," HA, depression, daytime sedation, dizziness **Interactions:** β-Blockers, steroids, NSAIDs, benzodiazepines

Milk Thistle (*Silybum marianum*) **Uses:** Prevent/Rx liver damage (eg, from alcohol, toxins, cirrhosis, chronic hepatitis); preventive w/chronic toxin exposure (painters, chemical workers, etc) **Efficacy:** Use before exposure more effective than use after damage has occurred **Dose:** 70–200 mg PO tid **SE:** GI intolerance **Interactions:** None

Saw Palmetto (*Serenoa repens*) **Uses:** Rx BPH (weak 5-α-reductase inhibitor) **Efficacy:** Small–significant benefit for prostatic Sx **Dose:** 320 mg qd **Caution:** Hormonal effects, avoid in PRG, w/women of childbearing years **SE:** Mild GI upset, mild HA, D w/large amounts **Interactions:** ↑ Iron absorption; ↑ estrogen replacement effects

St. John's Wort (*Hypericum perforatum*) **Uses:** Mild–moderate depression, anxiety, gastritis, insomnia, vitiligo; antiinflammatory; immune stimulant/anti-HIV/antiviral **Efficacy:** Variable; benefit in mild–moderate depression in several tri-

22

als, but not always seen in clinical practice **Dose:** 2–4 g of herb or 0.2–1 mg of total hypericin (standardized extract) qd. *Common preps:* 300 mg PO tid (0.3% hypericin) **Caution:** Excessive doses may potentiate MAOI, cause allergic reaction, not OK in PRG **SE:** Photosensitivity, xerostomia, dizziness, constipation, confusion, fluctuating mood w/chronic use **Interactions:** Do not use w/prescription antidepressants, (especially MAOI); ↑ cyclosporine efficacy (may cause rejection), digoxin (may exacerbate CHF), protease inhibitors, theophylline, oral contraceptives; cytochrome P-450 3A4 enzyme inducer; potency can vary between products/batches

Valerian (*Valeriana officinalis*) **Uses:** Anxiolytic, sedative, restlessness, dysmenorrheal **Efficacy:** Probably effective sedative (reduces sleep latency) **Dose:** 2–3 g extract PO qd–bid (Combined w/OTC sleep product Alluna) **Caution:** None known **SE:** Sedation, hangover effect, HA, cardiac disturbances, GI upset **Interactions:** Caution w/other sedating agents (eg, alcohol, or prescription sedatives): may cause drowsiness w/impaired Fxn

Yohimbine (*Pausinystalia yohimbe*) **Uses:** Improve sexual vigor, Rx ED **Efficacy:** Variable **Dose:** 5 mg PO tid (use w/physician supervision) **Caution:** Do not use w/renal/hepatic Dz; may exacerbate schizophrenia/mania (if pt predisposed). α_2-Adrenergic antagonist (↓ BP, abdominal distress, weakness w/ high doses), OD can be fatal; salivation, dilated pupils, arrhythmias **SE:** Anxiety, tremors, dizziness, high BP, ↑ heart rate **Interactions:** Do not use w/antidepressants (eg, MAOIs or similar agents)

Unsafe Herbs with Known Toxicity

Agent	Toxicities
Aconite	Salivation, N/V, blurred vision, cardiac arrhythmias
Aristolochic acid	Nephrotox
Calamus	Possible carcinogenicity
Chaparral	Hepatotox, possible carcinogenicity, nephrotox
"Chinese herbal mixtures"	May contain ma huang or other dangerous herbs
Coltsfoot	Hepatotox, possibly carcinogenic
Comfrey	Hepatotox, carcinogenic
Ephedra/ma huang	Adverse cardiac events, stroke, Sz
Juniper	High allergy potential, D, Sz, nephrotox
Kava kava	Hepatotox
Licorice	Chronic daily amounts (> 30 g/mo) can result in ↓ K^+, Na/fluid retention w/HTN, myoglobinuria, hyporeflexia
Life root	Hepatotox, liver CA
Ma huang/ephedra	Adverse cardiac events, stroke, Sz
Pokeweed	GI cramping, N/D/V, labored breathing, ↓ BP, Sz
Sassafras	V, stupor, hallucinations, dermatitis, abortion, hypothermia, liver CA
Usnic acid	Hepatotox
Yohimbine	Hypotension, abdominal distress, CNS stimulation (mania & psychosis in predisposed individuals)

TABLE 22–1
Quick Guide to Dosing of Acetaminophen Based on the Tylenol Product Line

	Suspension[a] Drops and Original Drops 80 mg/0.8 mL Dropperful	Chewable[a] Tablets 80-mg tabs	Suspension[a] Liquid and Original Elixir 160 mg/5 mL	Junior[a] Strength 160-mg Caplets/Chewables	Regular[b] Strength 325-mg Caplets/Tablets	Extra Strength[b] 500-mg Caplets/Gelcaps
Birth–3 mo/6–11 lb/2.5–5.4 kg	½ dppr[c] (0.4 mL)					
4–11 mo/12–17 lb/5.5–7.9 kg	1 dppr[c] (0.8 mL)		½ tsp			
12–23 mo/18–23 lb/8.0–10.9 kg	1½ dppr[c] (1.2 mL)		¾ tsp			
2–3 y/24–35 lb/11.0–15.9 kg	2 dppr[c] (1.6 mL)	2 tab	1 tsp			
4–5 y/36–47 lb/16.0–21.9 kg		3 tab	1½ tsp			
6–8 y/48–59 lb/22.0–26.9 kg		4 tab	2 tsp	2 cap/tab		
9–10 y/60–71 lb/27.0–31.9 kg		5 tab	2½ tsp	2½ cap/tab		
11 y/72–95 lb/32.0–43.9 kg		6 tab	4 tsp	3 cap/tab		
Adults & children 12 y and over/96 lb and over/44.0 kg and over				4 cap/tab	1 or 2 caps/tabs	2 caps/gel

[a]Doses should be administered 4 or 5 times daily. Do not exceed 5 doses in 24 h.
[b]No more than 8 dosage units in any 24-h period. Not to be taken for pain for more than 10 days or for fever for more than 3 days unless directed by a physician.
[c]Dropperful.

22

TABLE 22-2
Common Drug Levels[a]

Drug	When to Sample	Therapeutic Levels	Usual Half-life	Potentially Toxic Levels
ANTIBIOTICS				
Gentamicin	Peak: 30 min after 30-min infusion (peak level not necessary if extended-interval dosing: 6 mg/kg/dose)	Peak: 5–8 mcg/mL	2 h	Peak: >12 mcg/mL
	Trough: <0.5 h before next dose	Trough <2 mg/mL <1.0 mg/mL for extended intervals (6 mg/kg/dose) (peak levels not needed with extended-interval dosing)		
Tobramycin	Same as above	Same as above	Same as above	Same as above
Amikacin	Same as above	Peak: 20–30 mcg/mL	2 h	Peak: >35 mcg/mL
Vancomycin	Peak: 1 h after 1-h infusion	Peak: 30–40 mcg/mL	6–8 h	Peak: >50 mcg/mL
	Trough: <0.5 h before next dose			Trough: >15 mcg/mL
ANTICONVULSANTS				
Carbamazepine	Trough: just before next oral dose	8–12 mcg/mL (monotherapy) 4–8 mcg/mL (polytherapy)	15–20 h	Trough: >12 mcg/mL
Ethosuximide	Trough: just before next oral dose	40–100 mcg/mL	30–60 h	Trough: >100 mcg/mL

(continued)

22

TABLE 22-2
(Continued)

Drug	When to Sample	Therapeutic Levels	Usual Half-life	Potentially Toxic Levels
Phenobarbital	Trough: just before next dose	15–40 mcg/mL	40–120 h	Trough: >40 mcg/mL
Phenytoin	May use free phenytoin to monitor[b] Trough: just before next dose	10–20 mcg/mL	Concentration-dependent	>20 mcg/mL
Primidone	Trough: just before next dose (primidone is metabolized to phenobarb; order levels separately)	5–12 mcg/mL	10–12 h	>12 mcg/mL
Valproic acid	Trough: just before next dose	50–100 mcg/mL	5–20 h	>100 mcg/mL
BRONCHODILATORS				
Caffeine	Trough: just before next dose	Adults 5–15 mcg/mL Neonate 6–11 mg/mL	Adults 3–4 h Neonates 30–140 h	20 mcg/mL
Theophylline (IV)	IV: 12–24 h after infusion started	5–15 mcg/mL	Nonsmoking adults 8 h Children and smoking adults 4 h	>20 mcg/mL
Theophylline (PO)	Peak levels: not recommended Trough level: just before next dose	5–15 mcg/mL		

(continued)

22

TABLE 22-2
(Continued)

Drug	When to Sample	Therapeutic Levels	Usual Half-life	Potentially Toxic Levels
CARDIOVASCULAR AGENTS				
Amiodarone	Trough: just before next dose	1–2.5 mcg/mL	30–100 days	>2.5 mcg/mL
Digoxin	Trough: just before next dose (levels drawn earlier than 6 h after a dose will be artificially elevated)	0.8–2.0 ng/mL	36 h	>2 ng/mL
Disopyramide	Trough: just before next dose	2–5 mcg/mL	4–10 h	>5 mcg/mL
Flecainide	Trough: just before next dose	0.2–1.0 mcg/mL	11–14 h	>1.0 mcg/mL
Lidocaine	Steady-state levels are usually achieved after 6–12 h	1.2–5.0 mcg/mL	1.5 h	>6 mcg/mL
Procainamide	Trough: just before next oral dose	4–10 mcg/mL NAPA + Procaine: 5–30 mcg/mL	Procaine: 3–5 h NAPA: 6–10 h	>10 mcg/mL >30 mcg/mL (NAPA + Procaine)
Quinidine	Trough: just before next oral dose	2–5 mcg/mL	6 h	0.5 mcg/mL

(continued)

22

TABLE 22-2
(Continued)

Drug	When to Sample	Therapeutic Levels	Usual Half-life	Potentially Toxic Levels
OTHER AGENTS				
Amitriptyline plus nortriptyline	Trough: just before next dose	120–250 ng/mL		
Nortriptyline	Trough: just before next dose	50–140 ng/mL		
Lithium	Trough: just before next dose	0.5–1.5 mEq/mL	18–20 h	>1.5 mEq/mL
Imipramine plus desipramine	Trough: just before next dose	150–300 ng/mL		
Desipramine	Trough: just before next dose	50–300 ng/mL		
Methotrexate	By protocol	<0.5 μmol/L after 48 h		
Cyclosporine	Trough: just before next dose	Highly variable Renal: 150–300 ng/mL (RIA) Hepatic: 150–300 ng/mL	Highly variable	
Doxepin	Trough: just before next dose	100–300 ng/mL		
Trazodone	Trough: just before next dose	900–2100 ng/mL		

aResults of therapeutic drug monitoring must be interpreted in light of the complete clinical situation. For information on dosing or interpretation of drug levels contact the pharmacist or write an order for a pharmacokinetic consult in the patient's chart. Modified and reproduced with permission from the *Pharmacy and Therapeutics Committee Formulary*, 41st ed., Thomas Jefferson University Hospital, Philadelphia, PA.
bMore reliable in cases of uremia and hypoalbuminemia.

22

TABLE 22-3
Local Anesthetic Comparison Chart for Commonly Used Injectable Agents

Agent	Proprietary Names	Onset	Duration	Maximum Dose mg/kg	Maximum Dose Volume in 70-kg Adult[a]
Bupivacaine	Marcaine Sensorcaine	7–30 min	5–7 h	3	70 mL of 0.25% solution
Lidocaine	Xylocaine Anestacon	5–30 min	2 h	4	28 mL of 1% solution
Lidocaine with epinephrine (1:200,000)		5–30 min	2–3 h	7	50 mL of 1% solution
Mepivacaine	Carbocaine	5–30 min	2–3 h	7	50 mL of 1% solution
Procaine	Novocain	Rapid	30 min–1 h	10–15	70–105 mL of 1% solution

[a]To calculate the maximum dose if not a 70-kg adult, use the fact that a 1% solution has 10 mg of drug per milliliter.

TABLE 22–4
Comparison of Systemic Steroids

Drug	Relative Equivalent Dose (mg)	Mineralo-corticoid Activity	Duration (h)	Route
Betamethasone	0.75	0	36–72	PO, IM
Cortisone (Cortone)	25.00	2	8–12	PO, IM
Dexamethasone (Decadron)	0.75	0	36–72	PO, IV
Hydrocortisone (Solu-Cortef, Hydrocortone)	20.00	2	8–12	PO, IM, IV
Methylprednisolone acetate (Depo-Medrol)	4.00	0	36–72	PO, IM, IV
Methylprednisolone succinate (Solu-Medrol)	4.00	0	8–12	PO, IM, IV
Prednisone (Deltasone)	5.00	1	12–36	PO
Prednisolone (Delta-Cortef)	5.00	1	12–36	PO, IM, IV

TABLE 22-5
Topical Steroid Preparations

Agent	Common Trade Names	Potency	Apply
Aclometasone dipropionate	Aclovate, cream, oint 0.05%	Low	bid/tid
Amcinonide	Cyclocort, cream, lotion, oint 0.1%	High	bid/tid
Betamethasone			
Betamethasone valerate	Valisone cream, lotion 0.01%	Low	qd/bid
Betamethasone valerate	Valisone cream, 0.01, 0.1%, oint, lotion 0.1%	Intermediate	qd/bid
Betamethasone dipropionate	Diprosone cream (0.05%)	High	qd/bid
	Diprosone aerosol (0.1%)		
Betamethasone dipropionate augmented	Diprolene oint, gel 0.05%	Ultrahigh	qd/bid
Clobetasol propionate	Temovate cream, gel, oint, scalp, soln 0.05%	Ultrahigh	bid (2 wk max)
Clocortolone pivalate	Cloderm cream 0.1%	Intermediate	qd–qid
Desonide	DesOwen, cream, oint, lotion 0.05%	Low	bid–qid
Desoximetasone			
Desoximetasone 0.05%	Topicort LP cream, gel 0.05%	Intermediate	
Desoximetasone 0.25%	Topicort cream, oint	High	
Dexamethasone base	Aeroseb-Dex aerosol 0.01%	Low	bid–qid
	Decadron cream 0.1%		
Diflorasone diacetate	Psorcon cream, oint 0.05%	Ultrahigh	bid/qid

(continued)

TABLE 22-5
(Continued)

Agent	Common Trade Names	Potency	Apply
Fluocinolone			
Fluocinolone acetonide 0.01%	Synalar cream, soln 0.01%	Low	bid/tid
Fluocinolone acetonide 0.025%	Synalar oint, cream 0.025%	Intermediate	bid/tid
Fluocinolone acetonide 0.2%	Synalar-HP cream 0.2%	High	bid/tid
Fluocinonide 0.05%	Lidex, anhydrous cream, gel, soln 0.05%	High	bid/tid oint
	Lidex-E aqueous cream 0.05%		
Flurandrenolide	Cordran cream, oint 0.025%	Intermediate	bid/tid
	cream, lotion, oint 0.05%	Intermediate	bid/tid
	tape, 4 mcg/cm²	Intermediate	qd
Fluticasone propionate	Cultivate cream 0.05%, oint 0.005%	Intermediate	bid
Halobetasol	Ultravate cream, oint 0.05%	Very high	bid
Halcinonide	Halog cream 0.025%, emollient base 0.1% cream, oint, solution 0.1%	High	qd/tid
Hydrocortisone			
Hydrocortisone	Cortisone, Caldecort, Hycort, Hytone, etc. aerosol 1%, cream: 0.5, 1, 2.5%, gel 0.5% oint 0.5, 1, 2.5%, lotion 0.5, 1, 2.5%, paste 0.5% soln 1%	Low	tid/qid

(continued)

22

TABLE 22–5
(Continued)

Agent	Common Trade Names	Potency	Apply
Hydrocortisone acetate	Corticaine cream, oint 0.5, 1%	Low	tid/qid
Hydrocortisone butyrate	Locoid oint, soln 0.1%	Intermediate	bid/tid
Hydrocortisone valerate	Westcort cream, oint 0.2%	Intermediate	bid/tid
Mometasone furoate	Elocon 0.1% cream, oint, lotion	Intermediate	qd
Prednicarbate	Dermatop 0.1% cream	Intermediate	bid
Triamcinolone			
Triamcinolone acetonide 0.025%	Aristocort, Kenalog cream, oint, lotion 0.025%	Low	tid/qid
Triamcinolone acetonide 0.1%	Aristocort, Kenalog cream, oint, lotion 0.1%	Intermediate	tid/qid
	Aerosol 0.2 mg/2–sec spray		
Triamcinolone acetonide 0.5%	Aristocort, Kenalog cream, oint 0.5%	High	tid/qid

22

TABLE 22–6
Comparison of Insulins

Type of Insulin	Onset (h)	Peak (h)	Duration (h)
ULTRA RAPID			
Humalog (lispro)	Immediate	0.5–1.5	3–5
NovoLog (insulin aspart)	Immediate	0.5–1.5	3–5
RAPID			
Regular Iletin II	0.25–0.5	2.0–4.0	5–7
Humulin R	0.5	2.5–4.0	6–8
Novolin R	0.5	2.0–5.0	5–8
Velosulin	0.5	2.0–5.0	6–8
INTERMEDIATE			
NPH Iletin II	1.0–2.0	6–12	18–24
Lente Iletin II	1.0–2.0	6–12	18–24
Humulin N	1.0–2.0	6–12	14–24
Novulin L	2.5–5.0	7–15	18–24
Novulin 70/30	0.5	7–12	24
Prolonged			
Ultralente	4.0–6.0	14–24	28–36
Humulin U	4.0–6.0	8–20	24–28
Lantus (insulin glargine)	4.0–6.0	No peak	24
COMBINATION INSULINS			
Humalog Mix (lispro protamine/lispro)	0.25–0.5	1–4	24

22

TABLE 22-7
Some Oral Contraceptives (see page 579)

Drug (Manufacturer)[a]	Estrogen (mcg)	Progestin (mg)
Alesse 21, 28 (Wyeth)	Ethinyl estradiol (20)	Levonorgestrel (0.1)
Apri 28 (Barr)	Ethinyl estradiol (30)	Desogestrel (0.15)
Aviane 28 (Barr)	Ethinyl estradiol (20)	Levonorgestrel (0.1)
Brevicon 28 (Watson)	Ethinyl estradiol (35)	Norethindrone (0.5)
Cryselle 28 (Barr)	Ethinyl estradiol (30)	Norgestrel (0.3)
Demulen 1/35 21, 28 (Pfizer)	Ethinyl estradiol (35)	Ethynodiol diacetate (1)
Demulen 1/50 21, 28 (Pfizer)	Ethinyl estradiol (50)	Ethynodiol diacetate (1)
Desogen 28 (Organon)	Ethinyl estradiol (30)	Desogestrel (0.15)
Estrostep 28 (Warner Chilcott)[b]	Ethinyl estradiol (20, 20, 35)	Norethindrone acetate (1)
Junel Fr 1/20, 21, 28 (Barr)	Ethinyl estradiol (20)	Norethindrone acetate (1)
Junel Fe 1.5/30, 21, 28 (Barr)	Ethinyl estradiol (30)	Norethindrone acetate (1.5)
Kariva 28 (Barr)	Ethinyl estradiol (20, 0, 10)	Desogestrel (0.15)
Lessina 28 (Barr)	Ethinyl estradiol (20)	Levonorgestrel (0.1)
Levlen 28 (Berlex)	Ethinyl estradiol (30)	Levonorgestrel (0.15)
Levlite 28 (Berlex)	Ethinyl estradiol (20)	Levonorgestrel (0.1)
Levora 28 (Watson)	Ethinyl estradiol (30)	Levonorgestrel (0.15)
Loestrin Fe 1.5/30 21, 28 (Warner Chilcott)	Ethinyl estradiol (30)	Norethindrone acetate (1.5)
Loestrin Fe 1/20 21, 28 (Warner Chilcott)	Ethinyl estradiol (20)	Norethindrone acetate (1)
Lo/Ovral (Wyeth)	Ethinyl estradiol (30)	Norgestrel (0.3)
Low-Ogestrel (Watson)	Ethinyl estradiol (30)	Norgestrel (0.3)
Microgestin Fe 1/20 21, 28 (Watson)	Ethinyl estradiol (20)	Norethindrone acetate (1)

(continued)

22

TABLE 22–7
(Continued)

Drug (Manufacturer)[a]	Estrogen (mcg)	Progestin (mg)
Microgestin Fe 1.5/30 21, 28 (Watson)	Ethinyl estradiol (30)	Norethindrone acetate (1.5)
Mircette 28 (Organon)	Ethinyl estradiol (20, 0, 10)	Desogestrel (0.15)
Modicon 28 (Ortho-McNeil)	Ethinyl estradiol (35)	Norethindrone (0.5)
MonoNessa 28 (Watson)	Ethinyl estradiol (35)	Norgestimate (0.25)
Necon 1/50 28 (Watson)	Mestranol (50)	Norethindrone (1)
Necon 0.5/35, 28 (Watson)	Ethinyl estradiol (35)	Norethindrone (0.5)
Necon 1/35 28 (Watson)	Ethinyl estradiol (35)	Norethindrone (1)
Nordette 21, 28 (King)	Ethinyl estradiol (30)	Levonorgestrel (0.15)
Nortrel 0.5/35 28 (Barr)	Ethinyl estradiol (35)	Norethindrone (0.5)
Nortel 1/35 21, 28 (Barr)	Ethinyl estradiol (3.5)	Norethindrone (1)
Norinyl 1/35 28 (Watson)	Ethinyl estradiol (35)	Norethindrone (1)
Norinyl 1/50 28 (Watson)	Mestranol (50)	Norethindrone (1)
Ogestrel 0.5/50	Ethinyl estradiol (50)	Norgestrel (0.5)
Ogestrel 28 (Watson)	Ethinyl estradiol (50)	Norgestrel (0.5)
Ortho-Cept 28 (Ortho-McNeil)	Ethinyl estradiol (30)	Desogestrel (0.15)
Ortho-Cyclen 28 (Ortho-McNeil)[c]	Ethinyl estradiol (35)	Norgestimate (0.25)
Ortho-Novum 1/35 28 (Ortho-McNeil)	Ethinyl estradiol (35)	Norethindrone (1)
Ortho-Novum 1/50 28 (Ortho-McNeil)[c]	Mestranol (50)	Norethindrone (1)
Ovcon 35 21, 28 (Warner Chilcott)	Ethinyl estradiol (35)	Norethindrone (0.4)
Ovcon 50 28 (Warner Chilcott)	Ethinyl estradiol (50)	Norethindrone (1)
Ovral 21, 28 (Wyeth-Ayerst)[c]	Ethinyl estradiol (50)	Norgestrel (0.5)

(continued)

22

**TABLE 22–7
(Continued)**

Drug (Manufacturer)[a]	Estrogen (mcg)	Progestin (mg)
Portia 28 (Barr)	Ethinyl estradiol (30)	Levongesrel (0.15)
Sprintec 28 (Barr)	Ethinyl estradiol (35)	Norgestimate (0.25)
Yasmin 28 (Berlex)	Ethinyl estradiol (30)	Drospirenone (3)
Yaz (Berlex)	Ethinyl estradiol (20)	Drospirenon (3)
Zovia 1/50E 28 (Watson)	Ethinyl estradiol (50)	Ethynodiol diacetate (1)
Zovia 1/35E 21, 28 (Watson)	Ethinyl estradiol (35)	Ethynodiol diacetate (1)
MULTIPHASICS		
Cyclessa 28 (Orgonon)	Ethinyl estradiol (25)	Desogestrel (0.1, 0.125, 0.15)
Enpresse 28 (Barr)	Ethinyl estradiol (30, 40, 30)	Levonorgestrel (0.05, 0.075, 0.125)
Estrostep 21 (Warner Chilcott)	Ethinyl estradiol (20, 30, 35)	Norethindrone (1)
Estrostep Fe (Warner Chilcott)	Ethinyl estradiol (20, 30, 35)	Norethindrone (1)
Necon 10/11 21, 28 (Watson)	Ethinyl estradiol (35)	Norethindrone (0.5, 1)
Necon 7/7/7 28 (Barr)	Ethinyl estradiol (35)	Norethindrone (0.5, 1)
Nortel 7/7/7 28 (Barr)	Ethinyl estradiol (35)	Norethindrone (0.5, 1)
Ortho Tri-Cyclen 21, 28 (Ortho-McNeil)[b]	Ethinyl estradiol (25)	Norgestimate (0.18, 0.215, 0.25)
Ortho Tri-Cyclen lo 21, 28 (Ortho-McNeil)	Ethinyl estradiol (35, 35, 35)	Norgestimate (0.18, 0.215, 0.25)
Ortho-Novum 10/11 21 (Ortho-McNeil)	Ethinyl estradiol (35, 35)	Norethindrone (0.5, 1.0)
Ortho-Novum 7/7/7 21 (Ortho-McNeil)	Ethinyl estadiol (35, 35, 35)	Norethindrone (0.5, 0.75, 1.0)
Tri-Levlen 28 (Berlex)	Ethinyl estradiol (30,40, 30)	Levonorgestrel (0.05, 0.075, 0.125)
Tri-Nessa 28 (Watson)	Ethinyl estradiol (35)	Norgestimate (0.18, 0.215, 0.25)

(continued)

TABLE 22-7
(Continued)

Drug (Manufacturer)[a]	Estrogen (mcg)	Progestin (mg)
Tri-Norinyl 21, 28 (Watson)	Ethinyl estradiol (35, 35, 35)	Norethindrone (0.5, 1.0, 0.5)
Triphosil 21, 28 (Wyeth)	Ethinyl estradiol (30, 40, 30)	Levonorgestrel (0.05, 0.075, 0.125)
Tri-Sprintec (Barr)	Ethinyl estradiol (35)	Norgstimate (0.18, 0.215, 0.25)
Trivora-28 (Watson)	Ethinyl estradiol (30, 40, 30)	Levonorgestrel (0.05, 0.075, 0.125)
Velivet (Barr)	Ethinyl estradiol (25)	Desogestrel (0.1, 0.125, 0.15)
PROGESTIN ONLY		
Camila (Barr)	None	Norethindrone (0.35)
Errin (Barr)	None	Norethindrone (0.35)
Jolivette 28 (Watson)	None	Norethindrone (0.35)
Micronor (Ortho-McNeil)	None	Norethindrone (0.35)
Nor-QD (Watson)	None	Norethindrone (0.35)
Nora-BE 2B (Ortho-McNeil)	None	Norethindrone (0.35)
Ovrette (Wyeth-Ayerst)	None	Norgestrel (0.075)
EXTENDED-CYCLE COMBINATION		
Seasonale (Duramed)[c]	Ethinyl estradiol (30)	Levonorgestrel (0.15)

[a]21 and 28 = number of days in the regimen.
[b]Also approved for acne.
[c]84 tablets of active hormone followed by 7 inert tablets.

Source: Gomella LG, et al. *Clinician's Pocket Drug Reference 2006* New York: McGraw-Hill, 2006. Based in part on data published in *Medical Letter August 2004*; 2, no. 24.

22

TABLE 22–8
Common Oral Potassium Supplements

Brand Name	Salt	Form	mEq Potassium/ Dosing Unit
Glu-K	Gluconate	Tablet	2 mEq/tablet
Kaochlor 10%	KCl	Liquid	20 mEq/15 mL
Kaochlor S-F 10% (sugar-free)	KCl	Liquid	20 mEq/15 mL
Kaochlor Eff	Bicarbonate/ KCl/citrate	Effervescent tablet	20 mEq/tablet
Kaon elixir	Gluconate	Liquid	20 mEq/15 mL
Kaon	Gluconate	Tablets	5 mEq/tablet
Kaon-Cl	KCl	Tablet, SR	6.67 mEq/tablet
Kaon-Cl 20%	KCl	Liquid	40 mEq/15 mL
KayCiel	KCl	Liquid	20 mEq/15 mL
K-Lor	KCl	Powder	15 or 20 mEq/ packet
Klorvess	Bicarbonate/KCl	Liquid	20 mEq/15 mL
Klotrix	KCl	Tablet, SR	10 mEq/tablet
K-Lyte	Bicarbonate/ citrate	Effervescent tablet	25 mEq/tablet
K-Tab	KCl	Tablet, SR	10 mEq/tablet
Micro-K	KCl	Capsules, SR	8 mEq/capsule
Slow-K	KCl	Tablet, SR	8 mEq/tablet
Tri-K	Acetate/bicarbonate and citrate	Liquid	45 mEq/15 mL
Twin-K	Citrate/gluconate	Liquid	20 mEq/5 mL

SR = sustained release.

TABLE 22–9
Tetanus Prophylaxis

History of Absorbed Tetanus Toxoid Immunization	Clean, Minor Wounds		All Other Wounds[a]	
	Td[b]	TIG[c]	Td[d]	TIG[c]
Unknown or <3 doses	Yes	No	Yes	No
<3 doses	No[e]	No	No[f]	No

[a]Such as, but not limited to, wounds contaminated with dirt, feces, soil, saliva, etc; puncture wounds; avulsions; and wounds resulting from missiles, crushing, burns, and frostbite.

[b]Td = tetanus–diptheria toxoid (adult type), 0.5 mL IM.
- For children < 7 y, DPT (DT, if pertussis vaccine is contraindicated) is preferred to tetanus toxoid alone.
- For persons > 7 y, Td is preferred to tetanus toxoid alone.
- DT = Diptheria–tetanus toxoid (pediatric), used for those who cannot receive pertussis.

[c]TIG = tetanus immune globulin, 250 U IM.

[d]If only 3 doses of fluid toxoid have been received, then a fourth dose of toxoid, preferably an absorbed toxoid, should be given.

[e]Yes, if > 10 y since last dose.

[f]Yes, if > 5 y since last dose.

Source: Based on guidelines from the Centers for Disease Control and Prevention and reported in MMWR.

TABLE 22–10
Oral Anticoagulant Standards of Practice

Thromboembolic Disorder	INR	Duration
DEEP VENOUS THROMBOSIS		
Prophylaxis (high-risk surgery)	10 mg night before surgery 5 mg night of surgery	Short term only
Treatment single episode	2–3	3–6 mo
Recurrent	2–3	Indefinite
PREVENTION OF SYSTEMIC EMBOLISM		
Atrial fibrillation (AF)[a]	2–3	Indefinite
AF: cardioversion	2–3	3 wk prior; 4 wk post sinus rhythm
Valvular heart disease	2–3	Indefinite
Cardiomyopathy	2–3	Indefinite
ACUTE MYOCARDIAL INFARCTION		
Prevention of systemic embolization	2–3	<3 mo
Prevention of recurrence	2.5–3.5	Indefinite
PROSTHETIC VALVES		
Tissue heart valves	2–3	3 mo
Bileaflet mechanical valve in aortic position	2–3	2–3 mo Indefinite
Other mechanical prosthetic valves[b]	2.5–3.5	Indefinite

[a]With high-risk factors or multiple moderate risk factors.
[b]May add aspirin 81 mg to warfarin in patients with ball–cage valves or with additional risk factors.
INR = international normalized ratio.
Source: Based on data published in *Chest* 2001;119 Supplement 1S–307S.

TABLE 22–11
Serotonin 5–HT$_1$ Receptor Agonists

Drug	Initial Dose	Repeat Dose	Max Dose/24h	Supplied
Almotriptan (Axert)	6.25 or 12.5 mg PO	× 1 in 2 h	25 mg	Tabs 6.25, 12.5 mg
Frovatriptan (Frova)	2.5 mg PO	in 2 h	7.5 mg	Tabs 2.5 mg
Naratriptan (Amerge)	1 or 2.5 mg PO[a]	in 4 h	5 mg	Tabs 1, 2.5 mg
Rizatriptan (Maxalt)	5 or 10 mg PO[b]	in 2 h	30 mg	Tabs 5, 10 mg Disintegrating tabs, 5, 10 mg
Sumatriptan (Imitrex)	25, 50, or 100 mg PO	in 2 h	200 mg	Tabs 25, 50 mg
	5–20 mg intranasally	in 2 h	40 mg	Nasal spray 5, 20 mg
	6 mg SC	in 1 h	12 mg	Inj 12 mg/mL
Zolmitriptan (Zomig)	2.5 or 5 mg PO	in 2 h	10 mg	Tabs 2.5, 5 mg

Precautions/contraindications: (C, M) ischemic heart disease, coronary artery vasospasm, Prinzmetal angina, uncontrolled HTN, hemiplegic or basilar migraine, ergots, use of another serotonin agonist within 24 h, use with MAOI. Side effects: dizziness, somnolence, paresthesias, nausea, flushing, dry mouth, coronary vasospasm, chest tightness, HTN, GI upset.
[a]Reduce dose in mild renal and hepatic insufficiency (2.5 mg/d max); contraindicated with severe renal (CrCl < 15 mL/min) or hepatic impairment.
[b]Initiate therapy at 5 mg PO (15 mg/d max) in patients receiving propanolol.

22

TABLE 22–12
Antiarrhythmics: Vaughn Williams Classification

CLASS I: Sodium Channel Blockade

A. **Class Ia:** Lengthens duration of action potential (↑ the refractory period in artrial and ventricular muscles, in SA and AV conduction systems, and in Purkinje fibers)
   1. Amiodarone (also class II, II, IV)
   2. Disopyramide (Norpace)
   3. Imipramine (MAO inhibitor)
   4. Procainamide (Pronestyl)
   5. Quinidine

B. **Class Ib:** No effect on action potential
   1. Lidocaine (Xylocaine)
   2. Mexiletine (Mexitil)
   3. Phenytoin (Dilantin)
   4. Tocainide (Tonocard)

C. **Class Ic:** Greater sodium current depression (blocks the fast inward Na^+ current in heart muscle and Purkinje fibers, and slows the rate of ↑ of phase 0 of action potential)
   1. Flecainide (Tambocar)
   2. Propafenone

CLASS II: Beta blocker

D. Amiodarone (also class Ia, III, IV)
E. Esmolol (Brevibloc)
F. Sotalol (also class III)

CLASS III: Prolong refractory period via action potential

G. Amidarone (also class Ia, II, IV)
H. Sotalol (also class III)

CLASS IV: Calcium channel blocker

I. Amidarone (also class Ia, II, III)
J. Diltiazem (Cardizem)
K. Verapamil (Calan)

TABLE 22–13
Cytochrome P-450 Isoenzymes and Drugs They Metabolize, Inhibit, and Induce[a]

CYP1A2

Substrates:	Acetaminophen, caffeine, clozapine, imipramine, theophylline, propranolol
Inhibitors:	Most fluoroquinolone antibiotics, fluvoxamine, cimetidine
Inducer:	Tobacco smoking, charcoal-broiled foods, cruciferous vegetables, omeprazole

CYP2C9

Substrates:	Most NSAIDs (including COX-2), warfarin, phenytoin
Inhibitors:	Fluconazole
Induced:	Barbiturates, rifampin

CYP2C19

Substrates:	Diazepam, lansoprazole, omeprazole, phenytoin, pantoprazole
Inhibitors:	Omeprazole, isoniazid, ketoconazole
Inducer:	Barbiturates, rifampin

CYP2D6

Substrates:	Most β-blockers, codeine, clomipramine, clozapine, codeine, encainide, flecainide, fluoxetine, haloperidol, hydrocodone, 4-methoxy-amphetamine, metoprolol, mexiletine, oxycodone, paroxetine, propafenone, propoxyphene, risperidone, selegiline (deprenyl), thioridazine, most tricyclic antidepressants, timolol
Inhibitors:	Fluoxetine, haloperidol, paroxetine, quinidine
Inducer:	Unknown

CYP3A

Substrates:	**Anticholinergics:** Darifenacin, oxybutynin, solifenacin, tolterodine
	Benzodiazepines: Alprazolam, midazolam, triazolam
	Ca channel blockers: Diltiazem, felodipine, nimodipine, nifedipine, nisoldipine, verapamil
	Chemotherapy: Cyclophosphamide, erlotinib, ifosfamide, paclitaxel, tamoxifen, vinblastine, vincristine

(continued)

22

TABLE 22–13
(Continued)

	HIV protease inhibitors: Amprenavir, atazanavir, indinavir, nelfinavir, ritonavir, saquinavir
	HMG-CoA reductase inhibitors: Atorvastatin, lovastatin, simvastatin
	Immunosuppressive agent: Cyclosporine, tacrolimus
	Macrolide-type antibiotics: Clarithromycin, erythromycin, telithromycin, troleandomycin
	Opioids: Alfentanyl, cocaine, fentanyl, sufentanil
	Steroids: Budesonide, cortisol, 17 β-estradiol, progesterone
	Others: Acetaminophen, amiodarone, carbamazepine, delavirdine, efavirenz, nevirapine, quinidine, repaglinide, sildenafil, tadalafil, trazodone, vardenafil
Inhibitors:	Amiodarone, amprenavir, atazanavir, ciprofloxacin, cisapride, clarithromycin, diltiazem, eruthromycin, fluconazole, fluvoxamine, grapefruit juice (in high ingestion), indinavir, itraconazole, ketoconazole, nefazodone, nelfidomycin, verapamil, voriconazole
Inducer:	Carbamazepine, efavirenz, glucocorticoids, macrolide antibiotics, nevirapine, phenytoin, Phenobarbital, rifabutin, rifapentine, rifampin, St. John's wort

ªIncreased or decreased (primarily hepatic cytochrome P-450) metabolism of medications may influence the effectiveness of drugs or result in significant drug–drug interactions. Understanding the common cytochrome P-450 isoforms (eg, CYP2CP, CYP2O9, CYP2C19, CYP3A4) and common drugs that are metabolized by (aka "substrates"), inhibit, or induce activity of the isoform helps minimize significant drug interaction. CYP3A is involved in the metabolism of >50% of drugs metabolized by the liver.

Source: Based on the data from Katzung B (ed): *Basic and Clinical Pharmacology*, 9th ed. McGraw-Hill, New York, 2004; *The Medical Letter*, Volume 47, July 4, 2004; http://www.fda.gov/cder/drug/drugreactions (accessed September 16, 2005).

APPENDIX

Apgar Scores
Body Surface Area for Adults and
    Children
Body Mass Index
Cancer Screening
Epidemiology Basics
Glasgow Coma Scale
Immunization Guidelines
    (Adults and Children)

Measurement Equivalents
Measurement Prefixes and
    Symbols
Performance Status Scales
Radiation Terminology
Temperature Conversion
Weight Conversion

APGAR SCORES

Apgar scores (Table A–1, page 650) are a numerical expression of a newborn infant's physical condition. Usually determined 1 min after birth and again at 5 min, the score is the sum of points gained on assessment of color, heart rate, reflex irritability, muscle tone, and respirations.

BODY SURFACE AREA FOR ADULTS AND CHILDREN

Figure A–1, page 651, is a nomogram for determining the body surface area of an adult. Figure A–2, page 652, is a nomogram for determining the body surface area of children.

BODY MASS INDEX

Table A–2, page 653 gives BMI useful in the determination of obesity and other health-related risks. It also provides useful information for counseling patients on target body weights. Underweight ≤ 18.5; normal weight = 18.5–24.9; overweight = 25–29.9; obesity = ≥ 30. (From the National Heart Lung and Blood Institute (NIH), Bethesda MD, 2003 http://www.nhlbisupport.com/bmi)

CANCER SCREENING

(See Table A–3, page 654)

EPIDEMIOLOGY BASICS

$$\text{Prevalance} = \frac{\text{Number of persons who have a disease at one point in time}}{\text{Number of persons at risk at that point}}$$

$$\text{Incidence} = \frac{\text{Number of new cases of a disease over a period of time}}{\text{Number of persons at risk during that period}}$$

Sensitivity = Proportion of subjects with the disease who have a positive test
    $= (a / a = c)$

Specificity = Proportion of subjects without the disease who have a negative test
    $= (d / b + d)$

Predictive value = Positive: likelihood of a positive test indicates disease
    $= (a / a + b)$
    = Negative: likelihood of a negative test indicates lack of disease
    $= (d / c + d)$

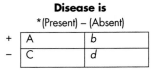

Disease is
*(Present) – (Absent)

+	A	b
–	C	d

GLASGOW COMA SCALE

The Glasgow Coma Scale (EMV Scale) is a fairly reliable, objective way to monitor changes in levels of consciousness. It is based on **Eye opening, Motor responses, and Verbal responses.** A person's EMV score is based on the total of the three responses. The score ranges from 3 (lowest) to 15 (highest) (Table A–4, page 656).

IMMUNIZATION GUIDELINES (ADULTS AND CHILDREN)

Figure A–3, page 657, indicates the currently recommended immunizations for adults. Figure A–4 indicates adult immunization recommendations by vaccine and other medical indications (*MMWR* October 14, 2005/Vol. 54/No. 40). Figure A–5, page 662, indicates childhood and adolescent immunization schedule recommended in the United States. (*MMWR* January 6, 2006;54, nos. 51 & 52)

MEASUREMENT EQUIVALENTS (APPROXIMATE)

Length
1 centimeter (cm) = 0.4 in
1 meter (m) = 39.4 in

Apothecary
1 grain (gr) = 60 mg
30 g = 1 oz
1 g = 15 gr

Household
1 teaspoon (tsp) = 5 mL
1 tablespoon (tbsp) = 15 mL
1 ounce (oz) = 30 mL
8 ounces (oz) = 1 cup = 240 mL
1 quart (qt) = 946 mL

(*Text continues on page 656.*)

TABLE A–1
Apgar Scores

	Score		
Sign	0	1	2
Appearance (color)	Blue or pale	Pink body with blue extremities	Completely pink
Pulse (heart rate)	Absent	Slow (< 100/min)	> 100/min
Grimace (reflex irritability)	No response	Grimace	Cough or sneeze
Activity (muscle tone)	Limp	Some flexion	Active movement
Respirations	Absent	Slow, irregular	Good, crying

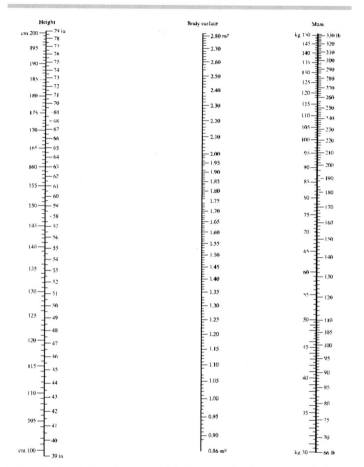

FIGURE A-1. Body surface area: Adult. Use a straight edge to connect the height and mass. The point of intersection on the body surface line gives the body surface area (in m²). (Reprinted, with permission, from: Lentner C [ed]: *Geigy Scientific Tables*, 8th ed. Ciba-Geigy, San Francisco, CA, 1981, Vol. 1, p. 226.)

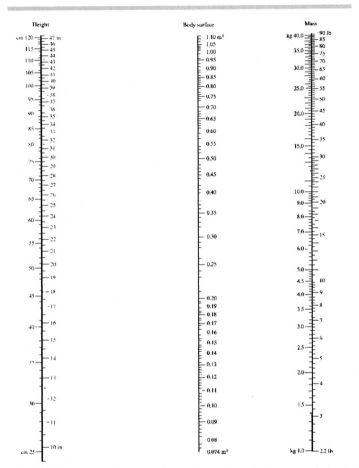

FIGURE A–2.   Body surface area: Child. Use a straight edge to connect the height and mass. The point of intersection on the body surface line gives the body surface area (in m²). (Reprinted, with permission, from: Lentner C [ed]: *Geigy Scientific Tables,* 8th ed. Ciba-Geigy, San Francisco, CA, 1981, Vol. 1, p. 226.)

TABLE A–2
Body Mass Index

Height↓ \ Weight→	120	130	140	150	160	170	180	190	200	210	220	230	240	250
4'6"	29	31	34	36	39	41	43	46	48	51	53	56	58	60
4'8"	27	29	31	34	36	38	40	43	45	47	49	52	54	56
4'10"	25	27	29	31	34	36	38	40	42	44	46	48	50	52
5'0"	23	25	27	29	31	33	35	37	39	41	43	45	47	49
5'2"	22	24	26	27	29	31	33	35	37	38	40	42	44	46
5'4"	21	22	24	26	28	29	31	33	34	36	38	40	41	43
5'6"	19	21	23	24	26	27	29	31	32	34	36	37	39	40
5'8"	18	20	21	23	24	26	27	29	30	32	34	35	37	38
5'10"	17	19	20	22	23	24	26	27	29	30	32	33	35	36
6'0"	16	18	19	20	22	23	24	26	27	28	30	31	33	34
6'2"	15	17	18	19	21	22	23	24	26	27	28	30	31	32
6'4"	15	16	17	18	20	21	22	23	24	26	27	28	29	30
6'6"	14	15	16	17	19	20	21	22	23	24	25	27	28	29
6'8"	13	14	15	17	18	19	20	21	22	23	24	25	26	28

TABLE A–3
American Cancer Society Recommendations for the Early Detection of Cancer in Average-Risk Asymptomatic Persons

Cancer Site	Population	Test or Procedure	Frequency
Breast	Women, age ≥ 20 y	Breast self-examination (BSE)	Beginning in their early 20s, women should be told about the benefits and limitations of BSE. The importance of prompt reporting of any new breast symptoms to a health professional should be emphasized. Women who choose to do BSE should receive instruction and have their technique reviewed on the occasion of a periodic health examination. It is acceptable for women to choose not to do BSE or to do BSE irregularly.
		Clinical breast examination (CBE)	For women in their 20s and 30s, it is recommended that CBE be part of a periodic health examination, preferably at least every 3 y. Asymptomatic women age 40 y and over should continue to receive a clinical breast examination as part of a periodic health examination, preferably annually.
		Mammography	Begin annual mammography at age 40 y (annual clinical breast exam should be performed before mammography).
Colorectal	Men and women, age ≥ 50 y	Fecal occult blood test (FOBT)ᵃ or fecal immunochemical test (FIT), or	Annual, starting at age 50 y
		Flexible sigmoidoscopy, or	Every 5 y, starting at age 50 y
		Fecal occult blood test (FOBT)ᵃ and flexible sigmoidoscopy,ᵇ or	Annual FOBT (or FIT) and flexible sigmoidoscopy every 5 y, starting at age 50 y
		Double contrast barium enema (DCBE) or	DCBE every 5 y, starting at age 50 y
		Colonoscopy	Colonoscopy every 10 y, starting at age 50 y

(continued)

TABLE A-3
(Continued)

Cancer Site	Population	Test or Procedure	Frequency
Prostate	Men, age ≥ 50 y	Digital rectal examination (DRE) and prostate-specific antigen test (PSA)	The PSA test and the DRE should be offered annually, starting at age 50 y, for men who have a life expectancy of at least 10 more y. (Information should be provided to men about the benefits and limitations of testing so that an informed decision about testing can be made with the clinician's assistance.)
Cervix	Women, age ≥ 18 y	Pap test	Screening should begin ~ 3 y after a woman begins having vaginal intercourse, but no later than 21 y. Screen every year with Pap tests or every 2 y using liquid-based Pap tests. At or after age 30, women w/3 normal test results in a row may be screened every 2–3 y with cervical cytology (either conventional or liquid-based Pap test) alone, or every 3 y with a human papillomavirus DNA test plus cervical cytology. Women ≥ 70 y w/ ≥3 normal Pap tests and no abnormal Pap in the last 10 y and women w/total hysterectomy may choose to stop cervical cancer screening.
Endometrial	Women, at menopause		At the time of menopause, women at average risk should be informed about risks and symptoms of endometrial cancer and strongly encouraged to report any unexpected bleeding or spotting to their physicians.
Cancer-related checkup	Men and women, ≥ 20 y		On the occasion of a periodic health examination, the cancer-related checkup should include examination for cancers of the thyroid, testicles, ovaries, lymph nodes, oral cavity, and skin, as well as health counseling about tobacco, sun exposure, diet and nutrition, risk factors, sexual practices, and environmental and occupational exposures.

aFOBT in physicians' offices, with the single stool sample collected on a fingertip during a rectal examination, is not an adequate substitute for the recommended at-home procedure of collecting two samples from three consecutive specimens. Toilet-bowl FOBT tests also are not recommended. In comparison with guaiac-based tests for the detection of occult blood, immunochemical tests are more patient-friendly and are likely to be equal or better in sensitivity and specificity. There is no justification for repeating FOBT in response to an initial positive finding.

bFlexible sigmoidoscopy together with FOBT is preferred compared with FOBT or flexible sigmoidoscopy alone.

Source: CA Cancer J Clin 2006;56:11–25.

TABLE A–4
Glasgow Coma Scale

Parameter	Response		Score
Eyes	Open: Spontaneously		4
		To verbal command	3
		To pain	2
		No response	1
Best motor response	To verbal command	Obeys	6
	To painful stimulus	Localized pain	5
		Flexion–withdrawal	4
		Decorticate (flex)	3
		Decerebrate (extend)	2
		No response	1
Best verbal response		Oriented, converses	5
		Disoriented, converses	4
		Inappropriate responses	3
		Incomprehensible sounds	2
		No response	1

(*Text continued from page 650.*)

MEASUREMENT PREFIXES AND SYMBOLS

Factor	Prefix	Symbol
10^9	giga	G
10^6	mega	M
10^3	kilo	k
10^2	hecto	h
Factor	**Prefix**	**Symbol**
10^1	deka	da
10^{-1}	deci	d
10^{-2}	centi	c
10^{-3}	milli	m
10^{-6}	micro	μ
10^{-9}	nano	n
10^{-12}	pico	p
10^{-15}	femto	f

PERFORMANCE STATUS SCALES

Table A–5, page 665, lists the most common performance scales used clinically.

(*Text continues on page 667.*)

FIGURE A–3. CDC adult recommended immunization schedule.

Vaccine ▼	Age group ▶ 19–49 years	50–64 years	≥ 65 years
Tetanus, diphtheria (Td)¹*	1-dose booster every 10 yrs		
Measles, mumps, rubella (MMR)²*	1 or 2 doses	1 dose	
Varicella³*	2 doses (0, 4–8 wks)		2 doses (0, 4–8 wks)
Influenza⁴*	1 dose annually	1 dose annually	
Pneumococcal (polysaccharide)⁵,⁶	1–2 doses		1 dose
Hepatitis A⁷*	2 doses (0, 6–12 mos, or 0, 6–18 mos)		
Hepatitis B⁸*	3 doses (0, 1–2, 4–6 mos)		
Meningococcal⁹	1 or more doses		

— Vaccines below broken line are for selected populations

For all persons in this category who meet the age requirements and who lack evidence of immunity (e.g., lack documentation of vaccination or have no evidence of prior infection)

Recommended if some other risk factor is present (e.g., based on medical, occupational, lifestyle, or other indications)

*Covered by the Vaccine Injury Compensation Program.

Note: These recommendations must be read in conjunction with the footnotes for Figure A–4; pages 659 through 661.

657

FIGURE A–4. CDC adult immunization based on vaccine and indications.

*Covered by the Vaccine Injury Compensation Program.

Legend:
- For all persons in this category who meet the age requirements and who lack evidence of immunity (e.g., lack documentation of vaccination or have no evidence of prior infection)
- Recommended if some other risk factor is present (e.g., based on medical, occupational, lifestyle, or other indications)
- Contraindicated

658

FIGURE A-4. *Notes:*

[a]Tetanus and diphtheria (Td) vaccination. Adults with uncertain histories of a complete primary vaccination series with diphtheria- and tetanus toxoid–containing vaccines should receive a primary series for adults using combined Td toxoid. A primary series for adults is 3 doses; administer the first 2 doses at least 4 wk apart and the third dose 6–12 mo after the second. Administer 1 dose if the person received the primary series and if the last vaccination was received > 10 y previously. Consult the ACIP statement for recommendations for administering Td as prophylaxis in wound management (http://www.cdc.gov/mmwr/preview/mmwrhtml/00041645.htm). The American College of Physicians Task Force on Adult Immunization supports a second option for Td use in adults: a single Td booster at age 50 y for persons who have completed the full pediatric series, including the teenage/young adult booster. A newly licensed tetanus–diphtheria–acellular pertussis vaccine is available for adults. ACIP recommendations for its use will be published.

[b]Measles, mumps, rubella (MMR) vaccination. Measles component: adults born before 1957 can be considered immune to measles. Adults born during or after 1957 should receive > 1 dose of MMR unless they have a medical contraindication, documentation of > 1 dose, history of measles based on health care provider diagnosis, or laboratory evidence of immunity. A second dose of MMR is recommended for adults who 1) were recently exposed to measles or in an outbreak setting; 2) were previously vaccinated with killed measles vaccine; 3) were vaccinated with an unknown type of measles vaccine during 1963–1967; 4) are students in postsecondary educational institutions; 5) work in a health care facility; or 6) plan to travel internationally. Withhold MMR or other measles-containing vaccines from HIV-infected persons with severe immunosuppression. Mumps component: 1 dose of MMR vaccine should be adequate for protection for those born during or after 1957 who lack a history of mumps based on health care provider diagnosis or who lack laboratory evidence of immunity. Rubella component: administer 1 dose of MMR vaccine to women whose rubella vaccination history is unreliable or who lack laboratory evidence of immunity. For women of childbearing age, regardless of birth year, routinely determine rubella immunity and counsel women regarding congenital rubella syndrome. Do not vaccinate women who are pregnant or who might become pregnant within 4 wk of receiving vaccine. Women who do not have evidence of immunity should receive MMR vaccine upon completion or termination of pregnancy and before discharge from the health care facility.

[c]Varicella vaccination. Varicella vaccination is recommended for all adults without evidence of immunity to varicella. Special consideration should be given to those who 1) have close contact with persons at high risk of severe disease (health care workers and family contacts of immunocompromised persons) or 2) are at high risk of exposure or transmission (eg, teachers of young children; child care employees; residents and staff members of institutional settings, including correctional institutions; college students; military personnel; adolescents and adults living in households with children; nonpregnant women of childbearing age; and international travelers). Evidence of immunity to varicella in adults includes any of the following: 1) documented age-appropriate varicella vaccination (ie, receipt of 1 dose before age 13 y or receipt of 2 doses [administered at least 4 wk apart] after age 13 y); 2) US-born before 1966 or history of varicella disease before 1966 for non-US-born persons; 3) history of varicella based on health care provider diagnosis or parental or self-report of typical varicella disease for persons born during 1966–1997 (for a patient reporting a history of an atypical, mild case, health care providers should seek either an epidemiologic link with a typical varicella case or evidence of laboratory confirmation, if it was performed at the time of acute disease); 4) history of herpes zoster based on health care provider diagnosis; or 5) laboratory evidence of immunity. Do not vaccinate women who are pregnant or who might become pregnant within 4 wk of receiving the vaccine. Assess pregnant women for evidence of varicella immunity. Women who do not have evidence of immunity should receive dose 1 of varicella vaccine upon completion or termination of pregnancy and before discharge from the health care facility. Dose 2 should be administered 4–8 wk after dose 1.

(continued)

FIGURE A-4. Continued

[d]Influenza vaccination. Medical indications: chronic disorders of the cardiovascular or pulmonary systems, including asthma; chronic metabolic diseases, including diabetes mellitus, renal dysfunction, hemoglobinopathies, or immunosuppression (including immunosuppression caused by medications or HIV); any condition (eg, cognitive dysfunction, spinal cord injury, seizure disorder, or other neuromuscular disorder) that compromises respiratory function or the handling of respiratory secretions or that can increase the risk for aspiration; and pregnancy during the influenza season. No data exist on the risk for severe or complicated influenza disease among persons with asplenia; however, influenza is a risk factor for secondary bacterial infections that can cause severe disease among persons with asplenia. Occupational indications: health care workers and employees of long-term care and assisted living facilities. Other indications: residents of nursing homes and other long-term care and assisted living facilities; persons likely to transmit influenza to persons at high risk (ie, in-home household contacts and caregivers of children age 0–23 mo, or persons of all ages with high-risk conditions), and anyone who wishes to be vaccinated. For healthy, nonpregnant persons age 5–49 y without high-risk conditions who are not contacts of severely immunocompromised persons in special care units, intranasally administered influenza vaccine (FluMist) may be administered in lieu of inactivated vaccine.

[e]Pneumococcal polysaccharide vaccination. Medical indications: chronic disorders of the pulmonary system (excluding asthma); cardiovascular diseases; diabetes mellitus; chronic liver disease, including liver disease as a result of alcohol abuse (eg, cirrhosis); chronic renal failure or nephrotic syndrome; functional or anatomic asplenia (eg, sickle cell disease or splenectomy [if elective splenectomy is planned, vaccinate at least 2 wk before surgery]); immunosuppressive conditions (eg, congenital immunodeficiency, HIV infection [vaccinate as close to diagnosis as possible when CD4 cell counts are highest], leukemia, lymphoma, multiple myeloma, Hodgkin disease, generalized malignancy, or organ or bone marrow transplantation); chemotherapy with alkylating agents, antimetabolites, or long-term systemic corticosteroids; and cochlear implants. Other indications: Alaska natives and certain American Indian populations; residents of nursing homes and other long-term care facilities.

[f]Revaccination with pneumococcal polysaccharide vaccine. One-time revaccination after 5 y for persons with chronic renal failure or nephritic syndrome; functional or anatomic asplenia (eg, sickle cell disease or splenectomy); immunosuppressive conditions (eg, congenital immunodeficiency, HIV infection, leukemia, lymphoma, multiple myeloma, Hodgkin disease, generalized malignancy, or organ or bone marrow transplantation); or chemotherapy with alkylating agents, antimetabolites, or long-term systemic corticosteroids. For persons age > 65 y, one-time revaccination if they were vaccinated > 5 y previously and were age < 65 y at the time of primary vaccination.

[g]Hepatitis A vaccination. Medical indications: persons with clotting-factor disorders or chronic liver disease. Behavioral indications: men who have sex with men or users of illegal drugs. Occupational indications: Persons working with hepatitis A virus (HAV)–infected primates or with HAV in a research laboratory setting. Other indications: persons traveling to or working in countries that have high or intermediate endemicity of hepatitis A (for list of countries, see http://www.cdc.gov/travel/diseases.htm#hepa) as well as any person wishing to obtain immunity. Current vaccines should be administered in a 2-dose series at either 0 and 6–12 mo, or 0 and 6–18 mo. If the combined hepatitis A and hepatitis B vaccine is used, administer 3 doses at 0, 1, and 6 mo.

[h]Hepatitis B vaccination. Medical indications: hemodialysis patients (use special formulation [40 mcg/ml] or two 20-mcg/ml doses) or patients who receive clotting-factor concentrates. Occupational indications: health care workers and public safety workers who have exposure to blood in the workplace and persons in training in schools of medicine, dentistry, nursing, laboratory technology, and other allied health professions. Behavioral indications: injection drug users; persons with more than one sex partner during the previous 6 mo; persons with a recently acquired sexually transmitted disease (STD); and men who have sex with men. Other indications: household contacts and sex partners of persons with chronic hepatitis B virus (HBV) infection; clients and staff members of institutions for developmentally disabled persons; all clients of STD clinics; inmates of correctional facilities; and international travelers who will be in countries with high or intermediate prevalence of chronic HBV infection for more than 6 mo (for list of countries, see http://www.cdc.gov/travel/diseases.htm#hepa).

FIGURE A–4. Continued

¹Meningococcal vaccination. Medical indications: adults with anatomic or functional asplenia or terminal complement component deficiencies. Other indications: first-year college students living in dormitories; microbiologists who are routinely exposed to isolates of Neisseria meningitidis; military recruits; and persons who travel to or reside in countries in which meningococcal disease is hyperendemic or epidemic (eg, the "meningitis belt" of sub-Saharan Africa during the dry season [December–June]), particularly if contact with local populations will be prolonged. Vaccination is required by the government of Saudi Arabia for all travelers to Mecca during the annual Hajj. Meningococcal conjugate vaccine is preferred for adults meeting any of the above indications who are age < 55 y, although meningococcal polysaccharide vaccine (MPSV4) is an acceptable alternative. Revaccination after 5 y may be indicated for adults previously vaccinated with MPSV4 who remain at high risk of infection (eg, persons residing in areas in which disease is epidemic).

²Selected conditions for which Haemophilus influenzae type b (Hib) vaccine may be used. Hib conjugate vaccines are licensed for children age 6–71 mo. No efficacy data are available on which to base a recommendation concerning use of Hib vaccine for older children and adults with the chronic conditions associated with an increased risk for Hib disease. However, study results suggest good immunogenicity in patients who have sickle cell disease, leukemia, or HIV infection or who have undergone splenectomy; administering vaccine to these patients is not contraindicated.

661

FIGURE A-5. CDC recommended immunization of children in the United States.

Vaccine ▼ / Age ▶	Birth	1 month	2 months	4 months	6 months	12 months	15 months	18 months	24 months	4–6 years	11–12 years	13–14 years	15 years	16–18 years
Hepatitis B[a]	HepB	HepB				HepB					HepB Series	HepB Series		
Diphtheria, Tetanus, Pertussis[b]			DTaP	DTaP	DTaP		DTaP	DTaP		DTaP	Tdap	Tdap	Tdap	
Haemophilus influenzae type b[c]			Hib	Hib	Hib[c]	Hib	Hib							
Inactivated Poliovirus			IPV	IPV	IPV	IPV	IPV			IPV				
Measles, Mumps, Rubella[d]						MMR	MMR			MMR	MMR	MMR	MMR	
Varicella[e]						Varicella	Varicella	Varicella			Varicella	Varicella		
Meningococcal[f]									MPSV4		MCV4		MCV4 / MCV4	
Pneumococcal[g]			PCV	PCV	PCV	PCV	PCV		PCV	PCV	PPV	PPV		
Influenza[h]					Influenza (Yearly)	Influenza (Yearly)					Influenza (Yearly)			
Hepatitis A[i]									HepA Series	HepA Series	HepA Series			

Vaccines within broken line are for selected populations

Legend:
- Range of recommended ages
- Catch-up immunization
- 11–12 year old assessment

This schedule indicates the recommended ages for routine administration of currently licensed childhood vaccines, as of December 1, 2005, for children through age 18 y. Any dose not administered at the recommended age should be administered at any subsequent visit, when indicated and feasible. ▇ Indicates age groups that warrant special effort to administer those vaccines not previously administered. Additional vaccines may be used whenever any components of the combination are indicated and other components of the vaccine are not contraindicated and if approved by the Food and Drug Administration for that dose of the series. Providers should consult respective Advisory Committee on Immunization Practice (ACIP) statements for detailed recommendations. Clinically significant adverse events that follow vaccination should be reported through the Vaccine Adverse Event Reporting System (VAERS). Guidance about how to obtain and complete a VAERS form is available at http://www.vaers.hhs.gov or by telephone, 800-822-7987.

▇ Range of recommended ages ▇ Catch up immunization ▇ Assessment at age 11–12 y

FIGURE A–5.   *Notes:*

^a**Hepatitis B vaccine (HepB).** *AT BIRTH:* All newborns should receive monovalent HepB soon after birth and before hospital discharge. **Infants born to mothers who are HBsAg-positive** should receive HepB and 0.5 mL of hepatitis B immune globulin (HBIG) within 12 hours of birth. **Infants born to mothers whose HBsAg status is unknown** should receive HepB within 12 hours of birth. The mother should have blood drawn as soon as possible to determine her HBsAg status; if the result is HBsAg-positive, the infant should receive HBIG as soon as possible (no later than age 1 wk). **For infants born to HBsAg-negative mothers,** the birth dose can be delayed in rare circumstances but only if a physician's order to withhold the vaccine and a copy of the mother's original HBsAg-negative laboratory report are documented in the infant's medical record. *FOLLOWING THE BIRTHDOSE:* The HepB series should be completed with either monovalent HepB or a combination vaccine containing HepB. The second dose should be administered at age 1–2 mo. The final dose should be administered at age ≥24 wks. It is permissible to administer 4 doses of HepB (eg, when combination vaccines are given after the birth dose); however, if monovalent HepB is used, a dose at age 4 mo is not needed. **Infants born to HBsAg positive mothers** should be tested for HBsAg and antibody to HBsAg after completion of the HepB series, at age 9–18 mo (generally at the next well-child visit after completion of the vaccine series).

^b**Diphtheria and tetanus toxoids and acellular pertussis vaccine (DTaP).** The fourth dose of DTaP may be administered as early as age 12 mo, provided 6 mo have elapsed since the third dose and the child is unlikely to return at age 15–18 mo. The final dose in the series should be given at age ≥4 y. **Tetanus and diphtheria toxoids and acellular pertussis vaccine (Tdap – adolescent preparation)** is recommended at age 11–12 y for those who have completed the recommended childhood DTP/DTaP vaccination series and have not received a Td booster dose. Adolescents 13–18 y who missed the 11–12-y Td/Tdap booster dose should also receive a single dose of Tdap if they have completed the recommended childhood DTP/DTaP vaccination series. Subsequent **tetanus and diphtheria toxoids (Td)** are recommended every 10 y.

^c**Haemophilus influenzae type b conjugate vaccine (Hib).** Three Hib conjugate vaccines are licensed for infant use. If PRP-OMP (PedvaxHIB or ComVax [Merck]) is administered at ages 2 and 4 mo, a dose at age 6 mo is not required. DTaP/Hib combination products should not be used for primary immunization in infants at ages 2, 4 or 6 mo but can be used as boosters after any Hib vaccine. The final dose in the series should be administered at age ≥12 mo.

^d**Measles, mumps, and rubella vaccine (MMR).** The second dose of MMR is recommended routinely at age 4–6 y but may be administered during any visit, provided at least 4 wk have elapsed since the first dose and both doses are administered beginning at or after age 12 mo. Those who have not previously received the second dose should complete the schedule by age 11–12 y.

^e**Varicella vaccine.** Varicella vaccine is recommended at any visit at or after age 12 mo for susceptible children (i.e., those who lack a reliable history of chickenpox). Susceptible persons aged ≥13 y should receive 2 doses administered at least 4 wk apart.

(continued)

663

FIGURE A-5. Continued.

[f]**Meningococcal vaccine.** Meningococcal conjugate vaccine (MCV4) should be given to all children at the 11–12 y old visit as well as to unvaccinated adolescents at high school entry (15 y of age). Other adolescents who wish to decrease their risk for meningococcal disease may also be vaccinated. All college freshmen living in dormitories should also be vaccinated, preferably with MCV4, although **meningococcal polysaccharide vaccine (MPSV4)** is an acceptable alternative. Vaccination against invasive meningococcal disease is recommended for children and adolescents aged ≥2 y with terminal complement deficiencies or anatomic or functional asplenia and certain other high risk groups (see MMWR 2005;54[RR-7]:1–21); use MPSV4 for children aged 2–10 y and MCV4 for older children, although MPSV4 is an acceptable alternative.

[g]**Pneumococcal vaccine.** The heptavalent **pneumococcal conjugate vaccine (PCV)** is recommended for all children aged 2–23 mo and for certain children aged 24–59 mo. The final dose in the series should be given at age ≥12 mo. **Pneumococcal polysaccharide vaccine (PPV)** is recommended in addition to PCV for certain high-risk groups. See MMWR 2000;49(RR-9):1–35.

[h]**Influenza vaccine.** Influenza vaccine is recommended annually for children aged ≥6 mo with certain risk factors (including, but not limited to, asthma, cardiac disease, sickle cell disease, HIV, diabetes, and conditions that can compromise respiratory function or handling of respiratory secretions or that can increase the risk for aspiration), healthcare workers, and other persons (including household members) in close contact with persons in groups at high risk (see MMWR 2005;54[RR-8]:1–55). In addition, healthy children aged 6–23 mo and close contacts of healthy children aged 0–5 mo are recommended to receive influenza vaccine because children in this age group are at substantially increased risk of influenza-related hospitalizations. For healthy persons aged 5–49 y, the intranasally administered, live, attenuated influenza vaccine (LAIV) is an acceptable alternative to the intramuscular trivalent inactivated influenza vaccine (TIV). See MMWR 2005;54(RR-8):1–55. Children receiving TIV should be administered a dosage appropriate for their age (0.25 mL if aged 6–35 mo or 0.5 mL if aged ≥3 y). Children aged ≤8 y who are receiving influenza vaccine for the first time should receive 2 doses (separated by at least 4 wk for TIV and at least 6 wk for LAIV).

[i]**Hepatitis A vaccine (HepA).** HepA is recommended for all children at 1 y of age (i.e.,12–23 mo). The 2 doses in the series should be administered at least 6 mo apart. States, counties, and communities with existing HepA vaccination programs for children 2–18 y of age are encouraged to maintain these programs. In these areas, new efforts focused on routine vaccination of 1-y-old children should enhance, not replace, ongoing programs directed at a broader population of children. HepA is also recommended for certain high-risk groups (see MMWR 1999;48[RR-12]:1–37).

TABLE A-5
Performance Status Scales

Karnofsky		ECOG		AJCC	
% Normal Status	Functional Status / Activity Level	Grade	Activity Level	Grade	Activity
100	Able to carry on normal activity; no special care needed / Normal; no complaints; no evidence of disease	0	Normal activity	H0	Normal activity
90	Able to carry on normal activity; minor signs or symptoms of disease				
80	Normal activity with effort; some signs or symptoms of disease	1	Symptoms but ambulatory	H1	Symptomatic and ambulatory; cares for self
70	Unable to work; able to live at home; cares for most personal needs, varying amount of assistance needed / Cares for self; unable to carry on normal activity or progressing rapidly to active work				
60	Requires occasional assistance but able to care for self	2	In bed 50% of time	H2	Ambulatory 50% of time; occasionally needs assistance
50	Requires considerable assistance and frequent medical care				

(continued)

TABLE A-5
(Continued)

Karnofsky		ECOG		AJCC	
Functional Status	% Normal Status	Activity Level	Grade	Activity Level	Grade	Activity

Functional Status	% Normal Status	Activity Level	Grade	Activity Level	Grade	Activity
Unable to care for self; requires equivalent of needed institutional or hospital care; may be progressing rapidly	40	Disabled; requires special care and assistance	3	In bed 50% of time	H3	Ambulatory 50% of time; nursing care
	30	Severely disabled; hospitalization indicated though death not imminent				
	20	Very sick; hospitalization necessary	4	100% bedridden	H4	Bedridden; may need hospitalization
	10	Moribund; fatal processes				
	0	Dead				

ECOG = Eastern Cooperative Oncology Group; AJCC = American Joint Committee on Cancer.
Source: Reprinted, with permission, from Cameron R (ed): *Practical Oncology.* Originally published by Appleton & Lange. Copyright © 1993. McGraw-Hill.

(Text continued from page 656.)

RADIATION TERMINOLOGY

Measure	Old Term	SI Unit
Activity	curie	becquerel (Bq)
Absorbed dose	rad	gray (Gy)

TEMPERATURE CONVERSION

Table A–6, below, gives information for converting temperature from the Fahrenheit (F) scale to the Celsius (C) scale and vice versa.

WEIGHT CONVERSION

Table A–7, page 668, gives information for converting weight in pounds (lb) to weight in kilograms (kg) and vice versa.

TABLE A–6
Temperature Conversion Table

F	C	C	F
0	–17.7	0	32.0
95.0	35.0	35.0	95.0
96.0	35.5	35.5	95.9
97.0	36.1	36.0	96.8
98.0	36.6	36.5	97.7
98.6	37.0	37.0	98.6
99.0	37.2	37.5	99.5
100.0	37.7	38.0	100.4
101.0	38.3	38.5	101.3
102.0	38.8	39.0	102.2
103.0	39.4	39.5	103.1
104.0	40.0	40.0	104.0
105.0	40.5	40.5	104.9
106.0	41.1	41.0	105.8
$C = (F-32) \times 5/9$		$F = (C \times 9/5) + 32$	

F = degrees Fahrenheit; C = degrees Celsius.

TABLE A-7
Weight Conversion Table

lb	kg	kg	lb
1	0.5	1	2.2
2	0.9	2	4.4
4	1.8	3	6.6
6	2.7	4	8.8
8	3.6	5	11.0
10	4.5	6	13.2
20	9.1	8	17.6
30	13.6	10	22.0
40	18.2	20	44.0
50	22.7	30	66.0
60	27.3	40	88.0
70	31.8	50	110.0
80	36.4	60	132.0
90	40.9	70	154.0
100	45.4	80	176.0
150	68.2	90	198.0
200	90.8	100	220.9

$kg = lb \times 0.454$ $lb = kg \times 2.2$

INDEX

Note: Page numbers followed by *t* indicate tables; those followed by *f* indicate figures.

A

Abacavir (Ziagen), 147*t,* 477
Abbokinase (urokinase), 618
Abciximab (ReoPro), 477
ABCs of emergency care, 456
Abdomen
 magnetic resonance imaging of, 350
 physical examination of, 5
Abdominal compartment syndrome, 445
Abdominal computed tomography, 347
Abdominal distention, 33
Abdominal pain, 34
Abdominal paracentesis, 304–306, 305*f,* 306*t*
Abdominal radiography, 341–342
Abdominal ultrasonography, 346
Abducens nerve, 5
Abelcet (amphotericin B lipid complex), 486–487
Abilify (aripiprazole), 489
Abraxane (paclitaxel), 582
Absorbable sutures, 361
Acalculous cholecystitis, 445
Acamprosate (Campral), 477
Acanthocyte, 99
Acarbose (Precose), 477
Accessory cephalic vein for intravenous access, 286*f*
Accidental needlestick, 242
Accolate (zafirkulast), 621
Accupril (quinapril), 594
Accutane (isotretinoin), 554
Acebutolol (Sectral), 477
Aceon (perindopril erbumine), 586
Acetadote (acetylcysteine), 478–479
Acetaminophen (Tylenol), 477–478, 627*t*
 for analgesia, 327*t*
 dosing guide for, 627*t*
 overdose of, 473*t*
Acetaminophen-butalbital-caffeine (Fioricet), 478
Acetaminophen-codeine, 334*t,* 478

Acetaminophen-hydrocodone (Lorcet, Vicodin), 546–547
Acetaminophen-oxycodone (Percocet, Tylox), 581
Acetaminophen-propoxyphene (Darvocet), 593
Acetaminophen-tramadol (Ultracet), 615
Acetate in parenteral formula, 234*t*
Acetazolamide (Diamox), 478
Acetic acid-aluminum acetate (Otic Domeboro), 478
Acetylcysteine (Mucomyst, Acetadote), 478–479
 for acetaminophen overdose, 473*t*
 in respiratory care, 382
Achromycin V (tetracycline), 610
Acid-base disorders, 165–177, 166*t,* 167*f*
 blood gas interpretation in, 167–168
 hypoxia and, 172–173, 173*f*
 metabolic acidosis in, 168–171, 169*f,* 170*t*
 metabolic alkalosis in, 171*f,* 171–172, 175, 176
 mixed, 165–167
 respiratory acidosis in, 172, 174
 respiratory alkalosis in, 172, 175
Acid-fast stain, 119
Acidemia, 165
Acidic urine, 109*f,* 110
Acidosis, 165
 metabolic, 168–171, 169*f,* 170*t*
 respiratory, 172, 174
Acinetobacter spp., 124*t,* 125*t*
Aciphex (rabeprazole), 595
Acitretin (Soriatane), 479
Aclometasone dipropionate (Aclovate), 634*t*
Acne, 137*t*
Acne rosacea, 137*t*
Aconite, 626
Acoustic nerve, 5
Acova (argatroban), 489

Actimmune (interferon-gamma-1b), 552
Actinomyces, 124*t*
Action tremor, 44
Actiq (fentanyl, transmucosal system), 534
Activase (alteplase, recombinant), 482–483
Activated charcoal, 503–504
Activated clotting time, 101
Activated partial thromboplastin time, 102–103
Activated protein C resistance, 101–102
Actonel (risedronate), 597
Actos (pioglitazone), 588
Acular (ketorolac), 555
Acupuncture, 338
Acute abdominal series, 342
Acute adrenal insufficiency, 445–446
Acute coronary syndromes, 466, 467–468*f*
Acute cough, 34
Acute diarrhea, 35
Acute intravascular hemolysis, 203, 204
Acute lung injury
    blood component therapy-related, 203, 204
    in septic shock, 444
Acute mastoiditis, 130*t*
Acute myocardial infarction, 644*t*
Acute pericarditis, 400*f*, 401
Acute renal failure
    complication in critical care, 444–445
    therapeutic diet in, 217*t*
Acute respiratory distress syndrome, 440, 441*t*
Acute retroviral syndrome, 156
Acyclovir (Zovirax), 479
Acyclovir-resistant herpes simplex virus, 144*t*
Adalat (nifedipine), 575
Adalimumab (Humira), 479
Adapin (doxepin), 522
Adefovir (Hepsera), 479
Adenosine (Adenocard), 479–480
    for pediatric tachycardia, 460*t*
    for tachycardia, 463*t*
Adjusted body weight, 213
Adrenal mass, 34
Adrenal scan, 350
Adrenergic receptors, 411*t*
Adrenocorticotropic hormone, 49
Adriamycin (doxorubicin), 522

Adrucil (fluorouracil), 536–537
Adult cardiopulmonary resuscitation, 456–458
Advair Diskus (fluticasone propionate-salmeterol xinafoate), 538
Advanced airways, 464
Advanced cardiac life support, 463, 463*t*
AeroBid (flunisolide), 536
Aeromonas hydrophilia, 125*t*
Aerosol therapy, 380–381
AFB smear, 119
Afrinol (pseudoephedrine), 593–594
Afterload, 409, 423
Agenerase (amprenavir), 487
Aggrastat (tirofiban), 613
Aggrenox (dipyridamole-aspirin), 520
Air-contrast barium enema, 345
Airborne precautions, 161
Airway
    cardiopulmonary resuscitation and, 456, 457*f*
    critical care and, 431–435, 432–434*f*
Airway management
    intubation in, 430–431, 431*t*
    in medical emergency, 463–464
AJCC scale, 665–666*t*
AK-Dex Ophthalmic (dexamethasone, ophthalmic), 515
Alamast (pemirolast), 584
Alanine aminotransferase, 50
Alavert (loratadine), 561
Albumin, 49, 84*t*, 201*t*
Albumin (Albuminar, Buminate, Albutein), 480
Albuminar (albumin), 480
Albutein (albumin), 480
Albuterol (Ventolin, Proventil, Volmax), 382, 469, 480
Albuterol-ipratropium (Combivent), 480
Aldactazide (hydrochlorothiazide-spironolactone), 546
Aldactone (spironolactone), 603
Aldara (imiquimod cream), 550
Aldesleukin (Proleukin), 480
Aldomet (methyldopa), 566–567
Aldosterone, 49
Alefacept (Amevive), 480
Alendronate (Fosamax), 481
Aleve (naproxen), 572
Alfentanil (Alfenta), 481
Alfuzosin (Uroxatral), 481
Alginic acid-aluminum hydroxide-magnesium trisilicate (Gaviscon), 481

Alimentum formula, 222*t*

Alimta (pemetrexed), 584

Alinia (nitazoxanide), 576

Alka-Mints (calcium carbonate), 497

Alkaline phosphatase, 50

Alkaline urine, 109*f,* 110

Alkalosis, 165

    metabolic, 171*f,* 171–172, 175, 176

    respiratory, 172, 175

Alkeran (melphalan), 564

Allegra (fexofenadine), 535

Allen test, 248

Allergic reaction

    to blood component therapy, 203, 204

    latex, 360

Allopurinol (Zyloprim, Lopurin,

        Aloprim), 481

Allowable blood loss, 197

Almotriptan (Axert), 645*t*

Alomide (lodoxamide), 560

Alopecia, 34

Aloprim (allopurinol), 481

Alosetron (Lotronex), 481

Aloxil (palonosetron), 582–583

Alpha-adrenergic receptors, 411*t*

Alpha-fetoprotein, 50

Alpha$_1$ globulin, 84*t*

Alpha$_1$-protease inhibitor (Prolastin),

    482

Alpha$_2$ globulin, 84*t*

Alphagan (brimonidine), 495

Alprazolam (Xanax), 482

Alprostadil (Prostin VR), 482

Alprostadil, intracavernosal (Caverject,

        Edex), 482

Alprostadil, urethral suppository (Muse),

    482

Altace (ramipril), 595

Alteplase, recombinant (Activase),

    482–483

AlternaGEL (aluminum hydroxide), 483

Altocor (lovastatin), 561

Altretamine (Hexalen), 483

Alum (ammonium aluminum sulfate),

    486

Aluminum hydroxide (Amphojel,

        AlternaGEL), 483

Aluminum hydroxide-magnesium

        carbonate (Gaviscon), 483

Aluminum hydroxide-magnesium

        hydroxide (Maalox), 483

Aluminum hydroxide-magnesium

        hydroxide-simethicone

        (Mylanta, Maalox Plus), 483

Aluminum hydroxide-magnesium

        trisilicate (Gaviscon), 483

Alupent (metaproterenol), 565

Alveolar hypoventilation, 173

Alveolar infiltrates, 354

Alveolar-to-arterial gradient, 428, 449*t*

    ventilator weaning and, 438*t*

Amantadine (Symmetrel), 483–484

Amaryl (glimepiride), 543

Ambien (zolpidem), 623

AmBisome (amphotericin B liposomal),

    487

Amcill (ampicillin), 487

Amcinonide (Cyclocort), 634*t*

Amebiasis, 150*t*

Amenorrhea, 34

Amerge (naratriptan), 572–573, 645*t*

American Joint Committee on Cancer

        performance scale, 665–666*t*

Amevive (alefacept), 480

Amicar (aminocaproic acid), 484

Amifostine (Ethyol), 484

Amikacin (Amikin), 484, 628*t*

Amiloride (Midamor), 484

Amino acid cervical cream, 484

Aminocaproic acid (Amicar), 484

Aminoglutethimide (Cytadren), 484

Aminophylline, 485

Amiodarone (Cordarone, Pacerone), 485,

    630*t*

    in pediatric advanced life support, 459*t*

    for pediatric tachycardia, 460*t*

    for tachycardia, 463*t*

Amitriptyline (Elavil), 485, 631*t*

Amlodipine (Norvasc), 485

Amlodipine-atorvastatin (Caduet), 485

Ammonia, 50

Amnesteem (isotretinoin), 554

Amniocentesis, 81

Amniotic fluid fern test, 245–246

Amoxicillin (Amoxil, Polymox), 159*t,*

    160*t,* 486

Amoxicillin-clavulanic acid (Augmentin),

    486

Amphojel (aluminum hydroxide), 483

Amphotec (amphotericin B cholesteryl),

    486

Amphotericin B (Fungizone), 486

Amphotericin B cholesteryl (Amphotec),

    486

Amphotericin B lipid complex (Abelcet),

    486–487

Amphotericin B liposomal (AmBisome),

    487

Ampicillin (Amcill, Omnipen), 159*t*, 160*t*, 487

Ampicillin-sulbactam (Unasyn), 487

Amprenavir (Agenerase), 487

Amrinone (Inocor), 550

Amyl nitrate for cyanide poisoning, 473*t*

Amylase, 50

Anakinra (Kineret), 487

Analgesia, 326–337, 327–336*t*
  in critical care, 406
  patient-controlled, 338–339, 339*t*

Anaphylaxis, 466–469
  blood component therapy-related, 203, 204

Anaprox (naproxen), 572

Anaspaz (hyoscyamine), 548

Anastrozole (Arimidex), 488

Anatomic scrub, 357

Ancef (cefazolin), 500

Anectine (succinylcholine), 605

Anergy screen, 310

Angiography, 344–345

Angiomax (bivalirudin), 495

Animal bite, 137*t*

Anion gap, 168, 169*f*

Anion gap acidosis, 169

Anisocytosis, 98, 99

Anistreplase (Eminase), 488

Ankle-arm index, 270–271

Ankle arthrocentesis, 251, 254*f*

Ankle-brachial index, 270–271

Anogenital warts, 145*t*

Anorexia, 34

Ansaid (flurbiprofen), 537–538

Anterior cutaneous nerve of neck, 6*f*

Anterior femoral cutaneous nerve, 6*f*, 7*f*

Anthralin (Anthra-Derm), 488

Anthrax, 124*t*

Anthropometric measurements, 209, 210*t*, 211*t*

Anti-activated factor X, 100–101

Anti-cyclic citrullinated polypeptide antibodies, 51

Anti-factor Xa, 100–101

Anti-neutrophil cytoplasmic antibodies, 52

Anti-SCL 70 antibody, 52

Anti-Xa test, 100–101

Antiarrhythmics, 646*t*

Antibiotics. *See* Antimicrobial therapy.

Anticentromere antibody, 52

Anticholinergic toxicity, 471

Anticholinesterase overdose, 473*t*

Anticoagulants, 644*t*

circulating anticoagulant screen and, 102
  for pulmonary embolism, 447

Anticonvulsants
  for analgesia, 337
  therapeutic levels of, 628–629*t*

Antidepressants
  for analgesia, 337
  overdose of, 473*t*

Antidotes, 473*t*

Antihemophilic factor (Monoclate), 488

Antilirium (physostigmine), 587–588

Antimicrobial resistance, 118–119

Antimicrobial therapy
  in bone and joint disorders, 129*t*
  in bronchitis, 129*t*
  in cervicitis, 130*t*
  in chancre, 130*t*
  in chlamydial infection, 130*t*
  in diverticulitis, 130*t*
  in ear infection, 130–131*t*
  empiric, 117
  in endocarditis, 131–132*t*
  in epiglottitis, 132*t*
  in fungal infections, 148–149*t*
  in gallbladder disease, 132*t*
  in gastroenteritis, 133*t*
  in gonorrhea, 133*t*
  in mastitis, 129*t*
  in meningitis, 133–134*t*
  in nocardiosis, 134*t*
  in parasitic infections, 150–151*t*
  in pelvic inflammatory disease, 134*t*
  in peritonitis, 135*t*
  in pharyngitis, 135*t*
  in pneumonia, 136*t*
  in septic shock, 443
  in sinusitis, 137*t*
  in skin and soft tissue infections, 137–138*t*
  in subacute bacterial endocarditis prophylaxis, 158–159, 159*t*, 160*t*
  in syphilis, 138*t*
  in tick-borne diseases, 152–153*t*
  in tuberculosis, 138*t*, 154–155
  in ulcer disease, 139*t*
  in urinary tract infection, 139–140*t*
  in vaginal infections, 140*t*
  in viral infections, 142–145*t*

Antimicrosomal antibody, 52

Antimitochondrial antibody, 52

Antinuclear antibody, 51–52

Antiretroviral therapy, 146–147*t*

Antistreptococcal O, 51
Antistreptolysin O, 51
Antithrombin III, 101
Antithymocyte globulin (Atgam, ATG), 562
Antivert (meclizine), 563
Anturane (sulfinpyrazone), 606
Anuria, 42–43
Anzemet (dolasetron), 521
Aortic insufficiency, 10*t*
Aortic stenosis, 10*t*
Apgar score, 640*t*, 649
Apheresis, 196
Apley test, 15
Apokyn (apomorphine), 488
Apomorphine (Apokyn), 488
Apraclonidine (Iopidine), 488
Aprepitant (Emend), 488–489
Apresoline (hydralazine), 546
Aprotinin (Trasylol), 489
Aquachloral (chloral hydrate), 504
AquaMEPHYTON (vitamin K), 588
ARA-C (cytarabine), 512
Aranesp (darbepoetin alfa), 514
Arava (leflunomide), 557
Aredia (pamidronate), 583
Argatroban (Acova), 489
Argyll Robertson pupil, 15
Arimidex (anastrozole), 488
Aripiprazole (Abilify), 489
Aristocort (triamcinolone), 636*t*
Aristolochic acid, 626
Arixtra (fondaparinux), 538–539
Aromasin (exemestane), 532
Arrhythmias
    atrial, 388–390, 388–390*f*
    ventricular, 391–392, 391–393*f*
Artane (trihexyphenidyl), 616–617
Arterial blood gases, 163–165, 164*t*, 167–168
Arterial carbon dioxide tension, 431*t*
Arterial hemoglobin saturation, 431*t*
Arterial line placement, 246–248, 247*f*
Arterial oxygen content, 428, 449*t*
Arterial puncture, 248–249
Arthritis
    arthrocentesis in, 249–253, 252*t*, 254*t*, 255*f*
    differential diagnosis in, 35
Arthrocentesis, 249–253, 252*t*, 254*f*, 255*f*
Artificial tears, 489
Asacol (mesalamine), 565
Ascariasis, 150*t*
Ascites, 35

Ascitic fluid analysis, 304–306, 305*f*, 306*t*
Ascorbic acid, 234*t*
Aseptic meningitis, 294*t*
ASO titer, 51
L-Asparaginase (Elspar, Oncaspar), 489
Aspartate aminotransferase, 51
Aspergillosis, 148*t*
Aspiration technique
    bone marrow, 253–256
    percutaneous suprapubic bladder, 316, 317*f*
Aspiration, tube feeding and, 230–231
Aspirin (Bayer, Ecotrin, St. Joseph's), 327*t*, 489
Aspirin-butalbital-caffeine-codeine, 490
Aspirin-butalbital compound (Fiorinal), 490
Aspirin-codeine (Empirin), 490
Aspirin-dipyridamole (Aggrenox), 520
Aspirin-hydrocodone (Lortab ASA), 547
Aspirin-oxycodone (Percodan), 581–582
Aspirin-propoxyphene (Darvon), 593
Assist-control ventilation, 435, 436*f*
Astelin (azathioprine), 491
Asthma, 469–471
Atacand (candesartan), 498
Atarax (hydroxyzine), 548
Ataxic tremor, 44
Atazanavir (Reyataz), 146*t*, 490
Atenolol (Tenormin), 490
Atenolol-chlorthalidone (Tenoretic), 490
ATG (antithymocyte globulin), 562
Atgam (antithymocyte globulin), 562
Ativan (lorazepam), 561
Atomoxetine (Strattera), 490–491
Atorvastatin (Lipitor), 491
Atorvastatin-amlodipine (Caduet), 485
Atovaquone (Mepron), 491
Atovaquone-proguanil (Malarone), 491
Atracurium (Tracrium), 491
Atrial arrhythmias, 388–390, 388–390*f*
Atrial fibrillation, 389, 390*f*
Atrial flutter, 389–390, 390*f*
Atrial hypertrophy, 395*f*, 395–396
Atrial septal defect, 11*t*
Atrioventricular junctional rhythm, 390, 390*f*
Atrophy, 13
Atropine, 491
    for anticholinesterase overdose, 473*t*
    for bradycardia, 463*t*
    for pediatric bradycardia, 460*t*
    in respiratory care, 382
Atrovent (ipratropium), 382, 469, 553

Atypical lymphocytes, 96
Auer rods, 99
Augmentin (amoxicillin-clavulanic acid), 486
Auralgan (benzocaine-antipyrine), 493
Auscultation of heart murmur, 409
Auspitz sign, 15
Austin Flint murmur, 16
Autoantibody, 51–52
Autoantibody test, 101
Autologous blood donation, 195–196
Automated external defibrillation, 464–466
Avandia (rosiglitazone), 598
Avapro (irbesartan), 553
Avastin (bevacizumab), 494
Avelox (moxifloxacin), 571
Aventyl (nortriptyline), 577–578, 630*t*
Avinza (morphine), 570
Avita (tretinoin), 615
Avlosulfon (dapsone), 513–514
Avodart (dutasteride), 523
Axid (nizatidine), 577
Axillary nerve, 6*f*, 7*f*
Axis deviation in electrocardiogram, 385*f*, 385–386
Axocet (acetaminophen-butalbital-caffeine), 478
Azactam (aztreonam), 492
Azathioprine (Astelin, Optivar), 491
Azithromycin (Zithromax), 159*t*, 491–492
Azmacort (triamcinolone), 615
Azopt (brinzolamide), 495
Aztreonam (Azactam), 492
Azulfidine (sulfasalazine), 605–606

B
B cell, 99
B-type natriuretic peptide, 78
Babesiosis, 152–153*t*
Babinski sign, 16
Bacille Calmette-Guérin (TheraCys, Tice BCG), 492
Back pain, 35
Baclofen (Lioresal), 492
Bacterial endocarditis, 158–159, 159*t*, 160*t*
Bacterial infection
    cerebrospinal fluid analysis in, 294*t*
    transfusion-related, 205
Bacterial vaginosis, 140*t*
Bacteroides fragilis, 125*t*

Bactocill (oxacillin), 580
Bactrim (trimethoprim-sulfamethoxazole), 617
Bactroban (mupirocin), 571
Bainbridge reflex, 16
Baker tube, 278
Balloon port of pulmonary artery catheter, 414, 414*f*
Balsalazide (Colazal), 492
Band neutrophils, 94*t*
Barium enema, 345
Barium swallow, 345
Base difference, 164*t*
Basic metabolic panel, 48
Basilic vein for intravenous access, 286*f*
Basiliximab (Simulect), 492
Bask mask ventilation, 464
Basophil, 94*t*, 96
Basophilic stippling, 99
Battle sign, 16
Bayer aspirin, 489
BCG (Bacille Calmette-Guérin), 492
BCNU (carmustine), 499
Beau lines, 16
Becaplermin (Regranex Gel), 493
Beck triad, 16
Beclomethasone (Beconase, Vancenase Nasal Inhaler, Qvar), 493
Bedside electrocardiography, 271–273, 272*f*
Bedside procedure note, 27–28
Beef tapeworm, 151*t*
Bell palsy, 16
Belladonna and opium suppositories, 493
Benadryl (diphenhydramine), 519
Benazepril (Lotensin), 493
Benemid (probenecid), 591
Bentyl (dicyclomine), 517
Benylin DM (dextromethorphan), 516
Benzamycin (erythromycin-benzoyl peroxide), 528
Benzocaine-antipyrine (Auralgan), 493
Benzodiazepines
    for analgesia, 337
    in critical care, 405
    overdose of, 473*t*
Benzonatate (Tessalon Perles), 493
Benztropine (Cogentin), 493
Beractant (Survanta), 493
Bergman triad, 16
Beta-adrenergic blockers, 646*t*
    overdose of, 473*t*
Beta-adrenergic receptors, 411*t*
Beta globulin, 84*t*

Beta-hydroxybutyrate, 52
Beta$_2$-microglobulin, 78, 111
Betadine hand scrub, 356–357
Betagan (levobunolol), 558
Betamethasone (Valisone, Diprolene, Diprosone), 633t, 634t
Betapace (sotalol), 602
Betaseron (interferon beta-1b), 552
Betaxolol (Kerlone), 494
Betaxolol, ophthalmic (Betoptic), 494
Bethanechol (Urecholine, Duvoid), 494
Bevacizumab (Avastin), 494
Bextra (valdecoxib), 618
Biaxin (clarithromycin), 507–508
Bicalutamide (Casodex), 494
Bicarbonate, 52, 55
    for septic shock, 444
Bicarbonate concentration, 163, 164t
Bicillin (penicillin G benzathine), 585
Bicitra (sodium citrate), 601
BiCNU (carmustine), 499
BIDA-scan, 351
Bigeminy, 391, 391f
Bilirubin, 52–53
    urine, 106
Bimanual pelvic examination, 298
Bioelectrical impedance analysis, 210t
Biopsy
    bone marrow, 253–256
    skin, 307–308
Biot breathing, 16
Bioterrorism, 158
Biotin, 234t
Bipolar leads, 383
Bisacodyl (Dulcolax), 494
Bisferious pulse, 16
Bismuth subsalicylate (Pepto-Bismol), 494
Bisoprolol (Zebeta), 494–495
Bite, 137t
Bitolterol (Tornalate), 495
Bitot spots, 16
Bivalirudin (Angiomax), 495
Black box precautions, 475
Black cohosh, 623
Bladder catheterization, 312–316, 314f, 317f
Blastomycosis, 148t
Bleeding scan, 350
Bleeding time, 101
Bleomycin sulfate (Blenoxane), 495
Blephamide (sulfacetamide-prednisolone), 605
Blocadren (timolol), 612

Blood
    total blood volume, 179
    in urine, 107
Blood alcohol, 64
Blood banking procedures, 195
Blood collection, 91
Blood component therapy, 195–205
    apheresis and, 196
    autologous blood donation and, 195–196
    blood banking procedures and, 195
    blood groups and, 196, 197t
    donor-directed blood products and, 196
    emergency transfusions and, 196
    indications and uses of, 198–201t
    irradiated blood components and, 196
    platelet transfusions in, 202
    red cell transfusions in, 197–202
    routine blood donation and, 195
    for septic shock, 443
    transfusion-associated infectious disease risk and, 204–205
    transfusion procedures in, 202–203
    transfusion reactions in, 203–204
    white cell transfusions in, 202
Blood culture, 119–120
Blood donation, 195–196
Blood gases, 163–165, 164t, 167–168
Blood glucose
    management in parenteral nutrition, 238–239
    metabolic syndrome and, 209, 211t
Blood groups, 196, 197t
Blood lead, 76
Blood loss
    hemorrhagic shock and, 442t
    red cell transfusion for, 197
Blood pressure
    critical care and, 404, 407–408
    guidelines for, 11–12, 12t
    hemorrhagic shock and, 442t
    metabolic syndrome and, 209, 211t
    orthostatic hypotension and, 296
Blood products, 198–201t
    donor-directed, 196
Blood smear, 91–92, 92f, 92t
Blood tests, 99–103, 100f
Blood urea nitrogen/creatinine ratio, 53
Blumberg sign, 16
Blumer shelf, 16
Body fluids, 181, 183t
Body mass index, 208, 209t, 210t, 649, 653t

Body surface area, 649, 651*f*, 652*f*
   rule of nines and, 183*t*, 185*f*
Body weight
   nutritional assessment and, 208, 210*t*
   rule of nines and, 183*t*
Bone densitometry, 343
Bone disease, 129*t*
Bone scan, 350–351
Boniva (ibandronate), 549
Bordetella pertussis, 125*t*
Bortezomib (Velcade), 495
Bouchard node, 16
Bradycardia, 386
   advanced cardiac life support in, 463,
      463*t*
   pediatric, 460*t*
Brain attack, 466, 469*t*, 470*f*
Brain scan, 351
Brand name drugs, 475
Branham sign, 16
Breast
   mass in, 35
   mastitis and, 129*t*
   physical examination of, 5
   screening for cancer, 654*t*
Breast feeding, 221
   drug use during, 476–477
Breast self-examination, 654*t*
Breathing, cardiopulmonary resuscitation
      and, 456, 457*f*
Brethine (terbutaline), 609
Brevibloc (esmolol), 528
Bricanyl (terbutaline), 609
Brimonidine (Alphagan), 495
Brinzolamide (Azopt), 495
Broad casts, 110
Bromocriptine (Parlodel), 495
Bronchial angiography, 345
Bronchiolitis, 145*t*
Bronchitis, 129*t*
Bronchodilators, 629*t*
Bronchopulmonary hygiene, 380–381
Broviac catheter, 263–264
Brucella, 125*t*
Brudzinski sign, 16
Budesonide (Rhinocort, Pulmicort), 495
Buffer deficiency, 170*t*
Bulla, 13
Bumetanide (Bumex), 496
Buminate (albumin), 480
Bundle branch block, 394*f*, 394–395
Bupivacaine (Marcaine, Sensorcaine),
      364*t*, 496, 632*t*
Buprenorphine (Buprenex), 496

Bupropion (Wellbutrin, Zyban), 496
Burns, 137*t*, 181–183
Burr cell, 99
Burrow, 13
Buspirone (BuSpar), 496
Busulfan (Myleran, Busulfex), 496
Butorphanol (Stadol), 496
Butterfly needle, 288*f*, 289
N-Butyl-2-cyanoacrylate, 373
Byetta (exenatide), 532–533

C

C-peptide, 53
C-reactive protein, 53–54, 210
CA-125 tumor marker, 54
Caduet (amlodipine-atorvastatin), 485
Caffeine, therapeutic levels of, 629*t*
Calamus, 626
Calan (verapamil), 620
Calcaneal nerve, 7*f*
Calcipotriene (Dovonex), 496
Calcitonin (Cibacalcin, Miacalcin), 54,
      190, 497
Calcitriol (Rocaltrol), 497
Calcium
   hypercalcemia and, 189–190
   hypocalcemia and, 190–191
   in parenteral formula, 234*t*
   requirements for, 180
   serum, 54–55
   urine, 113
Calcium acetate (Calphron, Phos-Ex,
      PhosLo), 497
Calcium carbonate (Tums, Alka-Mints),
      191, 497
Calcium channel blockers, 646*t*
   overdose of, 473*t*
Calcium chloride, 497
   for calcium channel blockers overdose,
      473*t*
   for hyperkalemia, 188
Calcium citrate, 191
Calcium glubionate (Neo-Calglucon),
      191, 497
Calcium gluceptate, 497
Calcium gluconate, 497
   for hypermagnesemia, 192
   for hypocalcemia, 191
Calcium lactate, 191
Calcium salts, 497
Caldecort (hydrocortisone, topical), 635*t*
Calfactant (Infasurf), 498
Caloric expenditure, 213

Calphron (calcium acetate), 497

Camphorated tincture of opium, 583

Campral (acamprosate), 477

Camptosar (irinotecan), 553

Cancer
cerebrospinal fluid analysis in, 295*t*
hypercalcemia in, 189
positron emission tomography in, 352
screening for, 654–655*t*

Cancidas (caspofungin), 499

Candesartan (Atacand), 498

Candidiasis
drug therapy for, 148*t*
testing for, 299
vaginal, 140*t*

Cantor tube, 277–278

Capillary blood gases, 164

Capillary blood sampling, 91, 280–282, 281*f*

Capnography, 404

Capoten (captopril), 498

Capsaicin (Capsin, Zostrix), 498

Captopril (Capoten), 498

Carafate (sucralfate), 605

Carbamazepine (Tegretol), 498, 628*t*

Carbidopa-levodopa (Sinemet), 498

Carbohydrate controlled diet, 216*t*

Carbohydrates in parenteral formula, 233

Carbon dioxide, 55

Carbon dioxide partial pressure, 164*t*
ventilator weaning and, 438*t*

Carbon monoxide, 55, 473*t*

Carboplatin (paraplatin), 498

Carboxyhemoglobin, 55

Carcinoembryonic antigen, 55

Cardene (nicardipine), 575

Cardiac angiography, 344

Cardiac arrest
advanced cardiac life support in, 463
cardiopulmonary resuscitation in, 456–462, 457*f*
adult, 456–458
child, 458–460, 459*t*, 460*t*, 461*f*
infant, 460–462
neonate, 462, 462*f*

Cardiac enzymes, 49

Cardiac hypertrophy, 395–396, 395–397*f*

Cardiac index, 419*t*, 448*t*

Cardiac output, 409, 448*t*
normal values of, 419*t*
pulmonary artery catheter measurement of, 421

Cardiac scan, 351

Cardiac-specific troponin, 89

Cardiac tamponade, 422*t*

Cardiogenic shock, 422*t*, 441–442

Cardiopulmonary resuscitation, 456–462, 457*f*
adult, 456–458
child, 458–460, 459*t*, 460*t*, 461*f*
infant, 460–462
neonate, 462, 462*f*

Cardiovascular agents, 630*t*

Cardiovascular system
adverse effects of pain on, 324*t*
critical care and, 406–410, 408*f*, 410*f*, 411*t*
review of systems and, 2
sympathetic nervous system influence on, 409–410, 411*t*

Cardioversion, 460*t*, 465–466

Cardizem (diltiazem), 518–519

Cardura (doxazosin), 522

Carisoprodol (Soma), 331*t*, 499

Carmustine (BiCNU, BCNU, Gliadel), 499

Carteolol (Cartrol, Ocupress Ophthalmic), 499

Cartia XT (diltiazem), 518–519

Cartrol (carteolol), 499

Carvedilol (Coreg), 499

Casodex (bicalutamide), 494

Caspofungin (Cancidas), 499

Casts, renal, 110

Cataflam (diclofenac), 517

Catapres (clonidine), 508–509

Catecholamines, fractionated, 55, 114

Catgut, 362*t*

Catheter-over-needle intravenous access, 287*f*, 287–288

Catheter-related sepsis, 239, 446

Catheterization
bladder, 312–316, 314*f*, 317*f*
central venous, 256–264
external jugular vein, 262
femoral vein, 262–263
indications and contraindications for, 256
left internal jugular vein, 261
materials for, 257
removal of catheter, 263–264
right internal jugular vein, 259–261, 260*f*
subclavian, 257–259, 258*f*
pulmonary artery, 412–424
catheter description of, 414*f*, 414–415

Catheterization (*cont.*)
    catheterization procedure in,
        415–419, 416–418*f,* 419*t*
    clinical applications of, 421–423
    complications of, 419–420
    continuous cardiac output
        measurement in, 421
    continuous mixed venous oxygen
        saturation monitoring in,
        423–424, 424*f*
    continuous pulse oximetry in, 424
    differential diagnosis of
        abnormalities in, 421, 422*t*
    indications for, 413
    measurements in, 420–421
    relative positioning of, 413*f*
Caverject (Alprostadil, intracavernosal),
    482
Cavitary lesion, 354
Ceclor (cefaclor), 499
Cedax (ceftibuten), 502
Cefaclor (Ceclor), 499
Cefadroxil (Duricef, Ultracef), 159*t,* 500
Cefazolin (Ancef, Kefzol), 159*t,* 500
Cefdinir (Spectracef), 500
Cefepime (Maxipime), 500
Cefixime (Suprax), 500
Cefizox (ceftizoxime), 502
Cefmetazole (Zefazone), 500–501
Cefobid (cefoperazone), 501
Cefonicid (Monocid), 501
Cefoperazone (Cefobid), 501
Cefotan (cefotetan), 501
Cefotaxime (Claforan), 501
Cefotetan (Cefotan), 501
Cefoxitin (Mefoxin), 501
Cefpodoxime (Vantin), 501–502
Cefprozil (Cefzil), 502
Ceftazidime (Fortaz, Ceptaz, Tazidime,
    Tazicef), 502
Ceftibuten (Cedax), 502
Ceftin PO (cefuroxime), 502–503
Ceftizoxime (Cefizox), 502
Ceftriaxone (Rocephin), 502
Cefuroxime (Ceftin PO, Zinacef
    parenteral), 502–503
Cefzil (cefprozil), 502
Celecoxib (Celebrex), 503
Celexa (citalopram), 507
CellCept (mycophenolate mofetil), 571
Cellophane tape test, 127
Cellulitis, 137*t*
Cenestin (estrogen, conjugated synthetic),
    531

Central cyanosis, 34
Central nervous system
    considerations in critical care,
        405–406
    dementia and, 37
    respiratory acidosis and, 172
Central nervous system infection, 155
Central parenteral nutrition, 235
Central venous catheterization, 256–264
    external jugular vein, 262
    femoral vein, 262–263
    indications and contraindications for,
        256
    left internal jugular vein, 261
    materials for, 257
    removal of catheter, 263–264
    right internal jugular vein, 259–261,
        260*f*
    subclavian, 257–259, 258*f*
Central venous pressure, 410–412, 412*t*
Cephalexin (Keflex, Keftab), 159*t,* 503
Cephalic vein for intravenous access, 286*f*
Cephradine (Velosef), 503
Cephulac (lactulose), 556
Ceptaz (ceftazidime), 502
Cerebellum examination, 5–6
Cerebral angiography, 344
Cerebral perfusion pressure, 449*t*
Cerebrospinal fluid analysis, 289–296,
        291*f,* 292*f,* 294–295*t*
Cerebrospinal fluid oligoclonal banding,
        79
Cerebyx (fosphenytoin), 540
Cerubidine (daunorubicin), 514
Cerumenex (triethanolamine), 616
Cervical cancer screening, 655*t*
Cervical spine radiography, 343
Cervicitis, 130*t,* 299
Cervidil vaginal insert (dinoprostone),
        519
Cetirizine (Zyrtec), 503
Cetuximab (Erbitux), 503
Chadwick sign, 16
Chagas disease, 151*t*
Chamomile, 623–624
Chancre, 130*t*
Chancroid, 130*t*
Chandelier sign, 16, 298
Chaparral, 626
Charcoal, activated, 503–504
Charcot triad, 16
Chartwork, 25–32
    bedside procedure note in, 27–28
    delivery note in, 29

discharge summary/note in, 26–27
night of surgery note in, 29
off-service note in, 27
on-service note in, 27
operative note in, 28–29
outpatient prescription writing and, 29–32, 30*f*
preoperative note in, 28
shorthand for laboratory values, 31*f*
SOAP note in, 26
writing orders, 25–26
Chem-7 panel, 48
Chemet (succimer), 604–605
Chemstrip 10, 105
Chest
magnetic resonance imaging of, 350
physical examination of, 3
Chest computed tomography, 347
Chest electrodes, 271–272, 272*f*
Chest pain, 35
Chest physiotherapy, 381
Chest radiography, 341, 342*f*, 343*f*, 353–354
Chest tube placement, 264–265, 266*f*
Cheyne-Stokes respiration, 16
Chief complaint, 1
Chilbroxin (norfloxacin), 577
Child
cardiopulmonary resuscitation in, 458–462, 459*t*, 460*t*, 461*f*
endotracheal tube for, 273*t*
eruption of teeth, 13, 14*f*
fever work-up in, 277
immunization guidelines for, 650, 657–664*f*
maintenance fluids for, 181, 183*t*
pneumonia in, 136*t*
protein needs of, 214
rule of nines and, 183*t*, 185*f*
septic shock in, 444
Chills, 35
Chinese herbal mixtures, 626
Chiropractic treatment for pain, 337–338
Chlamydial infection, 130*t*, 299
Chlor-Trimeton (chlorpheniramine), 504–505
Chloral hydrate (Aquachloral, Supprettes), 504
Chlorambucil (Leukeran), 504
Chlordiazepoxide (Librium, Mitran, Libritabs), 504
Chlorhexidine hand scrub, 356–357

Chloride
in parenteral formula, 234*t*
requirements for, 180
serum, 55–58
sweat, 86
urine, 111
Chlorothiazide (Diuril), 504
Chlorpheniramine (Chlor-Trimeton), 504–505
Chlorpromazine (Thorazine), 505
Chlorpropamide (Diabinase), 505
Chlorthalidone (Hygroton), 505
Chlorzoxazone (Paraflex, Parafon Forte DSC), 505
Cholangitis, 132*t*
Cholecalciferol, 505
Cholecystitis, 132*t*
acalculous, 445
Cholesterol, 56–59*t*, 58
metabolic syndrome and, 209, 211*t*
Cholesterol restricted diet, 218*t*
Cholestyramine (Questran, LoCHOLEST), 505
Choline magnesium trisalicylate (Trilisate), 328*t*
Chondroitin sulfate, 625
Chorionic villus sampling, 81
Chromic catgut, 362*t*
Chromium in parenteral formula, 235*t*
Chronic anemia, red cell transfusion in, 197
Chronic cough, 34
Chronic diarrhea, 35
Chronic hepatitis, 142*t*, 143*t*
Chronic mastoiditis, 130*t*
Chronulac (lactulose), 556
Chvostek sign, 16
Chylomicron, 77
Chylothorax, 43
Cialis (tadalafil), 606
Cibacalcin (calcitonin), 497
Ciclopirox (Loprox), 506
Cidofovir (Vistide), 506
Cilostazol (Pletal), 506
Ciloxan (ciprofloxacin, ophthalmic), 507
Cimetidine (Tagamet), 506
Cinacalcet (Sensipar), 506
Cincinnati Prehospital Stroke Scale, 469*t*
Ciprofloxacin, 506–507
Circulating anticoagulant screen, 102
Cisplatin (Platinol), 507
Citalopram (Celexa), 507
Citrobacter, 125*t*
Cladribine (Leustatin), 507

Claforan (cefotaxime), 501

Claravis (isotretinoin), 554

Clarinex (desloratadine), 515

Clarithromycin (Biaxin), 159*t*, 507–508

Claritin (loratadine), 561

Clean-catch urine specimen, 315

Clear liquid diet, 216*t*

Clemastine fumarate (Tavist), 508

Cleocin (clindamycin), 508

Climara (estradiol, transdermal), 529

Clindamycin (Cleocin), 159*t*, 508

Clinical breast examination, 654*t*

Clinoril (sulindac), 606

Clobetasol propionate (Temovate), 634*t*

Clocortolone pivalate (Cloderm), 634*t*

Cloderm (clocortolone pivalate), 634*t*

Clofarbine (Clolar), 508

Clofazimine (Lamprene), 508

Clolar (clofarbine), 508

Clonazepam (Klonopin), 508

Clonidine (Catapres), 508–509

Clopidogrel (Plavix), 509

Clopra (metoclopramide), 567

Clorazepate (Tranxene), 509

Closed thoracostomy, 264–265, 266*f*

Clostridium difficile, 124*t*, 156

    assay for, 60

    in colitis, 231

Clotrimazole (Lotrimin, Mycelex), 509

Clotrimazole-betametasone (Lotrisone), 509

Clozapine (Clozaril), 510

Clubbing, 36

Cluster headache, 39

Cluster of differentiation, 98–99

Coagulation factors, 100*f*

Coagulation tests, 99–103, 100*f*

Cobalamin, 234*t*

Cocaine, 510

Coccidioidomycosis, 148*t*

Cockcroft-Gault equation, 113

Codeine, 331*t*, 510

Codeine-acetaminophen, 334*t*, 478

Codeine-aspirin (Empirin), 490

Codeine-guaifenesin (Robitussin AC), 544

Cogentin (benztropine), 493

Cognex (tacrine), 606

Coin lesion, 354

Colace (docusate sodium), 521

Colazal (balsalazide), 492

Colchicine, 510

Cold agglutinins, 60

Colesevelam (Welchol), 510

Colestid (colestipol), 510–511

Colitis

    Clostridium difficile, 231

    cytomegalovirus, 142*t*

Colloids, 180

Colonoscopy, 654*t*

Colorectal cancer screening, 654*t*

CoLyte (polyethylene glycol), 590

Coma

    differential diagnosis in, 36

    emergency care in, 471

Combination analgesics, 334–336*t*

Combitube, 464

Combivent (albuterol-ipratropium), 480

Combivir (zidovudine-lamivudine), 622

Combunox (oxycodone-ibuprofen), 582

Comfrey, 626

Commercial infant formulas, 221, 222–223*t*

Compazine (prochlorperazine), 592

Complement C3, 60

Complement C4, 61

Complement CH$_{50}$, 61

Complement studies, 60–61

Complete blood count

    hematocrit and, 97–98

    normal values in, 92–95, 93*t*, 94*t*

    normal variations in, 95

    platelets and, 98

    red blood cells and, 97

    white blood cells and, 96–97

Complete bundle branch block, 394

Comprehensive metabolic panel, 48

Computed tomography, 347–348

Comtan (entacapone), 525

Condylox (podophyllin), 589

Conjugated bilirubin, 52

Conjunctivitis, 130*t*

Connecting peptide, 53

Constipation

    differential diagnosis in, 36

    enteral nutrition-related, 231

Contact precautions, 161

Contaminants in urine, 110

Continuous electrocardiography, 404

Continuous running suture, 367*f*

Contraceptives, 579, 638–641*t*

Contract reaction, 344

Contractility of heart, 409

    pulmonary artery catheter and, 423

Contrast nephropathy, 445

Contrast radiography, 344–346

Controlled mechanical ventilation, 435, 436*f*

Controlled substance classification, 476

Contusion, precordial, 407

Coombs test, 101

Copper, 235*t*

Cordarone (amiodarone), 485

Cordran (flurandrenolide), 635*t*

Coreg (carvedilol), 499

Corgard (nadolol), 571–572

Corlopam (fenoldopam), 533–534

Coronary CT angiography, 348

Corrigan pulse, 16

Cortef (hydrocortisone), 547–548

Corticosteroids
    for analgesia, 337
    urine, 114–115

Corticotropin, 49

Cortisol
    free, 114
    serum, 61

Cortisone, 633*t*, 635*t*

Cortrosyn stimulation test, 61

Corvert (ibutilide), 549

Corynebacterium spp., 125*t*

Cosmegen (dactinomycin), 513

Cosopt (dorzolamide-timolol), 522

Cotazym (pancrelipase), 583

Cotrimazole (trimethoprim-
        sulfamethoxazole), 617

Coudé catheter, 313, 314*f*

Cough, 36

Coumadin (warfarin), 447, 621

COX-2 inhibitors, 331*t*

Cozaar (losartan), 561

CPT code, 49

Cranberry, 624

Cranial nerves, 5

Creatine kinase, 61–62

Creatine phosphokinase isoenzymes,
        61–62

Creatinine clearance, 112–113

Creatinine, serum, 62

Creon (pancrelipase), 583

Crestor (rosuvastatin), 598

Cricothyroidotomy, 268–269

Critical care, 403–453
    analgesia and, 406
    cardiovascular instability and,
        406–410, 408*f*, 410*f*, 411*t*
    central venous pressure and, 410–412,
        412*t*
    common ICU equations for, 448–449*t*
    complications in, 440–447

        abdominal compartment syndrome
            in, 445
        acalculous cholecystitis in, 445
        acute adrenal insufficiency in,
            445–446
        acute renal failure in, 444–445
        acute respiratory distress syndrome
            in, 440, 441*t*
        deep venous thrombosis in, 447
        infection in, 446
        pulmonary embolism in, 447
        shock in, 441–444, 442*t*
        upper gastrointestinal hemorrhage
            in, 440–441
    drug infusions in, 450–453*t*
    ICU progress note in, 403–404
    intubation and, 430–431, 431*t*
    mechanical ventilation in, 435–439,
        436*f*, 438*t*
    nutrition and, 440
    oxygenation and, 428–430, 428–430*f*
    pulmonary artery catheter and,
        412–424, 413*f*
        catheter description of, 414*f*,
            414–415
        catheterization procedure in,
            415–419, 416–418*f*, 419*t*
        clinical applications of, 421–423
        complications of, 419–420
        continuous cardiac output
            measurement in, 421
        continuous mixed venous oxygen
            saturation monitoring in,
            423–424, 424*f*
        continuous pulse oximetry in, 424
        differential diagnosis of
            abnormalities in, 421, 422*t*
        indications for, 413
        measurements in, 420–421
    routine monitoring in, 404
    securing airway in, 431–435,
        432–434*f*
    sedation and, 405–406
    transport of patient in, 404–405
    ventilation in, 424–428, 425–427*f*

Critical closing volume, 426, 427*f*

Crixivan (indinavir), 551

Cromolyn sodium (Intal, NasalCrom,
        Opticrom), 511

Cross-table lateral abdominal
        radiography, 342

Crust, 13

Cryocrit, 62

Cryoglobulins, 62

Cryoprecipitated antihemophilic factor, 200*t*
Cryptococcosis, 148*t*
Cryptosporidiosis, 150*t*
Crystalloids, 181, 182*t*
Crystals in urine, 110
Cubicin (daptomycin), 514
Culdocentesis, 269–270
Cullen sign, 16
Culture
    blood, 119–120
    gonorrhea, 120–121
    nasal, 127
    sputum, 154
    stool, 155–156
    throat, 127–128
    urine, 141, 154
    in viral infection, 128, 154
Cushing triad, 16
Cutaneous innervation patterns, 6–7*f*
Cutaneous larva migrans, 150*t*
Cutting needle, 363
Cyanide poisoning, 473*t*
Cyanocobalamin, 89, 511
Cyanosis, 36
Cyclic antidepressants overdose, 473*t*
Cyclobenzaprine (Flexeril), 331*t*, 511
Cyclopentolate (Cyclogyl), 511
Cyclophosphamide (Cytoxan, Neosar), 511–512
Cyclospora, 150*t*
Cyclosporine (Sandimmune, NeOral), 512, 631*t*
Cyclosporine, ophthalmic (Restasis), 512
Cymbalta (duloxetine), 523
Cyproheptadine (Periactin), 512
Cysteine, 114
Cysticercosis, 151*t*
Cystitis, 139*t*, 148*t*
Cystogram, 345
Cystospaz (hyoscyamine), 548
Cytadren (aminoglutethimide), 484
Cytarabine (ARA-C, Cytosar-U), 512
Cytarabine liposome (DepoCyt), 512
Cytochrome P-450 isoenzymes, 647–648*t*
CytoGam (cytomegalovirus immune globulin), 512–513
Cytomegalovirus, 142*t*
    transfusion-related, 205
Cytomegalovirus antibodies, 62
Cytomegalovirus immune globulin (CytoGam), 512–513
Cytomel (liothyronine), 560

Cytosar-U (cytarabine), 512
Cytotec (misoprostol), 569
Cytovene (ganciclovir), 541
Cytoxan (cyclophosphamide), 511–512

D
D-Dimer, 62–63
Dacarbazine (DTIC), 513
Daclizumab (Zenapax), 513
Dactinomycin (Cosmegen), 513
Daily progress note, 26
Dalmane (flurazepam), 537
Dantrolene (Dantrium), 513
Dapsone (Avlosulfon), 513–514
Daptomycin (Cubicin), 514
Darbepoetin alfa (Aranesp), 514
Darier sign, 16
Darifenacin (Enablex), 514
Darkfield examination, 120
Darvocet (propoxyphene-acetaminophen), 593
Darvon (propoxyphene-aspirin), 593
Daunorubicin (Daunomycin, Cerubidine), 514
Daypro (oxaprozin), 580
DDAVP (desmopressin), 515
ddI (didanosine), 517–518
de Musset sign, 18
DEA number, 29
Decadron (dexamethasone), 515, 633*t*
Declomycin (demeclocycline), 515
Decubitus infection, 138*t*
Deep breathing exercises, 381
Deep peroneal nerve, 6*f*
Deep venous thrombosis, 447, 644*t*
Defibrillation, 465
Dehydration, enteral nutrition-related, 231
Dehydroepiandrosterone, 63
Delavirdine (Rescriptor), 514
Delayed type hypersensitivity, 308–309
Delirium, 36
Delivery note, 29
Delta-Cortef (prednisolone), 633*t*
Delta D (vitamin D$_3$), 505
Deltasone (prednisone), 633*t*
Deltoid muscle injection, 284
Demadex (torsemide), 614
Demeclocycline (Declomycin), 515
Dementia, 37
Demerol (meperidine), 564
Denavir (penciclovir), 584
Dennis tube, 278

Dental emergency, 471
Dental examination, 12–13, 14*f*
Depakene (valproic acid), 618–619
Depakote (valproic acid), 618–619
Depo-Provera (medroxyprogesterone), 563
DepoCyt (cytarabine liposome), 512
Dermabond, 373
Dermalon suture, 363*t*
Dermatologic descriptions, 13–15
Dermatomes, 6–7*f*
Dermatop (prednicarbate), 636*t*
Desipramine (Norpramin), 515, 631*t*
Desloratadine (Clarinex), 515
Desmopressin (DDAVP, Stimate), 515
Desonide (DesOwen), 634*t*
Desoximetasone (Topicort), 634*t*
Desyrel (trazodone), 615, 630*t*
Detrol (tolterodine), 614
Detussin (hydrocodone-pseudephedrine), 547
Dexamethasone, 515, 633*t*
Dexamethasone-neomycin, 573
Dexamethasone suppression test, 63
Dexamethasone-tobramycin, 613
Dexferrum (iron dextran), 553
Dexon suture material, 362*t*
Dexpanthenol (Ilopan), 516
Dexrazoxane (Zinecard), 516
Dextran 40 (Rheomacrodex), 516
Dextromethorphan (Mediquell, Benylin DM, PediaCare 1), 516
Dextromethorphan-guaifenesin, 544
DiaBeta (glyburide), 543
Diabetes mellitus
  enteral formula for, 229*t*
  parenteral nutrition and, 238–239
Diabetic ketoacidosis, 176
Diabinase (chlorpropamide), 505
Diagnostic arthrocentesis, 249
Diagnostic peritoneal lavage, 303, 304*t*
Dialose (docusate potassium), 521
Dialysis, therapeutic diet in, 217*t*
Diamox (acetazolamide), 478
Diaphragm, 353
Diarrhea
  differential diagnosis in, 37
  enteral nutrition-related, 231
  infectious, 155–156
  replacement fluids in, 181
Diastolic hypertension, 407–408
Diazepam (Valium), 474*t*, 516
Diazoxide (Hyperstat, Proglycem), 516–517

Dibucaine (Nupercainal), 517
Diclofenac (Cataflam, Voltaren), 517
Dicloxacillin (Dynapen, Dycill), 517
Didanosine (ddI, Videx), 517–518
Didronel (etidronate disodium), 532
Diet
  modifying nutrient content of, 220
  therapeutic, 214–221, 215–219*t*
Differential diagnosis, 33–45
  abdominal distention and, 33
  abdominal pain and, 34
  adrenal mass and, 34
  alopecia and, 34
  amenorrhea and, 34
  anorexia and, 34
  anuria and, 42–43
  arthritis and, 35
  ascites and, 35
  back pain and, 35
  breast lump and, 35
  chest pain and, 35
  chills and, 35
  clubbing and, 36
  coma and, 36
  constipation and, 36
  cough and, 36
  cyanosis and, 36
  delirium and, 36
  dementia and, 37
  diarrhea and, 37
  diplopia and, 37
  dizziness and, 37–38
  dysphagia and, 38
  dyspnea and, 38
  dysuria and, 38
  earache and, 38
  edema and, 38
  epistaxis and, 38
  failure to thrive and, 38
  fever and, 39
  fever of unknown origin and, 39
  flatulence and, 39
  frequency and, 39
  galactorrhea and, 39
  gynecomastia and, 39
  headache and, 39–40
  heartburn and, 40
  hematemesis and, 40
  hematochezia and, 40
  hematuria and, 40
  hemoptysis and, 41
  hepatomegaly and, 41
  hiccups and, 41
  hirsutism and, 41

Differential diagnosis (*cont.*)
  impotence and, 41
  incontinence and, 41
  jaundice and, 41–42
  lymphadenopathy and, 42
  melena and, 40
  melenemesis and, 40
  nausea and vomiting and, 42
  nystagmus and, 42
  oliguria and, 42–43
  pleural effusion and, 43
  pruritus and, 43
  seizures and, 43
  splenomegaly and, 42
  syncope and, 44
  tremors and, 44
  vaginal bleeding and, 44
  vaginal discharge and, 44
  vertigo and, 44
  vomiting and, 42
  weight loss and, 45
  wheezing and, 45
Differential white blood cell count,
    91–92, 92*f*, 92*t*
Diffuse abdominal pain, 34
Diffusion capacity, 377
Diflucan (fluconazole), 536
Diflunisal (Dolobid), 328*t*, 518
Digibind (digoxin immune Fab), 518
Digital rectal examination, 655*t*
Digital subtraction angiography, 344
Digitalis effect, 401
Digitalis toxicity, 401
Digoxin (Lanoxin, Lanoxicaps), 473*t*,
    518, 630*t*
Digoxin immune Fab (Digibind), 473*t*,
    518
Dilacor XR (diltiazem), 518–519
Dilantin (phenytoin), 587
Dilatrate-SR (isosorbide dinitrate), 554
Dilaudid (hydromorphone), 548
Diltiazem (Cardizem, Cartia XT, Dilacor
    XR, Diltia XT, Tiamate,
    Tiazac), 450*t*, 518–519
Dilutional hyponatremia, 187
Dimenhydrinate (Dramamine), 519
Dimethyl sulfoxide (DMSO, Rimso-50),
    519
Dinoprostone, 519
Diovan (valsartan), 619
Dipentum (olsalazine), 578
Diphenhydramine, 469
Diphenhydramine (Benadryl), 519
Diphenoxylate-atropine (Lomotil), 519

Diphtheria, tetanus, pertussis vaccine,
    520, 662–664*t*
Diphyllobothrium latum, 151*t*
Dipivefrin (Propine), 520
Diplopia, 37
Diprivan (propofol), 592–593
Diprolene (betamethasone), 634*t*
Diprosone (betamethasone), 634*t*
Dipyridamole (Persantine), 520
Dipyridamole-aspirin (Aggrenox), 520
Direct antiglobulin test, 101
Direct Coombs test, 101
Dirithomycin (Dynabac), 520
Discharge summary/note, 26–27
Disopyramide (Norpace, NAPamide),
    520, 630*t*
Distal port of pulmonary artery catheter,
    414, 414*f*
Distal renal tubular acidosis, 170*t*
Ditropan (oxybutynin), 581
Diuril (chlorothiazide), 504
Diverticulitis, 130*t*
Dizziness, 37–38
DMSO (dimethyl sulfoxide), 519
DNA probes, 126
Dobbhoff tube, 278
Dobutamine (Dobutrex), 520–521
  in critical care, 450*t*
  effects on adrenergic receptors, 411*t*
Docetaxel (Taxotere), 521
Docusate calcium (Surfak), 521
Docusate potassium (Dialose), 521
Docusate sodium (DOSS, Colace), 521
Dofetilide (Tikosyn), 521
Dog tapeworm, 151*t*
Döhle inclusion bodies, 99
Dolasetron (Anzemet), 521
Doll eyes, 17
Dolobid (diflunisal), 518
Dolophine (methadone), 566
Dong quai, 624
Donnatal (hyoscyamine-atropine-
    scopolamine-phenobarbital),
    548–549
Donor-directed blood products, 196
Dopamine (Intropin), 521–522
  for bradycardia, 463*t*
  in critical care, 450*t*
  effects on adrenergic receptors, 411*t*
Doppler echocardiography, 347
Doppler pressures, 270–271
Doral (quazepam), 594
Dornase alfa (Pulmozyme), 522
Dorsal nerve of penis, 6*f*

Dorzolamide (Trusopt), 522

Dorzolamide-timolol (Cosopt), 522

DOSS (docusate sodium), 521

Double contrast barium enema, 654t

Dovonex (calcipotriene), 496

Doxazosin (Cardura), 522

Doxepin (Sinequan, Adapin), 522, 631t

Doxepin, topical (Zonalon), 522

Doxorubicin (Adriamycin, Rubex), 522

Doxycycline (Vibramycin), 522–523

Dramamine (dimenhydrinate), 519

Draping of patient, 359

Drawer sign, 17

Dronabinol (Marinol), 523

Droplet precautions, 161

Drotrecogin alfa (Xigris), 523

Droxia (hydroxyurea), 548

Drug abuse screen, 115

Drug-induced disorders, 34–35

Drug therapy. *See also* Antimicrobial
        therapy.
   black box precautions and, 475
   breast feeding and, 476–477
   controlled substance classification and,
       476
   in critical care, 450–453t
   cytochrome P-450 isoenzymes and,
       647–648t
   in emergency care, *inside covers*
   empiric, 117
   FDA fetal risk categories and, 476
   for fungal infections, 148–149t
   for human immunodeficiency virus
       infection, 146–147t
   natural and herbal agents and,
       623–626
   for pain, 326–337, 327–336t
   for parasitic infections, 150–151t

DTIC (dacarbazine), 513

Dual-energy x-ray absorptiometry
       (DEXA), 210t, 343

Dual-lumen feeding tube, 227

Dulcolax (bisacodyl), 494

Duloxetine (Cymbalta), 523

Duo-Tube, 278

Duodenal ulcer, 139t

Dupuytren contracture, 17

Duragesic (fentanyl, transdermal), 534

Duramorph (morphine), 570

Duricef (cefadroxil), 500

Duroziez sign, 17

Dutasteride (Avodart), 523

Duvoid (bethanechol), 494

Dwarf tapeworm, 151t

Dyazide (hydrochlorothiazide-
       triamterene), 546

Dycill (dicloxacillin), 517

Dynabac (dirithomycin), 520

DynaCirc (isradipine), 554

Dynamic compliance, 427

Dynapen (dicloxacillin), 517

Dyrenium (triamterene), 616

Dysmorphic red cells, 111

Dysphagia, 38

Dyspnea, 38

Dysuria, 38

E

E-Mycin (erythromycin), 527–528

Ear
   infection of, 130–131t
   physical examination of, 3
   review of systems and, 2

Earache, 38

Eastern Cooperative Oncology Group
       performance scale, 665–666t

Ecchymosis, 13

Echinacea, 624

Echocardiography, 346–347

Echothiophate iodine (Phospholine
       Ophthalmic), 523–524

ECOG performance scale, 665–666t

Econazole (Spectazole), 524

Ecotrin (aspirin), 327t, 489

Edema, 38

Edex (Alprostadil, intracavernosal), 482

Edrophonium (Tensilon), 524

Efalizumab (Raptiva), 524

Efavirenz (Sustiva), 146t, 524

Effexor (venlafaxine), 620

Efudex (fluorouracil, topical), 537

Elavil (amitriptyline), 485

Eldepryl (selegiline), 599

Elderly patient, fever work-up in, 277

Electrical alternans, 17

Electrical stimulation for pain
       management, 338

Electrocardiography, 383–402, 384f
   atrial arrhythmias and, 388–390,
       388–390f
   axis deviation in, 385f, 385–386
   bedside, 271–273, 272f
   cardiac hypertrophy and, 395–396,
       395–397f
   continuous, 404
   electrolyte and drug effects on, 399,
       399f

Electrocardiography (*cont.*)
    equipment in, 383–385
    heart blocks and, 393*f*, 393–395, 394*f*
    heart rate and, 386, 386*f*
    hypothermia and, 401, 401*f*
    myocardial infarction and, 396–399,
        397–399*f*, 398*t*
    nodal rhythm and, 390, 390*f*
    pericarditis and, 400*f*, 401
    sinus rhythm and, 387*f*, 387–388, 388*f*
    ventricular arrhythmias and, 391–392,
        391–393*f*
    Wolff-Parkinson-White syndrome
        and, 401*f*, 402
Electrodes in electrocardiography,
    271–272, 272*f*
Electrolyte(s), 179–193
    baseline requirements for, 180
    body fluids and, 181, 183*t*
    disturbances of, 185–193
        hypercalcemia in, 189–190
        hyperkalemia in, 187–188
        hypermagnesemia in, 191–192
        hypernatremia in, 185–193, 186
        hyperphosphatemia in, 192–193
        hypocalcemia in, 190–191
        hypokalemia in, 188–189
        hypomagnesemia in, 192
        hyponatremia in, 186–187
        hypophosphatemia in, 193
        parenteral nutrition-related, 239
    effects on electrocardiogram, 399, 399*f*
    ordering intravenous fluids, 181–185,
        183*t*, 184–185*f*
    parenteral fluids and, 180–181, 182*t*
    in parenteral formula, 233, 234*t*
    spot urine for, 111
Electrolyte panel, 48
Electromyography, 326
Elemental formula, 228*t*
Elestat (epinastine), 526
Eletriptan (Relpax), 524
Elidel (pimecrolimus), 588
Eligard (leuprolide), 557–558
Elimate (permethrin), 586
Elitek (rasburicase), 595
Ellence (epirubicin), 526
Elmiron (pentosan polysulfate sodium),
    586
Elocon (mometasone furoate), 636*t*
Eloxatin (oxaliplatin), 580
Elspar (L-Asparaginase), 489
Emadine (emedastine), 524
Embolism prevention, 644*t*

Emcyt (estramustine phosphate), 530
Emedastine (Emadine), 524
Emend (aprepitant), 488–489
Emergency, 455–474
    in acute coronary syndromes, 466,
        467–468*f*
    advanced cardiac life support in, 463,
        463*t*
    airway and ventilatory support in,
        463–464
    in anaphylaxis, 466–469
    in anticholinergic toxicity, 471
    in asthma attack, 469–471
    automated external defibrillation in,
        464–466
    cardiopulmonary resuscitation in,
        456–462, 457*f*
        adult, 456–458
        child, 458–462, 459*t*, 460*t*, 461*f*
        neonate, 462, 462*f*
        care medications, *inside covers*
    in coma, 471
    dental, 471
    emergency cardiac care in, 455–456
    in hypertensive crisis, 472
    in hypoglycemia, 472
    medications for, *inside covers*
    in opioid overdose, 472
    in poisoning, 472, 473*t*
    in status epilepticus, 473–474, 474*t*
    in stroke, 466, 469*t*, 470*f*
Emergency transfusion, 196
Emesis, replacement fluids in, 181
Eminase (anistreplase), 488
EMLA (lidocaine-prilocaine), 559
Empiric antibiotics, 117
Empirin (aspirin-codeine), 490
Empyema endocarditis, 131–132*t*
Emtricitabine (Emtriva), 146*t*, 524–525
Enablex (darifenacin), 514
Enalapril (Vasotec), 525
Enbrel (etanercept), 531
Encephalitis, herpes, 144*t*
Endocarditis, 131–132*t*, 158–159, 159*t*,
    160*t*
Endocrine system
    adverse effects of pain on, 324*t*
    review of systems and, 2
Endometrial cancer screening, 655*t*
Endoscopic retrograde
            cholangiopancreatography,
        345
Endotracheal intubation, 273*t*, 273–275,
    274*f*, 464

Endovaginal ultrasonography, 347
Energy requirements, 213–214
Enfamil formula, 222*t*
Enfuvirtide (Fuzeon), 525
Enoxaparin (Lovenox), 525
Entacapone (Comtan), 525
Entamoeba histolytica, 150*t*
Enteral access devices, 227
Enteral formulas, 227–230, 228–229*t*
Enteral nutrition, 225–231, 228–229*t*
Enterobacter spp., 124*t*
Enterobius vermicularis, 150*t*
Enteroclysis, 345
Enterococcus spp., 124*t*
Enulose (lactulose), 556
Environmental failure to thrive,
        38
Enzone (hydrocortisone-pramoxine), 591
Enzyme-linked immunosorbent assay, 74
Eosinophils, 94*t*
Ephedra, 624, 626
Ephedrine, 525
Epidemiology basics, 649
Epiglottitis, 132*t*
Epinastine (Elestat), 526
Epinephrine (Adrenalin, Sus-Phrine,
        EpiPen), 526
    for anaphylaxis, 466–469
    for bradycardia, 463*t*
    in critical care, 451*t*
    effects on adrenergic receptors, 411*t*
    in pediatric advanced life support, 459*t*
    for pediatric bradycardia, 460*t*
    racemic, 382
Epirubicin (Ellence), 526
Epistaxis, 38
Epithelial cells in urine, 109, 110
Epivir (lamivudine), 146*t*, 556
Eplerenone (Inspra), 526
Epoetin alfa (Epogen, Procrit), 526
Epoprostenol (Flolan), 526–527
Eprosartan (Teveten), 527
Epstein-Barr virus, 142*t*
Eptifibatide (Integrillin), 527
Equinil (meprobamate), 564
Equipment
    for bedside procedures, 243, 243*t*,
        244–245*f*
    for central venous catheterization, 257
    for lumbar puncture, 290
Erbitux (cetuximab), 503
Erectile dysfunction, 41
Ergamisol (levamisole), 558
Ergocalciferol, 234*t*

Erlotinib (Tarceva), 527
Erosion, 13
Ertaczo (sertaconazole), 599
Ertapenem (Invanz), 527
Erthyrocytapheresis, 196
Eruption of teeth, 13, 14*f*
Erysipelas, 138*t*
Erythrocyte morphology, 111
Erythrocyte sedimentation rate, 103
Erythromycin (E-Mycin, E.E.S., Ery-Tab,
        EryPed, Ilotycin), 527–528
Erythromycin-benzoyl peroxide
        (Benzamycin), 528
Erythromycin-sulfisoxazole (Eryzole,
        Pediazole), 528
Erythropoietin, 64, 526
Escherichia coli, 124*t*
Escitalopram (Lexapro), 528
Esidrix (hydrochlorothiazide), 546
Eskalith (lithium), 560, 630*t*
Esmolol (Brevibloc), 451*t*, 528
Esomeprazole (Nexium), 528–529
Esophagitis
    cytomegalovirus, 142*t*
    fungal, 148*t*
Esophagogram, 345
Esophagotracheal airway, 464
Esterified estrogens (Estratab, Menest),
        529
Esterified estrogens-methyltestosterone
        (Estratest), 529
Estimated creatinine clearance, 113
Estinyl (ethinyl estradiol), 531
Estrace (estradiol), 529
Estracyt (estramustine phosphate), 530
Estraderm (estradiol, transdermal), 529
Estradiol
    serum, 64
    transdermal, 529
Estradiol cypionate-medroxyprogesterone
        acetate (Lunelle), 529–530
Estramustine phosphate (Estracyt,
        Emcyt), 530
Estratab (esterified estrogens), 529
Estratest (esterified estrogens-
        methyltestosterone), 529
Estrazolam (ProSom), 529
Estrogen
    conjugated (Premarin), 530–531
    conjugated-medroxyprogesterone
        (Prempro, Premphase),
        530–531
    conjugated synthetic (Cenestin), 531
Estrogen-progesterone receptors, 64

Eszopiclone (Lunesta), 531
Etanercept (Enbrel), 531
Ethambutol (Myambutol), 531
Ethanol, 64
    for methanol poisoning, 473t
Ethibond suture material, 363t
Ethilon suture, 363t
Ethinyl estradiol (Estinyl, Feminone), 531
Ethinyl estradiol-levonorgestrel (Preven),
        531
Ethinyl estradiol-norelgestromin (Ortho
        Evra), 531
Ethosuximide (Zarontin), 531–532, 628t
Ethylene glycol poisoning, 473t
Ethyol (amifostine), 484
Etidronate disodium (Didronel), 532
Etodolac (Lodine), 532
Etonogestrel-ethinyl estradiol
        (NuvaRing), 532
Etoposide (VePesid, Toposar), 532
Eubacterium spp., 125t
Eulexin (flutamide), 538
Eumorphic red cells, 111
Evening primrose oil, 624
Evista (raloxifene), 595
Ewaid tube, 278
Ewart sign, 17
Excess water intake, 187
Excoriation, 14
Exelon (rivastigmine), 597
Exemestane (Aromasin), 532
Exenatide (Byetta), 532–533
Expiratory chest radiography, 341
Expiratory reserve volume, 425, 425f
External jugular vein catheterization, 262
Extra heart sounds, 8, 10–11t
Extracellular fluid, 179
Extremity
    perfusion of, 407
    suturing of, 363–365, 364t
Extrinsic factor, 89
Extubation, ventilator weaning and,
        439
Exudative pleural effusion, 43
Eye
    physical examination of, 3
    review of systems and, 2
Ezetimibe (Zetia), 533
Ezetimibe-simvastatin (Vytorin), 533

F

Face, suturing of, 363
Facial nerve, 5

Factive (gemifloxacin), 541–542
Factor IX concentrate, 201t
Factor V mutation, 101–102
Factor VIII, 201t, 488
Failure to thrive, 38
Famciclovir (Famvir), 533
Family history, 2
Famotidine (Pepcid), 533
Famvir (famciclovir), 533
Faslodex (fulvestrant), 540
Fast catgut, 362t
Fasting blood glucose, 209, 211t
Fat
    fecal, 65
    in parenteral formula, 233
Fat restricted diet, 218t
Fatty casts, 110
FDA fetal risk categories, 476
Fecal *Clostridium difficile* toxin assay, 60
Fecal fat, 65
Fecal *Helicobacter pylori* antigen, 68
Fecal leukocytes, 156
Fecal occult blood test, 65, 654t
Feeding enterostomy, 227
Feeding tube, 278–280
Feldene (piroxicam), 589
Felodipine (Plendil), 533
Femara (letrozole), 557
Feminone (ethinyl estradiol), 531
Femoral vein catheterization, 262–263
Fenofibrate (Tricor), 533
Fenoldopam (Corlopam), 533–534
Fenoprofen (Nalfon), 534
Fentanyl (Sublimaze), 534
    in critical care, 406
    in patient-controlled analgesia, 339t
Fentanyl, transdermal (Duragesic), 534
Fentanyl, transmucosal (Actiq), 534
Fergon (ferrous gluconate), 534
Fern test, 245–246
Ferritin, 65
Ferrous gluconate, 534
Ferrous sulfate, 534–535
Fetal risk categories of drugs, 476
Fetal scalp monitoring, 282–283
Fever, 39
Fever of unknown origin, 39
Fever work-up, 275–277
Feverfew, 624
Fexofenadine (Allegra), 535
Fibrillation
    atrial, 389, 390f
    ventricular, 392, 392f
Fibrin degradation products, 102

Fibrin D-dimers, 102
Fibrin split products, 102
Fibrinogen, 102
Filariasis, 150*t*
Filgrastim (Neupogen), 535
Finasteride (Proscar, Propecia), 535
Fingerstick technique, 281
Fioricet (acetaminophen-butalbital-caffeine), 478
Fiorinal (aspirin-butalbital compound), 490
First-degree atrioventricular block, 393, 393*f*
First trimester screening, 81
Fish tapeworm, 151*t*
Fissure, 14
Fistulography, 345
FK 506, 606
Flagyl (metronidazole), 567–568
FLAMP (fludarabine phosphate), 536
Flatulence, 39
Flavoxate (Urispas), 535
Flecainide (Tambocor), 535, 630*t*
Flexeril (cyclobenzaprine), 511
Flexible sigmoidoscopy, 654*t*
Flolan (epoprostenol), 526–527
Flomax (tamsulosin), 607
Flonase (fluticasone), 538
Florinef (fludrocortisone acetate), 536
Flovent (fluticasone), 538
Floxin (ofloxacin), 578
Floxuridine (FUDR), 535
Fluconazole (Diflucan), 536
Fludarabine phosphate (FLAMP, Fludara), 536
Fludrocortisone acetate (Florinef), 536
Fluid compartments, 179
Fluids and electrolytes, 179–193
    baseline requirements for, 180
    body fluids and, 181, 183*t*
    determination of intravenous infusion rate, 185
    disturbances of, 185–193
        hypercalcemia in, 189–190
        hyperkalemia in, 187–188
        hypermagnesemia in, 191–192
        hypernatremia in, 185–193, 186
        hyperphosphatemia in, 192–193
        hypocalcemia in, 190–191
        hypokalemia in, 188–189
        hypomagnesemia in, 192
        hyponatremia in, 186–187
        hypophosphatemia in, 193
    parenteral nutrition-related, 239

ordering intravenous fluids, 181–185, 183*t*, 184–185*f*
    parenteral fluids and, 180–181, 182*t*
    for septic shock, 443
Flumadine (rimantadine), 596
Flumazenil (Romazicon), 473*t*, 536
Flunisolide (AeroBid, Nasalide), 536
Fluocinolone (Synalar, Lidex), 635*t*
Fluorescent treponemal antibody-absorbed, 66
Fluorouracil (Adrucil), 536–537
Fluorouracil, topical (Efudex), 537
Fluoxetine (Prozac, Sarafem), 537
Fluoxymesterone (Halotestin), 537
Fluphenazine (Prolixin, Permitil), 537
Flurandrenolide (Cordran), 635*t*
Flurazepam (Dalmane), 537
Flurbiprofen (Ansaid), 537–538
Flutamide (Eulexin), 538
Fluticasone (Flonase, Flovent), 538, 635*t*
Fluticasone propionate-salmeterol xinafoate (Advair Diskus), 538
Fluvastatin (Lescol), 538
Fluvoxamine (Luvox), 538
Folate, 65–66
Folex (methotrexate), 566
Foley catheter, 313, 314*f*
Folic acid, 65–66, 234*t*, 538
Follicle-stimulating hormone, 66
Folstein Mini-Mental State Examination, 8, 9*t*
Fomepizole, 473*t*
Fondaparinux (Arixtra), 538–539
Fong lesion, 17
Foradil Aerolizer (formoterol), 539
Forced expiratory volume in 1 second, 378, 378*t*, 379*t*
Forced vital capacity, 378, 378*t*, 379*t*
Formoterol (Foradil Aerolizer), 539
Formulas
    enteral, 227–230, 228–229*t*
    infant, 221, 222–223*t*
    parenteral, 232–235, 234*t*, 235*t*
Fortaz (ceftazidime), 502
Forteo (teriparatide), 609
Fortovase (saquinavir), 598
Fosamax (alendronate), 481
Fosamprenavir (Lexiva), 146*t*, 539
Foscarnet (Foscavir), 539
Fosfomycin (Monurol), 539
Fosinopril (Monopril), 539–540
Fosphenytoin (Cerebyx), 474*t*, 540
Fosrenol (lanthanum carbonate), 557

Fourth heart sound, 11*t*
Fraction of inspired oxygen, 437
Fractional excreted sodium, 116*t*
Fractionated catecholamines, 55, 114
Fragmin (dalteparin), 513
Frank sign, 17
Free cortisol, 114
Free prostate-specific antigen, 82
Free thyroxine, 88
French catheter scale, 243, 244*t*
Frequency, 39
Fresh frozen plasma, 200*t*
Frovatriptan (Frova), 645*t*
FUDR (floxuridine), 535
Full liquid diet, 215*t*
Fulvestrant (Faslodex), 540
Functional residual capacity, 378, 378*t*,
    426, 426*f*, 427*f*
Functional status scales, 665–666*t*
Fungal infection, 138*t*
    cerebrospinal fluid analysis in, 294*t*
    drug therapy for, 148–149*t*
    serology in, 66
Fungizone (amphotericin B), 486
Furadantin (nitrofurantoin), 576
Furosemide (Lasix), 540
Fusobacterium spp., 124*t*
Fuzeon (enfuvirtide), 525

G

G-Mycitin (gentamicin), 542
Gabapentin (Neurontin), 540
Gabitril (tiagabine), 611
Galactorrhea, 39
Galantamine (Razadyne), 540
Gallbladder disease, 132*t*
Gallium nitrate (Ganite), 190, 540–541
Gallium scan, 351
Gamimune (intravenous immune
    globulin), 550
Gamma globulins, 84*t*
Gamma-glutamyltransferase, 67
Gammar IV (intravenous immune
    globulin), 550
Ganciclovir (Cytovene, Vitrasert), 541
Ganite (gallium nitrate), 190, 540–541
Garamycin (gentamicin), 542
Garlic, 624
Gas exchange impairment, 431*t*
Gastric residual volume, 227, 231
Gastric ulcer, 139*t*
Gastrin, serum, 66
Gastroenteritis, 133*t*

Gastrografin enema, 345
Gastrointestinal function assessment,
    211–213
Gastrointestinal intubation, 277–280
Gastrointestinal system
    adverse effects of pain on, 324*t*
    review of systems and, 2
Gatifloxacin (Tequin, Zymar
    Ophthalmic), 541
Gaviscon, 481, 483
Gefitinib (Iressa), 541
Gemcitabine (Gemzar), 541
Gemfibrozil (Lopid), 541
Gemifloxacin (Factive), 541–542
Gemtuzumab ozogamicin (Mylotarg),
    542
Gemzar (gemcitabine), 541
Gen-Probe, 121
General appearance, physical
    examination and, 3
Generalized seizure, 43
Generic drugs, 475
Genital herpes, 143–144*t*
Genitofemoral nerve, 6*f*
Genitourinary system
    adverse effects of pain on, 324*t*
    review of systems and, 2
Genoptic (gentamicin), 542
Genotyping, 158
Gentamicin (Garamycin, G-Mycitin,
    Genoptic), 542
    for subacute bacterial endocarditis
        prophylaxis, 160*t*
    therapeutic levels of, 628*t*
Gentamicin-prednisolone, ophthalmic
    (Pred-G Ophthalmic),
    542
Geodon (ziprasidone), 622
Gestational diabetes, 67
Giardiasis, 150*t*
Gibbus, 17
Giemsa stain, 120
Ginger, 624
Ginkgo biloba, 624–625
Ginseng, 625
Glasgow Coma scale, 650, 656*t*
Gleevec (imatinib), 549–550
Gliadel (carmustine), 499
Glimepiride (Amaryl), 543
Glipizide (Glucotrol), 543
Glitter cell, 110
Globulin, 84*t*
Glossopharyngeal nerve, 5
Gloving, 358–359

Glucagon, 473t, 543
Glucophage (metformin), 565
Glucosamine sulfate, 625
Glucose
    control in septic shock, 444
    laboratory values of, 66–67
    requirements for, 180
    urine, 107
Glucose tolerance test, 67
Glucotrol (glipizide), 543
Glucovance (glyburide-metformin), 543
Glutamyl transferase, 67
Gluteus muscle injection, 284
Glyburide (DiaBeta, Micronase, Glynase), 543
Glyburide-metformin (Glucovance), 543
Glycated hemoglobin, 67–68
Glycerin suppository, 543
Glycet (miglitol), 568–569
Glycohemoglobin, 67–68
Glycosylated hemoglobin, 67–68
Glynase (glyburide), 543
GoLYTELY (polyethylene glycol), 590
Gonadorelin (Lutrepulse), 543
Gonococcal antigen assay, 121
Gonorrhea, 133t
    antimicrobial therapy for, 133t
    smear and culture for, 120–121
    testing for, 299
Gore-Tex suture material, 363t
Goserelin (Zoladex), 544
Gowning, 358–359
Graft-*versus*-host disease, transfusion-associated, 196
Gram-negative organisms, 123f, 124–126t
Gram-positive organisms, 122f, 124–126t
Gram stain, 121, 122f, 123f, 124–126t, 299
Granisetron (Kytril), 544
Granulocyte, 199t
Granulocyte colony stimulating factor, 535
Granulocyte-macrophage colony stimulating factor, 598
Granuloma inguinale, 133t
Granulomatous infection, 294t
Great occipital nerve, 7f
Greater auricular nerve, 7f
Gregg triad, 17
Grey Turner sign, 17
Grocco sign, 17
Guaifenesin (Robitussin), 544

Guaifenesin-codeine (Robitussin AC), 544
Guaifenesin-dextromethorphan, 544
Guaifenesin-hydrocodone (Hycotuss Expectorant), 547
Guillain-Barré syndrome, 295t
Gynecologic system, 2
Gynecomastia, 39

H
HAART (highly active antiretroviral therapy), 157
Habitrol (nicotine transdermal), 575
Haemophilus ducreyi, 124t
Haemophilus influenzae, 124t
Haemophilus influenzae type b vaccine, 544, 662–664t
Hairworm infection, 151t
Halbetasol (Ultravate cream), 635t
Halcinonide (Halog cream), 635t
Halcion (triazolam), 616
Haloperidol (Haldol), 406, 544–545
Haloprogin (Halotex), 545
Halotestin (fluoxymesterone), 537
Halotex (haloprogin), 545
Hand scrub, surgical, 356–357
Handrub, 357
Haptoglobin, 68
Head
    computed tomography of, 348
    magnetic resonance imaging of, 350
    physical examination of, 3
    review of systems and, 2
Headache, 39–40
Health Screen-12, 49
Heart
    adverse effects of pain on, 324t
    chest radiography and, 353
    emergency cardiac care and, 455–456
    nuclear scan of, 351
    physical examination of, 4, 4f
Heart block, 393f, 393–395, 394f
Heart murmur, 4, 4f, 8, 10–11t, 409
Heart rate
    electrocardiography and, 386, 386f
    hemorrhagic shock and, 442t
    pulmonary artery catheter and, 421
Heart rhythm, 387–395
    atrial arrhythmias and, 388–390, 388–390f
    heart block and, 393f, 393–395, 394f
    nodal rhythms and, 390, 390f

Heart rhythm (*cont.*)
   sinus rhythms and, 387*f,* 387–388,
         388*f*
   ventricular arrhythmias and, 391–392,
         391–393*f*
Heart sounds, 8, 10–11*t*
Heartburn, 40
Heberden node, 17
Heelstick, 91, 280, 281*f*
Hegar sign, 17
Heinz bodies, 99
Helical computed tomography, 348
Helicobacter pylori, 68
Helmet cell, 99
Helper T cell, 99
Hematemesis, 40
Hematochezia, 40
Hematocrit, 93*t,* 95, 97–98
Hematology, 91–103
   blood collection and, 91
   blood smears and, 91–92, 92*f,* 92*t*
   coagulation tests and, 99–103, 100*f*
   complete blood count values and,
         92–95, 93*t,* 94*t*
   hematocrit and, 95, 97–98
   left shift and, 95
   lymphocyte subsets and, 98–99
   platelets and, 98
   red blood cells and, 97, 99
   reticulocyte count and, 95–96
   review of systems and, 3
   white blood cells and, 96–97, 99
Hematuria, 40, 107
Hemodialysis
   for septic shock, 444
   therapeutic diet in, 217*t*
Hemoglobin, 93*t,* 95
Hemoglobin A$_{1c}$, 67–68
Hemoptysis, 41
Hemorrhagic shock, 441, 442*t*
Henderson-Hasselbalch equation,
         164–165
Heparin, 444, 447, 545
Hepatic function panel, 48
Hepatitis
   blood component therapy-related, 204
   testing for, 68–72, 69–71*t,* 71*f,* 72*f,*
         157–158
Hepatitis A vaccine, 545, 657–661*t,*
         662–664*t*
Hepatitis A virus, 68, 71*f,* 142*t,* 157
Hepatitis B immune globulin, 545
Hepatitis B vaccine, 520, 545–546,
         657–661*t,* 662–664*t*

Hepatitis B virus, 70, 72*f,* 142*t*
   blood component therapy-related, 204
   testing for, 157
Hepatitis C virus, 72, 143*t*
   blood component therapy-related,
         204
   testing for, 157–158
Hepatobiliary scan, 351
Hepatobiliary system, 239
Hepatomegaly, 41
Hepsera (adefovir), 479
Herbal agents, 623–626
Herceptin (trastuzumab), 615
Herpes culture, 299
Herpes simplex virus, 143–144*t*
Herpes zoster, 145*t*
Hetastarch (Hespan), 546
Hexalen (altretamine), 483
Hibiclens hand scrub, 356–357
Hiccups, 41
Hickman catheter, 263–264
HIDA-scan, 351
High-density lipoprotein cholesterol, 60
High-density lipoproteins, 59*t,* 209,
         211*t*
High-dose dexamethasone suppression
         test, 63
High-frequency positive pressure
         ventilation, 436*f*
Highly active antiretroviral therapy
         (HAART), 157
Hill sign, 17
Hiprex (methenamine), 566
Hirsutism, 41
Histoplasmosis, 149*t*
History, 1–3
   in nutritional assessment, 210–211
   psychiatric, 8, 9*t*
History of present illness, 1
Histussin-D (hydrocodone-
         pseudoephedrine), 547
HIV (human immunodeficiency virus
         infection)
   antiretroviral therapy for, 146–147*t*
   cryptococcal meningitis in, 134*t*
   testing for, 73*f,* 73–75, 156–157
   transfusion-related, 205
Hivid (zalcitabine), 621
HLA typing, 72
Hoffmann reflex, 17
Hollenhorst plaque, 17
Holoxan (ifosfamide), 549
Homan sign, 17
Homocysteine, serum, 72–73

Hookworm infection, 150*t*

Horizontal interrupted mattress sutures, 368*f*

Horner syndrome, 17

Hospital diets, 214–221, 215–219*t*

Hounsfield units, 347

House diet, 215*t*

Howell-Jolly bodies, 99

Humalog, 637*t*

Human bite, 137*t*

Human chorionic gonadotropin, 73

Human granulocyte ehrlichiosis, 152–153*t*

Human immunodeficiency virus infection (HIV)
 antiretroviral therapy for, 146–147*t*
 cryptococcal meningitis in, 134*t*
 testing for, 73*f*, 73–75, 156–157
 transfusion-related, 205

Human leukocyte antigen, 72

Human milk, 222*t*

Human papillomavirus, 145*t*

Human T-cell leukemia virus, transfusion-related, 205

Humidity supplementation, 380*t*

Humira (adalimumab), 479

Humulin, 637*t*

Hyaline casts, 110

Hycamtin (topotecan), 614

Hycodan (hydrocodone-homatropine), 547

Hycomine compound (hydrocodone-chlorpheniramine-phenylephrine-acetaminophen-caffeine), 547

Hycort (hydrocortisone, topical), 635*t*

Hycotuss Expectorant (hydrocodone-guaifenesin), 547

Hydatid cyst, 151*t*

Hydralazine (Apresoline), 546

Hydrochlorothiazide (Esidrix, HydroURICIL), 546

Hydrochlorothiazide-amiloride (Moduretic), 546

Hydrochlorothiazide-spironolactone (Aldactazide), 546

Hydrochlorothiazide-triamterene (Dyazide, Maxzide), 546

Hydrocodone-acetaminophen (Hydrocet, Lorcet, Lortab, Vicodin), 334*t*, 546–547

Hydrocodone-aspirin (Lortab ASA), 547

Hydrocodone-chlorpheniramine-phenylephrine-acetaminophen-caffeine (Hycomine compound), 547

Hydrocodone-guaifenesin (Hycotuss Expectorant), 547

Hydrocodone-homatropine (Hycodan, Hydromet), 547

Hydrocodone-ibuprofen (Vicoprofen), 335*t*, 547

Hydrocodone-pseudoephedrine (Detussin, Histussin-D), 547

Hydrocortisone, 547–548
 for hypercalcemia, 190
 for septic shock, 443
 systemic, 633*t*
 topical, 635–636*t*

Hydrocortisone-polymyxin B, 590

Hydrocortisone-pramoxine (Enzone, Proctofoam-HC), 591

HydroDIURIL (hydrochlorothiazide), 546

Hydromet (hydrocodone-homatropine), 547

Hydromorphone (Dilaudid), 332*t*, 339*t*, 548

Hydrothorax, 43

5-Hydroxyindoleacetic acid, 114

Hydroxyurea (Hydrea, Droxia), 548

Hydroxyzine (Atarax, Vistaril), 548

Hygroton (chlorthalidone), 505

Hyoscyamine (Anaspaz, Cystospaz, Levsin), 548

Hyoscyamine-atropine-scopolamine-phenobarbital (Donnatal), 548–549

Hypercalcemia, 189–190, 399

Hyperglycemia, parenteral nutrition-related, 237–238

Hyperglycemic, hyperosmolar, nonketotic syndrome, 237–238

Hyperkalemia, 187–188, 399, 399*f*

Hypermagnesemia, 191–192

Hypernatremia, 186

Hyperparathyroidism, 189

Hyperphosphatemia, 192–193

Hypersegmentation of white blood cells, 99

Hyperstat (diazoxide), 516–517

Hypertension, 11–12, 12*t*, 407–408

Hypertensive crisis, 472

Hypertonic hyponatremia, 187

Hypertrophy
  atrial, 395*f,* 395–396
  ventricular, 396, 396*f,* 397*f*
Hyperventilation syndrome, 172
Hypervolemic hyponatremia, 187
Hypocalcemia, 190–191, 399
Hypoglossal nerve, 5
Hypoglycemia
  emergency care in, 472
  parenteral nutrition-related, 238
Hypokalemia, 188–189, 399, 399*f*
Hypomagnesemia, 192
Hyponatremia, 186–187
Hypophosphatemia, 193
Hypothermia, 401, 401*f*
Hypotonic hyponatremia, 187
Hypovolemic hypernatremia, 186
Hypovolemic hyponatremia, 187
Hypovolemic shock, 422*t,* 441, 442*t*
Hypoxia, 172–173, 173*f*
Hysterosalpingography, 345
Hytone (hydrocortisone, topical), 635*t*
Hytrin (terazosin), 608–609

I
Ibandronate (Boniva), 549
Ibuprofen (Advil, Motrin, Nuprin,
      Mediprin, Rufen), 328*t,* 549
Ibuprofen-hydrocodone (Vicoprofen),
      547
Ibuprofen-oxycodone (Combunox), 582
Ibutilide (Corvert), 549
ICU progress note, 403–404
Idarubicin (Idamycin), 549
Ideal body weight, 208
Ifosfamide (Ifex, Holoxan), 549
Iliohypogastric nerve, 6*f,* 7*f*
Ilioinguinal nerve, 6*f*
Iliopsoas sign, 19
Ilopan (dexpanthenol), 516
Iloprost (Ventavis), 549
Ilotycin (erythromycin), 527–528
Imaging studies, 341–354
  computed tomography in, 347–348
  magnetic resonance imaging in,
      348–350
  nuclear scans in, 350–352
  positron emission tomography in,
      352–353
  radiography in, 341–346, 342*f,* 343*f,*
      353–354
  spiral computed tomography in, 348
  ultrasonography in, 346–347

Imatinib (Gleevec), 549–550
Imdur (isosorbide mononitrate), 554
Imipenem-cilastatin (Primaxin), 550
Imipramine (Tofranil), 550, 631*t*
Imiquimod cream (Aldara), 550
Imitrex (sumatriptan), 606, 645*t*
Immune globulin (Gamimune,
      Sandoglobulin, Gammar IV),
      550
Immune modulation, enteral formula for,
      229*t*
Immune serum globulin, 201*t*
Immune system, adverse effects of pain
      on, 324*t*
Immunization guidelines, 650, 657–664*f*
Immunoglobulins, 75, 84*t*
Imodium (loperamide), 560–561
Impaired glucose tolerance, 67
Impetigo, 138*t*
Impotence, 41
In-and-out catheterized urine, 315
Inactivated poliovirus vaccine, 520,
      662–664*t*
Inamrinone, 550
Inapsine (droperidol), 523
Incentive spirometry, 381
Incontinence, 41
Inderal (propranolol), 593
Indermil, 373
India ink preparation, 121
Indinavir (Crixivan), 47*t,* 551
Indirect antiglobulin test, 101
Indirect Coombs test, 101
Indium-111 octreotide scan, 351
Indomethacin (Indocin), 329*t,* 551
Indopamide (Lozol), 550–551
Inducer T cell, 99
Infant
  cardiopulmonary resuscitation in,
      460–462
  endotracheal tube for, 273*t*
  feeding of, 221–224, 222–223*t*
  fever work-up in, 277
  heelstick technique in, 280, 281*f*
  pneumonia in, 136*t*
Infasurf (calfactant), 498
Infection
  complication in critical care, 446
  contamination and colonization
      versus, 118
Infectious disorders, 129–140*t*
  bone and joint, 129*t*
  breast, 129*t*
  bronchitis, 129*t*

cervicitis, 130*t*

chancroid, 130*t*

chlamydial, 130*t*

dementia in, 35

diarrhea, 155–156

diverticulitis, 130*t*

ear, 130–131*t*

empyema endocarditis, 131–132*t*

epiglottitis, 132*t*

gallbladder, 132*t*

gastroenteritis, 133*t*

gonorrhea, 133*t*

granuloma inguinale, 133*t*

meningitis, 133–134*t*

nocardiosis, 134*t*

pelvic inflammatory disease, 134*t*

peritonitis, 135*t*

pharyngitis, 135*t*

pneumonia, 136*t*

sinusitis, 137*t*

skin and soft tissue, 137–138*t*

syphilis, 138*t*

transfusion-associated, 204–205

tuberculosis, 138*t*

ulcer disease, 139*t*

urinary tract, 139–140*t*

vaginal, 140*t*

Infectious mononucleosis, 142*t*

INFeD (iron dextran), 553

Infergen (interferon alfacon-1), 552

Infiltrates, 354

Infliximab (Remicade), 551

Influenza, 144*t*

Influenza vaccine, 551–552, 657–661*t*, 662–664*t*

Informed consent, 242

INH (isoniazid), 553–554

Injection techniques, 283–284

Innohep (tinzaparin), 612

Inocor (amrinone), 550

Inotropes, 409, 443

Insensible fluid loss, 179

Inspiratory capacity, 426

Inspiratory force, ventilator weaning and, 438*t*

Inspiratory reserve volume, 425, 425*f*

Inspiratory to expiratory ratio, 438

Inspra (eplerenone), 526

Instrument tie, 374*f*

Instruments for bedside procedures, 243, 244*t*, 244–245*f*

Insulins, 552, 637*t*

Intake and output, 179

Intal (cromolyn sodium), 511

Integrillin (eptifibatide), 527

Intensive care unit, 403–453

analgesia and, 406

cardiovascular instability and, 406–410, 408*f*, 410*f*, 411*t*

central venous pressure and, 410–412, 412*f*

common ICU equations for, 448–449*t*

complications in, 440–447

abdominal compartment syndrome in, 445

acalculous cholecystitis in, 445

acute adrenal insufficiency in, 445–446

acute renal failure in, 444–445

acute respiratory distress syndrome in, 440, 441*t*

deep venous thrombosis in, 447

infection in, 446

pulmonary embolism in, 447

shock in, 441–444, 442*t*

upper gastrointestinal hemorrhage in, 440–441

drug infusions in, 450–453*t*

ICU progress note in, 403–404

intubation and, 430–431, 431*t*

mechanical ventilation in, 435–439, 436*f*, 438*t*

nutrition and, 440

oxygenation and, 428–430, 428–430*f*

pulmonary artery catheter and, 412–424, 413*f*

catheter description of, 414*f*, 414–415

catheterization procedure in, 415–419, 416–418*f*, 419*t*

clinical applications of, 421–423

complications of, 419–420

continuous cardiac output measurement in, 421

continuous mixed venous oxygen saturation monitoring in, 423–424, 424*f*

continuous pulse oximetry in, 424

differential diagnosis of abnormalities in, 421, 422*t*

indications for, 413

measurements in, 420–421

routine monitoring in, 404

securing airway in, 431–435, 432–434*f*

sedation and, 405–406

transport of patient in, 404–405

ventilation in, 424–428, 425–427*f*

Interferon alfa (Roferon-A, Intron A), 552
Interferon alfa-2b-ribavirin combo
    (Rebetron), 552
Interferon alfacon-1 (Infergen), 552
Interferon beta-1b (Betaseron), 552
Interferon-gamma-1b (Actimmune),
    552
Interleukin-2 (Proleukin), 480
Internal fetal scalp monitoring, 282–283
Interrupted suturing, 366*f,* 367*f*
Interstitial fluid, 179
Interstitial infiltrates, 354
Intestinal decompression tube, 277–278
Intracavernosal alprostadil (Caverject,
    Edex), 482
Intracellular fluid, 179
Intracerebral stimulation for pain
    management, 338
Intracranial pressure, 449*t*
Intradermal injection, 283–284
Intramuscular injection, 284
Intrauterine pressure monitoring,
    284–285
Intravenous fluids
    composition of, 180–181, 182*t*
    ordering of, 181–185, 183*t,*
        184–185*f*
Intravenous immune globulin
    (Gamimune, Sandoglobulin,
    Gammar IV), 550
Intravenous infusion rate, 185
Intravenous pyelography, 345
Intravenous techniques, 285–289,
    286–288*f*
Intron A (interferon alfa), 552
Intropin (dopamine), 521–522
Intubation
    critical care and, 430–431, 431*t*
    endotracheal, 273*t,* 273–275, 274*f,*
        464
    gastrointestinal, 277–280
Invanz (ertapenem), 527
Iodine-125 fibrinogen scanning, 351
Ipecac syrup, 553
Ipratropium (Atrovent), 382, 469, 553
Ipratropium-albuterol (Combivent), 480
Iquix Ophthalmic (levofloxacin), 558
Irbesartan (Avapro), 553
Iressa (gefitinib), 541
Irinotecan (Camptosar), 553
Iron, 75
Iron-binding capacity, 75
Iron dextran (Dexferrum, INFeD), 553
Iron sucrose (Venofer), 553

Irradiated blood components, 196
Ischemia, myocardial, 396–398, 397*f,*
    398*f*
Ismo (isosorbide mononitrate),
    554
Isoenzymes
    creatine phosphokinase, 61–62
    lactate dehydrogenase, 76
Isolation protocols, 159–161
Isomil formula, 222*t*
Isoniazid (INH), 553–554
Isoosmolar formulas, 223*t*
Isoproterenol (Isuprel), 554
    in critical care, 451*t*
    effects on adrenergic receptors,
        411*t*
Isoptin (verapamil), 620
Isosorbide dinitrate (Isordil, Sorbitrate,
    Dilatrate-SR), 554
Isosorbide mononitrate (Ismo, Imdur),
    554
Isosporiasis, 150*t*
Isotonic hyponatremia, 186–187
Isotretinoin (Accutane, Amnesteem,
    Claravis, Sotret), 554
Isovolemic hypernatremia, 186
Isovolemic hyponatremia, 187
Isradipine (DynaCirc), 554
Isuprel (isoproterenol), 554
Itching, 43
Itraconazole (Sporonox), 554–555
IV techniques, 285–289, 286–288*f*

J
Janeway lesion, 17
Jaundice, 41–42
Joffroy reflex, 17
Joint disorders, 129*t*
Jugular vein catheterization
    external, 262
    left internal, 261
    right internal, 259–261, 260*f*
Jugular venous distention, 407
Junctional rhythm, 390, 390*f*
Juniper, 626

K
Kabikinase (streptokinase), 604
Kaletra (lopinavir-ritonavir), 561
Kaolin-pectin (Kaodene, Kao-Spen,
    Kapectolin), 555
Karnofsky performance scale, 665–666*t*

Kava kava, 625, 626
Kayexalate (sodium polystyrene
    sulfonate), 188, 601–602
Kayser-Fleischer ring, 17
Keflex (cephalexin), 503
Keftab (cephalexin), 503
Kefzol (cefazolin), 500
Kehr sign, 17
Keloid, 15
Keogh tube, 278
Keppra (levetiracetam), 558
Keratoconjunctivitis, 144t
Kerley B lines, 354
Kerlone (betaxolol), 494
Kernig sign, 17
Ketek (telithromycin), 607–608
Ketoconazole (Nizoral), 555
17-Ketogenic steroids, 114–115
Ketones, 107
Ketoprofen (Orudis, Oruvail), 555
Ketorolac (Toradol, Acular), 329t,
    555
17-Ketosteroids, 115
Ketotifen (Zaditor), 555
Kidney
    adverse effects of pain on, 324t
    Modification of Diet in Renal Disease,
        113
    nuclear scan of, 351–352
    oliguria and anuria, 42–43
    renal failure and
        enteral formula for, 228t
        hypercalcemia in, 190
        patient-controlled analgesia in,
            339
        therapeutic diet in, 217t
        urinary indices in, 115, 116t
Kidney, ureter, and bladder radiography
    (KUB), 342
Kineret (anakinra), 487
Kinyoun stain, 119
Klebsiella spp., 124t
Klonopin (clonazepam), 508
Knee arthrocentesis, 251, 253f
Knot-tying techniques, 365–366,
    370–374f
KOH preparation, 123
Koplik spots, 17
Korotkoff sounds, 11, 18
Kussmaul respiration, 18
Kussmaul sign, 18
Kwell (lindane), 559–560
Kyphosis, 18
Kytril (granisetron), 544

L

Labetalol (Trandate, Normodyne), 472,
    555–556
Labor
    amniotic fluid fern test and, 245–246
    internal fetal scalp monitoring during,
        282–283
    intrauterine pressure monitoring
        during, 284–285
Laboratory diagnosis
    clinical hematology in, 91–103
        blood collection and, 91
        blood smears and, 91–92, 92f,
            92t
        coagulation tests and, 99–103, 100f
        complete blood count values and,
            92–95, 93t, 94t
        hematocrit and, 95, 97–98
        left shift and, 95
        lymphocyte subsets and, 98–99
        platelets and, 98
        red blood cells and, 97, 99
        reticulocyte count and, 95–96
        white blood cells and, 96–97, 99
    in fever work-up, 276
    in nutritional assessment, 209–210
    principles of laboratory testing and,
        48–49
    urine studies in, 104–116
        creatinine clearance in, 112–113
        differential diagnosis in, 106–108
        drug abuse screen in, 115
        normal values in, 106
        spot or random, 110–112
        twenty-four hour, 113–115
        urinalysis procedure in, 105–106
        urinary indices in renal failure and,
            115, 116t
        urine output in, 116
        urine sediment in, 108–110, 109f
        xylose tolerance test in, 115
Laboratory values, shorthand for, 31f, 32
Lactate, 76
Lactate dehydrogenase, 75–76
Lactic acid-ammonium hydroxide-
    ammonium lactate (Lac-
    Hydrin), 556
Lactic acidosis, 174
Lactin acid, 76
Lactobacillus (Lactinex), 125t, 231, 556
Lactose-free diet, 218t
Lactulose (Chronulac, Cephulac,
    Enulose), 556
Lamictal (lamotrigine), 556

Lamisil (terbinafine), 609
Lamivudine (Epivir), 146t, 556
Lamotrigine (Lamictal), 556
Lamprene (clofazimine), 508
Lanoxicaps (digoxin), 518
Lanoxin (digoxin), 518
Lansoprazole (Prevacid), 556–557
Lanthanum carbonate (Fosrenol), 557
Lantus, 637t
LAP score, 76
Large-bore feeding tube, 227
Laryngeal mask airway, 464
Laryngoscope for endotracheal
        intubation, 274, 274f
Lasègue sign, 18
Lasix (furosemide), 540
Latanoprost (Xalatan), 557
Lateral cutaneous nerve of calf, 7f
Lateral cutaneous nerve of forearm, 6f,
        7f
Lateral decubitus chest radiography, 341
Lateral femoral cutaneous nerve, 6f, 7f
Lateral film, 354
Lateral plantar nerve, 6f, 7f
Latex allergy, 242–243, 360
Lawsium (magaldrate), 562
Lead, blood, 76
Leflunomide (Arava), 557
Left atrial enlargement, 395f, 395–396
Left axis deviation, 386
Left bundle branch block, 394f, 394–395
Left internal jugular vein catheterization,
        261
Left lower quadrant abdominal pain, 34
Left shift, 95
Left upper quadrant abdominal pain, 34
Left ventricular end-diastolic pressure,
        420
Left ventricular end-diastolic volume,
        409
Left ventricular hypertrophy, 396, 397f
Legionella antibody, 76
Legionella pneumophila, 124t
Lente Iletin, 637t
Leonard tube, 278
Lepirudin (Refludan), 557
Leptocyte, 99
Lescol (fluvastatin), 538
Lesser occipital nerve, 7f
Letrozole (Femara), 557
Leucovorin (Wellcovorin), 557
Leukapheresis, 196
Leukeran (chlorambucil), 504
Leukine (sargramostim), 598

Leukocyte, 96–97
Leukocyte alkaline phosphatase score, 76
Leukocyte esterase, 107, 141
Leukocyte-poor red cells, 198t
Leukocyte-reduced platelets, 199t
Leuprolide (Lupron, Viadur, Eligard),
        557–558
Leustatin (cladribine), 507
Levalbuterol (Xopenex), 382, 469, 558
Levamisole (Ergamisol), 558
Levaquin (levofloxacin), 558
Levatol (penbutolol), 584
Levetiracetam (Keppra), 558
Levin tube, 277
Levine sign, 18
Levitra (vardenafil), 619
Levobunolol (Betagan), 558
Levocabastine (Livostin), 558
Levofloxacin (Levaquin, Quixin, Iquix
        Ophthalmic), 558
Levonorgestrel (Norplant), 558–559
Levophed (norepinephrine), 577
Levorphanol (Levo-Dromoran), 559
Levothyroxine (Synthroid, Levoxyl),
        559
Levoxyl (levothyroxine), 559
Levsin (hyoscyamine), 548
Lexapro (escitalopram), 528
Lexiva (fosamprenavir), 539
Lhermitte sign, 18
Libritabs (chlordiazepoxide), 504
Librium (chlordiazepoxide), 504
Lice, 150t
Lichenification, 15
Licorice, 626
Lidex (fluocinolone), 635t
Lidocaine (Xylocaine, Anestacon), 364t,
        559, 630t
    with epinephrine, 632t
    in pediatric advanced life support, 459t
Lidocaine-prilocaine (EMLA, LMX), 559
Life root, 626
Limb electrodes, 271
Lindane (Kwell), 559–560
Line sepsis, 446
Linezolid (Zyvox), 560
Lioresal (baclofen), 492
Liothyronine (Cytomel), 560
Lipase, 76–77
Lipid panel, 48
Lipid profile, 77, 209
Lipitor (atorvastatin), 491
Lipoprotein profile, 77
Lipoproteins, 59t

Lisinopril (Prinivil, Zestril), 560
List, 18
Listeria monocytogenes, 125*t*
Lithium (Eskalith, Lithobid), 560, 630*t*
Lithobid (lithium), 560, 630*t*
Liver
    complications of parenteral nutrition,
        239
    hepatitis and
        blood component therapy-related,
            204
        testing for, 68–72, 69–71*t,* 71*f,* 72*f,*
            157–158
    therapeutic diet for disease of, 218*t*
Liver-spleen scan, 351
Livostin (levocabastine), 558
LMX (lidocaine-prilocaine), 559
Local anesthetics, 337, 364*t,* 632*t*
LoCHOLEST (cholestyramine), 505
Lodine (etodolac), 532
Lodoxamide (Alomide), 560
Löffler methylene blue stain, 156
Lomefloxacin (Maxaquin), 560
Lomotil (diphenoxylate-atropine), 519
Loniten (minoxidil), 569
Loperamide (Imodium), 560–561
Lopid (gemfibrozil), 541
Lopidine (apraclonidine), 488
Lopinavir, 147*t*
Lopinavir-ritonavir (Kaletra), 561
Lopressor (metoprolol), 567
Loprox (ciclopirox), 506
Lopurin (allopurinol), 481
Lorabid (loracarbef), 561
Loracarbef (Lorabid), 561
Loratadine (Claritin, Alavert), 561
Lorazepam (Ativan), 405, 561
Lorcet (hydrocodone-acetaminophen),
    546–547
Lordosis, 18
Lordotic chest radiography, 341
Lortab ASA (hydrocodone-aspirin),
    547
Los Angeles Prehospital Stroke Screen,
    469*t*
Losartan (Cozaar), 561
Lotensin (benazepril), 493
Lotrimin (clotrimazole), 509
Lotrisone (clotrimazole-betamethasone),
    509
Lotronex (alosetron), 481
Louvel sign, 18
Lovastatin (Mevacor, Altocar), 561
Lovenox (enoxaparin), 525

Low-density lipoprotein cholesterol, 58*t,*
    60
Low-density lipoproteins, 59*t*
Low-dose dexamethasone suppression
    test, 63
Low-fat diet, 218*t*
Low-fiber diet, 216*t*
Low lactose diet, 218*t*
Low-molecular-weight heparin
    for deep venous thrombosis, 447
    for DVT prophylaxis in septic shock,
        444
    for pulmonary embolism, 447
Low-sodium diet, 219*t*
Lower abdominal pain, 34
Lozol (indapamide), 550–551
Lugol solution (potassium iodide), 590
Lumbar puncture, 289–296, 291*f,* 292*f,*
    294–295*t*
Lumbar radiography, 344
Lunelle (estradiol cypionate-
        medroxyprogesterone
        acetate), 529–530
Lunesta (eszopiclone), 531
Lung
    adverse effects of pain on, 324*t*
    chest radiography and, 353–354
    clinical physiology of, 424–430,
        425*f*
    complications of parenteral nutrition,
        239
    infection of, 154–155
    pulmonary function tests and,
        377–378, 378*f,* 379*t*
    pulmonary infiltrates and, 354
Lung capacity, 426
Lung compliance, 426, 427*f*
    ventilator weaning and, 438*t*
Lung scan, 351
Lung volumes, 377, 378*t,* 425, 425*f*
Lupron (leuprolide), 557–558
Lupus erythematosus preparation, 76
Luteinizing hormone, 77
Lutrepulse (gonadorelin), 543
Lutropin alfa (Luveris), 562
Luvox (fluvoxamine), 538
Lyme disease, 77, 126, 152–153*t*
Lymph node examination, 3
Lymphadenopathy, 42
Lymphangiography, 345–346
Lymphocyte, 94*t,* 96
Lymphocyte immune globulin, 562
Lymphocyte subsets, 98–99
Lymphogranuloma venereum, 130*t*

Lyrica (pregabalin), 591

M

M-mode echocardiography, 346
Ma huang, 624, 626
Maalox (aluminum hydroxide-
    magnesium hydroxide), 483
Maalox Plus (aluminum hydroxide-
    magnesium hydroxide-
    simethicone), 483
Macroalbuminuria, 111
Macrobid (nitrofurantoin), 576
Macrodantin (nitrofurantoin), 576
Macule, 15
Magaldrate (Riopan, Lawsium), 562
Magnesium, 77–78
    hypermagnesemia and, 191–192
    hypomagnesemia and, 192
    in parenteral formula, 234t
    in pediatric advanced life support, 459t
    requirements for, 180
Magnesium citrate, 562
Magnesium hydroxide (Milk of
    Magnesia), 562
Magnesium oxide, 192, 562
Magnesium sulfate, 192, 562
Magnetic resonance imaging, 348–350
Maintenance fluids, 181, 183t
Malaria, 126, 150–151t
Malarone (atovaquone-proguanil), 491
Male genitalia, 5
Malnutrition, 207
Mammography, 343–344, 654t
Mandibular branch of trigeminal nerve, 6f
Manganese, 235t
Mannitol, 562–563
Mantoux test, 309–310
Marcaine (bupivacaine), 496
Marcus Gunn pupil, 18
Marinol (dronabinol), 523
Mass
    adrenal, 34
    breast, 34
Mastitis, 129t
Mastoiditis, 130t
Matulane (procarbazine), 592
Mavik (trandolapril), 615
Maxair (pirbuterol), 589
Maxalt (rizatriptan), 645t
Maxaquin (lomefloxacin), 560
MAXI drip chamber, 185
Maxillary branch of trigeminal nerve, 6f
Maxipime (cefepime), 500

Maxitrol (neomycin-polymyxin B-
    dexamethasone), 574
Maxzide (hydrochlorothiazide-
    triamterene), 546
McBurney point, 18
McGill Pain Questionnaire, 325
McMurray test, 18
MDRD (Modification of Diet in Renal
    disease equation), 113
Mean arterial pressure, 408, 448
Mean corpuscular hemoglobin, 93t, 97
Mean corpuscular hemoglobin
    concentration, 93t, 98
Mean corpuscular volume, 93t, 98
Mean pulmonary artery pressure, 448t
Measles, 144t
Measles, mumps, rubella vaccine, 563,
    657–661t, 662–664t
Measurement equivalents, 650
Mechanical soft diet, 215t
Mechanical ventilation, 435–439, 436f,
    438t
    indications for, 431t
    in sepsis-induced acute lung injury,
    444
Mechlorethamine (Mustargen), 563
Meclizine (Antivert), 563
Medial cutaneous nerve of arm, 7f
Medial cutaneous nerve of forearm, 6f, 7f
Medial femoral cutaneous nerve, 6f, 7f
Medial plantar nerve, 6f, 7f
Median cubital vein for intravenous
    access, 286f
Median nerve, 6f, 7f
Mediastinal computed tomography, 348
Mediastinal radiography, 353
Medical emergency, 455–474
    in acute coronary syndromes, 466,
    467–468f
    advanced cardiac life support in, 463,
    463t
    airway and ventilatory support in,
    463–464
    in anaphylaxis, 466–469
    in anticholinergic toxicity, 471
    in asthma attack, 469–471
    automated external defibrillation in,
    464–466
    cardiopulmonary resuscitation in,
    456–462, 457f
        adult, 456–458
        child, 458–462, 459t, 460t, 461f
        neonate, 462, 462f
    in coma, 471

dental, 471
emergency cardiac care in, 455–456
in hypertensive crisis, 472
in hypoglycemia, 472
medications for, *inside covers*
in opioid overdose, 472
in poisoning, 472, 473*t*
in status epilepticus, 473–474, 474*t*
in stroke, 466, 469*t*, 470*f*
Medications. *See* Drug therapy; specific drugs.
Medigesic (acetaminophen-butalbital-caffeine), 478
Mediquell (dextromethorphan), 516
Medroxyprogesterone (Provera, Depo-Provera), 563
Mefoxin (cefoxitin), 501
Megestrol acetate (Megace), 563
Melatonin, 625
Melena, 40
Melenemesis, 40
Mellaril (thioridazine), 611
Meloxicam (Mobic), 563
Melphalan (Alkeran), 564
Memantine (Namenda), 564
Menest (esterified estrogens), 529
Meningitis, 133–134*t*
cerebrospinal fluid analysis in, 294*t*
testing for, 155
Meningococcal vaccine, 564, 657–661*t*, 662–664*t*
Mental status examination, 5, 8
Meperidine (Demerol, Mepergan), 564
for analgesia, 332*t*
in patient-controlled analgesia, 339*t*
Mepivacaine (Carbocaine), 364*t*, 632*t*
Meprobamate (Equinil, Miltown), 564
Mepron (atovaquone), 491
Mercaptopurine (Purinethol), 564
Meridia (sibutramine), 599
Meropenem (Merrem), 564–565
Mesalamine (Rowasa, Asacol, Pentasa), 565
Mesna (Mesnex), 565
Mesoridazine (Serentil), 565
Metabolic acidosis, 166*t*, 168–171, 169*f*, 170*t*
Metabolic alkalosis, 166*t*, 171*f*, 171–172, 175, 176
Metabolic disorders
delirium in, 34
dementia in, 35
Metabolic gap acidosis, 176
Metabolic nongap acidosis, 176–177

Metabolic syndrome, 209, 211*t*
Metamucil (psyllium), 594
Metanephrines, 114
Metaprel (metaproterenol), 565
Metaproterenol (Alupent, Metaprel), 565
Metastron scan, 352
Metaxalone (Skelaxin), 565
Metered-dose inhaler, 382
Metformin (Glucophage), 565
Metformin-pioglitazone (ActoPlus Met), 588
Methadone (Dolophine), 332*t*, 566
Methanol poisoning, 473*t*
Methenamine (Hiprex, Urex), 566
Methergine (methylergonovine), 567
Methimazole (Tapazole), 566
Methocarbamol (Robaxin), 566
Methotrexate (Folex, Rheumatrex), 566, 630*t*
Methyldopa (Aldomet), 566–567
Methylene blue stain, 156
Methylergonovine (Methergine), 567
Methylprednisolone, 633*t*
for anaphylaxis, 469
for asthma attack, 469–471
Metoclopramide (Reglan, Clopra, Octamide), 567
Metolazone (Mykrox, Zaroxolyn), 567
Metoprolol (Lopressor, Toprol XL), 567
Metronidazole (Flagyl, MetroGel), 567–568
Mevacor (lovastatin), 561
Mexiletine (Mexitil), 568
Mezlocillin (Mezlin), 568
Miacalcin (calcitonin), 497
Micardis (telmisartan), 608
Miconazole (Monistat), 568
Microalbuminuria, 111
Microbiology, 117–161
acid-fast stain and, 119
antimicrobial resistance and, 118–119
bioterrorism and, 158
blood culture and, 119–120
in bone and joint disorders, 129*t*
in bronchitis, 129*t*
in central nervous system infection, 155
in cervicitis, 130*t*
in chancre, 130*t*
in chlamydial infection, 130*t*
darkfield examination and, 120
in diverticulitis, 130*t*
in ear infection, 130–131*t*

Microbiology (*cont.*)
  in endocarditis, 131–132*t*
  in epiglottitis, 132*t*
  in fungal infections, 148–149*t*
  in gallbladder disease, 132*t*
  in gastroenteritis, 133*t*
  general principles of, 117–118
  Giemsa stain and, 120
  in gonorrhea, 133*t*
  gonorrhea smear and culture and,
      120–121
  Gram stain and, 121, 122*f,* 123*f,*
      124–126*t*
  in hepatitis, 157–158
  in human immunodeficiency virus
      infection, 156–157
  India ink preparation and, 121
  in infectious diarrhea, 155–156
  isolation protocols and, 159–161
  Lyme disease testing and, 126
  malaria smear and, 126
  in mastitis, 129*t*
  in meningitis, 133–134*t*
  molecular, 126
  nasal culture and, 127
  in nocardiosis, 134*t*
  ova and parasites and, 127
  in parasitic infections, 150–151*t*
  in pelvic inflammatory disease, 134*t*
  in peritonitis, 135*t*
  in pharyngitis, 135*t*
  pinworm preparation and, 127
  in pneumonia, 136*t*
  potassium hydroxide preparation and,
      123
  in pulmonary infections, 154–155
  in sinusitis, 137*t*
  in skin and soft tissue infections,
      137–138*t,* 155
  in subacute bacterial endocarditis,
      158–159, 159*t,* 160*t*
  in syphilis, 138*t*
  throat culture and, 127–128
  in tick-borne diseases, 152–153*t*
  in tuberculosis, 138*t,* 154–155
  Tzanck smear and, 128
  in ulcer disease, 139*t*
  in urinary tract infection, 139–140*t,*
      141, 154
  in vaginal infections, 140*t*
  in viral infections, 128, 142–145*t*
Microglobulin, 78, 111
Microhemagglutination, *Treponema
      pallidum,* 78

Micronase (glyburide), 543
Midamor (amiloride), 484
Midazolam (Versed), 405, 568
Mifepristone (RU 486, Mifeprex), 568
Miglitol (Glycet), 568–569
Migraine, 40
Milk of Magnesia (magnesium
      hydroxide), 562
Milk thistle, 625
Miller-Abbott tube, 278
Milrinone (Primacor), 451*t,* 569
Miltown (meprobamate), 564
Mineral oil, 569
MINI drip chamber, 185
Mini-Mental State Examination, 8, 9*t*
Minipress (prazosin), 591
Minnesota tube, 278
Minoxidil (Loniten, Rogaine), 569
Minute ventilation, 437
    ventilator weaning and, 438*t*
MiraLax (polyethylene glycol), 589
Mirapex (pramipexole), 590
Mirtazapine (Remeron), 569
Misoprostol (Cytotec), 569
Mitomycin (Mutamycin), 569
Mitoxantrone (Novantrone), 569–570
Mitral insufficiency, 10*t*
Mitral stenosis, 10*t*
Mitran (chlordiazepoxide), 504
Mixed acid-base disorders, 165–167
Mixed monoclonal cryoglobulins, 62
Mixed polyclonal cryoglobulins, 62
Mixed venous oxygen content, 449*t*
Mixed venous oxygen saturation, 419*t,*
      423–424, 424*f*
Mixing studies, 102
Moban (molindone), 570
Mobic (meloxicam), 563
Mobitz type I block, 393, 393*f*
Mobitz type II block, 393
Möbius sign, 18
Modification of Diet in Renal disease
      equation, 113
Modofinil (Provigil), 570
Moduretic (hydrochlorothiazide-
      amiloride), 546
Moexipril (Univasc), 570
Molecular microbiology, 126
Molindone (Moban), 570
Mometasone furoate (Elocon), 636*t*
Monistat (miconazole), 568
Monitoring
    in critical care, 404
    fetal scalp, 282–283

intrauterine pressure, 284–285
of parenteral nutrition, 237
Monocid (cefonicid), 501
Monoclate (antihemophilic factor), 488
Monoclonal cryoglobulins, 62
Monocytes, 94*t*, 97
Monopril (fosinopril), 539–540
Monospot, 78
Montelukast (Singulair), 570
Monurol (fosfomycin), 539
Moraxella catarrhalis, 124*t*
Morganella morganii, 124*t*
Moro reflex, 18
Morphine (Roxanol, Kadian, MS Contin,
  Oramorph SR, Avinza),
  570–571
  for analgesia, 333*t*
  in critical care, 406
  in patient-controlled analgesia, 339*t*
Motor examination, 5
Moxifloxacin (Avelox, Vigamox
  ophthalmic), 571
MS Contin (morphine), 570
Mucin clot test, 250
Mucomyst (acetylcysteine), 382, 478–479
Mucormycosis, 149*t*
Mucus in urine, 110
MUGA scan, 351
Multifocal atrial tachycardia, 389, 389*f*
Multifocal premature ventricular
  contractions, 391, 391*f*
Multiple sclerosis, 295*t*
Mupirocin (Bactroban), 571
Muromonab-CD3 (Orthoclone, OKT3),
  571
Murphy sign, 18
Muscle wasting, 212*t*
Musculoskeletal system
  magnetic resonance imaging of, 350
  physical examination of, 5
  review of systems and, 3
Muse (alprostadil, urethral suppository),
  482
Musset sign, 18
Mustargen (mechlorethamine), 563
Mutamycin (mitomycin), 569
Myambutol (ethambutol), 531
Mycelex (clotrimazole), 509
Mycobacterium spp., 125*t*
Mycobutin (rifabutin), 596
Mycolog-II (triamcinolone-nystatin), 616
Mycophenolate mofetil (CellCept), 571
Mycophenolic acid (Myfortic), 571
Mycostatin (nystatin), 578

Myelography, 346
Myfortic (mycophenolic acid), 571
Mykrox (metolazone), 567
Mylanta (aluminum hydroxide-
  magnesium hydroxide-
  simethicone), 483
Myleran (busulfan), 496
Mylicon (simethicone), 600
Mylotarg (gemtuzumab ozogamicin), 542
Myocardial infarction
  electrocardiography in, 396–399,
    397–399*f*, 398*t*
  emergency care in, 466, 467–468*f*
  oral anticoagulants for, 644*t*
Myocardial ischemia, 396–398, 397*f*,
  398*f*
Myoglobin, 78, 112

N
N-telopeptide, 86–87
Nabumetone (Relafen), 329*t*, 571
Nadolol (Corgard), 571–572
Nafcillin (Nallpen), 572
Naftifine (Naftin), 572
Nalbuphine (Nubain), 572
Nalfon (fenoprofen), 534
Nallpen (nafcillin), 572
Naloxone (Narcan), 472, 572
Naltrexone (ReVia), 572
Namenda (memantine), 564
NAPamide (disopyramide), 520
Naphazoline, 572
Naproxen (Aleve, Anaprox, Naprosyn),
  330*t*, 572
Naratriptan (Amerge), 572–573, 645*t*
Narcan (naloxone), 572
Nardil (phenelzine), 587
Nasal cannula, 380*t*
Nasal culture, 127
NasalCrom (cromolyn sodium), 511
Nasalide (flunisolide), 536
Nasogastric tube, 277–280
Nasopharyngeal airway, 464
Natalizumab (Tysabri), 573
National Cholesterol Education Program,
  56–58*t*
Natrecor (nesiritide), 574
Natriuretic peptide, B-type, 78
Nausea, 42
Navane (thiothixene), 611
Navelbine (vinorelbine), 620
Nebcin (tobramycin), 613
Nebulizer therapy, 380–381

NebuPent (pentamidine), 585
Neck
    computed tomography of, 348
    physical examination of, 3
Nedocromil (Tilade), 573
Needle cricothyroidotomy, 268–269
Needle gauge reference, 243, 244*t*
Needlestick, accidental, 242
Nefazodone (Serzone), 573
Neisseria gonorrhoeae, 120–121, 124*t,*
    299
Neisseria meningitidis, 124*t*
Nelfinavir (Viracept), 147*t,* 573
Neo-Calglucon (calcium glubionate), 497
Neo-Synephrine (phenylephrine), 587
Neomycin, 573–574
Neomycin-polymyxin B (Neosporin
    cream), 573
Neomycin-polymyxin B-dexamethasone
    (Maxitrol), 574
Neonatal bilirubin, 53
Neonatal ophthalmia, 130*t*
Neonate. *See* Newborn.
NeOral (cyclosporine), 512
Neosar (cyclophosphamide), 511–512
Nephropathy, contrast, 445
Nephrotomogram, 345
Nerve conduction studies, 326
Nesiritide (Natrecor), 574
Neteglinide (Starlix), 573
Neulasta (pegfilgrastim), 583–584
Neumega (oprelvekin), 579
Neupogen (filgrastim), 535
Neural blockade
    for analgesia, 337
    in pain assessment, 326
    in septic shock, 444
Neurogenic shock, 422*t,* 444
Neuroleptics, 337
Neurologic disorders
    delirium in, 34
    dementia in, 35
    mechanical ventilation in, 431*t*
Neurologic examination, 5–7
Neurologic system
    considerations in critical care,
        405–406
    dementia and, 37
    imaging of, 352–353
Neurolysis, 337
Neurontin (gabapentin), 540
Neuropathic pain, 323
Neuropsychiatric system, 3
Neutrexin (trimetrexate), 617

Neutron activation analysis, 210*t*
Neutrophils, 94*t*
Nevirapine (Viramune), 146*t,* 574
Newborn
    cardiopulmonary resuscitation in, 462,
        462*f*
    cerebrospinal fluid analysis and, 294*t*
    endotracheal tube for, 273*t*
    herpes simplex virus in, 144*t*
    neonatal ophthalmia and, 130*t*
    pneumonia in, 136*t*
Newborn screening panel, 79
Nexium (esomeprazole), 528–529
Niacin, 234*t,* 575
Nicardipine (Cardene), 452*t,* 575
Nicotine gum, 575
Nicotine nasal spray, 575
Nicotine transdermal (Habitrol, Nicoderm
    CQ, Nicotrol), 575
Nifedipine (Procardia, Adalat), 575
Night of surgery note, 29
Nilutamide (Nilandron), 575–576
Nimodipine (Nimotop), 576
Nisoldipine (Sular), 576
Nitazoxanide (Alinia), 576
Nitrate, urine, 107
Nitrazine paper, 245
Nitrofurantoin (Macrodantin, Furadantin,
    Macrobid), 576
Nitrogen balance, 214
Nitroglycerin (Tridil), 452*t,* 576
Nitroprusside (Nipride, Nitropress), 452*t,*
    576–577
Nix (permethrin), 586
Nizatadine (Axid), 577
Nizoral (ketoconazole), 555
Nocardiosis, 125*t,* 134*t*
Nodal rhythm, 390, 390*f*
Nodule, 15
Nolvadex (tamoxifen), 607
Non-anion gap acidosis, 169
Nonabsorbable sutures, 361, 363*t*
Nonhemolytic febrile reaction, 203,
    204
Nonopioid analgesics, 326
Nonpharmacologic management of pain,
    337–338
Nonrebreathing face mask, 380*t*
Nonsteroidal antiinflammatory drugs
    (NSAIDs), 326, 328–330*t*
Norcuron (vecuronium), 619–620
Norepinephrine (Levophed), 577
    in critical care, 453*t*
    effects on adrenergic receptors, 411*t*

Norethindrone acetate-ethinyl estradiol (FemHRT), 577
Norflex (orphenadrine), 580
Norfloxacin (Noroxin, Chilbroxin), 577
Norgestrel (Ovrette), 577
Normal sinus rhythm, 387, 387*f*
Normoalbuminuria, 111
Normodyne (labetalol), 472, 555–556
Norpace (disopyramide), 520
Norplant (levonorgestrel), 558–559
Norpramin (desipramine), 515
Nortriptyline (Aventyl, Pamelor), 577–578, 630*t*
Norvasc (amlodipine), 485
Norvir (ritonavir), 597
Nose, 2, 3
Novafed (pseudoephedrine), 593–594
Novantrone (mitoxantrone), 569–570
Novolin, 637*t*
Novolog, 637*t*
Novulin, 637*t*
NPH Iletin, 637*t*
NT-Pro B-type natriuretic peptide, 78–79
Nubain (nalbuphine), 572
Nuclear scan, 350–352
Nucleated red blood cells, 99
5'-Nucleotidase, 79
Numeric pain intensity scale, 325*f*
Numorphan (oxymorphone), 582
Nupercainal (dibucaine), 517
Nurolon suture, 363*t*
Nursoy formula, 222*t*
Nutramigen formula, 222*t*
Nutritional assessment, 208–213, 209–212*t*
Nutritional support, 225–239
  candidates for, 224
  critical care and, 440
  enteral nutrition in, 225–231, 228–229*t*
  illness and, 207
  parenteral nutrition in, 231–239
    blood glucose management in, 238–239
    central *versus* peripheral, 235
    complications of, 237–238
    formulas for, 232–235, 234*t*, 235*t*
    indications for, 231–232, 232*t*
    initiation and maintenance of, 235–237, 237*t*
    monitoring of, 237
    termination of, 239
NuvaRing (etonogestrel-ethinyl estradiol), 532

Nylon suture, 363*t*
Nystagmus, 42
Nystatin (Mycostatin), 578

O
Obesity
  metabolic syndrome and, 209, 211*t*
  nutritional status and, 212*t*
Obstructive pulmonary diseases, 377, 379*t*
Obturator nerve, 6*f*, 7*t*
Obturator sign, 18
Octamide (metoclopramide), 567
Octreotide (Sandostatin), 578
Octyl cyanoacrylate, 373
Oculomotor nerve, 5
Ocupress Ophthalmic (carteolol), 499
Odor of urine, 107
Off-service note, 27
Ofloxacin (Floxin, Ocuflox Ophthalmic), 578
OKT3 (muromonab-CD3), 571
Olanzapine (Zyprexa, Zydis), 578
Older adult, fever work-up in, 277
Olfactory nerve, 5
Oligoclonal banding, 79
Oliguria, 42–43, 116*t*
Olopatadine (Pantanol), 578
Olsalazine (Dipentum), 578
Omalozumab (Xolair), 579
Omeprazole (Prilosec, Zegerid), 579
Omnipen (ampicillin), 487
On-service note, 27
Oncaspar (L-Asparaginase), 489
Oncovin (vincristine), 620
Ondansetron (Zofran), 579
One-handed tie, 372–373*f*
Operating room, 355–360
  draping of patient, 359
  entering, 355–356
  gowning and gloving, 358–359
  latex allergy and, 360
  patient preparation and, 357–358
  position in, 359–360
  sterile technique in, 355
  surgical hand scrub and, 356–357
  universal precautions and, 360
Operative note, 28–29
Ophthalmic branch of trigeminal nerve, 6*f*
Opioids
  for analgesia, 331–334*t*, 337
  overdose of, 472, 473*t*
Opium, tincture of, 583

Oprelvekin (Neumega), 579
Optic nerve, 5
Opticrom (cromolyn sodium), 511
Optivar (azathioprine), 491
Oral anticoagulants, 644*t*
Oral cholecystography, 346
Oral contraceptives, 579, 638–641*t*
Oral glucose tolerance test, 67
Oral nutritional supplements, 220–221
Oral potassium supplements, 642*t*
Oral rehydration solutions, 221–223
Oral thrush, 148*t*
Orders, writing of, 25–26
Organic failure to thrive, 38
Orinase (tolbutamide), 613
Orlistat (Xenical), 580
Orolabial herpes, 143*t*
Oropharyngeal airway, 464
Orphenadrine (Norflex), 580
Ortho Evra (ethinyl estradiol-
        norelgestromin), 531
Orthoclone (muromonab-CD3), 571
Orthostatic blood pressure measurement,
        296
Orthostatic syncope, 44
Ortolani test, 18
Orudis (ketoprofen), 555
Osborne wave, 401, 401*f*
Oseltamivir (Tamiflu), 580
Osler node, 18
Osmolality
    serum, 79
    urine, 112, 116*t*
Osteomyelitis, 129*t*
Osteopathic treatment for pain
        management, 337–338
Otic Domeboro (acetic acid-aluminum
        acetate), 478
Otitis externa, 131*t*
Otitis media, 131*t*
Outpatient prescription writing, 29–32,
        30*f*
Ova and parasites, 127
Ovrette (norgestrel), 577
Oxacillin (Bactocill, Prostaphlin), 580
Oxaliplatin (Eloxatin), 580
Oxaprozin (Daypro), 330*t*, 580
Oxazepam (Serax), 580
Oxcarbazepine (Trileptal), 580–581
Oxiconazole (Oxistat), 581
Oximetric pulmonary artery catheter, 415
Oxybutynin (Ditropan, Oxytrol), 581
Oxycodone (OxyContin, Roxicodone),
        333–334*t*, 581–582

Oxycodone-acetaminophen (Percocet,
        Roxicet, Tylox), 334*t*
Oxygen carrying capacity, 449*t*
Oxygen consumption, 449*t*
Oxygen delivery, 428
Oxygen partial pressure, 164*t*, 448*t*
    mechanical ventilation and, 431*t*
    ventilator weaning and, 438*t*
Oxygen saturation, 164*t*
Oxygen supplementation, 379, 380*t*
Oxygenation
    critical care and, 428–430, 428–430*f*
    ventilator weaning and, 438*t*
Oxyhemoglobin dissociation curve, 173*f*
Oxytocin (Pitocin), 582

P
P wave, 384*f*, 385
Pacerone (amiodarone), 485
Pacing pulmonary artery catheter, 414
Packed red blood cells, 198*t*
Paclitaxel (Taxol, Abraxane), 582
PAD programs, 455
Pain, 323–339
    adverse physiologic effects of, 323,
        324*t*
    assessment of, 323–326, 325*f*
    back, 34
    chest, 34
    classification of, 323
    nonpharmacologic management of,
        337–338
    patient-controlled analgesia for,
        338–339, 339*t*
    pharmacologic management of,
        326–337, 327–336*t*
Palifermin (Synagis), 582
Palonosetron (Aloxil), 582–583
Pamelor (nortriptyline), 577–578, 630*t*
Pamidronate (Aredia), 190, 583
Panacryl suture material, 362*t*
Pancoast syndrome, 18
Pancrelipase (Pancrease, Cotazym,
        Creon, Ultrase), 583
Pancuronium (Pavulon), 583
Pantanol (olopatadine), 578
Pantoprazole (Protonix), 583
Pap smear, 298–299, 655*t*
Papilloma virus, 145*t*
Papule, 15
Paracentesis, 304–306, 305*f*, 306*t*
Paracoccidioidomycosis, 149*t*
Paradoxical pulse, 306–307, 408, 408*f*

Paraflex (chlorzoxazone), 505
Parafon Forte DSC (chlorzoxazone), 505
Paraldehyde, 474*t*
Paranasal sinus radiography, 344
Paraplatin (carboplatin), 498
Parasites in urine, 109
Parasitic infection, 150–151*t*
    transfusion-related, 205
Parathyroid hormone, 80
Parathyroid hormone deficiency, 190
Paregoric, 583
Parenteral fluids, 180–181, 182*t*
Parenteral nutrition, 231–239
    blood glucose management in,
        238–239
    central *versus* peripheral, 235
    complications of, 237–238
    formulas for, 232–235, 234*t*, 235*t*
    indications for, 231–232, 232*t*
    initiation and maintenance of,
        235–237, 237*t*
    monitoring of, 237
    termination of, 239
Parenteral nutrition formulas, 232–235,
        234*t*, 235*t*
Parkland Formula, 181
Parlodel (bromocriptine), 495
Paroxetine (Paxil), 583
Paroxysmal atrial tachycardia, 388, 389*f*
Partial rebreathing face mask, 380*t*
Partial seizure, 43
Partial thromboplastin time, 102–103
Past medical history, 1–2
Pastia lines, 19
Patch, 15
Patent ductus arteriosus, 11*t*
Pathogens, 121, 122*f*, 123*f*, 124–126*t*,
        129–140*t*
    in bone and joint disease, 129*t*
    in breast disease, 129*t*
    in bronchitis, 129*t*
    in cervicitis, 130*t*
    in chancroid, 130*t*
    chlamydial, 130*t*
    in diverticulitis, 130*t*
    in ear infection, 130–131*t*
    in empyema endocarditis, 131–132*t*
    in epiglottitis, 132*t*
    in gallbladder infection, 132*t*
    in gastroenteritis, 133*t*
    in gonorrhea, 133*t*
    in granuloma inguinale, 133*t*
    in infectious diarrhea, 155–156
    in meningitis, 133–134*t*

    in nocardiosis, 134*t*
    in pelvic inflammatory disease, 134*t*
    in peritonitis, 135*t*
    in pharyngitis, 135*t*
    in pneumonia, 136*t*
    in sinusitis, 137*t*
    in skin and soft tissue infections,
        137–138*t*
    in syphilis, 138*t*
    in tuberculosis, 138*t*
    in ulcer disease, 139*t*
    in urinary tract infections, 139–140*t*
    in vaginal infections, 140*t*
Patient-controlled analgesia (PCA),
        338–339, 339*t*
Patient preparation, 357–358
Pavulon (pancuronium), 583
Paxil (paroxetine), 583
PediaCare 1 (dextromethorphan), 516
Pediarix, 519
Pediatric advanced life support, 459*t*
Pediazole (erythromycin-sulfisoxazole),
        528
Pediculosis, 150*t*
Peg interferon alfa-2a (Pegasys), 584
Peg interferon alfa-2b (PEG-Intron), 584
PEG tube, 227
Pegfilgrastim (Neulasta), 583–584
Pelvic computed tomography, 348
Pelvic examination, 296–299
Pelvic inflammatory disease, 134*t*
Pelvic ultrasonography, 347
Pelvis, magnetic resonance imaging of,
        350
Pemetrexed (Alimta), 584
Penbutolol (Levatol), 584
Penciclovir (Denavir), 584
Penicillin G, 585–586
Penicillin G benzathine (Bicillin), 585
Penicillin G procaine (Wycillin), 585
Penicillin V (Pen-Vee, Veetids), 585
Pentamidine (Pentam 300, NebuPent),
        585
Pentasa (mesalamine), 565
Pentazocine (Talwin), 585
Pentobarbital (Nembutal), 586
Pentoxifylline (Trental), 586
Pentozocine-aspirin (Talwin), 335*t*
Pepcid (famotidine), 533
Pepto-Bismol (bismuth subsalicylate),
        494
Peptostreptococcus spp., 124*t*
Percocet (oxycodone-acetaminophen),
        581

Percodan (oxycodone-aspirin), 581–582
Percussion and postural drainage, 381
Percutaneous endoscopic gastrostomy
    tube, 227
Percutaneous nephrostography, 346
Percutaneous suprapubic bladder
        aspiration, 316, 317*f*
Percutaneous transhepatic
        cholangiography, 346
Performance status scales, 665–666*t*
Pergolide (Permax), 586
Periactin (cyproheptadine), 512
Pericardiocentesis, 299–301, 300*f*
Pericarditis, 400*f*, 401
Perindopril erbumine (Aceon), 586
Perineal nerve, 6*f*
Peripheral cyanosis, 34
Peripheral parenteral nutrition, 235
Peripheral vascular system
    physical examination of, 5
    review of systems and, 3
Peripheral venography, 346
Peripherally inserted central catheter,
        301–302
Peritoneal dialysis, 217*t*
Peritoneal dialysis-related peritonitis,
        135*t*
Peritoneal lavage, 303, 304*t*
Peritoneal paracentesis, 304–306, 305*f*,
        306*t*
Peritonitis, 135*t*
Permax (pergolide), 586
Permethrin (Nix, Elimite), 586
Permitil (fluphenazine), 537
Perphenazine (Trilafon), 586
Persantine (dipyridamole), 520
Petechiae, 15
pH, 163, 164*t*
    of urine, 107–108
Phalen test, 19
Pharmacologic management of pain,
        326–337, 327*–336t*
Pharyngitis, 135*t*
Phenazopyridine (Pyridium), 586–587
Phenelzine (Nardil), 587
Phenergan (promethazine), 592
Phenobarbital, 587
    for status epilepticus, 474*t*
    therapeutic levels of, 629*t*
Phenylephrine (Neo-Synephrine), 587
    in critical care, 453*t*
    effects on adrenergic receptors, 411*t*
Phenytoin (Dilantin), 587
    for status epilepticus, 474*t*

therapeutic levels of, 629*t*
Pheresis, 199*t*
Phlebotomy, 316–321, 318–320*t*
Phos-Ex (calcium acetate), 497
PhosLo (calcium acetate), 497
Phosphate
    hyperphosphatemia and, 192–193
    hypophosphatemia and, 193
    in parenteral formula, 234*t*
Phospholine Ophthalmic (echothiophate
        iodine), 523–524
Phosphorus, 80
Phrenilin Forte (acetaminophen-
        butalbital-caffeine), 478
Phthirus pubis, 150*t*
Physical examination, 3–24
    blood pressure guidelines in, 11–12,
        12*t*
    dental, 12–13, 14*f*
    dermatologic descriptions for, 13–15
    example of, 20–24
    heart murmurs and extra heart sounds
        in, 4, 4*f*, 8, 10–11*t*
    mental status examination and, 8, 9*t*
    in nutritional assessment, 211, 212*t*
    signs and symptoms in, 15–20
Physical therapy for pain management,
        337
Physostigmine (Antilirium), 471,
        587–588
Phytonadione (vitamin K), 588
PICC line, 301–302
Pick-up note, 27
Pimecrolimus (Elidel), 588
Pindolol (Visken), 588
Pinworms, 127, 150*t*
Pioglitazone (Actos), 588
Piperacillin (Pipracil), 588
Piperacillin-tazobactam (Zosyn),
        588–589
Pirbuterol (Maxair), 589
Piroxicam (Feldene), 330*t*, 589
Pitocin (oxytocin), 582
Pitressin (vasopressin), 453*t*, 619
Plain catgut, 362*t*
Plaque, 15
Plasma, 179
Plasma B-type natriuretic peptide, 78–79
Plasma protein fraction (Plasmanate),
        201*t*, 589
Plasma renin activity, 85
Plasma viral load test, 74–75
Platelet, 98
Platelet count, 94*t*

Platelet transfusion, 199*t,* 202

Plateletpheresis, 196

Platinol (cisplatin), 507

Plavix (clopidogrel), 509

Plendil (felodipine), 533

Pletal (cilostazol), 506

Pleural effusion, 43

Pleural fluid analysis, 310–312, 311*f,* 313*t*

Pleurodesis, 267–268

Plicamycin, 190

Pneumococcal vaccine, 589, 657–661*t,* 662–664*t*

Pneumocystis carinii pneumonia, 151*t*

Pneumonia, 136*t*

    chlamydial, 130*t*

    Pneumocystis carinii, 151*t*

    ventilator-associated, 446

Podophyllin (Condylox), 589

Poikilocytosis, 99

Poisoning, 472, 473*t*

Pokeweed, 626

Poliglecaprone 25 suture material, 362*t*

Poliovirus vaccine, 520, 662–664*t*

Polychromasia, 99

Polydioxanone suture material, 362*t*

Polyester suture material, 363*t*

Polyethylene glycol (MiraLax, GoLYTELY, CoLyte), 589–590

Polyglactin suture material, 362*t*

Polyglycolic acid suture material, 362*t*

Polyglyconate suture material, 362*t*

Polymorphonuclear neutrophil, 97

Polymox (amoxicillin), 486

Polymyxin B-hydrocortisone, 590

Polypropylene suture material, 363*t*

Polytetrafluoroethylene suture material, 363*t*

Pork tapeworm, 151*t*

Portable chest radiography, 341

Portagen formula, 222*t*

Positive end-expiratory pressure, 437–438

    in acute respiratory distress syndrome, 440, 441*t*

    functional residual capacity and, 427*f*

Positron emission tomography, 352–353

Posterior femoral cutaneous nerve, 7*f*

Posterior rami of cervical nerves, 7*f*

Postop note, 29

Postoperative pulmonary care, 379–380

Postrenal oliguria, 43

Postural drainage, 381

Potassium

    hyperkalemia and, 187–188

    hypokalemia and, 188–189

    in parenteral formula, 234*t*

    requirements for, 180

    serum, 80

    supplemental, 590, 642*t*

    urine, 111

Potassium chloride for hypokalemia, 189

Potassium citrate, 590

Potassium citrate-citric acid, 590

Potassium hydroxide prep, 123, 299

Potassium iodide (Lugol solution, SSKI, Thyro-Block), 590

Povidone iodine hand scrub, 356–357

Pramipexole (Mirapex), 590

Pramoxine, 590–591

Prandin (repaglinide), 595

Pravastatin (Pravachol), 591

Prazosin (Minipress), 591

Precordial contusion, 407

Precordial leads, 385

Precose (acarbose), 477

Pred-G Ophthalmic (gentamicin-prednisolone, ophthalmic), 542

Prednicarbate (Dermatop), 636*t*

Prednisolone (Delta-Cortef), 633*t*

Prednisone (Deltasone), 633*t*

Prefixes, 651–652

Pregabalin (Lyrica), 591

Pregestimil formula, 222*t*

Pregnancy

    FDA fetal risk categories of drugs and, 476

    human immunodeficiency virus infection and, 156–157

    screening for, 80–81

Prehypertension, 12*t*

Preload, 409, 410*f*

    pulmonary artery catheter and, 421

Premarin (estrogen, conjugated), 530–531

Premature atrial contraction, 388, 388*f*

Premature infant

    endotracheal tube for, 273*t*

    formulas for, 223*t*

    oral feeding of, 224

Premature ventricular contraction, 391*f,* 391–392

Premphase (estrogen, conjugated-medroxyprogesterone), 530

Prempro (estrogen, conjugated-medroxyprogesterone), 530

Preoperative note, 28

Prepidil vaginal gel (dinoprostone), 519

Preprocedure patient assessment, 242

Prerenal oliguria, 42
Prescription writing, 29–32, 30*f*
Pressure-controlled ventilation, 435, 436*f*
Pressure-regulated volume control,
    435–437
Pressure-support ventilation, 435, 436*f*,
    437
Prevacid (lansoprazole), 556–557
Preven (ethinyl estradiol-levonorgestrel),
    531
Prialt (ziconotide), 622
Priftin (rifapentine), 596
Prilosec (omeprazole), 579
Primacor (milrinone), 569
Primaxin (imipenem-cilastatin), 550
Primidone, 629*t*
Prinivil (lisinopril), 560
Priscoline (tolazoline), 613
Pro-Banthine (propantheline), 592
Probenecid (Benemid), 591
Problem list, 8
Procainamide (Pronestyl, Procan),
    591–592, 630*t*
    for pediatric tachycardia, 460*t*
    toxicity of, 401
Procaine (Novocain), 364*t*, 632*t*
Procan (procainamide), 591–592
Procarbazine (Matulane), 592
Procardia (nifedipine), 575
Prochlorperazine (Compazine), 592
Procrit (epoetin alfa), 526
Proctitis, 130*t*
Progesterone, 81
Proglycem (diazoxide), 516–517
Prograf (tacrolimus), 606
Prokine (sargramostim), 598
Prolactin, 81
Prolastin (alpha$_1$-protease inhibitor), 482
Prolene suture material, 363*t*
Proleukin (aldesleukin), 480
Prolixin (fluphenazine), 537
Proloprim (trimethoprim), 617
Promethazine (Phenergan), 592
Pronestyl (procainamide), 591–592
Propafenone (Rhythmol), 592
Propantheline (Pro-Banthine), 592
Propecia (finasteride), 535
Prophylaxis
    for subacute bacterial endocarditis,
        158–159, 159*t*, 160*t*
    tetanus, 366*t*, 609–610, 643*t*
Propine (dipivefrin), 520
Propionibacterium acnes, 125*t*
Propofol (Diprivan), 406, 592–593

Propoxyphene (Darvon), 334*t*, 593
Propoxyphene-acetaminophen
        (Darvocet), 334*t*
Propranolol (Inderal), 593
Propylthiouracil (PTU), 593
Proscar (finasteride), 535
ProSobee formula, 222*t*
ProSom (estrazolam), 529
Prostaglandin E$_1$, 482
Prostaphlin (oxacillin), 580
Prostate cancer screening, 655*t*
Prostate-specific antigen, 82, 655*t*
Prostatitis, 139–140*t*
Prosthetic joint disease, 129*t*
Prosthetic valve endocarditis, 132*t*
Prostin VR (alprostadil), 482
Protamine, 593
Protein
    in parenteral formula, 232–233
    requirements for, 213–214
    serum, 82
    spot urine for, 112
    twenty-four hour urine for, 114
Protein electrophoresis, 82, 83*f*, 84*t*
Protein hydrolysate formulas, 222*t*
Proteinuria, 108
Proteus mirabilis, 124*t*
Proteus vulgaris, 124*t*
Prothrombin complex, 201*t*
Prothrombin time, 103
Protonix (pantoprazole), 583
Proventil (albuterol), 382, 480
Provera (medroxyprogesterone), 563
Providencia spp., 124*t*
Provigil (modofinil), 570
Proximal port of pulmonary artery
        catheter, 414, 414*f*
Proximal renal tubular acidosis, 170*t*
Prozac (fluoxetine), 537
Pruritus, 43
Pseudoephedrine (Sudafed, Novafed,
        Afrinol), 593–594
Pseudoephedrine-hydrocodone (Detussin,
        Histussin-D), 547
Pseudohyperkalemia, 188
Pseudohyponatremia, 187
Pseudotumor cerebri, 295*t*
Psoas sign, 19
Psychiatric disorders, 35
Psychiatric history, 8, 9*t*
Psychiatric status examination, 8
Psychological evaluation in pain
        assessment, 325
Psychosocial history, 2

Psyllium (Metamucil, Serutan, Effer-syllium), 594
PTU (propylthiouracil), 593
Pulmicort (budesonide), 495
Pulmonary angiography, 345
Pulmonary artery catheter, 412–424
    catheter description of, 414f, 414–415
    catheterization procedure in, 415–419, 416–418f, 419t
    clinical applications of, 421–423
    complications of, 419–420
    continuous cardiac output measurement in, 421
    continuous mixed venous oxygen saturation monitoring in, 423–424, 424f
    continuous pulse oximetry in, 424
    differential diagnosis of abnormalities in, 421, 422t
    indications for, 413
    measurements in, 420–421
    relative positioning of, 413f
Pulmonary artery occlusion pressure, 419t, 420, 448t
Pulmonary artery pressure, 419t, 420
Pulmonary artery systolic pressure, 448t
Pulmonary capillary oxygen content, 449t
Pulmonary capillary wedge pressure, 448t
Pulmonary consolidation, 429, 429f
Pulmonary embolism, 422t, 447
Pulmonary function tests, 377–378, 378f, 379t
Pulmonary infection, 154–155
Pulmonary infiltrates, 354
Pulmonary system
    clinical physiology of, 424–430, 425f
    complications of parenteral nutrition, 239
Pulmonary vascular resistance, 448t
Pulmonary vascular resistance index, 448t
Pulmonary viral culture, 154
Pulmonic insufficiency, 10t
Pulmonic stenosis, 10t
Pulmozyme (dornase alfa), 522
Pulse oximetry, 173
    critical care and, 404
    pulmonary artery catheter in, 424
Pulse pressure, 408
Pulseless electrical activity, 459t, 461f
Pulsus alternans, 19
Pulsus paradoxus, 306–307
Pureed diet, 215t
Purified antihemophilic factor, 201t
Purified protein derivative, 309–310

Purinethol (mercaptopurine), 564
Purpura, 15
Pustule, 15
Pyelonephritis, 140t
Pyrazinamide, 594
Pyridium (phenazopyridine), 586–587
Pyridoxine, 234t, 594
Pyrosis, 40

Q
Q wave, 384f, 385
QRS complex, 384f, 385
Quantitative immunoglobulins, 75
Quazepam (Doral), 594
Queckenstedt test, 19
Questran (cholestyramine), 505
Quetiapine (Seroquel), 594
Quinapril (Accupril), 594
Quincke sign, 19
Quinidine, 401, 594–595, 630t
Quinupristin-dalfopristin (Synercid), 595
Quixin (levofloxacin), 558
Qvar (beclomethasone), 493

R
R wave, 384f, 385
Rabeprazole (Aciphex), 595
Racemic epinephrine, 382
Radial nerve, 6f, 7f
Radiation terminology, 656
Radiation therapy for cancer pain, 338
Radiography, 341–346, 342f, 343f
    abdominal, 341–342
    chest, 353–354
Radovici sign, 19
Raloxifene (Evista), 595
Ramipril (Altace), 595
Random urine studies, 110–112
Ranitidine (Zantac), 469, 595
Rapamycin (Rapamune), 600
Rapid influenza test, 154
Rapid plasma reagin test, 83–85
Raptiva (efalizumab), 524
Rasburicase (Elitek), 595
RASS scale, 405–406
Raynaud phenomenon, 19
Razadyne (galantamine), 540
Rebetron (interferon alfa-2b-ribavirin combo), 552
Recombinant human activated protein C, 443

Recombinant immunoblot assay (RIBA),
158
Rectovaginal examination, 298
Rectum, 5
Red blood cell, 97, 99
transfusion of, 197–202
in urine, 108
Red blood cell casts, 110
Red blood cell count, 93*t*
Red blood cell mass, 179
Red blood cell morphology, 99
Red cell distribution width, 93*t*, 98
Red rubber catheter, 314, 314*f*
Reducing substances, urine, 108
Refeeding syndrome, 236
Reflexes, 7
Refludan (lepirudin), 557
Regional Poison Center, 472
Reglan (metoclopramide), 567
Regranex Gel (becaplermin), 493
Regular diet, 215*t*
Relafen (nabumetone), 571
Relenza (zanamivir), 622
Relpax (eletriptan), 524
Remeron (mirtazapine), 569
Remicade (infliximab), 551
Remodulin (treprostinil sodium), 615
Removal of sutures, 367–372, 375*f*
Renagel (sevelamer), 599
Renal casts, 110
Renal failure
enteral formula for, 228*t*
hypercalcemia in, 190
patient-controlled analgesia in,
339
therapeutic diet in, 217*t*
urinary indices in, 115, 116*t*
Renal failure index, 116*t*
Renal function panel, 48
Renal replacement therapy, 444
Renal scan, 351–352
Renal tubular acidosis, 170*t*
Renin, 85
Renova (tretinoin), 615
ReoPro (abciximab), 477
Repaglinide (Prandin), 595
Repan (acetaminophen-butalbital-
caffeine), 478
Requip (ropinirole), 598
Rescriptor (delavirdine), 514
Residual volume, 378, 378*t*, 379*t*, 425,
425*f*
Respiratory acidosis, 166*t*, 172, 174
Respiratory alkalosis, 166*t*, 172, 175

Respiratory care, 377–382
bronchopulmonary hygiene in,
380–381
metered-dose inhalers in, 382
oxygen supplements in, 379, 380*t*
postoperative, 379–380
pulmonary function tests and,
377–378, 378*f*, 379*t*
respiratory therapy and, 377
topical medications in, 382
Respiratory failure
enteral formula for, 229*t*
mechanical ventilation in, 431*t*
Respiratory rate
hemorrhagic shock and, 442*t*
ventilator weaning and, 438*t*
Respiratory syncytial virus, 145*t*
Respiratory system
adverse effects of pain on, 324*t*
review of systems and, 2
Respiratory therapy, 377
Restasis (cyclosporine, ophthalmic), 512
Resting tremor, 44
Restoril (temazepam), 608
Restrictive pulmonary diseases, 377, 379*t*
Reteplase (Retavase), 595–596
Reticulocyte count, 95–96
Retin-A (tretinoin), 615
Retinitis, cytomegalovirus, 142*t*
Retinoic acid, 554
Retinol, 234*t*
Retinol-binding protein, 85
Retrograde urethrography, 346
Retroperitoneal computed tomography,
348
Retrovir (zidovudine), 146*t*, 622
Revatio (sildenafil), 600
ReVia (naltrexone), 572
Review of systems, 2–3
Reyataz (atazanavir), 490
Rheomacrodex (Dextran 40), 516
Rheumatoid factor, 85
Rheumatrex (methotrexate), 566
Rhinocort (budesonide), 495
Rho D immune globulin, 200*t*
Rhythmol (propafenone), 592
Rib, chest radiography of, 341
RIBA (recombinant immunoblot assay),
158
Ribavirin (Virazole), 596
Riboflavin, 234*t*
Rifabutin (Mycobutin), 596
Rifampin (Rifadin), 596
Rifapentine (Priftin), 596

Rifaximin (Xifaxan), 596
Right atrial pressure, 419*t*, 448*t*
Right axis deviation, 386
Right bundle branch block, 394, 394*f*
Right internal jugular vein catheterization, 259–261, 260*f*
Right lower quadrant abdominal pain, 34
Right shift, 95
Right-to-left shunt, 173
Right upper quadrant abdominal pain, 34
Right ventricular ejection fraction, 420–421
Right ventricular ejection fraction catheter, 415
Right ventricular end-diastolic volume index, 420–421
Right ventricular hypertrophy, 396, 396*f*
Right ventricular pressure, 419*t*
Right ventricular systolic pressure, 448*t*
Rimantadine (Flumadine), 596
Rimexolone (Vexol Ophthalmic), 596–597
Rimso-50 (dimethyl sulfoxide), 519
Ringworm, 138*t*
Riopan (magaldrate), 562
Risedronate (Actonel), 597
Risperidone (Risperdal), 597
Ritonavir (Norvir), 146*t*, 147*t*, 597
Rivastigmine (Exelon), 597
Rizatriptan (Maxalt), 645*t*
Robaxin (methocarbamol), 566
Robinson catheter, 314, 314*f*
Robitussin (guaifenesin), 544
Rocaltrol (calcitriol), 497
Rocephin (ceftriaxone), 502
Rocky Mountain spotted fever, 85, 152–153*t*
Rocuronium (Zemuron), 597
Roferon-A (interferon alfa), 552
Rogaine (minoxidil), 569
Romazicon (flumazenil), 536
Romberg test, 19
Ropinirole (Requip), 598
Rosiglitazone (Avandia), 598
Rosuvastatin (Crestor), 598
Roth spot, 19
Rovsing sign, 19
Rowasa (mesalamine), 565
Roxanol (Morphine), 570
Roxicodone (oxycodone), 581
RU 486, 568
Rubex (doxorubicin), 522
Rule of nines, 183, 183*t*, 184–185*f*

S
S wave, 384*f*, 385
Sacral vertebral radiography, 344
Safety, preprocedure, 242
St. John's wort, 625–626
St. Joseph's aspirin, 489
Salem sump, 277
Salicylates, 327–328*t*
Salmeterol (Serevent), 598
Salmonella spp., 124*t*
Salsalate (Disalcid), 328*t*
Sanctura (trospium chloride), 618
Sandimmune (cyclosporine), 512
Sandoglobulin (intravenous immune globulin), 550
Sandostatin (octreotide), 578
Saphenous nerve, 6*f*, 7*f*
Saquinavir (Fortovase), 147*t*, 598
Sarafem (fluoxetine), 537
Sarcoptes scabiei, 151*t*
Sargramostim (Prokine, Leukine), 598
Sassafras, 626
Saw palmetto, 625
Scabies, 151*t*
Scales, 15
Scalp, suturing of, 363
Scalp vein needle, 288*f*, 289
Scalpel blades, 245*f*
Scar, 15
Schistocyte, 99
Schmorl node, 19
Schwartz equation, 113
Scoliosis, 19
Scopolamine, 598
Scotch tape test, 127
Screening
    cancer, 654–655*t*
    drug abuse, 115
    newborn, 79
    pregnancy, 80–81
Secobarbital (Seconal), 599
Second-degree atrioventricular block, 393, 393*f*
Second trimester screening, 81
Sectral (acebutolol), 477
Sedapap-10 (acetaminophen-butalbital-caffeine), 478
Sedation
    critical care and, 405–406
    in septic shock, 444
Sedimentation rate, 103
Segmented neutrophil, 94*t*
Seizure
    differential diagnosis in, 43

Seizure (*cont.*)
  in hypomagnesemia, 192
  in status epilepticus, 473–474, 474*t*
Seldinger technique
  in arterial line placement, 247–248
  in central venous catheterization,
    256–257
  in chest tube placement, 267
Selegiline (Eldepryl), 599
Selenium, 235*t*
Selenium sulfide, 599
Self shielding device, 288*f*, 288–289
Semen analysis, 86
Sengstaken-Blackmore tube, 278
Sensipar (cinacalcet), 506
Sensory examination, 6–7*f*
Sentinel loop, 19
Sepsis, 442
  acute lung injury and, 444
  blood component therapy-related, 203,
    204
  catheter-related, 446
Septic arthritis, 129*t*
Septic shock, 422*t*, 442
Septra (trimethoprim-sulfamethoxazole),
  617
Serax (oxazepam), 580
Serentil (mesoridazine), 565
Serevent (salmeterol), 598
Serology
  for fungal infection, 66
  for Lyme disease, 77
  for viral hepatitis, 71
  for viral infection, 128
Seroquel (quetiapine), 594
Serotonin 5-HT₁ receptor agonists, 645*t*
Serratia spp., 124*t*
Sertaconazole (Ertaczo), 599
Sertraline (Zoloft), 599
Serum calcium, 54–55
Serum catecholamines, 55
Serum chloride, 55–58
Serum cortisol, 61
Serum creatinine, 62, 116*t*
Serum estradiol, 64
Serum gastrin, 66
Serum homocysteine, 72–73
Serum human chorionic gonadotropin, 73
Serum luteinizing hormone, 77
Serum N-telopeptide, 86–87
Serum osmolality, 79
Serum osmolarity, 116*t*
Serum potassium, 80
Serum protein, 82

Serum protein electrophoresis, 82, 83*f*,
  84*t*
Serum sodium, 86
Serzone (nefazodone), 573
Sevelamer (Renagel), 599
Shift-to-left, 95
Shift-to-right, 95
Shigella spp., 126*t*
Shock
  complication in critical care, 441–444,
    442*t*
  hemodynamic parameters in, 422*t*
Shorthand for laboratory values, 31*f*, 32
Shunt fraction, 428, 428*f*, 438*t*, 449*t*
Sibutramine (Meridia), 599
Sickling, 99
Sildenafil (Viagra, Revatio), 600
Silhouette sign, 354
Silk suture, 363*t*
Silver nitrate, 600
Silver sulfadiazine (Silvadene), 600
Simethicone (Mylicon), 600
Similac formula, 222*t*
Simple acid-base disorders, 165–167,
  166*t*
Simple descriptive pain intensity scale,
  325*f*
Simple face mask, 380*t*
Simple interrupted suturing, 366*f*, 367*f*
Simulect (basiliximab), 492
Simvastatin (Zocor), 600
Sinemet (carbidopa-levodopa), 498
Sinequan (doxepin), 522
Single donor plasma, 200*t*
Single photon emission computed
  tomography, 352
Singulair (montelukast), 570
Singultus, 41
Sinogram, 345
Sinus bradycardia, 387, 388*f*, 401*f*
Sinus film, 344
Sinus rhythms, 387*f*, 387–388, 388*f*
Sinus tachycardia, 387, 387*f*
Sinusitis, 137*t*
Sirolimus, 600
Sister Mary Joseph sign, 19
Six-minute hand scrub, 356–357
Sjögren syndrome antibody, 52
Skelaxin (metaxalone), 565
Skin
  biopsy of, 307–308
  cutaneous innervation patterns of, 6–7*f*
  infection of, 137–138*t*, 155
  lesions of, 13–15

nutritional status and, 212*t*
physical examination of, 3
pruritus and, 43
review of systems and, 2
Skin staples, 375*f*
Skin testing, 308–310
Skull film, 344
Small-bore feeding tube, 227
Small bowel follow-through, 346
Smallpox vaccine, 600–601
Smear
    AFB, 119
    gonorrhea, 120–121
    malaria, 126
    Tzanck, 128
SMX (trimethoprim-sulfamethoxazole), 617
SOAP note, 26
Social history, 2
Sodium
    hypernatremia and, 186
    hyponatremia and, 186–187
    in parenteral formula, 234*t*
    requirements for, 180
    serum, 86
    urine, 111, 116*t*
Sodium bicarbonate, 601
    for antidepressant overdose, 473*t*
    for hyperkalemia, 188
Sodium channel blockers, 646*t*
Sodium citrate (Bicitra), 601
Sodium nitrite for cyanide poisoning, 473*t*
Sodium oxybate (Xyrem), 601
Sodium phosphate (Visicol), 193, 601
Sodium polystyrene sulfonate (Kayexalate), 188, 601–602
Sodium-potassium phosphate, 193
Sodium thiosulfate for cyanide poisoning, 473*t*
Soft tissue
    infections of, 137–138*t,* 155
    radiography of, 353
Solifenacin (VESIcare), 602
Solu-Cortef (hydrocortisone), 547–548
Soma (carisoprodol), 499
Somatic pain, 323
Sonata (zaleplon), 621–622
Sorbitol, 602
Sorbitrate (isosorbide dinitrate), 554
Sore throat, 135*t*
Soriatane (acitretin), 479
Sotalol (Betapace), 602
Sotret (isotretinoin), 554

Soy formulas, 222*t*
Sparfloxacin (Zagam), 602
Specific gravity, 108
Spectazole (econazole), 524
Spectracef (cefdinir), 500
Speculum examination, 297
Spermatozoa in urine, 109
Spherocyte, 99
Spin echo, 349
Spinal accessory nerve, 5
Spinal computed tomography, 348
Spinal cord stimulators, 338
Spinal headache, lumbar puncture-related, 292
Spinal tap, 289–296, 291*f,* 292*f,* 294–295*t*
Spine, magnetic resonance imaging of, 350
Spiral computed tomography, 348
Spiriva (tiotropium), 613
Spirometry, 377
Spironolactone (Aldactone), 603
Splenomegaly, 42
Sporonox (itraconazole), 554–555
Sporotrichosis, 149*t*
Spot urine studies, 110–112
Sputum culture and stain, 154
Square knot, 370–371*f*
SSKI (potassium iodide), 590
Stadol (butorphanol), 496
Stain
    acid-fast, 119
    Giemsa, 120
    Gram, 121, 122*f,* 123*f,* 124–126*t*
    Kinyoun, 119
    sputum, 154
    stool leukocyte, 156
Stainless steel suture, 363*t*
Standard catheter-over-needle intravenous access, 287*f,* 287–288
Staphylococcus spp., 124*t*
Starling law, 409, 410*f*
Starlix (nateglinide), 573
Startle reflex, 18
Static compliance, 427–428
Status epilepticus, 473–474, 474*t*
Stavudine (Zerit), 603
Stelazine (trifluoperazine), 616
Stellwag sing, 19
Stenotrophomonas maltophilia, 126*t*
Sterile technique, 355
Steroids
    for analgesia, 337
    for septic shock, 443

Steroids (*cont.*)
    systemic, 603–604, 633*t*
    topical, 634–636*t*
Stimate (desmopressin), 515
Stomatitis, 148*t*
Stool culture, 155–156
Stool for ova and parasites, 127
Stool leukocyte stain, 156
Straight-leg-raising sign, 18
Strattera (atomoxetine), 490–491
Streptococcus spp., 124*t*
Streptokinase (Streptase, Kabikinase), 604
Streptomycin, 604
Streptozocin (Zanosar), 604
Streptozyme, 51
Stress ulcer, 444
Strict precautions, 161
Stroke, 466, 469*t*, 470*f*
Stroke volume, pulmonary artery catheter and, 421
Strongyloidiasis, 151*t*
Strontium-89 scan, 352
Subacute bacterial endocarditis, 158–159, 159*t*, 160*t*
Subarachnoid hemorrhage, 295*t*
Subclavian vein catheterization, 257–259, 258*f*
Subcutaneous injection, 283–284
Subcutaneous tissue loss, 212*t*
Subcuticular closure, 369*f*
Subendocardial myocardial infarction, 398
Sublimaze (fentanyl), 534
Succimer (Chemet), 604–605
Succinylcholine (Anectine, Quelicin, Sucostrin), 605
Sucralfate (Carafate), 605
Sudafed (pseudoephedrine), 593–594
Sular (nisoldipine), 576
Sulfacetamide-prednisolone (Blephamide), 605
Sulfasalazine (Azulfidine), 605–606
Sulfinpyrazone (Anturane), 606
Sulindac (Clinoril), 606
Sumatriptan (Imitrex), 606, 645*t*
Sumycin (tetracycline), 610
Superficial peroneal nerve, 6*f*, 7*f*
Suppressor T cell, 99
Supprettes (chloral hydrate), 504
Supraclavicular nerves, 6*f*, 7*f*
Suprax (cefixime), 500
Sural nerve, 6*f*, 7*f*
Surfak (docusate calcium), 521

Surgical cricothyroidotomy, 268, 269
Surgical hand scrub, 356–357
Surgical knots, 365–366, 370–374*f*
Survanta (beractant), 493
Sustiva (efavirenz), 524
Suturing, 361–375
    materials for, 361–363, 362*t*, 363*t*
    patterns in, 365, 366–369*f*
    procedure in, 363–365, 364*t*
    removal of sutures, 367–372, 375*f*
    surgical knots in, 365–366, 370–374*f*
    tissue adhesives and, 373–375
    vacuum-assisted closure and, 361
    wound healing and, 361
Sweat chloride, 86
Symbols, 651–652
Symmetrel (amantadine), 483–484
Sympathetic nervous system, 409–410, 411*t*
Sympathomimetic drugs, 411*t*
Synagis (palifermin), 582
Synalar (fluocinolone), 635*t*
Synchronized intermittent mandatory ventilation, 435, 436*f*
Syncope, 44
Synercid (quinupristin-dalfopristin), 595
Synovial fluid interpretation, 251, 252*t*
Synthroid (levothyroxine), 559
Syphilis, 83–85, 138*t*
Systemic inflammatory response syndrome, 442
Systemic steroids, 603–604, 633*t*
Systemic vascular resistance, 448*t*
Systemic vascular resistance index, 448*t*
Systolic hypertension, 407

T
T-1 weighted image, 349
T-2 weighted image, 349
T cell, 99
T-tube cholangiography, 346
T wave, 384*f*, 385
Tachycardia, 386
    advanced cardiac life support in, 463, 463*t*
    atrial, 388–389, 389*f*
    pediatric, 460*t*
    sinus, 387, 387*f*
    ventricular, 392, 392*f*
Tachypnea, 431*t*
Tacrine (Cognex), 606
Tadalafil (Cialis), 606
Taenia saginata, 151*t*

Taenia solium, 151*t*
Tagamet (cimetidine), 506
Talc, 607
Talwin (pentazocine), 585
Tambocor (flecainide), 535
Tamiflu (oseltamivir), 580
Tamoxifen (Nolvadex), 607
Tamsulosin (Flomax), 607
Tapazole (methimazole), 566
Tapered needle, 363
Tapeworm infection, 151*t*
Tarceva (erlotinib), 527
Target cell, 99
Tasmar (tolcapone), 613–614
Tavist (clemastine fumarate), 508
Taxol (paclitaxel), 582
Taxotere (docetaxel), 521
Tazarotene (Tazorac), 607
Tazicef (ceftazidime), 502
Tazidime (ceftazidime), 502
Teeth, eruption of, 13, 14*f*
Tegaserod (Zelnorm), 607
Tegretol (carbamazepine), 498
Telangiectasia, 15
Telithromycin (Ketek), 607–608
Telmisartan (Micardis), 608
Temazepam (Restoril), 608
Temovate (clobetasol propionate), 634*t*
Temperature conversion table, 667*t*
Tenecteplase (TNKase), 608
Tenofivir (Viread), 146*t,* 608
Tenofivir-emtricitabine (Truvada), 608
Tenoretic (atenolol-chlorthalidone), 490
Tenormin (atenolol), 490
Tensilon (edrophonium), 524
Tension headache, 40
Tequin (gatifloxacin), 541
Terazosin (Hytrin), 608–609
Terbinafine (Lamisil), 609
Terbutaline (Brethine, Bricanyl), 609
Terconazole (Terazol 7), 609
Teriparatide (Forteo), 609
Tespa (triethylenethiophosphamide), 616
Tessalon Perles (benzonatate), 493
Testosterone, 87, 609
Tetanus, diphtheria vaccine, 657–661*t*
Tetanus prophylaxis, 366*t,* 609–610, 643*t*
Tetany, 192
Tetracycline (Achromycin V, Sumycin), 610
Teveten (eprosartan), 527
Thalidomide (Thalomid), 610
Thallium-201 scan, 351
Thayer-Martin medium, 299

Theophylline, 610, 629*t*
TheraCys (Bacille Calmette-Guérin), 492
Therapeutic apheresis, 196
Therapeutic arthrocentesis, 249
Therapeutic diets, 214–221, 215–219*t*
Thermistor, 414, 414*f*
Thermography, 326
Thiamine, 610
    in parenteral formula, 234*t*
    for status epilepticus, 473
Thiethylperazine (Torecan), 610
Thio-Tepa (triethylene-thiophosphamide), 616
6-Thioguanine (Tabloid), 611
Thioridazine (Mellaril), 611
Thiothixene (Navane), 611
Third-degree atrioventricular block, 394, 394*f*
Third heart sound, 11*t*
Thoracentesis, 310–312, 311*f,* 313*t*
Thoracic radiography, 344
Thorazine (chlorpromazine), 505
Throat
    physical examination of, 3
    review of systems and, 2
Throat culture, 127–128
Thrombin time, 103
Thromboembolism prevention, 644*t*
Thrush, 148*t*
Thyro-Block (potassium iodide), 590
Thyrocalcitonin, 54
Thyroglobulin, 87
Thyroid scan, 352
Thyroid-stimulating hormone, 87
Thyroid ultrasonography, 347
Thyroxine, free, 88
Tiagabine (Gabitril), 611
Tiazac (diltiazem), 518–519
Ticarcillin (Ticar), 611
Ticarcillin-potassium clavulanate (Timentin), 611
Tice BCG (Bacille Calmette-Guérin), 492
Tick-borne diseases, 152–153*t*
Ticlopidine (Ticlid), 612
Tidal volume, 378, 378*t,* 425, 425*f*
    ventilator weaning and, 438*t*
Tigan (trimethobenzamide), 617
Tigecycline (Tygacil), 612
Tikosyn (dofetilide), 521
Tilade (nedocromil), 573
Timate (diltiazem), 518–519
Timed scrub, 356
Timentin (ticarcillin-potassium clavulanate), 611

Timolol (Blocadren, Timoptic), 612
Tinactin (tolnaftate), 614
Tincture of opium, 583
Tine test, 309
Tinea capitis, 138*t*
Tinea corporis, 138*t*
Tinea unguium, 138*t*
Tinel sign, 19
Tinidazole (Tindamax), 612
Tinzaparin (Innohep), 612
Tioconazole (Vagistat), 612–613
Tiotropium (Spiriva), 613
Tirofiban (Aggrastat), 613
Tissue adhesives, 373–375
TMP (trimethoprim-sulfamethoxazole), 617
TNKase (tenecteplase), 608
Tobramycin (Nebcin, Tobrex), 613, 628*t*
Tobramycin-dexamethasone ophthalmic (TobraDex), 613
Tocopherol, 234*t*
Tofranil (imipramine), 550
Tolazamide (Tolinase), 613
Tolazoline (Priscoline), 613
Tolbutamide (Orinase), 613
Tolcapone (Tasmar), 613–614
Tolmetin (Tolectin), 614
Tolnaftate (Tinactin), 614
Tolterodine (Detrol), 614
Topical medications in respiratory care, 382
Topical steroid preparations, 634–636*t*
Topicort (desoximetasone), 634*t*
Topiramate (Topamax), 614
Toposar (etoposide), 532
Topotecan (Hycamtin), 614
Toprol XL (metoprolol), 567
Toradol (ketorolac), 555
TORCH battery, 88
Torecan (thiethylperazine), 610
Tornalate (bitolterol), 495
Torsemide (Demadex), 614
Total blood volume, 179
Total body water, 179
Total carbon dioxide, 55
Total complement CH$_{50}$, 61
Total creatine kinase, 61–62
Total iron-binding capacity, 75
Total 17-ketosteroids, 115
Total lung capacity, 378, 378*t*, 379*t*, 425, 425*f*
Total lymphocytes, 99
Total nutrient admixture, 232
Total prostate-specific antigen, 82

Toxic granulation, 99
Toxin-induced disorders, 34–35
Toxocara canis, 151*t*
Toxoplasmosis, 151*t*
Trace minerals, 234–235, 235*t*
Tracrium (atracurium), 491
Tramadol (Ultram), 327*t,* 614
Tramadol-acetaminophen (Ultracet), 615
Trandate (labetalol), 555–556
Trandolapril (Mavik), 615
Transcutaneous electrical nerve stimulation (TENS), 338
Transferrin, 88
Transfusion, 195–205
    apheresis and, 196
    autologous blood donation and, 195–196
    blood banking procedures and, 195
    blood groups and, 196, 197*t*
    donor-directed blood products and, 196
    emergency, 196
    indications and uses of, 198–201*t*
    infectious disease risk and, 204–205
    irradiated blood components and, 196
    platelet, 202
    procedure in, 202–203
    reactions to, 203–204
    red cell, 197–202
    routine blood donation and, 195
    for septic shock, 443
    white cell, 202
Transfusion reactions, 203–204
Transmural myocardial infarction, 398, 398*t*
Transport of critically ill patient, 404–405
Transrectal ultrasonography, 347
Transudative pleural effusion, 43
Tranxene (clorazepate), 509
Trastuzumab (Herceptin), 615
Trasylol (aprotinin), 489
Traube sign, 19
Trauma
    dementia in, 35
    lumbar puncture-related, 293–296
Traumatic tap, 295*t*
Trazodone (Desyrel), 615, 630*t*
Trelstar (triptorelin), 617–618
Tremors, 44
Trendelenburg test, 19
Trental (pentoxifylline), 586
Treponema pallidum
    microhemagglutination, 78
Treprostinil sodium (Remodulin), 615

Tretinoin (Retin-A, Avita, Renova), 615

Triamcinolone (Aristocort, Azmacort), 615, 636*t*

Triamcinolone-nystatin (Mycolog-II), 616

Triamterene (Dyrenium), 616

Triaprin (acetaminophen-butalbital-caffeine), 478

Triazolam (Halcion), 616

Trichinosis, 151*t*

Trichomoniasis, 140*t*, 151*t*

Trichuriasis, 151*t*

Tricor (fenofibrate), 533

Tricuspid insufficiency, 11*t*

Tricyclic antidepressants overdose, 473*t*

Triethanolamine (Cerumenex), 616

Triethylenethiophosphamide (Thio-Tepa, Tespa, TSPA), 616

Trifluoperazine (Stelazine), 616

Trifluridine (Viroptic), 616

Trigeminal nerve, 5, 6*f*

Trigeminy, 391, 391*f*

Triglycerides, 58*t*, 59*t*, 88
    metabolic syndrome and, 209, 211*t*

Trihexyphenidyl (Artane), 616–617

Triiodothyronine, 88

Trilafon (perphenazine), 586

Trileptal (oxcarbazepine), 580–581

Trimethobenzamide (Tigan), 617

Trimethoprim (Trimpex, Proloprim), 617

Trimethoprim-sulfamethoxazole (TMP, SMX, Cotrimazole, Bactrim, Septra), 617

Trimetrexate (Neutrexin), 617

Triptorelin (Trelstar), 617–618

Trochlear nerve, 5

Troponin, cardiac-specific, 89

Trospium chloride (Sanctura), 618

Trousseau sign, 19

Trovafloxacin (Trovan), 618

Trunk, suturing of, 363–365, 364*t*

Trusopt (dorzolamide), 522

Truvada (tenofivir-emtricitabine), 608

Trypanosoma cruzi, 151*t*

Tube feeding, 225–231, 228–229*t*

Tube thoracostomy, 264–265, 266*f*

Tuberculosis, 138*t*, 154–155
    cerebrospinal fluid analysis in, 294*t*
    testing for, 154–155

Tubular casts, 110

Tumor, 15
    cerebrospinal fluid analysis in, 295*t*

Tumor markers, 54

Tums (calcium carbonate), 497

Tunneled catheter removal, 263–264

Turner sign, 19

Twenty-four hour urine studies, 113–115

Two-dimensional echocardiography, 347

Two-Dyne (acetaminophen-butalbital-caffeine), 478

Two-handed square knot, 370–371*f*

Tycron suture material, 363*t*

Tylenol (acetaminophen), 477–478, 627*t*

Tylox (oxycodone-acetaminophen), 581

Tysabri (natalizumab), 573

Tzanck smear, 128

U

Ulcer, 15, 139*t*

Ulnar nerve, 6*f*, 7*f*

Ultracef (cefadroxil), 500

Ultralente, 637*t*

Ultram (tramadol), 614

Ultrase (pancrelipase), 583

Ultrasonography, 346–347

Ultravate cream (halbetasol), 635*t*

Unasyn (ampicillin-sulbactam), 487

Unconjugated bilirubin, 52–53

Unifocal premature ventricular contractions, 391, 391*f*

Univasc (moexipril), 570

Universal donor, 196, 197*t*

Universal Pedi-Packs, 198*t*

Universal precautions, 241–242, 360

Universal recipient, 196, 197*t*

Upper gastrointestinal hemorrhage, 440–441

Upper gastrointestinal series, 346

Urate, 89

Urecholine (bethanechol), 494

Urethritis, 130*t*, 139*t*

Urex (methenamine), 566

Uric acid, 89

Urinalysis, 141

Urinary incontinence, 41

Urinary indices in renal failure, 115, 116*t*

Urinary sodium, 111, 116*t*

Urinary system, adverse effects of pair on, 324*t*

Urinary tract infection, 139–140*t*, 1 154

Urinary tract procedures, 312–3 317*f*

Urine calcium, 113

Urine chloride, 171, 171*f*

Urine creatinine, 116*t*

Urine culture, 141, 154

Urine N-telopeptide, 86
Urine osmolality, 112, 116*t*
Urine osmolarity, 116*t*
Urine output, 116
  hemorrhagic shock and, 442*t*
Urine protein electrophoresis, 82, 83*f*,
  84*t*
Urine sediment, 108–110, 109*f*
Urine studies, 104–116
  creatinine clearance in, 112–113
  differential diagnosis in, 106–108
  drug abuse screen in, 115
  normal values in, 106
  spot or random, 110–112
  twenty-four hour, 113–115
  urinalysis procedure in, 105–106
  urinary indices in renal failure and,
    115, 116*t*
  urine output in, 116
  urine sediment in, 108–110, 109*f*
  xylose tolerance test in, 115
Urine urea nitrogen, 214
Urispas (flavoxate), 535
Urobilinogen, 108
Urokinase (Abbokinase), 618
Uroxatral (alfuzosin), 481
Usnic acid, 626
Uterine cancer screening, 655*t*

V

Vacutainer system, 318–320*t*, 321
Vacuum-assisted closure, 361
Vagal nerve, 5
Vaginal bleeding, 44
Vaginal discharge, 44
Vaginal infection
  bacterial, 140*t*
  ~~al~~, 148*t*
  ~~for~~, 299
  ~~prep~~, 299
  ~~examination~~, 297
  ~~612–613~~
  ~~8~~

~~1,~~
~~, 314f,~~

Vancomycin (Vancocin, Vancoled), 619
  for subacute bacterial endocarditis
    prophylaxis, 160*t*
  therapeutic levels of, 628*t*
Vanillylmandelic acid, 115
Vantin (cefpodoxime), 501–502
Vardenafil (Levitra), 619
Varicella vaccine, 563, 619, 657–661*t*,
  662–664*t*
Varicella zoster virus, 145*t*
Vasopressin (Pitressin), 453*t*, 619
Vasopressors, 409
  for septic shock, 443
Vasotec (enalapril), 525
Vasovagal syncope, 44
Vastus lateralis muscle injection, 284
Vaughn Williams classification of
  antiarrhythmics, 646*t*
Vecuronium (Norcuron), 619–620
Veetids (penicillin V), 585
Veillonella spp., 124*t*
Velban (vinblastine), 620
Velcade (bortezomib), 495
Velosef (cephradine), 503
Velosulin, 637*t*
Venereal Disease Research Laboratory,
  89
Venipuncture, 316–321, 318–320*t*
Venlafaxine (Effexor), 620
Venofer (iron sucrose), 553
Venography, 346
Venous blood gases, 164, 164*t*
Ventavis (iloprost), 549
Ventilation-perfusion abnormalities, 173
Ventilator-associated pneumonia, 446
Ventilator orders, 437
Ventilatory support
  critical care and, 424–428, 425–427*f*
  in medical emergency, 463–464
Ventolin (albuterol), 382, 480
Ventricular arrhythmias, 391–392,
  391–393*f*
Ventricular fibrillation, 392, 392*f*, 459*t*
Ventricular hypertrophy, 396, 396*f*, 397*f*
Ventricular septal defect, 11*t*
Ventricular tachycardia, 392, 392*f*, 459*t*
Venturi mask, 380*t*
VePesid (etoposide), 532
Verapamil (Calan, Isoptin), 620
Versed (midazolam), 568
Vertical interrupted mattress sutures, 368*f*
Vertigo, 44
VESIcare (solifenacin), 602
Vesicle, 15